Cardiac Drug Therapy

Contemporary Cardiology

Christopher P. Cannon, MD
Series Editor
Annemarie M. Armani, MD
Executive Editor

Nuclear Cardiology: *The Basics: How to Set Up and Maintain a Laboratory, Second Edition,* by *Frans Wackers, MD, PhD, Barry L. Zaret, MD, PhD, and Wendy Bruni, CNMT, 2008*

Rapid ECG Interpretation, Third Edition, by *M. Gabriel Khan, MD, FRCP, 2007*

Therapeutic Lipidology, edited by *Michael H. Davidson, MD, Kevin C. Maki, PhD, and Peter P. Toth, MD, PhD, 2007*

Essentials of Restenosis: *For the Interventional Cardiologist,* edited by *Henricus J. Duckers, PhD, MD, Patrick W. Serruys, MD, and Elizabeth G. Nabel, MD, 2007*

Cardiac Drug Therapy, *Seventh Edition,* by *M. Gabriel Khan, MD, FRCP(LONDON), FRCP(C), FACP, FACC, 2007*

Cardiovascular Magnetic Resonance Imaging, edited by *Raymond Y. Kwong, MD, 2007*

Essential Echocardiography: *A Practical Handbook With DVD,* edited by *Scott D. Solomon, MD, 2007*

Management of Acute Pulmonary Embolism, edited by *Stavros Konstantinides, MD, 2007*

Stem Cells and Myocardial Regeneration, edited by *Marc S. Penn, MD, PhD, 2007*

Handbook of Complex Percutaneous Carotid Intervention, edited by *Jacqueline Saw, MD, Jose Exaire, MD, David S. Lee, MD, Sanjay Yadav, MD, 2007*

Preventive Cardiology: *Insights Into the Prevention and Treatment of Cardiovascular Disease, Second Edition,* edited by *JoAnne Micale Foody, MD, 2006*

The Art and Science of Cardiac Physical Examination: *With Heart Sounds and Pulse Wave Forms on CD,* by *Narasimhan Ranganathan, MD, Vahe Sivaciyan, MD, and Franklin B. Saksena, MD, 2006*

Cardiovascular Biomarkers: *Pathophysiology and Disease Management,* edited by *David A. Morrow, MD, 2006*

Cardiovascular Disease in the Elderly, edited by *Gary Gerstenblith, MD, 2005*

Platelet Function: *Assessment, Diagnosis, and Treatment,* edited by *Martin Quinn, MB BCh BAO, PhD, and Desmond Fitzgerald, MD, FRCPI, FESC, APP, 2005*

Diabetes and Cardiovascular Disease, Second Edition, edited by *Michael T. Johnstone, MD, CM, FRCP(C), and Aristidis Veves, MD, DSc, 2005*

Angiogenesis and Direct Myocardial Revascularization, edited by *Roger J. Laham, MD, and Donald S. Baim, MD, 2005*

Interventional Cardiology: *Percutaneous Noncoronary Intervention,* edited by *Howard C. Herrmann, MD, 2005*

Principles of Molecular Cardiology, edited by *Marschall S. Runge, MD, and Cam Patterson, MD, 2005*

Heart Disease Diagnosis and Therapy: *A Practical Approach, Second Edition,* by *M. Gabriel Khan, MD, FRCP(LONDON), FRCP(C), FACP, FACC, 2005*

Cardiovascular Genomics: *Gene Mining for Pharmacogenomics and Gene Therapy,* edited by *Mohan K. Raizada, PhD, Julian F. R. Paton, PhD, Michael J. Katovich, PhD, and Sergey Kasparov, MD, PhD, 2005*

Surgical Management of Congestive Heart Failure, edited by *James C. Fang, MD and Gregory S. Couper, MD, 2005*

Cardiopulmonary Resuscitation, edited by *Joseph P. Ornato, MD, FACP, FACC, FACEP and Mary Ann Peberdy, MD, FACC, 2005*

CT of the Heart: *Principles and Applications,* edited by *U. Joseph Schoepf, MD, 2005*

Coronary Disease in Women: *Evidence-Based Diagnosis and Treatment,* edited by *Leslee J. Shaw, PhD and Rita F. Redberg, MD, FACC, 2004*

Cardiac Transplantation: *The Columbia University Medical Center/New York-Presbyterian Hospital Manual,* edited by *Niloo M. Edwards, MD, Jonathan M. Chen, MD, and Pamela A. Mazzeo, 2004*

Heart Disease and Erectile Dysfunction, edited by *Robert A. Kloner, MD, PhD, 2004*

Complementary and Alternative Cardiovascular Medicine, edited by *Richard A. Stein, MD and Mehmet C. Oz, MD, 2004*

Nuclear Cardiology, The Basics: *How to Set Up and Maintain a Laboratory,* by *Frans J. Th. Wackers, MD, PhD, Wendy Bruni, BS, CNMT, and Barry L. Zaret, MD, 2004*

CARDIAC DRUG THERAPY

Seventh Edition

by

M. GABRIEL KHAN, MD, FRCP, FACC

Associate Professor of Medicine, University of Ottawa, and
Cardiologist, The Ottawa Hospital,
Ottawa, Ontario, Canada

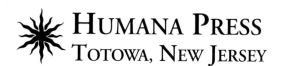

999 Riverview Drive, Suite 208
Totowa, New Jersey 07512

www.humanapress.com

For additional copies, pricing for bulk purchases, and/or information about other Humana titles, contact Humana at the above address or at any of the following numbers: Tel.: 973-256-1699; Fax: 973-256-8341, E-mail: orders@humanapr.com; or visit our Website: www.humanapress.com

This publication is printed on acid-free paper. ∞
ANSI Z39.48-1984 (American National Standards Institute) Permanence of Paper for Printed Library Materials.

Printed in the United States of America. 10 9 8 7 6 5 4 3 2 1

eISBN 1-59745-238-6 ISBN13 978-1-58829-904-8
Library of Congress Cataloging-in-Publication Data
Khan, M. I. Gabriel.
Cardiac drug therapy / by M. Gabriel Khan. — 7th ed.
p. ; cm. — (Contemporary cardiology)
Includes bibliographical references and index.
ISBN-13: 978-1-58829-904-8 (alk. paper)
ISBN-10: 1-58829-904-X (alk. paper)
1. Cardiovascular agents. 2. Heart—Diseases—Chemotherapy. I. Title. II. Series: Contemporary cardiology (Totowa, N.J. : Unnumbered)
[DNLM: 1. Heart Diseases—drug therapy—Handbooks. 2. Cardiovascular Agents—therapeutic use—Handbooks. WG 39 K45c 2007]
RC684.C48K437 2007
616.1'2061—dc22 2006032373

Dedication

To My wife Brigid
and
To our children
Susan, Christine, Yasmin, Stephen, Jacqueline, and Natasha

PREFACE

The impetus to provide a seventh edition of *Cardiac Drug Therapy* was generated by the positive comments received from readers worldwide, and from favorable reviews of earlier editions. The seventh edition updates and revises the sixth edition in several respects. In particular, the text includes: Six new chapters that deal with ongoing important controversies regarding the use of several widely used cardiac drugs.

Controversies have arisen regarding the use of beta blockers for the treatment of hypertension. The front cover of *The Lancet* November 4, 2005 highlighted "beta blockers should not remain first choice in the treatment of primary hypertension." Is this statement true or false? In addition Trialists have indicated that beta blockers and diurectics cause an increased incidence of new diabetes; it appears that most experts in the field have endorsed this information. In the *Lancet*, January 2007, another faulty metaanalysis provides the same misleading information.

- The chapter Beta-Blocker Controversies gives substantial evidence that indicates to Clinicians that both preceding statements are false. In the chapter Beta-blockers, a section is given entitled "Which Beta Blocker is Best for Your Patients?"

New chapters include:

- ACE Inhibitor Controversies.
- Calcium Antagonist Controversies: The controversies regarding the use of calcium antagonists are further analyzed and clear directions are given to clinicians regarding when to choose a calcium antagonist, and which one to choose.
- Hypertension Controversies. There are more than one billion hypertensive individuals requiring drug therapy and only four classes of antihypertensive agents are available: diuretics, beta blockers, ACE inhibitors/angiotensin receptor blockers, and calcium antagonists. Alpha blockers and centrally acting agents have limited use. If it is true that both beta blockers and diuretics cause an increased incidence of new onset diabetes, then patient treatment would be compromised. Physicians worldwide are perplexed. This important area is clarified and treatment algorithms are given for the choice of drug based on the age and ethnicity of the hypertensive patient.
- The chapter Heart Failure Controversies discusses : heart failure preserved ejection fraction; is the combination of ACE inhibitor or ARB genuinely beneficial ? Recommended heart failure agents all cause bothersome lowering of blood pressure. Digoxin has been discarded by most who fail to recall that this is the only heart failure drug that does not lower blood pressure, and it can be used without causing toxicity because salutary effects are obtained with low serum digoxin levels 0.5–0.9 ng/mL particularly in patients with class III-IV heart failure.
- The chapter Statin Controversies explores rhabdomyolysis , interactions, and other issues.
- The chapter Hallmark Clinical Trials has been expanded to accommodate the wealth of practical information derived from these studies.

As in all previous editions, therapeutic strategies and advice are based on a thorough review of the scientific literature, applied logically:

- Scientific documentation regarding which drugs are superior.
- Information on which cardiovascular drugs to choose and which agents to avoid in various clinical situations.
- Information that assists with the rapid writing of prescriptions. To write a prescription accurately, a practitioner needs to know how a drug is supplied and its dosage. Thus, supply and dosage are given first, followed by action and pharmacokinetics, then advice as to efficacy and comparison with other drugs, indications, adverse effects, and interactions.
- The name of each drug, the formulation, and the dosage have been put in tabular format; this allows quick retrieval of the information required when writing prescriptions.
- An appendix provides a global table of cardioactive drugs with their generic and tradenames in North America, the UK, Europe, and Japan.
- The text contains practical advice, such as the following:

  The life-saving potential of 75–160 mg chewable aspirin is denied to many individuals who succumb to an acute coronary syndrome because of poor dissemination of clinically proven, documented facts. The text advises: two ~ 80 mg chewable aspirins should be placed in the cap of a nitrolingual spray container to be used before proceeding to an emergency room. Clinicians should inform patients that rapidly acting chewable aspirin may prevent a heart attack or death but that nitroglycerin does not.

  The dosages of drugs given in the text apply to the adult and are standard. Often, a lower dose than the manufacturer's recommended maximum is advised because in clinical practice a lesser dose suffices and results in fewer adverse effects, especially when medications are combined.

The information provided in the seventh edition should serve as a refresher for cardiologists and internists. The information should improve the prescribing skills of medical residents, general practitioners, and all who care for patients with cardiac problems.

Acknowedgments: First to Paul Dolgert Publishing Director at Humana Press, whom I sought to publish this work because he is without equal at his craft. He has made my book *Heart Disease Diagnosis and Therapy* a success and has agreed to do more for *Rapid ECG Interpretation* to be published in 2008. I thank him particularly for agreeing to display my material in a more user friendly format than that of the sixth edition. The pages are wider and the font enlarged. Now, crucial information can be rapidly retrieved and I feel fulfilled.

Also, to James Geronimo who expertly guided me through the production concerns and to Lisa Bargeman. *Lastly, a special, thank you, to my wife Brigid, who has allowed me to be a student of the science of Medicine to this day.*

M. Gabriel Khan, MD

CONTENTS

About the Author

Dr. M. Gabriel Khan is a cardiologist at the Ottawa Hospital and an Associate Professor of Medicine, at the University of Ottawa. Dr. Khan graduated MB, BCh, with First-Class Honours at The Queen's University of Belfast. He was appointed Staff Physician in charge of a Clinical Teaching Unit at the Ottawa General hospital and is a Fellow of the American College of Cardiology, the American College of Physicians, and the Royal College of Physicians of London and Canada. He is the author of *On Call Cardiology*, 3rd ed., Elsevier, Philadelphia (2006); *Heart Disease Diagnosis and Therapy,* 2nd ed., Humana Press (2006); *Rapid ECG Interpretation*, 2nd ed., Elsevier, Philadelphia, PA (2003); and *Cardiac and Pulmonary Management* (1993), *Medical Diagnosis and Therapy* (1994), *Heart Attacks, Hypertension and Heart Drugs* (1986), *Heart Trouble Encyclopedia* (1996), and *Encyclopedia of Heart Diseases* (2006), Academic Press/ Elsevier, San Diego.

Dr. Khan's books have been translated into Chinese, Czech, Farsi, French, German, Greek, Italian, Japanese, Polish, Portuguese, Russian, Spanish, and Turkish. He has built a reputation as a clinician-teacher and has become an internationally acclaimed cardiologist through his writings.

His peers have acknowledged the merits of his books by their reviews of *Cardiac Drug Therapy*: Review of the 5th edition in *Clinical Cardiology*: "this is an excellent book. It succeeds in being practical while presenting the major evidence in relation to its recommendations. Of value to absolutely anyone who prescribes for cardiac patients on the day-to-day basis. From the trainee to the experienced consultant, all will find it useful. The author stamps his authority very clearly throughout the text by very clear assertions of his own recommendations even when these recommendations are at odds with those of official bodies. In such situations the 'official' recommendations are also stated but clearly are not preferred."

And for the fourth edition a cardiologist reviewer states that it is "by far the best handbook on cardiovascular therapeutics I have ever had the pleasure of reading. The information given in each chapter is up-to-date, accurate, clearly written, eminently readable and well referenced."

1 Beta-Blockers

The Cornerstone of Cardiac Drug Therapy

NEW CONCEPTS

This chapter tells you

- Which beta-blocker is best for your patients.
- The pharmacodynamic reasons why atenolol is a relatively ineffective beta-blocker and why the use of atenolol should be curtailed.
- More about the important indication for heart failure (HF), New York Heart Association (NYHA) class II–III and now compensated class IV, and for all with left ventricular (LV) dysfunction regardless of functional class; thus, in class I patients with an ejection fraction (EF) < 40% and in those with myocardial infarction (MI) with HF or LV dysfunction without HF, beta-blockers are recommended at the same level as angiotensin-converting enzyme (ACE) inhibitors.
- *Why beta-blockers should be recommended for diabetic patients with hypertension with or without proteinuria* and for diabetic patients with coronary heart disease (CHD). From about 1990 to 2002, most internists proclaimed in editorials and to trainees that these agents were a poor choice in this setting.
- More recently, their use as initial agents for the treatment of primary hypertension has been criticized, particularly for diabetics with hypertension; do beta-blocking drugs cause diabetes or is the condition observed, simply, benign glucose intolerance in some? (*See* Chapter 2, Beta-Blocker Controversies.)
- Why is it incorrect to say that *beta-blockers are not advisable for hypertensive patients over age 65*, as many teachers, textbooks, and editorials state. This was reiterated in an editorial by Cruickshank entitled "Beta-blockers continue to surprise us" *(1)*.
- The results of randomized clinical trials (RCTs) that prove the lifesaving properties of these agents.
- All their indications.
- Salient points that relate to each beta-blocker and show the subtle and important differences confirming that beta-blockers are not all alike. Beta-blockade holds the key, but lipophilic versus hydrophilic features may be important, and brain concentration may enhance cardioprotection.

Four classes of oral agents have been shown in RCTs to decrease cardiovascular morbidity and mortality:

- Beta-blockers.
- Aspirin and clopidogrel.
- ACE inhibitors or angiotensin II receptor blockers (ARBs).
- Statins.

From: *Contemporary Cardiology: Cardiac Drug Therapy, Seventh Edition*
M. Gabriel Khan © Humana Press Inc., Totowa, NJ

Beta-blockers are now recommended and used by virtually all cardiologists because they are necessary for the management of acute and chronic ischemic syndromes, manifestations of CHD. The statins have been added to the list of proven agents.

The approximate lifesaving potentials of these agents are as follows:

- Beta-blockers: approx 33%; **they enhance the salutary effects of ACE inhibitors**; in mild to moderate HF, average mortality reduction for beta-blockers is 36% versus 21% for ACE inhibitors.
- Aspirin: 23%.
- ACE inhibitors: 20%.
- Statins: approx 15%.

Many internists and family physicians, however, remain reluctant to prescribe beta-blockers in many cardiovascular situations including HF, in hypertension in patients aged >65 years, and in diabetic patients. Other agents, particularly calcium antagonists, are used in preference mainly because of fears engendered by the pharmaceutical firms that market calcium antagonists and ACE inhibitors.

- It is noteworthy that a body as illustrious as the Joint National Committee on Prevention, Detection, Evaluation, and Treatment of High Blood Pressure (JNC) advised against the use of beta-blockers in hypertensive patients with diabetes or dyslipidemia *(2)*. It appears that these views are similar to those of most internists and family physicians.
- For many years (1989–2002), the JNC advised physicians to use alpha-blockers for the treatment of hypertension in patients with dyslipidemia because these agents do not alter lipid levels unfavorably *(2)*. The JNC only advised in 2002 against the use of alpha-blockers after it was shown that the alpha-blocker doxazosin caused a marked increase in the incidence of HF in treated hypertensive patients. In 1988, the second edition of the present text issued a warning regarding the use of alpha-blockers.

In the setting of dyslipidemia, editorials, textbooks, internists, and committee guidelines of the World Health Organization (WHO) and the JNC have recommended agents other than beta-blockers, but beta-blockers are *not* contraindicated in dyslipidemia.

Fears that beta-blockers influence lipid levels unfavorably are unfounded. Beta-blocking drugs do not alter low-density lipoprotein (LDL) levels; they may cause a mild increase in levels of triglycerides and may produce a 1% to approx 6% lowering of high-density lipoprotein cholesterol (HDL-C) in fewer than 10% of patients treated *(3)*. The alteration in HDL-C levels is of minimal clinical concern because the effect is so small, if it occurs at all *(4)*. The clinical importance of this mild disturbance in lipid levels is of questionable significance and should not submerge the prolongation of life and other salutary effects obtained with the administration of beta-blocking drugs (Fig. 1-1).

Since their original discovery by Sir James Black at Imperial Chemical Industries in the United Kingdom *(5)* and the introduction of the prototype, propranolol, for the treatment of hypertension in 1964 by Prichard and Gillam *(6)*, more than 12 beta-blocking drugs have become available.

The first edition of *Cardiac Drug Therapy* in 1984 included a table entitled "Beta-blockers: first-line oral drug treatment in angina pectoris" (Table 1-1); this table indicated the superiority of beta-blockers over calcium antagonists and nitrates. Calcium antagonists were downrated because they decreased blood flow to subendocardial areas; in addition, in the condition for which they were developed, coronary artery spasm (CAS), they were not shown to decrease mortality. This table has never been altered. The 1990s have shown the possible adverse effects and potential dangers of dihydropyridine

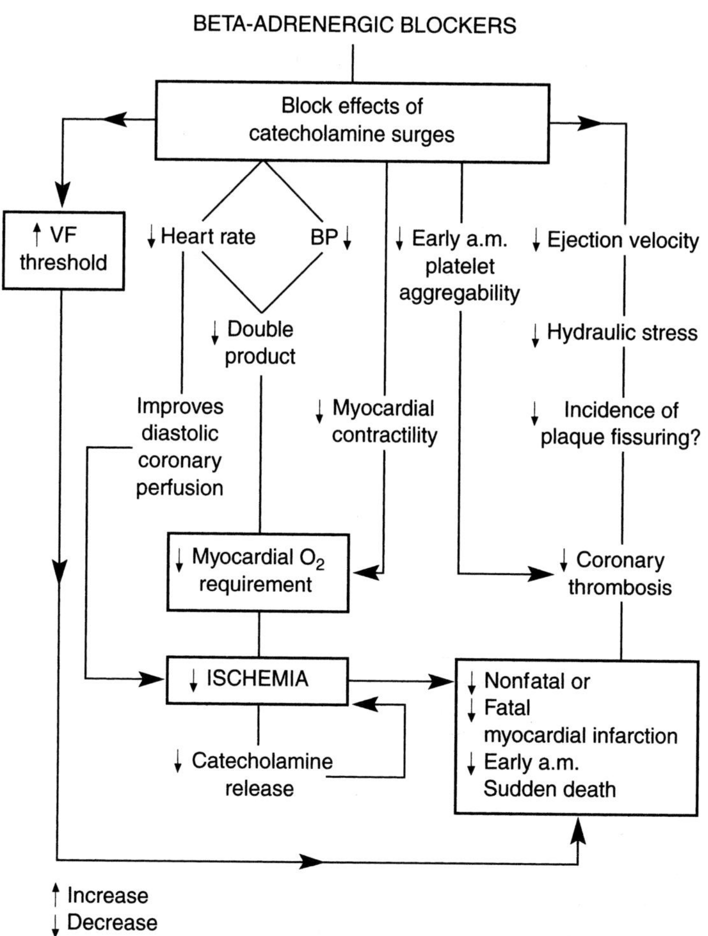

Fig. 1-1. Salutary effects of beta-adrenergic blockade. (From Khan M Gabriel, Topol EJ. Acute myocardial infarction diagnosis and therapy, a practical approach. Philadelphia, PA, Williams and Wilkins, 1996.)

Table 1-1
Beta-Blockers: First-Line Oral Drug Treatment in Angina Pectoris

Effect on	*Beta-blocker*	*Calcium antagonist*	*Oral nitrate*
Heart rate	↓	↑↓	↓
Diastolic filling of coronary arteries	↑	—	—
Blood pressure	↓↓	↓↓	—
Rate pressure product (RPP)	↓	—[a]	—
Relief of angina	Yes	Yes	Variable
Blood flow (subendocardial ischemic area)[b]	↑	↓	Variable
First-line treatment for angina pectoris	Yes	No	No
Prevention of recurrent ventricular fibrillation	Proven	No	No
Prevention of cardiac death	Proven	No	No
Prevention of pain owing to CAS	No	Yes	Variable
Prevention of death in patient with CAS	No	No	No

[a]RPP variable decrease on exercise, but not significant at rest or on maximal exercise.
[b]Distal to organic obstruction *(40)*.
CAS, coronary artery spasm; ↓, decrease; ↑, increase; —, no significant change.

Table 1-2
Beta-Blockers: Randomized Controlled Trials Showing Significant Reduction in Mortality Rate

		Mortality		*Relative risk reduction*	
Trial	*Drug*	*Placebo*	*Drug*	*%*	*P*
APSI *(39)*	Acebutolol	34/309 11.0%	17/298 5.7%	48	0.019
BHAT *(31)*	Propranolol	188/1921 9.8%	138/1916 7.2%	26.5	<0.01
Norwegian Postinfarction Study *(16)*	Timolol	152/939 16.2%	98/945 10.4%	35.8	<0.001
Salathia	Metoprolol	43/364 11.8%	27/391 6.9%	41.5	<0.05
Hjalmarson et al. *(69)*	Metoprolol Post MI	62/679 8.9%	40/698 5.7%	36.0	<0.03
COPERNICUS					
CAPRICORN					
CIBIS-II					
MERIT-HF					

calcium antagonists. Dihydropyridines increase the risk of death in patients with unstable angina; these agents are not approved for use in unstable angina in the absence of beta-blockade. Diltiazem and verapamil have been shown to increase mortality in patients with acute MI with LV dysfunction *(7)*. After more than 25 yr of use, calcium antagonists have not been shown in RCTs to prolong life significantly in patients with CHD. Beta-blockers have been shown to prolong life in more than four RCTs (Table 1-2). Because calcium antagonists have been shown to increase cardiovascular mortality in hypertensive diabetic patients *(8)*, the author strongly recommends the use of beta-blockers except in diabetic patients prone to hypoglycemia. This recommendation is in accordance with those of most cardiologists and differs from that of the JNC. Diabetic patients can be given a cardioselective beta-blocker *(4)* or an ACE inhibitor.

This chapter provides information that includes

- Sound reasons and results of RCTs that document the salutary effects of beta-blockers in many cardiovascular settings (Tables 1-1, 1-2, and 1-3).
- The appropriate indications as advocated by virtually all cardiologists.

The many approved cardiovascular indications (Table 1-3) allow the author to proclaim that beta-blockers are the cornerstone of cardiac drug therapy. As a class, beta-blockers represent one of the five all-time major breakthroughs in clinical drug development *(4)*. Virtually all cardiologists now concur with the author's views on the salutary effects of beta-blockers.

BETA-RECEPTORS

The beta-receptors are subdivided into

- The $beta_1$-receptors, present mainly in the heart, intestine, renin-secreting tissues of the kidney, those parts of the eye responsible for the production of aqueous humor, adipose tissue, and, to a limited degree, bronchial tissue.

Table 1-3
Cardiovascular Indications for Beta-Blockers

1. Ischemic heart disease
   Stable angina
   Unstable angina
   Acute MI
   MI, long-term prevention
   Silent ischemia
2. Arrhythmias
   VPBs
   AVNRT
   Atrial fibrillation
   Nonsustained VT
   VT
   Recurrent VF
3. Hypertension
   Isolated
   With IHD, diabetes*, LVH, dyslipidemia[a]
   With arrhythmias
   Perioperative and on intubation
   Severe, urgent
   Pheochromocytoma (on alpha-blocker)
4. Heart failure: new indication class I–III
5. Prolonged QT syndrome
6. Aortic dissection
7. Valvular heart disease
   Mitral stenosis? tachycardia in pregnancy*
   Mitral valve prolapse
   Mitral regurgitation
8. To decrease perioperative mortality
9. Cardiomyopathy
   Hypertrophic
   Dilated
10. Marfan's syndrome
11. Neurocardiogenic syncope
12. Tetralogy of Fallot
13. Aneurysm

[a]*See* text; 10-yr CHD event risk score > 20%; *see* Chapter 17.

AVNRT, atrioventricular node reentry tachycardia; CHD, coronary heart disease; IHD, ischemic heart disease; LVH, left ventricular hypertrophy; VPB, ventricular premature beat; VF, ventricular fibrillation; VT, ventricular tachycardia.

- The beta$_2$-receptors, predominating in bronchial and vascular smooth muscle, gastrointestinal tract, the uterus, insulin-secreting tissue of the pancreas, and, to a limited degree, the heart and large coronary arteries. Metabolic receptors are usually beta$_2$. In addition, it should be noted that
  a. None of these tissues contains exclusively one subgroup of receptors.
  b. The beta-receptor population is not static, and beta-blockers appear to increase the number of receptors during long-term therapy. The number of cardiac beta$_2$-receptors increases after beta$_1$-blockade *(9)*.
  c. The population density of receptors decreases with age.

The beta-receptors are situated on the cell membrane and are believed to be a part of the adenyl cyclase system. An agonist acting on its receptor site activates adenyl cyclase to produce cyclic adenosine-5'-monophosphate, which is believed to be the intracellular messenger of beta-stimulation.

The heart contains $beta_1$- and $beta_2$-adrenergic receptors in the proportion 70:30. Normally, cardiac $beta_1$-adrenergic receptors appear to regulate heart rate and/or myocardial contractility, but in situations of stress, with the provocation of epinephrine release, stimulation of cardiac $beta_2$-receptors may contribute to additional increases in heart rate and/or contractility *(10)*. In HF, cardiac $beta_1$- but not $beta_2$-adrenergic receptors are reduced in number and population, and the myocardium may be less responsive to $beta_1$-inotropic agents.

MECHANISM OF ACTION

By definition, beta-blockers block beta-receptors. Structurally, they resemble the catecholamines. Beta-blockers are competitive inhibitors, their action depending on the ratio of beta-blocker concentration to catecholamine concentration at beta-adrenoceptor sites.

- Blockade of cardiac $beta_1$-receptors causes a decrease in heart rate, myocardial contractility, and velocity of cardiac contraction. The heart rate multiplied by the systolic blood pressure (i.e., the rate pressure product [RPP]) is reduced at rest and during exercise, and this action is reflected in a reduced myocardial oxygen demand (which is an important effect in the control of angina).
- The main in vitro antiarrhythmic effect of beta-blockers is the depression of phase 4 diastolic depolarization. Beta-blockers are effective in abolishing arrhythmias produced by increased catecholamines. Maximum impulse traffic through the atrioventricular (AV) node is reduced, and the rate of conduction is slowed. Paroxysmal supraventricular tachycardia (PSVT) caused by AV nodal reentry is often abolished by beta-blockers, which also slow the ventricular rate in atrial flutter and atrial fibrillation. There is a variable effect on ventricular arrhythmias, which may be abolished if induced by increased sympathetic activity, as is often seen in myocardial ischemia.
- Beta-blockers reduce the activity of the renin-angiotensin system by reducing renin release from the juxtaglomerular cells. Also, beta-blockade augments atrial and brain natriuretic peptide (see next section and Suggested Reading).
- Beta-blockers interfere with sympathetic vasoconstrictor nerve activity; this action is partly responsible for their antihypertensive effect. Cardiac output usually falls and remains slightly lower than normal with administration of nonintrinsic sympathomimetic activity (ISA) agents. Systemic vascular resistance increases acutely but falls to near normal with long-term administration *(14)*.

Other Important Clinically Beneficial Mechanisms

Beta-blockers

- Lower plasma endothelin-1 levels, as shown for carvedilol *(11)*, and inhibit catecholamine-induced cardiac necrosis (apoptosis) *(12)*.
- Stimulate the endothelial-*arginine/nitric oxide pathway*, as shown for the interesting vasodilatory beta-blocker nebivolol *(13)*. (*See* last section "Which Beta-Blocker Is Best for Your Patients?".)
- Augment atrial and brain natriuretic peptide, upregulate cardiac $beta_1$-receptors, and inhibit stimulatory anti-$beta_1$-receptor autoantibodies.

Beta-Blocker Effect on Calcium Availability

The slow channels represent two of the mechanisms by which calcium gains entry into the myocardial cell. At least two channels exist *(15)*, namely,

- A voltage-dependent channel blocked by calcium antagonists (*see* Chapter 8).
- A receptor-operated channel blocked by beta-receptor blockers that therefore decrease calcium availability inside the myocardial cell. The negative inotropic effect of beta- blockers is probably based on this effect.

DOSAGE CONSIDERATIONS

- The **beta-blocking effect** is manifest as a blockade of tachycardia when induced by exercise or isoproterenol. The therapeutic response to beta-blockers does not correlate in a linear fashion with the oral dose or plasma level. Differences in the degree of absorption and variation in hepatic metabolism give rise to unpredictable plasma levels, but in addition the same blood level may elicit a different cardiovascular response in patients, depending on the individual's sympathetic and vagal tone and the population of beta-receptors.
- The **dose** of beta-blocker is titrated to achieve control of angina, hypertension, or arrhythmia. The dose is usually adjusted to achieve a heart rate of 50–60/min and an exercise heart rate < 110/min. The dosage of propranolol varies considerably (120–480 mg daily) because of the marked but variable first-pass hepatic metabolism. There is a 20-fold variation in plasma level from a given dose of this drug. The proven **cardioprotective** (CP) dose may be different from the dose necessary to achieve control of angina or hypertension. The effective CP dose (i.e., the dose shown to prevent cardiac deaths in the post-MI patient) for timolol is 10–20 mg daily *(16)*, and for propranolol it is within the range 160–240 mg daily. When possible, the dosage of beta-blocker should be kept within the CP range. Other experts are in agreement with this concern for use of the CP dose when possible *(17)*.
- An **increase in the dose** beyond the CP dosage (e.g., timolol > 30 mg or propranolol > 240 mg daily), for better control of angina, hypertension, or arrhythmia, may have a poor reward, that is, there could be an increase in side effects, especially dyspnea, HF, and distressing fatigue.
- A review of the clinical literature reveals that too large a dose of beta-blockers may be not only nonprotective but also positively harmful, and this is supported by studies on animals *(18)*. In some patients, one should be satisfied with 75% control of symptoms and, if necessary, the addition of a further therapeutic agent. The patient is not fearful of anginal pain or high blood pressure—what the patient fears is death. *Beta-blockers do prevent cardiac deaths, but they have been shown to do so only at certain doses*. In addition, beta-blockers are not all alike; subtle differences can be of importance. Only bisoprolol, carvedilol, metoprolol, propranolol, and timolol have been shown to prolong life in RCTs (*see* Table 1-2).
- Patients may require different drug concentrations to achieve adequate beta-blockade because of different levels of sympathetic tone (circulating catecholamines and active beta-adrenoceptor binding sites). However, **plasma levels** do not indicate active metabolites, and the effect of the drug may last longer than is suggested by the half-life.
- Propranolol may take 4–6 wk to achieve stable plasma levels because of the extensive hepatic metabolism, but timolol and pindolol undergo less than 60% metabolism, and constant plasma concentrations are more readily achieved. Therefore, **propranolol** should be given three times daily for about 6 wk and then twice daily, or propranolol long-acting (LA) 160–240 mg once daily.
- **Atenolol**, **nadolol**, and **sotalol** are excreted virtually unchanged by the kidneys and require alteration of the dosage in severe renal dysfunction, as follows:

Table 1-4
Dosage of Commonly Used Beta-Blockers

Beta-blocker	*Daily starting dose (mg)*	*Maintenance dose (mg)*	*Maximum suggested dose (mg)*
Atenolol*	50	50–100	100
Acebutolol	100–400	600–1000	1200
Bisoprolol	5	5–15	20
Carvedilol	12.5	25–50	50
Metoprolol	50–100	100–300	400
Nadolol	20–80	20–160	160
Propranolol	40–120	40–240	320
Sotalol	80–160	60–320	320
Timolol	5–10	20–30	40

*Not recommended by the author; *see* Chapter 2, Controversies.

a. Creatinine clearance of 30–50 mL/min, half the average dose per 24 h.
b. Creatinine clearance less than 30 mL/min, half the usual dose every 48 h.

The **oral doses** of commonly used beta-blockers are given in Table 1-4. The **intravenous (IV) doses** are as follows:

Esmolol: 3–6 mg over 1 min, then 1–5 mg/min.
Propranolol: up to 1 mg, at a rate of 0.5 mg/min, repeated if necessary at 2–5-min intervals to a maximum of 5 mg (rarely 10 mg): 0.1 mg/kg.
Metoprolol: up to 5 mg, at a rate of 1 mg/min, repeated if necessary at 5-min intervals to a maximum of 10 mg (rarely 15 mg).
Atenolol: up to 2.5 mg, at a rate of 1 mg/min, repeated if necessary at 5-min intervals to a maximum of 10 mg.
By IV infusion (atenolol): 150 mg/kg over 20 min repeated every 12 h if required.

PHARMACOLOGIC PROPERTIES AND CLINICAL IMPLICATIONS

A clinically useful classification of beta-blockers is given in Figure 1-2, and their pharmacologic properties are summarized in Table 1-5.

Cardioselectivity

Cardioselectivity implies that the drug blocks chiefly the $beta_1$-receptors and therefore partially spares $beta_2$-receptors in the lungs and blood vessels. A small quantity of $beta_1$-receptors is present in the lungs. Large doses of all beta-blocking drugs block $beta_2$-receptors. Selectivity holds only for small doses and may be lost at the doses necessary for the relief of angina or for the control of hypertension. Atenolol, betaxolol, bisoprolol, metoprolol, bevantolol, esmolol, and, to a lesser degree, acebutolol, have less of a blocking effect on $beta_2$-receptors in the lungs, so they are not cardiospecific. They can precipitate bronchospasm in susceptible individuals. Nebivolol is the most $beta_1$-selective, followed by bisoprolol, which is highly selective; the others are moderately to weakly selective.

1. **Bronchospasm.** Cardioselective agents may precipitate bronchospasm in a susceptible patient, and this is no different from that of nonselective drugs, **except** when bronchospasm

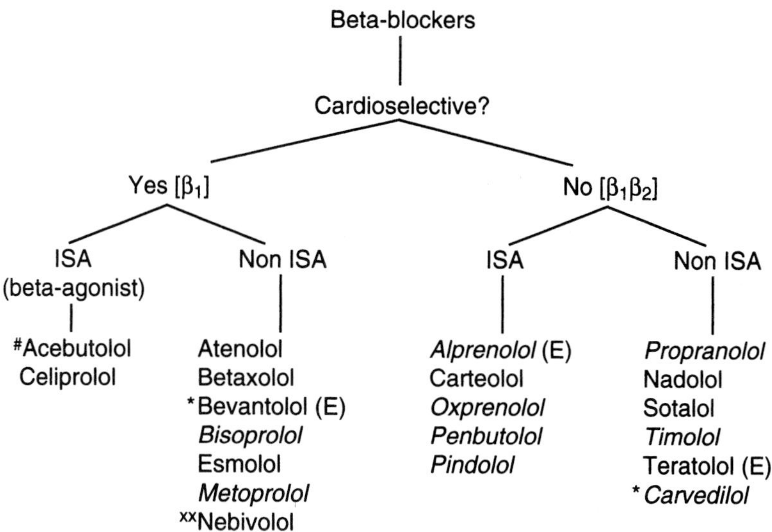

Fig. 1-2. Classification of beta-blockers.

occurs the patient will **respond to a beta$_2$-stimulant** such as albuterol (salbutamol) if a cardioselective drug was administered. When bronchospasm occurs with the use of nonselective drugs, including pindolol, the spasm may be more resistant to beta-stimulants. Beta-blockers should not be given to patients with **bronchial asthma** or severe chronic bronchitis or emphysema. It is wise in such patients to choose alternative therapeutic agents. *Mild chronic bronchitis* is indicated by the following:

- Forced expiratory volume greater than 1.5 L.
- No hospital emergency room or office treatments for bronchospastic disease.

If a patient with mild chronic bronchitis requires treatment with a beta-blocker for angina, treatment should begin with bisoprolol or metoprolol. If bronchospasm occurs, albuterol (salbutamol) should be added, or the beta-blocker should be discontinued. Bisoprolol is the most cardioselective beta-blocker available and is safer than metoprolol for patients with chronic obstructive pulmonary disease (COPD). In humans, the drug has a twofold higher beta$_1$-selectivity than atenolol.

2. **Peripheral vascular disease** (PVD). If a beta-blocker is necessary in a patient with PVD, some clinical trials indicate that it is safer to use a cardioselective drug, atenolol or metoprolol; agents such as carvedilol or bucindolol that cause vasodilation may have a role. Analysis of 11 randomized trials of beta-blockers in patients with PVD showed no worsening of intermittent claudication. Patients with PVD are at high risk for CHD events, and beta-blockers are recommended for all indications. In the United Kingdom Prospective Diabetes Study Group (UKPDS) *(19), atenolol did not worsen PVD, and there was a nonsignificant 48% excess of amputations in the captopril group.*

Table 1-5
Pharmacologic Properties of Beta-Adrenoceptor Blockers

Beta-blocker	*Propranol*	*Timolol*	*Metoprolol*	*Nadolol*	*Atenolol*	*Carvedilol*	*Bisoprolol*	*Acebutolol*	*Sotalol*
Equivalent dose (mg)	80	10	100	60	50	12.5	10	400	80
Potency ratio	1	6–8	1	1–1.5	1–2	?		0.3	0.5–1
Relative cardioselectivity	No	No	Yes Moderate	No	Yes Strong	No	Strong	Yes Mild	No
Partial agonist activity (ISA)	0	0	0	0	0	0	Nil	Mild	0
Half life (h)	2–6	2–6	2–6	14–24	7–20		14	2–6	7–20
Variation in plasma level	20-fold	7-fold	7-fold	7-fold	4-fold			?	4-fold
Lipid solubility	Strong	Moderate	Strong	Nil	Nil	Moderate	Moderate	Weak	Nil
Absorption (%)	90	90	95	30	50			75	90
Bioavailability (%)	30	75	50	30	50			40	90
Hepatic metabolism (HM)	HM	60% HM	HM	No	No	HM	50%	HM	No
Renal excretion (RE)		40% RE		RE	RE		50% RE	60% RE	RE

ISA, intrinsic sympathomimetic activity.

3. **Hypoglycemia** stimulates an increase in catecholamine release, which increases blood glucose. The recovery from hypoglycemia may be delayed by nonselective beta-blockers. The incidence of hypoglycemia is higher in insulin-dependent diabetic patients treated with nonselective beta-blockers, whereas both selective and nonselective varieties modify the symptoms of hypoglycemia (with the exception of sweating). Glycolysis and lipolysis in skeletal muscles are mediated mainly by beta$_2$-receptors. Hypoglycemia induced by exercise is more likely to occur with a nonselective beta-blocker. However, evidence to support a greater benefit of selective beta-blockers in joggers is lacking *(20)*. **Insulin** secretion is probably beta$_2$-mediated. Glucose-sulfonylurea-stimulated insulin secretion is inhibited by beta-blockers. Beta-blockers may increase blood glucose by 1.0–1.5 mmol/L, but this glucose intolerance is not type 2 diabetes.

   The following points deserve consideration:

- Catecholamine stimulation of beta$_2$-receptors produces transient hypokalemia. Thus, cardioselective drugs that spare beta$_2$-receptors may fail to maintain constancy of serum potassium in response to increase in epinephrine and norepinephrine during acute MI *(21)*.
- *Noncardioselective agents are superior to selective agents in preventing fluctuations of serum potassium concentration during stress and possibly during acute MI.*
- *Nonselective drugs should confer a greater degree of cardioprotection; carvedilol, propranolol, and timolol have been shown to prevent total mortality and cardiac death in well-controlled RCTs.*
- *Carvedilol, therefore should replace the commonly used metoprolol in patients with acute MI and in heart failure patients post-MI.*

Intrinsic Sympathomimetic Activity (ISA)

ISA indicates partial agonist activity, the primary agonists being epinephrine and isoproterenol. Beta-blockers that cause a small agonist response (i.e., stimulate as well as block the beta-receptors) include pindolol, alprenolol, acebutolol, celiprolol, carteolol, oxprenolol, and practolol. The last drug has been removed from medical practice because it produced the oculomucocutaneous syndrome. Beta-blockers with ISA cause a slightly lower incidence of bradycardia compared with non-ISA drugs. In practice, this is a minor advantage in the choice of a beta-blocker. The heart rate at rest may be only slightly lowered or unchanged; in patients with angina, a slower heart rate is conducive to less pain on activity.

The RPP at rest is not significantly reduced. Myocardial oxygen consumption is therefore not usually reduced at rest by ISA beta-blockers. Beta-blockers with ISA, therefore, carry **no advantage** in angina at rest or in angina occurring at low exercise levels; in particular, they do not have a beneficial effect on cardioprotection. The ISA of beta-blockers produces adverse effects on ventricular fibrillation (VF) threshold *(22)*. Acebutolol with weak ISA, however, has been shown to prevent cardiac death. Because they limit exercise tachycardia, these drugs do have a **minor role** to play in the treatment of patients who have a relatively low resting heart rate (50–60/min) and in whom further bradycardia may not be acceptable. Even in this subgroup, it is still important to exclude patients with sick sinus syndrome because all beta-blockers are contraindicated here. **Renin** secretion may remain unaltered or may even be increased by agents with ISA. There may be added sodium and water retention, causing edema. There is no clear-cut evidence that peripheral vascular complications are less frequent when beta-blockers with partial agonist activity are used. *Agents with ISA, except acebutolol (very weak ISA) are not recommended by the author because of the aforementioned points; these are not CP drugs.*

Membrane-Stabilizing Activity

The quinidine-like or local anesthetic action, membrane-stabilizing activity (MSA), is of no clinical importance, except perhaps for its effect on platelets and in the treatment of glaucoma. It is not related to the antiarrhythmic, antianginal, or CP properties of beta-blockers. Unlike most available beta-blockers, timolol and betaxolol have no MSA. Because of high potency and lack of anesthetic effect, these drugs are the only beta-blockers that have been proved safe and effective in the treatment of glaucoma when used topically.

MSA appears to be important in the management of thyrotoxic crisis, and propranolol has been shown to be more effective than nadolol in this condition.

Effects on Renin

Renin release from the juxtaglomerular cells is suppressed by $beta_1$-receptor blockade; this results in reduced activity of the renin-angiotensin system. Beta-blockers enhance the lifesaving effects of ACE inhibitors in patients with HF or MI *(23)*.

Lipid Solubility

- Highly lipid-soluble, lipophilic beta-blockers—carvedilol, propranolol, timolol, and metoprolol—reach high concentrations in the brain and are metabolized in the liver.
- Atenolol, nadolol, and sotalol are lipid insoluble, show poor brain concentration, and are not metabolized by the liver; they are water soluble, are excreted by the kidneys, and have a long half-life. Pindolol and timolol are about 50% metabolized and about 50% excreted by the kidney.
- Brain:plasma ratios are 15:1 for propranolol, 3:1 for metoprolol, and 1:8 for atenolol.
- Lipid-insoluble, hydrophilic beta-blockers appear to have a lower incidence of central nervous system (CNS) side effects such as vivid dreams, significant effects on sleep *(24)*, impairment of very fast mental reactions *(25)*, depression, fatigue, and impotence. Depending on dosage, even the lipid-insoluble drugs can achieve sufficient brain concentration to impair very fast mental reactions. There is little doubt, however, that atenolol causes fewer central side effects than propranolol *(25)*. Timolol has been shown to cause less bizarre dreams than pindolol or propranolol in small groups of patients.
- **Lipid-soluble beta-blocking agents with high brain concentrations block sympathetic discharge in the hypothalamus better than water-soluble agents *(26)*, and they are more effective in the prevention of cardiac deaths.**
- Bisoprolol is 50% lipophilic and liver metabolized but does not involve the cytochrome P-450 3A4 pathway; renal elimination is approx 50%.

Plasma Volume

A reduction in cardiac output is usually followed by an increase in plasma volume. Beta-blockers cause a reduction in plasma volume; the exact reason for this is unknown. Pindolol (ISA) may increase plasma volume.

Hepatic Metabolism

Propranolol, oxprenolol, and metoprolol have high first-pass liver metabolism. Timolol and acebutolol have modest lipid solubility and undergo major hepatic metabolism. Acebutolol is metabolized to an active metabolite, diacetolol, which is water soluble and is excreted by the kidneys. Atenolol, nadolol, and sotalol are not metabolized in the liver. First-pass metabolism varies greatly among patients and can alter the dose of drug required, especially with propranolol. Cigarette smoking interferes with drug metabolism in the liver and reduces the efficacy of propranolol, other hepatically metabolized beta-blockers, and calcium antagonists *(27)*.

Effects on Blood and Arteries

1. **Platelets.** Platelet hyperaggregation seen in patients with angina or induced by catecholamines can be normalized by propranolol. The second stage of platelet aggregation, induced by adenosine diphosphate, catecholamines, collagen, or thrombin, can be abolished or inhibited by propranolol. Propranolol is able to block [^{14}C]serotonin released from platelets and inhibits platelet adherence to collagen; these favorable effects can be detected with the usual clinical doses of propranolol and other beta-blocking drugs.
2. **HDL-C.** It has been suggested that beta-blockers may increase atherosclerosis by decreasing HDL levels. Propranolol causes a mild decrease in HDL levels of approx 7%. There is at present no proof that decreasing HDL values from, for example, 55 to 50 mg/dL (i.e., from 1.4 to 1.3 mmol/L), will have any adverse effect on the progression of atherosclerosis. Some studies suggest that HDL_2 remains unaltered *(28,29)*. There is little doubt that in some patients HDL_2 is slightly lowered. In one study, there was an 8% lowering of HDL_2 and a rise in triglycerides produced by both propranolol and pindolol at 6 wk. Beta-blockers do not decrease total serum cholesterol. The effect of beta-blockers on triglycerides is variable, and the evidence associating raised triglycerides with ischemic heart disease (IHD) is weak. Acebutolol with weak ISA causes no significant disturbance of lipid levels. **Bisoprolol**, being highly $beta_1$-selective, does not significantly decrease HDL-C.
3. **Arteries.** Beta-blockers decrease the force and velocity of cardiac contraction, decrease, RPP and heart rate × peak velocity, and therefore decrease hemodynamic stress on the arterial wall, especially at the branching of arteries. This action may decrease the atherosclerotic process and *plaque rupture*. This beneficial hemodynamic effect, and that described on blood coagulation, may favorably influence atherosclerotic CHD and subsequent occlusion by platelets or thrombosis.
4. **Coronary blood flow.** Beta-blockers increase diastolic coronary perfusion time and coronary blood flow because bradycardia lengthens the diastolic filling time. Thus, these agents produce beneficial effects in angina and IHD by increasing coronary blood supply while reducing myocardial oxygen demands; the reduction of hydraulic stress in the coronary arteries appears to *provide protection from plaque fissuring and rupture* (*see* Fig. 1-1).

Effect on Serum Potassium

- Beta-blockade causes a mild increase in serum potassium because of blockade of the $beta_2$-mediated epinephrine activation of the Na^+, K^+-ATPase pump, which transports potassium from extracellular fluid into cells.
- During stress, serum potassium has been observed to decrease up to 1.0 mEq (mmol)/L; this fall in serum potassium concentration can be prevented by blockade of $beta_2$-receptors.
- *Noncardioselective agents are superior to selective agents in preventing fluctuations of serum potassium concentration during stress and possibly during acute MI.*

SALUTARY EFFECTS OF BETA-ADRENERGIC BLOCKADE

These beneficial effects *(30)* are outlined in Fig. 1-1 and include the following:

- A decrease in heart rate increases the diastolic interval and allows for improved diastolic filling of the coronary arteries. This effect is especially important during exercise in patients with angina.

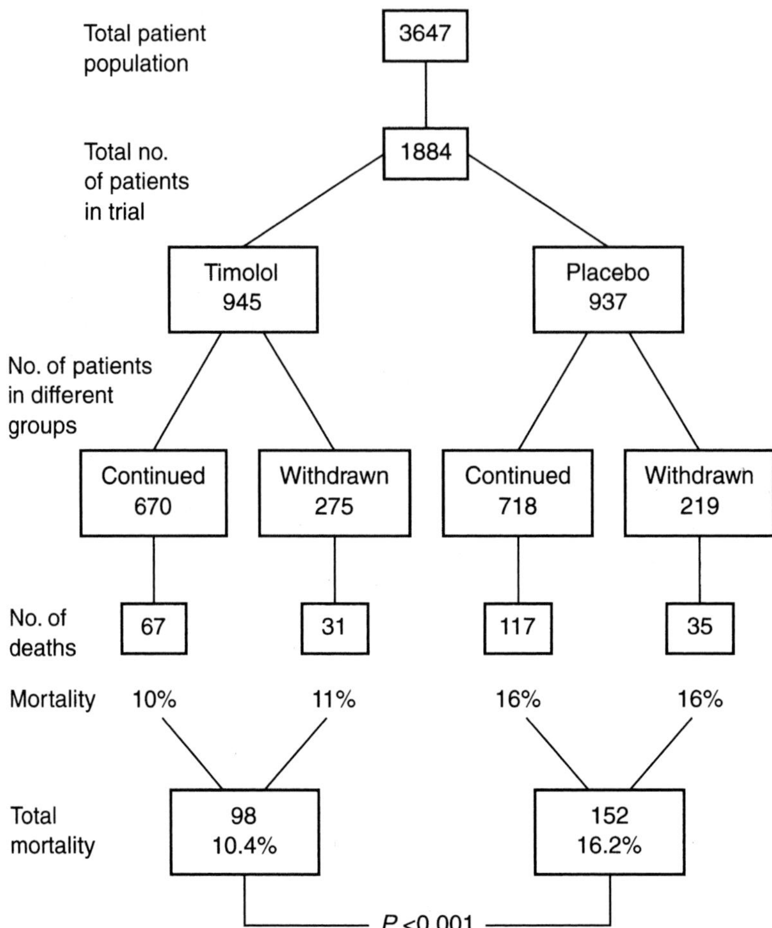

Fig. 1-3. Results of the Norwegian Multicenter Postinfarction Trial of timolol. Timolol was administered at a dosage of 10 mg twice daily from 7 to 28 d. Patients were followed for a mean duration of 17 mo. The age range was 20 to 75 yr. (From Am J Cardiol 1990;66:4C; with permission of Excerpta Medica, Inc. [Elsevier].)

- The RPP is decreased, so there is less myocardial demand for oxygen, resulting in an improvement of ischemia.
- A decrease in sudden cardiac death has been documented in several studies. *An impressive 67% reduction in sudden death was observed in smokers and nonsmokers in the Timolol Norwegian Reinfarction Study (16)*: timolol decreased the overall mortality rate by 36%, $p < 0.001$ (Fig. 1-3).
- This beneficial effect of beta-blockers in postinfarction patients was reconfirmed in the Beta-Blocker Heart Attack Trial (BHAT) *(31)*. This well-run trial randomized 16,400 post-MI patients to propranolol or placebo and after 2-yr follow-up showed a 26% reduction in the mortality rate with propranolol *(31)*.
- A decrease in fatal arrhythmias and an increase in VF threshold, as well as amelioration of bothersome benign ventricular and supraventricular arrhythmias, have been established by several clinical studies.
- A decrease in the velocity and force of myocardial contraction results in a decrease in myocardial oxygen requirement and also reduces the rate of rise of aortic pressure, which is

important in the prevention and treatment of aortic dissection. Beta-blockade is effective in slowing the rate of aortic dilation and reducing the development of aortic complications in patients with Marfan's syndrome *(32)*.

- A decrease in ejection velocity reduces hydraulic stress on the arterial wall that could be crucial at the site of atheroma. This mechanism of action may reduce the incidence of plaque rupture and may thus protect patients from coronary thrombosis and fatal or nonfatal infarction *(31)*.
- Beta-blockers may prevent early morning platelet aggregation induced by catecholamines and may decrease the early morning peak incidence of acute MI *(33)*.
- Low heart rate variability predicts mortality in postinfarction patients *(34,35)*. Metoprolol and atenolol enhance heart rate variability in patients with CHD *(36)*.

The favorable effect of beta-blockade on sudden death relative to reduction in heart rate is observed only with the use of beta-blockers that reduce heart rate *(37,38)*. Beta-blockers such as pindolol with marked ISA and no bradycardic response at rest cause no reduction in sudden death or mortality rates Acebutolol with mild ISA, however, caused a 48% reduction in overall mortality rate and a 58% reduction in cardiovascular mortality rate in postinfarction patients *(39)*.

BETA-BLOCKERS VERSUS CALCIUM ANTAGONISTS AND ORAL NITRATES

The clinical effects of beta-blockers compared with calcium antagonists and oral nitrates are shown in Table 1-1.

1. **A decrease in heart rate** by beta-blockers allows for a **longer diastolic filling** time and therefore **greater coronary perfusion**.
2. It is often stated that beta-blockers may decrease coronary blood flow, but this is secondary to the reduction in myocardial work; in practice, this effect is not harmful. A decrease in blood flow does not occur if there is ischemia, and therefore it is not of importance in occlusive coronary disease. If you need less oxygen, you will need less blood flow; this fact is often misinterpreted. The RPP at rest and on maximal exercise is reduced by beta-blockers, but it is not decreased by calcium antagonists or oral nitrates.
3. Both beta-blockers and calcium antagonists have been proved to be more effective than nitrates when they are used alone in the relief of angina pectoris.
4. In animals, **blood flow** to the subendocardial ischemic myocardium distal to an organic obstruction is improved by beta-blockers, and it may be decreased by calcium antagonists *(40)*. Beta-blockers divert blood from the epicardium to the ischemic subendocardium by activation of autoregulatory mechanisms. Calcium antagonists may have the opposite effect and can cause deterioration in patients with critical coronary artery stenosis *(41)*. Unfortunately, calcium antagonists, when used without a beta-blocker in patients with unstable angina, can increase chest pain and infarction, and they appeared to increase mortality in the largest subgroup of patients with unstable angina. Oral nitrates have an effect similar to that of calcium antagonists.
5. Beta-blockers can prevent **recurrent VF** in animals and in patients *(42–44)*, whereas calcium antagonists do not significantly alter VF threshold.
6. Beta-blockers have been shown to prevent cardiac death in patients after MI, followed for 2 yr *(16,31,39)*. There is no reason to suppose that the same favorable effect is absent in the patient with angina pectoris or hypertension, provided an appropriate beta-blocker is used at CP doses (metoprolol, timolol, or propranolol, the last drug in nonsmokers). In

contrast, calcium antagonists provide only symptomatic relief. There are good reasons, therefore, for employing beta-blockers as first-line drugs in the treatment of **angina pectoris**, and this should remain the case until other therapeutic maneuvers are proved conclusively to prevent sudden and other cardiac deaths. Current evidence clearly indicates that calcium antagonists do not prevent cardiac deaths. *There has been a misguided tendency to replace beta-blockers in the management of angina pectoris with calcium antagonists because they are just as effective for the relief of cardiac pain in patients with angina pectoris. Calcium antagonists cannot be regarded as alternative therapy; they constitute suitable therapy when beta-blockers are contraindicated.*

7. Occasionally, **CAS** can be made worse in allowing unopposed alpha-vasoconstriction. It is emphasized that variant angina resulting from CAS is rare, and only the occasional patient may have an increase in chest pain secondary to beta-blockers *(40,45)*. Usually, this is not dangerous, and it gives an indication that CAS may be present. In patients in whom the mechanism of unstable angina is unclear, beta-blockers should be used combined with calcium antagonists or nitrates *(45)*.

INDICATIONS FOR BETA-BLOCKERS

Angina

The use of beta-blockers in the management of angina pectoris and silent ischemia is discussed in Chapter 10 (*see* Table 1-3).

Arrhythmias

- Ventricular premature beats that are symptomatic in patients with normal hearts and in those with a history of cardiac disease benefit from treatment with a beta-blocker. In the acute phase of MI, ventricular premature beats and ischemia caused by catecholamine surge respond favorably.
- AV nodal reentrant tachycardia may be aborted by beta-blocker therapy.
- Atrial fibrillation: rate control is best achieved with a small dose of a beta-blocking drug, particularly because digoxin does not decrease heart rate adequately in patients during exercise. Sotalol may decrease the recurrence of paroxysmal atrial fibrillation. Other beta-blockers do not possess class III activity and are not recommended for the maintenance of sinus rhythm in patients with paroxysmal atrial fibrillation. In patients converted to sinus rhythm by DC shock, maintenance of sinus rhythm with the use of sotalol is as good as quinidine.
- Esmolol IV may be used instead of diltiazem or verapamil, particularly in the perioperative period for most supraventricular tachycardias (SVTs) including atrial fibrillation.
- Nonsustained ventricular tachycardia (VT) is more appropriately treated with a beta-blocker than with antiarrhythmic agents. The use of most antiarrhythmics has dwindled because of the increased mortality attributed to these agents.
- Recurrent episodes of VT may be prevented in some patients. In the management of life-threatening arrhythmias in patients after cardiac arrest, metoprolol has been shown to be as good as amiodarone. When amiodarone and a beta-blocker combination is used, it appears that the prolongation of life observed is caused mainly by the addition of the beta-blocker. A European trial has shown that empiric use of metoprolol was as effective as electrophysiologically guided antiarrhythmic therapy *(46)*. Sotalol has been shown to be more effective than class I antiarrhythmics for VT. In the Canadian Amiodarone Myocardial Infarction Arrhythmia Trial (CAMIAT), all the good effects observed were in patients taking a beta-blocker along with amiodarone.

- Recurrent VF is unique among cardiac arrhythmias because the management is immediate countershock. Antifibrillatory drugs can be useful in the prevention of recurrent VF. Beta-blockers have long been known to have a role in the management of patients with persistently recurring VF *(42,43)*. Beta-blockers decrease the incidence of VF in patients with acute MI *(44)*. Beta-blockers increase VF threshold and should be given by the IV route in patients with recurrent VF if lidocaine or bretylium fails. IV beta-blockers are given by some before the use of bretylium.
- The importance of beta-blockade in the management of patients with sustained VT has been demonstrated in a prospective study *(47)*.

Hypertension

- **Young patients.** A beta-blocker is the drug of choice in younger and older white patients with or without comorbid conditions, particularly IHD, MI, diabetes, and hyperlipidemia. Beta-blockers are generally known to be effective in white people aged less than 65 yr. In a study by Matterson and colleagues *(48)* in African-American patients younger than 60 yr, atenolol was, surprisingly, the second most effective drug, after diltiazem, and it was more effective than hydrochlorothiazide (HCTZ). *See* treatment algorithms in Chapter 9, Hypertension Controversies.
- **Elderly patients.** *Contrary to common opinion, beta-blockers have been proved effective in older white patients (48).* The statement that beta-blockers are not advisable in elderly hypertensive patients, as given in textbooks and excellent editorials, review articles *(1)*, and JNC and WHO guidelines, is **false because it is based on the results of the Medical Research Council (MRC) trial in the elderly** *(49)* (*see* Chapters 8 and 9). Unfortunately, of the 4396 elderly hypertensive patients in this trial, 25% were lost to follow-up, and the 63% randomized to a beta-blocker either withdrew or were lost to follow-up. More than half the patients were not taking their assigned therapy by the end of the study. Cruickshank's review *(1)* quotes these relevant statistics and yet states "certainly beta-blockers should not be first-line therapy for elderly hypertensives." *The misleading MRC trial rings out this statement: elderly hypertensive patients respond best to diuretic-based rather than beta-blocker-based therapy in terms of fewer heart attacks.* If this poorly conducted MRC trial carries so much credibility, then diuretics should be used instead of beta-blockers to prevent heart attacks in all cardiac patients (hypertensive and normotensive) with high risk for CHD events. However, every practitioner knows that diuretics are not prescribed for prevention of CHD events in patients at risk for CHD events. Why prescribe them in place of beta-blockers in elderly hypertensive patients based on one unsound RCT? In the HANE (HCTZ, atenolol, nitrendipine, enalapril) study *(50)*, at 8 wk the blood pressure response rate was significantly higher for atenolol (64%) than for enalapril (50%), HCTZ (46%), or nitrendipine (45%). Effectivity was maintained at the end of 1 yr. **A beta-blocker was as effective in elderly patients as in younger ones.**
- In patients with hypertension or angina with LV dysfunction, a beta-blocker used in combination with an ACE inhibitor improves outcome.
- For prevention and regression of LVH, a beta-blocker or ACE inhibitor is more effective than a diuretic or calcium antagonist *(23,51)*.

Acute Myocardial Infarction

For the **first 7 d**, beta-blockers given within 4 h of an acute MI slightly reduce the 7-d mortality rate. There is evidence that beta-blockers can lower the incidence of acute MI, decrease the size of infarction, reduce the incidence of VF, and reduce the incidence of early cardiac rupture. Reduction of infarct size has been documented with the early use of timolol in acute MI *(52)*. Beta-blockers are recommended from d 1 and for 2 yr or more; their combination with ACE inhibitors is superior to ACE inhibitors alone *(23)*. During this period, these agents prevent sudden death and nonfatal and fatal MI and reduce overall mortality.

In the **CAPRICORN** study *(53)*, carvedilol produced an outstanding reduction in cardiac deaths and events in early post-MI patients (*see* the discussion of study results in Chapter 22).

- Caution is needed because beta-blockers may increase cardiac mortality when used indiscriminately in patients in whom the drugs are contraindicated, particularly IV use in patients who are hemodynamically unstable, with impending cardiogenic shock, pulmonary edema, or acute MI with HF (*see* COMMIT, Chapter 22).

Heart Failure

The potentially deleterious effects of overactivation of the sympathetic nervous system in HF are now well established; beta-blockers curb this sympathetic overactivation, hence the rationale for the judicious use of titrated doses of beta-blockers in patients with impaired LV function (*see* Chapter 12 for a discussion of the Second Cardiac Insufficiency Bisoprolol Study [CIBIS II] *(54)* and COPERNICUS *(55)*, which showed a significant reduction in overall mortality with bisoprolol and carvedilol therapy).

- Carvedilol has been shown in an RCT in patients with class II–III HF to decrease mortality and the risk of hospitalization for recurrent HF. Thus, approved beta-blockers have a new indication for the management of patients with LV dysfunction or class I–III HF.
- In **COPERNICUS** *(55)*, carvedilol produced a significant reduction in serious events in patients with compensated class IV HF, and the indication has been extended from class I to *compensated class IV* patients (*see* Chapters 12 and 22).
- *Most important, in MERIT-HF (56), only a small dose of a beta-blocking drug administered to patients in the low-dose subgroup achieved risk reduction similar to that observed in the high-dose subgroup.*

Elective Percutaneous Coronary Intervention (PCI)

Beta-blocker therapy is associated with a marked long-term survival benefit among patients undergoing successful PCI *(57)*; beta-blocker therapy was associated with a reduction from 6.0% to 3.9% at 1 yr ($p = 0.0014$).

Prolonged QT Interval Syndromes

- Congenital syndromes are rare, but they do respond to beta-blockers. These agents appear to restore an imbalance between the left and right stellate ganglia. If recurrent episodes of torsades de pointes develop in a patient with a prolonged QT interval, the condition usually responds to propranolol and acutely to pacing. Propranolol has been proved to be useful in the congenital long-QT syndromes (*see* Chapter 14).
- Beta-blockers have a variable effect in the acquired idiopathic long-QT syndromes.

Dissecting Aneurysm

A beta-blocker is the drug of choice to reduce the rate of rise of aortic pressure, which increases dissection. Even if the systolic blood pressure is 100–120 mmHg, propranolol or another IV preparation should be commenced. If the blood pressure exceeds 130 mmHg, a careful infusion of nitroprusside, or trimethaphan along with furosemide, is given to maintain systolic blood pressure at 100–120 mmHg. Labetalol has both beta- and alpha-blocking properties and has a role in therapy.

Note: The important effect of a beta-blocker in the treatment of dissecting aneurysm is not to lower blood pressure, but to decrease the force and velocity of myocardial contraction (*dp/dt*) and thus to arrest the progress of the dissection *(58)*. The drug decreases the reflex tachycardia provoked by nitroprusside. The aforementioned beneficial effects of beta-blocking drugs can be translated to protection of arteries in patients with moderate to severe hypertension and in those with aneurysms. These agents are useful during the surgical clipping of intracranial aneurysms.

Mitral Valve Prolapse

Patients who have palpitations respond favorably to beta-blockers. These drugs should not be prescribed routinely, however, if the patient has only the occasional brief episode of palpitations. Asymptomatic atrial or ventricular ectopic beats require no medication. Chest pain in mitral valve prolapse syndrome is usually noncardiac. Care should be taken not to overtreat with medications and to avoid cardiac neurosis because this syndrome is usually benign. A beta-blocker can be tried if symptoms are distressing.

Mitral Regurgitation and Mitral Stenosis

Clinical trials with the use of carvedilol in patients with mitral regurgitation have shown salutary effects that include improved geometry of the left ventricle. Beta-blockers are the cornerstone of treatment for pregnant patients with mitral stenosis. These agents may prevent fulminant pulmonary edema.

Tetralogy of Fallot

Propranolol, by inhibiting right ventricular contractility, is of value in the acute treatment and prevention of prolonged hypoxic spells *(59)*.

- IV propranolol is used only for severe hypoxic spells.
- Oral propranolol for the prevention of hypoxic episodes is useful in centers where surgical correction is not available or the surgical mortality rate is greater than 10% *(59)*.

Hypertrophic Cardiomyopathy

Medical management remains poor and does not significantly alter the mortality rate. Propranolol is effective for the relief of symptoms such as dizziness, presyncope, angina, and dyspnea, but the dose may need to be as high as 160–480 mg daily. Beta-blockers possessing ISA do not have a role here. **Verapamil** is a useful alternative if beta-blockers are contraindicated or have failed to relieve symptoms. **Disopyramide** appears to be of value in patients with hypertrophic cardiomyopathy, but it needs further randomized studies for confirmation. **Amiodarone** is useful for the control of arrhythmias associated with this condition, but it must not be combined with verapamil.

Marfan's Syndrome

Progressive dilation of the aorta, culminating in aortic dissection, is the most dreaded complication in patients with Marfan's syndrome. Prophylactic beta-blockade slows the rate of aortic dilation and retards the development of aortic complications *(32)*. Propranolol has been shown to increase crosslinking of collagen in animals known to have a higher rate of aortic dissection *(60,61)*.

Subarachnoid Hemorrhage

Arrhythmias and other electrocardiographic abnormalities, LV dysfunction with reduced EF *(62)*, and myocardial damage including subendocardial necrosis have been documented in patients with subarachnoid hemorrhage. These changes are believed to be caused by the release of sympathetic outflow that occurs with CNS damage and by local norepinephrine release from sympathetic nerves in the heart. Beta-blockers are indicated in individual patients with subarachnoid hemorrhage in conjunction with nimodipine therapy.

Perioperative Mortality

Optimization of cardiac medications in cardiac patients undergoing noncardiac surgery requires the addition of a beta-blocker. Beta-blockade allows safer induction of anesthesia and prevents the hypertensive response to endotracheal intubation; also, these agents prevent recurrent arrhythmias and have been shown to improve morbidity and mortality. Atenolol has been shown in an RCT to decrease morbidity and mortality when given before operation and for up to 1 wk postoperatively *(63)*.

Neurocardiogenic Syncope (Vasovagal/Vasodepressor Syncope)

If syncopal episodes are bothersome, a beta-blocking drug is advisable. Cardiac sympathetic overstimulation, vigorous LV contraction, and stimulation of intramyocardial mechanoreceptors (C fibers) are underlying mechanisms in the causation of unexplained syncope in patients with a normal heart *(64)*; a beta-blocker or disopyramide is the logical therapy and appears to be beneficial in patients with disabling syncope. Esmolol IV can be used to predict the outcome of oral beta-blocker therapy. Although a small trial has shown no beneficial effect for some beta-blockers, a noncardioselective agent with greater vasoconstrictive properties such as timolol should be tested in RCTs.

Diabetic Patients

Diabetic patients at risk are a new indication for beta-blockers.

The UKPDS results *(19)* confirm that in type 2 diabetes, beta-blockers significantly reduced all-cause mortality, risk for MI, stroke, PVD, and microvascular disease (Fig. 1-4). In addition, over the 9-yr follow-up, the change in albuminuria and serum creatinine was the same in the captopril and beta-blocker groups. Also, *in the SOLVD (65) HF study, surprisingly, in contrast to enalapril, beta-blockers were renoprotective in both the ACE inhibitor and placebo groups;* see *Chapter 2, Beta-Blocker Controversies.*

Noncardiac Indications

Noncardiac indications for beta-blockers are given in Table 1-6.

ADVICE AND ADVERSE EFFECTS

Warnings

Beta-blockers are relatively safe if the *warnings and contraindications* are carefully respected.

1. Beta-blockers are not advisable in patients with decompensated class IV HF (see discussions on the special use of these drugs in Chapter 12). (HF in the presence of acute MI with

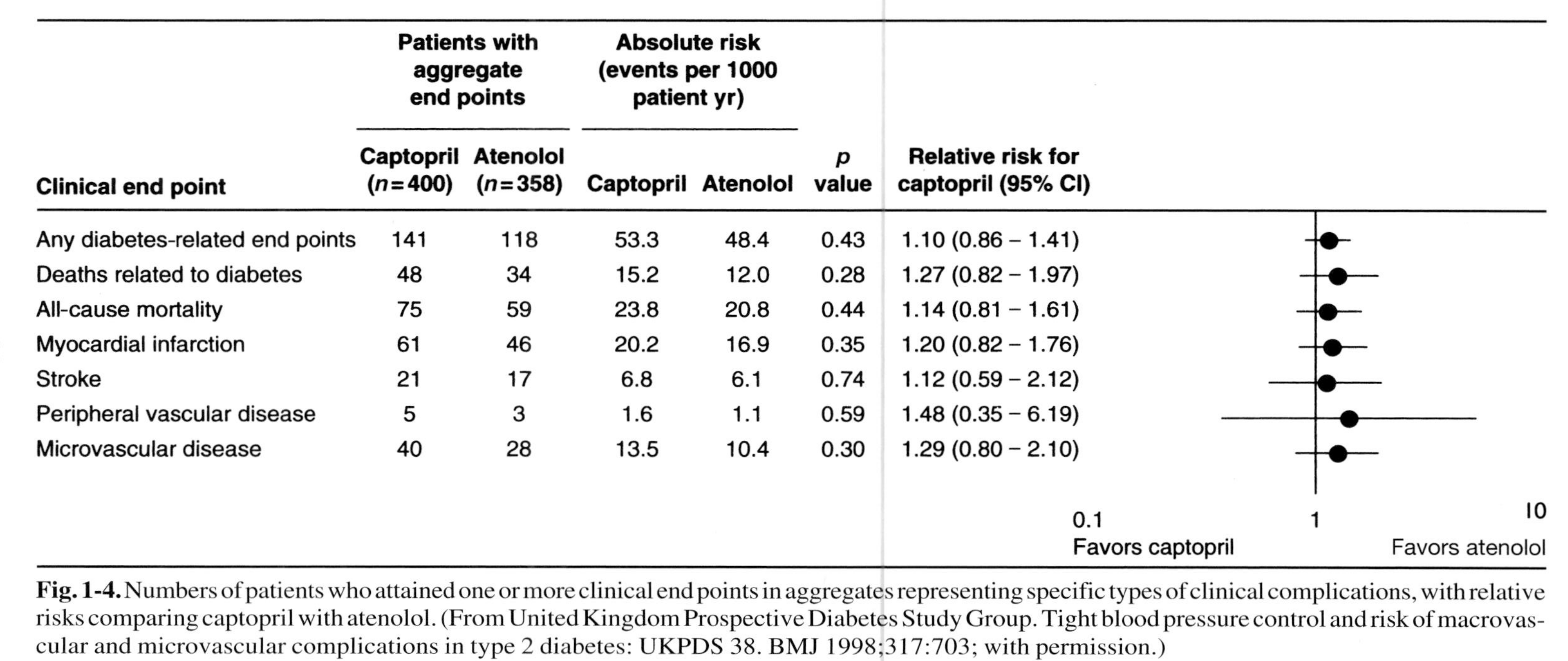

Clinical end point	Patients with aggregate end points		Absolute risk (events per 1000 patient yr)			
	Captopril ($n=400$)	Atenolol ($n=358$)	Captopril	Atenolol	p value	Relative risk for captopril (95% CI)
Any diabetes-related end points	141	118	53.3	48.4	0.43	1.10 (0.86 – 1.41)
Deaths related to diabetes	48	34	15.2	12.0	0.28	1.27 (0.82 – 1.97)
All-cause mortality	75	59	23.8	20.8	0.44	1.14 (0.81 – 1.61)
Myocardial infarction	61	46	20.2	16.9	0.35	1.20 (0.82 – 1.76)
Stroke	21	17	6.8	6.1	0.74	1.12 (0.59 – 2.12)
Peripheral vascular disease	5	3	1.6	1.1	0.59	1.48 (0.35 – 6.19)
Microvascular disease	40	28	13.5	10.4	0.30	1.29 (0.80 – 2.10)

Fig. 1-4. Numbers of patients who attained one or more clinical end points in aggregates representing specific types of clinical complications, with relative risks comparing captopril with atenolol. (From United Kingdom Prospective Diabetes Study Group. Tight blood pressure control and risk of macrovascular and microvascular complications in type 2 diabetes: UKPDS 38. BMJ 1998;317:703; with permission.)

Table 1-6
Noncardiac Indications for Beta-Blockers?

- Situational anxiety (e.g., preoperative)
- Essential tremor
- Alcohol withdrawal: delirium tremens
- Bartter's syndrome (juxtaglomerular hyperplasia)
- Insulinoma
- Glaucoma
- Migraine prophylaxis
- Narcolepsy
- Thyrotoxicosis (arrhythmias)
- Portal hypertension
- Tetanus

complete clearing of failure in a few days is not a contraindication.) RCTs have established that these agents save lives in patients with class I–III HF and are strongly indicated.

2. **Severe cardiomegaly** is a relative contraindication.
3. They are not advisable in patients with EF < 20%.
4. They are not advisable in symptomatic bradycardia or chronotropic incompetence.
5. They are not advisable in conduction defects, or second- or third-degree AV block.
6. Bronchial asthma is a contraindication. Chronic bronchitis and emphysema are relative contraindications depending on their severity and the necessity for beta-blockade.
7. Severe allergic rhinitis is a relative contraindication.
8. **Avoid abrupt cessation** of therapy. A worsening of angina or precipitation of acute MI has occurred on abrupt withdrawal of therapy. Although this happens only rarely, the patient must be warned. The incidence of this syndrome is said to be infrequent with pindolol because of ISA. Do not discontinue suddenly before surgery. When it is necessary to discontinue beta-blockers, the dosage should be reduced gradually over 2–3 wk, and the patient should be advised to minimize exertion during this period. Added therapy or nitrates and/or calcium antagonists are required during the withdrawal phase.
9. Insulin-dependent diabetes prone to hypoglycemia represents a relative contraindication.
10. Severe PVD, including Raynaud's disease, is a contraindication.

Side Effects

Cardiovascular

Precipitation of HF, AV block, hypotension, severe bradycardia, intermittent claudication, cold extremities, Raynaud's phenomenon, and dyspnea may occur.

Central Nervous System

Depression may occur, especially with propranolol, and psychosis can occur *(66)*. Dizziness, weakness, fatigue, vivid dreams, insomnia, and rare loss of hearing may occur.

Gastrointestinal

Nausea, vomiting, and epigastric distress are possible.

Respiratory

Bronchospasm, laryngospasm, respiratory distress, respiratory arrest (rare—with overdose) may occur.

Skin, Genitourinary

Rashes, exacerbation of psoriasis *(67)*, reduction of libido, and impotence (a clinical trial comparing propranolol with diuretics showed that impotence was significantly more common in the diuretic-treated group *[68]*) are possible. Based on studies of 39,745 patients, 149 (0.4%) reported impotence. The true incidence of sexual dysfunction is in the 1–5% range. Reportedly, problems with erection occurred in 5.5% of patients administered a beta-blocker versus 19.6% for patients who received a diuretic *(69)*.

Very rare cases of retroperitoneal fibrosis have been reported with oxprenolol, atenolol, metoprolol, timolol, propranolol, sotalol, pindolol, and acebutolol. The mucocutaneous syndrome observed with practolol has not been reported with other beta-blockers. Positive antinuclear factor has been reported, however, with acebutolol, pindolol, and labetalol. A lupus-like syndrome has been seen rarely with the use of practolol, and a case has been reported with the use of acebutolol. Labetalol can cause a lupus syndrome and hepatic necrosis *(70)*.

Large-scale clinical trials with timolol and propranolol in post-MI patients followed for 1–2 yr showed that these two drugs do not cause an increased incidence of HF. If patients are selected carefully, HF is not usually precipitated by beta-blockers.

Drug Interactions

Cimetidine, chlorpheniramine, hydralazine, and other drugs that decrease hepatic blood flow increase the bioavailability of hepatic metabolized beta-blockers.

Systemic hypertension may be precipitated by combined beta-blocker and epinephrine or by timolol and phenylephrine ophthalmic therapy. Close monitoring of the blood pressure is therefore necessary when a beta-blocker is combined with phenylephrine or other alpha-adrenergic agonists.

INDIVIDUAL BETA-BLOCKERS

Drug name:	**Acebutolol**
Trade names:	Monitan, Sectral
Supplied:	100, 200, 400 mg
Dosage:	100–400 mg twice daily, max. 1000 mg daily

Acebutolol is a relatively cardioselective and hydrophilic agent that possesses mild ISA and mild membrane-stabilizing activities (*see* Table 1-5). The very mild ISA activity prevents undue symptomatic bradycardia. Also, no significant decrease in HDL cholesterol occurs with long-term administration. In the Treatment of Mild Hypertension Study, acebutolol caused no significant change in HDL after 1 yr of therapy.

Weak cardioselectivity and moderate lipid solubility are CP features. Mild ISA does not appear to negate the CP potential of acebutolol. It is possible that strongly cardioselective, water-soluble agents render less cardioprotection, and moderate or strong ISA is counterproductive.

The drug appears to have CP properties and caused about a 48% decrease in cardiac deaths in a randomized post-MI study *(39)*. Clearly, a moderate degree of ISA is a disadvantage and destroys several salutary effects of beta-blockade *(30)*, but mild ISA is an advantage in patients who require beta-blockade and demonstrate bothersome sinus bradycardia when they are given small doses of a non-ISA beta-blocker.

Drug name:	**Atenolol**
Trade name:	Tenormin
Supplied:	25, 50, 100 mg
Dosage:	Initial: 25–50 mg once daily

This drug was a favorite of trialists from 1980 to 2005 but has often proved ineffective in decreasing CVD outcomes compared with newer agents. One notable exception is the UKPDS study *(19)*. In these diabetic patients, renal dysfunction may have increased the serum levels of the drug, thus increasing effectiveness. In this small but long-term follow-up study in high-risk patients, atenolol was as effective as captopril in reducing CVD outcomes.

The drug is almost totally excreted by the kidney. There is only a fourfold variation in plasma level, and the main difference from nadolol is that it is a beta$_1$-cardioselective drug. Atenolol is a long-acting preparation and can be used once daily. Atenolol has not caused the mucocutaneous syndrome; indeed, patients who developed the syndrome while taking practolol were cleared of the syndrome when treated with atenolol. Blood levels are maintained in heavy smokers, the opposite of the effect of propranolol and hepatically metabolized (HM) beta-blockers. In smokers who will not stop, bisoprolol, carvedilol, metoprolol, or timolol should be used.

The author has discontinued use of atenolol since 2001 because the drug has lower CVD protective effects compared with other proven beta-blockers.

Drug name:	**Bisoprolol**
Trade names:	Zebeta, Monocor, Emcor
Supplied:	5–10 mg
Dosage:	5–10 mg daily, max. 20 mg Ziac, Monozide: bisoprolol and hydrochlorothiazide 6.25 mg

This agent is highly beta$_1$-selective, and it is more cardioselective than metoprolol; in humans, the drug has a twofold higher beta$_1$-selectivity than atenolol. A 10-mg dose is equivalent to atenolol 100 mg. The drug has a half-life of 12–14 h and thus has a long duration of action beyond 24 h. Bisoprolol is 50% lipophilic, metabolized by the liver, and 50% hydrophilic, excreted by the kidney. The concentration of unchanged bisoprolol in rat brain is lower than that of metoprolol or propranolol but higher than that of atenolol after dosing. A study *(54)* in patients with LV dysfunction, CIBIS II, showed a markedly significant reduction in overall mortality with bisoprolol therapy; the study was stopped because of significant favorable effects. Bisoprolol treatment reduced all-cause mortality by 32% ($p = 0.00005$) and sudden death by 45% ($p = 0.001$). There was a 30% reduction in hospitalization caused by worsening HF (*see* Chapter 12).

The combination of bisoprolol and 6.25 mg HCTZ (Ziac) has been approved by the U.S. Food and Drug Administration (FDA) as first-line initial therapy for hypertension (Monozide 10 in the United Kingdom).

The blood pressure-lowering effect is superior to that of atenolol (Fig. 1-5). The 5-mg dose seems equipotent to atenolol 50 mg. Most important, this is a genuine 24-h acting, once-daily drug.

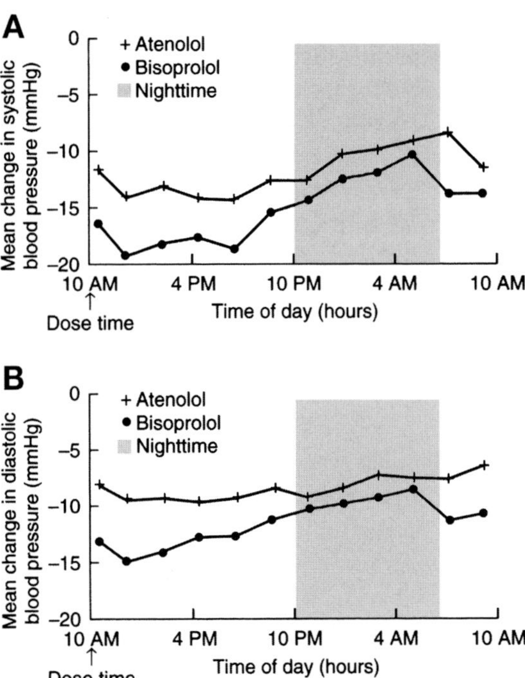

Fig. 1-5. Mean changes from baseline to end of treatment in ambulatory systolic (**A**) and diastolic (**B**) blood pressures over the 24-h monitoring period in patients receiving bisoprolol ($n = 107$) or atenolol ($n = 96$). (From Neutel JM, Smith DHG, Ram CVS. Application of ambulatory blood pressure monitoring in differentiating between antihypertensive agents. Am J Med 1993;94:181; with permission.)

Bisoprolol has been shown to *reduce ambulatory systolic and diastolic pressures by 43% and 49%, respectively, more than atenolol* (*see* Fig. 1-5) *during the early morning hours during which catecholamine surge causes an increased risk of ischemia and sudden death.* In response to pressure stimuli and increased catecholamines, there is less rise in blood pressure, *and excessive increase in exercise blood pressure is controlled.* Renal blood flow is enhanced. Coldness of the fingers and toes appears to be less than that observed with atenolol, metoprolol, and propranolol.

Perioperative Protection

Bisoprolol, in an RCT of 1351 high-risk patients undergoing vascular surgery, significantly reduced events ($p < 0.001$). Bisoprolol was started 1 wk preoperatively and continued for 30 d postoperatively; there were two deaths and no MIs versus nine deaths and nine MIs in the untreated group *(71)*.

Drug name:	**Carvedilol**
Trade names:	Coreg, Eucardic
Supplied:	6.25, 12.5, 25 mg
Dosage:	Heart failure: 3.125 mg, then 6.25 mg twice daily; titrate over weeks to 25 mg twice daily; see text for further advice Hypertension: 12.5 mg daily; titrate over weeks to 25–50 mg daily, max. 50 mg Angina: 12.5 mg twice daily; titrate over days to weeks to 25 mg twice daily

For the beneficial results observed in the CAPRICORN and COPERNICUS trials, *see* Chapter 22. **Carvedilol is one of the most effective beta-blockers available and is rated by the author as the best choice for use in acute MI and post-MI prophylaxis particularly if LV dysfunction is present.** It is also recommended for hypertension, particularly in diabetics or prediabetics, because it has been shown to improve insulin sensitivity compared with metoprolol *(72)* (*see* Chapter 2, Beta-Blocker Controversies and also the last section of this chapter, Which Beta-Blocker Is Best for Your Patients?).

Dosage (Further Advice)

The dosage must be individualized during up-titration. Titration also depends on the occurrence of hypotension and bradycardia. The dose of digoxin, diuretic, and ACE inhibitor or angiotensin II receptor blocker must be stabilized before commencing carvedilol. The initial dose is 3.125 mg twice daily for 2 wk and then, if tolerated, 6.25 mg twice daily. The dose can be doubled every 4 wk to the highest level tolerated by the patient. Observe the patient for dizziness, light-headedness, and hypotension for 1 h after the initiation of each new dose. The maximum dose is 25 mg twice daily in patients weighing less than 85 kg and 50 mg twice daily in those weighing over 85 kg. Carvedilol should be administered with food to slow the rate of absorption and to reduce the incidence of orthostatic effects. If symptoms of vasodilation occur (e.g., dizziness and lightheadedness), reduce the dose of diuretic and then, if necessary, the ACE inhibitor. If symptoms do not resolve, reduce the carvedilol dosage. Symptoms of worsening HF (e.g., edema, weight gain, and shortness of breath) should be treated with increased doses of diuretic. The carvedilol dose should be reduced if symptoms persist.

Action

The ratio of $alpha_1$- to beta-blockade for carvedilol is 1:10, compared with 1:4 for labetalol, a more powerful $alpha_1$-blocker that causes a greater degree of vasodilation and orthostatic hypotension; antioxidant and antiproliferative properties have been reported. The drug improves ventricular function without upregulating downregulated myocardial beta-receptors in the failing heart.

Indications

The drug is approved by the FDA for the management of class I–III HF. The U.S. Carvedilol Heart Failure Study *(73)* in patients with NYHA class II and III HF showed a 27% reduction in hospitalization and a 65% reduction in mortality risk.

- The drug is contraindicated in patients with decompensated class IV HF.
- As with other beta-blockers, the drug is contraindicated in patients with asthma, severe COPD, second-or third-degree AV block, and sick sinus syndrome. Carvedilol is not advisable in patients with clinically manifest *hepatic impairment. Mild hepatic injury has been noted.* Stop the drug and do not restart if the patient has evidence of liver injury.
- *Class IV patients,* when stabilized and *free of fluid overload*, can be started on 3.125 mg, a dose titrated slowly up over several weeks.
- Ejection fraction and myocardial energetics take about 8 wk to improve as a biologic effect with beta-blocker therapy. The ventricle goes from a more spherical shape to a more normal elliptical shape, and LV mass decreases; these changes indicate that the pathologic remodeling process is being attenuated and in many cases reverts back to normal. It is important to initiate therapy as early as possible while there is myocardial viability left and it is possible to recover a biologic effect on myocytes.

- End-diastolic volume decreases; myocardial contractility increases, after about 3 mo of therapy; mechanical work improves, as reflected by stroke work; and myocardial O_2 consumption decreases.
- Myocardial efficiency increases in patients who receive a beta-blocker as well as an ACE inhibitor. Plasma norepinephrine increases over time in patients treated with an ACE inhibitor. *The combination of a beta-blocker and ACE inhibitor is complementary and cardioprotective in patients with MI, HF, diabetes, hypertension, and LVH.*

Drug name:	**Esmolol**
Trade name:	Brevibloc
Dosage:	IV infusion within range 50–200 μg/kg/min; *see* text for further advice

Dosage (Further Advice)

The dose is 5–40 mg, usually 3–6 mg IV infusion over 1 min (30–300 μg to maximum of 500 μg/kg over 1 min) and then maintenance infusion 1–5 mg/min (maximum 50 μg/kg/min). If control of the clinical situation is not achieved and more rapid titration is necessary, a further bolus may be given followed by an increase in the maintenance infusion rate. If mild hypotension is present, the maintenance dose should be reduced to 1–3 mg/min. Hypotensive effects of the drug usually disappear within minutes of cessation of the infusion.

Esmolol IV 50–200 μg/kg/min has an effect equivalent to that of propranolol 3–6 mg IV.

Action

Esmolol is a cardioselective ultrashort-acting beta-blocker that is quickly converted by esterases of red blood cells to inactive metabolites *(74)*. The drug has a short half-life of about 9 min *(74)* that is stable in patients with mild HF, hepatic dysfunction, or renal failure. The drug action dissipates within 20–30 min of administration.

Indications

1. The drug is used for SVT in the perioperative period *(75)* and for SVT not terminated by adenosine or in patients with contraindications to the use of adenosine or verapamil, especially during acute MI or other ischemic syndromes.
2. Esmolol is superior to verapamil in the management of recent-onset atrial fibrillation or flutter *(76)*.

The drug is given only under continuous monitoring of cardiac rhythm and blood pressure under close supervision. Hypotension is the major adverse effect, and in one study this occurred more often with esmolol than with IV propranolol *(77)*, but, with careful titration, esmolol is superior, given that adverse effects dissipate rapidly.

Contraindications include

- Severe hypotension or cardiogenic shock.
- Asthma or severe COPD.
- Other contraindications to the use of beta-blocking agents.

Drug name:	**Labetalol**
Trade names:	Normodyne, Trandate
Supplied:	50, 100, 200, 400 mg
Dosage:	50–100 mg twice daily; titrate over weeks to 200–400 mg twice daily; *see* text for IV dosage

A combined alpha- and beta-blocker, this drug is useful in the management of hypertension of all grades including hypertensive emergencies.

Disadvantages: Labetalol causes significant postural hypotension and must be given two or three times daily in large doses. Side effects include a lupus-like illness, a lichenoid rash, impotence *(70)*, and, very rarely, hepatotoxicity manifesting as raised levels of transaminases, abnormal liver function test results, hepatitis, and fatal or nonfatal hepatic necrosis *(78)*.

Drug name:	**Metoprolol**
Trade names:	Betaloc, Betaloc SR, Lopressor, Toprol-XL
Supplied:	50, 100 mg Betaloc SR: 200 mg Toprol-XL: 50, 100, 200 mg
Dosage:	50–200 mg twice daily Long-acting: 50–200 g once daily, max. 300 mg

Toprol XL, with its 24-h duration of action, is important for coverage of early morning catecholamine surge and early morning fatal MI. **This drug is superior to other sustained-release metoprolol tartrate formulations, whose action may not continue throughout the 24-h period.**

Metoprolol is beta$_1$-cardioselective. In patients with bronchospastic disease, metoprolol, in doses lower than 150 mg daily, causes less bronchospasm than a nonselective beta-blocker at equivalent beta-blocking dose. If bronchospasm is precipitated, it will respond to beta$_2$-stimulants, whereas there would be a poor response if a nonselective beta-blocker were used. Cardioselectivity confers advantages when beta-blockers are given to patients with labile diabetes.

Metoprolol has been shown to reduce the incidence of VT during acute MI *(44)*. The Göteborg metoprolol trial has documented the beneficial effect of metoprolol on survival during the early phase of MI (from d 1 for 90 d). Metoprolol caused a 36% reduction in mortality rate during the 90 d of therapy, and benefit was maintained for 1 yr.

Metoprolol causes less sedation and drowsiness than atenolol. In addition, *metoprolol is lipid soluble and appears to be more cardioprotective than water-soluble beta-blockers, which achieve lower concentration in the brain.*

The MERIT-HF study *(56,79)* has established metoprolol as indicated in patients with class I–III HF. It is most important to start with small doses: metoprolol succinate (CR/XL) controlled-release 12.5 mg once daily, and titrate up slowly over 4–8 wk to a target dose of 150–200 mg.

Drug name:	**Nadolol**
Trade name:	Corgard
Supplied:	40, 80, 120, 160 mg
Dosage:	40–80 mg once daily, max. 160 mg; *see* text for further advice

Dosage (Further Advice)

The manufacturers suggest a maximum of 240 mg for angina and 320 mg for hypertension. These high doses are not recommended by the author. Because the drug has a very long half-life and is excreted entirely by the kidneys, accumulation commonly occurs in patients with mild renal dysfunction and in patients over 65 yr of age. In practice, a dose of 80 mg is equivalent to approximately 160 mg of propranolol. The dose must be reduced in renal failure and in the elderly. Also, the time interval between doses should be increased, that is, one tablet every 36 or 48 h may suffice in renal failure. Use a nonrenally excreted beta-blocker in the presence of severe renal failure.

Like propranolol, nadolol is a nonselective beta-blocker. It has a weak lipid solubility and therefore is almost completely excreted by the kidney. No large RCT has been done to prove its effectiveness in reducing CVD mortality or morbidity. Because of its long half-life it is given as a one-a-day tablet; this may be important when compliance is a problem.

Insomnia and **vivid dreams** occur much less frequently with nadolol and atenolol compared with propranolol and other lipid-soluble beta-blockers, but they can occur with sotalol.

The dose of atenolol, nadolol, and sotalol should be reduced in renal failure, and with severe renal failure, the time interval between doses should be increased.

Drug name:	**Propranolol**
Trade name:	Inderal
Supplied:	Inderal: 10, 20, 40, 80, 120 mg Inderal LA: 80, 120, 160 mg capsules
Dosage:	40–80 mg twice daily; titrate over weeks to 80–120 mg twice daily LA: 80–160 mg once daily, max. 240 mg; *see* text for further advice

Indications

In the new millennium, **it is no longer justifiable to prescribe propranolol** because bisoprolol, carvedilol, and metoprolol have less severe side effects and have been proved to reduce morbidity and mortality in a wide range of cardiac patients including those with very sick hearts (HF class II–III and some class IV patients). Propranolol is contraindicated in patients with HF or EF < 35%.

This beta-blocker has been in use since 1964 and is still the most frequently prescribed beta-blocker worldwide. Unlike other beta-blockers, the drug is approved by the FDA for many indications: angina, acute MI, postinfarction prevention, arrhythmias, hypertension, IV use, anesthetic arrhythmias, hypertrophic cardiomyopathy, syncope, anxiety and essential tremor, migraine prophylaxis, and thyrotoxicosis.

The long-acting preparation provides full 24-h coverage. The BHAT study *(33)* proved the beneficial effects of propranolol in post-MI patients for the prevention of reinfarction, sudden death, and fatal and nonfatal MIs. Cigarette smoking alters blood levels of propranolol and may mask CP effects. In nonsmokers, however, the drug has been proved effective, whereas only timolol has been proved effective in RCTs and in the post-MI patient.

The drug is strongly lipid soluble and therefore has a high uptake in the brain; this may be the reason for fatigue, the rare occurrence of depression, and vivid dreams. Lipid solubility, brain concentration, and $beta_1$- and $beta_2$-blockade provide cardioprotection. In smokers, the salutary effects of propranolol are masked *(27)*.

If depression, fatigue, or mild memory impairment occurs, switch to bisoprolol, metoprolol, or timolol.

Drug name:	**Sotalol**
Trade names:	Sotacor, Betapace, Beta-Cardone
Supplied:	80, 160, 240 mg
Dosage:	40–80 mg once daily; increase over days to weeks to 80–160 mg once or twice daily

Indications

In the United States, this drug is approved for oral use in patients with life-threatening ventricular arrhythmias (sustained VT). This agent is not recommended for the treatment of asymptomatic ventricular premature beats. In the United Kingdom and Canada, the drug is indicated for hypertension and for the management of arrhythmias, including paroxysmal atrial fibrillation, or for the maintenance of sinus rhythm in place of quinidine *(80)*. The response to sotalol predicts the response to amiodarone during serial drug testing in patients with sustained VT.

Sotalol is unique among the approved beta-blockers. The drug has all the effects of a nonselective beta-blocker plus an added class III antiarrhythmic effect: the drug lengthens the duration of the cardiac action potential and prolongs the QTc interval of the surface electrocardiogram.

The drug appears to be more effective than other beta-blockers in the control of numerous bothersome ventricular premature beats and sustained VT. However, some studies indicate no difference in efficacy. The drug has been shown to cause an 88% reduction in ventricular ectopic beat frequency at the optimal titrated dosage.

Torsades de pointes have been precipitated as a rare complication, mainly in patients with hypokalemia. Torsades occurred, however, despite therapeutic plasma sotalol concentration and normal serum potassium level in the absence of diuretics. **Caution** is necessary: do not administer sotalol with nonpotassium-sparing diuretics and drugs that cause QT prolongation.

The drug represents a significant advance in the management of some ventricular tachyarrhythmias, including recurrent VT tachycardia or VF.

Contraindications

Congenital or acquired long QT syndromes are contraindications, as well as other contraindications to beta-blockade.

Drug name:	**Timolol**
Trade names:	Blocadren, Betim
Supplied:	5, 10 mg
Dosage:	5–10 mg twice daily, max. 20 mg twice daily

This noncardioselective drug has some advantages over propranolol. First-pass hepatic metabolism is 60%, and 40% of the drug is excreted unchanged in the urine. Variation in plasma level is only sevenfold. The drug is six times more potent than propranolol, so for a given dose, a better plasma level is achieved with less variation. It has moderate lipid solubility.

Timolol can be given twice a day with a fair certainty that plasma levels will be adequate. It has proved to be efficacious and safe in the reduction of raised intraocular pressure when used topically.

Timolol is the first beta-blocker to have been shown beyond reasonable doubt to reduce cardiac mortality in the post-MI patient. A remarkable 67% reduction in sudden cardiac deaths was achieved by timolol in the post-MI study *(16)*.

Newer Beta-Blocker

NEBIVOLOL

Nebivolol is the most highly beta$_1$-selective agent to be tested. *The drug stimulates the endothelial L-arginine/nitric oxide pathway* and thus causes vasodilation *(13)*. Results of trials in HF and in hypertension are awaited.

Indications: essential hypertension.

Dosage: 5 mg daily; for the **elderly**, initially 2.5 mg daily, increased if necessary to 5 mg daily.

Cautions: reduce dose in renal impairment, in the elderly, and with hepatic dysfunction.

WHICH BETA-BLOCKER IS BEST FOR YOUR PATIENTS?

- More than 12 beta-blockers are available worldwide. As emphasized earlier, there are subtle and, fortunately, important differences among them *(30)*.
- Agents with ISA are not cardioprotective drugs and do not enter the contest.
- Cardioselective agents (*see* Fig. 1-2) cause fewer adverse effects, and, particularly in diabetic patients, they are usually the agents of choice but carvedilol, a nonselective agent, exhibited improved insulin sensitivity compared with metoprolol in GEMINI *(72)* and is recommended by the author provided that the patient is not hypoglycemia prone and postural hypotension is not a problem.
- Of the **cardioselective agents**, *only bisoprolol and metoprolol (both lipophilic)* have been shown to reduce CHD mortality and events significantly in the following well-conducted RCTs: CIBIS II, MERIT-HF, and SOLVD (beta-blocker renoprotection as good as ACE inhibitor) (also *see* Tables 1–2 and 1-7, and Chapter 22). **The noncardioselective** agent *carvedilol* was studied in the successful CAPRICORN and COPERNICUS trials. *See* earlier discussion of the beta$_2$ effect on K^+ homeostasis. The common threads are beta$_1$ and lipophilicity, which augment brain concentration and may protect from sudden death. In the timolol study, there was a 67% reduction in sudden death *(16)*. (Timolol is beta$_1$- and beta$_2$-selective and lipophilic; it appears to be a forgotten beta-blocker in North America.)
- Of the agents—bisoprolol, carvedilol, and metoprolol—that should be recommended based on the aforementioned logical approach, bisoprolol carries some advantages for the hypertensive patient: genuine one-a-day administration, quelling of early morning catecholamine surge, and better control of early morning and exercise-induced excessive-rise in blood pressure than atenolol *(81)*. It does not cause postural hypotension, as does carvedilol. **Bisoprolol** is the most highly cardioselective (of the three) and is therefore relatively safe to use in diabetes, COPD, and perioperatively, as is Toprol XL, a proven 24-h metoprolol formulation that has been well tested in the United States for hypertension.
- Bisoprolol, carvedilol, and timolol followed by metoprolol succinate (sustained release) appear to be the winners overall for the management of hypertension.
- Carvedilol showed marked benefit and safety in the CAPRICORN post-MI study and the COPERNICUS HF study and is the beta-blocker of choice for patients with HF and post MI with LV dysfunction. For hypertension, Toprol XL or bisoprolol, given once daily, has advantages over carvedilol, which usually should be administered twice daily.
- The older beta-blocking drugs including atenolol, pindolol, oxprenolol, and nadolol should become obsolete.

Table 1-7
Which Beta-Blocker is Best?

Feature	*Bisoprolol*	*Carvedilol*	*Metoprolol succinate*	*Atenolol*
$Beta_1$ selectivity[a]	++++	0 ($\beta_1\beta_2$)	+	++
Lipophilic	++	++	+++	0 (lipophilic)
Mortality ↓ Post MI	Not tried	Yes (CAPRICORN)	Yes	Modest effect
Mortality ↓ HF	Yes (CIBBIS II)	Yes (COPERNICUS)	Yes (MERIT-HF)	Not tried
Mortality ↓ Hypertensives	No large RCT	No large RCT	Yes	Yes[b]
Mortality ↓ Diabetics	No RCT	No RCT *See* GEMINI	No RCT	Yes (UKPDS)
Perioperative mortality ↓	Yes		No RCT	↓ Morbidity
Adverse effects	Low	Postural hypotension	Low	Low
Dosing	Once/24 h	Twice/24 h	Once	Once or twice[d]
Overall rating	++++ for hypertension	++++ (not in diabetics)[d] for HF and post MI	+++	

[a]For nebivolol, selectivity is twofold higher than for bisoprolol, and selectivity for the latter is twofold greater than for atenolol.

[b]*See* text, Chapters 8 and 9.

[c]Carvedilol improves insulin sensitivity compared with metoprolol *(72)*.

[d]May not be full 24 h in some patients.

REFERENCES

1. Cruickshank JM. Beta-blockers continue to surprise us. Eur Heart J 2000;21:355.
2. Sixth Report of Joint National Committee on Prevention, Detection, Evaluation and Treatment of High Blood Pressure. Arch Intern Med 1997;157:2413.
3. Khan M Gabriel. Hyperlipidemia. In: Heart Disease, Diagnosis and Therapy. Baltimore, Williams & Wilkins, 1996, p. 384.
4. Frishman WH. Beta-adrenergic blocking drugs. Am Coll Cardiol Curr J Rev 1997;23.
5. Black JW, Crowther AF, Shanks RG, et al. A new adrenergic beta-receptor-antagonist. Lancet 1964; 2:1080.
6. Pritchard BNC, Gillam PMS. The use of propranolol in the treatment of hypertension. BMJ 1964;2:725.
7. Multi Center Diltiazem Postinfarction Trial Research Group. The effect of diltiazem on mortality and reinfarction after myocardial infarction. N Engl J Med 1988;319:385.
8. Estacio RO, Barrett WJ, Hiatt WR. The effect of nisoldipine as compared with enalapril on cardiovascular outcomes in patients with non-insulin dependent diabetes and hypertension. N Engl J Med 1998;338:645.
9. Kaumann AJ. Some aspects of heart beta adrenoceptor function. Cardiovasc Drugs Ther 1991;5:549.
10. Motomura S, Zerkowski HR, Daul A, et al. On the physiologic role of beta-2 adrenoceptors in the human heart: in vitro and in vivo studies. Am Heart J 1990;119:608.
11. Krum H, Gu A, Wiltshire-Clement M, et al. Changes in plasma endothelin-1 levels reflects clinical response to β-blockade in chronic heart failure. Am Heart J 1996;131:337.
12. Cruickshank JM, Degaute JP, Kuurne T, et al. Reduction of stress/catecholamine induced cardiac necrosis by B1 selective blockade. Lancet 1987;2:585.

13. Cockcroft JR, Chowienczyk PJ, Brett SE, et al. Nebivolol vasodilates human forearm vasculature: Evidence for a L-arginine/No-dependent mechanism. J Pharmacol Exp Ther 1995;274:1067.
14. Man in't Veld AJ, Van den Meiracker AH, Schalekamp MA. Do beta-blockers really increase peripheral vascular resistance? Review of the literature and new observations under basal conditions. Am J Hypertens 1988;1:91.
15. Braunwald E. Mechanism of action of calcium-channel-blocking agents. N Engl J Med 1982;307:1618.
16. The Norwegian Multicenter Study Group. Timolol-induced reduction in mortality and reinfarction in patients surviving acute myocardial infarction. N Engl J Med 1981;304:801.
17. Pratt CM, Roberts R. Chronic beta-blockade therapy in patients after myocardial infarction. Am J Cardiol 1983;52:661.
18. Khan MI, Hamilton JT, Manning GW. Protective effect of beta adrenoceptor blockade in experimental coronary occlusion in conscious dogs. Am J Cardiol 1972;30:832.
19. United Kingdom Prospective Diabetes Study Group. Tight blood pressure control and risk of macrovascular and microvascular complications in type 2 diabetes: UKPDS 38. BMJ 1998;317:703.
20. Breckenridge A. Jogger's blockade. BMJ 1982;284:532.
21. Johansson BW. Effect of beta-blockade on ventricular fibrillation and tachycardia induced circulatory arrest in acute myocardial infarction. Am J Cardiol 1986;57:34F.
22. Raeder EA, Verrier RL, Lown B. Intrinsic sympathomimetic activity and the effects of beta-adrenergic blocking drugs on vulnerability to ventricular fibrillation. J Am Coll Cardiol 1983;1:1442.
23. Pitt B. Regression of left ventricular hypertrophy in patients with hypertension: Blockade of the renin-angiotensin-aldosterone system. Circulation 1998;98:1987.
24. Kostis JB, Rosen RC. Central nervous system effects of beta-adrenergic blocking drugs: The role of ancillary properties. Circulation 1987;75:204.
25. Engler RL, Conant J, Maisel A, et al. Lipid solubility determines the relative CNS effects of beta-blocking agents. J Am Coll Cardiol 1986;7:25A.
26. Pitt B. The role of beta-adrenergic blocking agents in preventing sudden cardiac death. Circulation 85(Suppl I): 1992;I107.
27. Deanfield J, Wright C, Krikler S. Cigarette smoking and the treatment of angina with propranolol, atenolol and nifedipine. N Engl J Med 1984;310:951.
28. Valimaki ML, Harno K. Lipoprotein lipids and apoproteins during beta-blocker administration: Comparison of penbutolol and atenolol. Eur J Clin Pharmacol 1986;30:17.
29. Pasotti C, Zoppi A, Capra A. Effect of beta-blockers on plasma lipids. Int J Clin Pharmacol Ther Toxicol 1986;24:448.
30. Khan M Gabriel. Angina. In: Heart Disease, Diagnosis and Therapy. Baltimore, Williams & Wilkins, 1996.
31. Beta-Blocker Heart Attack Study Group. The beta-blocker heart attack trial. JAMA 1981;246:2073.
32. Shore SJ, Berger KR, Murphy EA, et al. Progression of aortic dilation and the benefit of long-term beta-adrenergic blockade in Marfan's syndrome. N Engl J Med 1994;330:1335.
33. BHAT: Peters RW, Muller JE, Goldstein S, et al. for the BHAT Study Group. Propranolol and the morning increase in the frequency of sudden cardiac deaths (BHAT Study). Am J Cardiol 1990;63:1518.
34. Kleiger RE, Miller JP, Bigger JT, et al. Decreased heart rate variability and its association with increased mortality after acute myocardial infarction. Am J Cardiol 1987;59:256.
35. Malik M, Farrell T, Camm J. Circadian rhythm of heart rate variability with clinical and angiographic variables and late mortality after coronary angiography. Am J Cardiol 1990;66:1049.
36. Niemelä MJ, Juhani Airaksinen KE, Huikuri HV, et al. Effect of beta-blockade on heart rate variability in patients with coronary artery disease. J Am Coll Cardiol 1994;23:1370.
37. Kjekshus JK. Importance of heart rate in determining beta-blocker efficacy in acute and long-term myocardial infarction intervention trials. Am J Cardiol 1986;57:43F.
38. Singh BN. Advantages of beta-blockers versus antiarrhythmic agents and calcium antagonists in secondary prevention after myocardial infarction. Am J Cardiol 1990;66:9C.
39. Boissel JP, Leizorovicz A, Picolet H, et al. Efficacy of acebutolol after acute myocardial infarction (the APSI Trial). Am J Cardiol 1990;66:24C.
40. Weintraub WS, Akizuki S, Agarwal JB, et al. Comparative effects of nitroglycerin and nifedipine on myocardial blood flow and contraction during flow-limiting coronary stenosis in the dog. Am J Cardiol 1982;50:281.
41. Warltier DC, Hardman HJ, Brooks HL, et al. Transmural gradient of coronary blood flow following dihydropyridine calcium antagonists and other vasodilator drugs. Basic Res Cardiol 1983;78:644.
42. Sloman G, Robinson JS, McLean K. Propranolol (Inderal) in persistent ventricular fibrillation. BMJ 1965;5439:895.

43. Rothfield EL, Lipowitz M, Zucker IR, et al. Management of persistently recurring ventricular fibrillation with propranolol hydrochloride. JAMA 1968;204:546.
44. Ryden L, Ariniego R, Arnman K, et al. A double-blind trial of metoprolol in acute myocardial infarction: Effects on ventricular tachyarrhythmias. N Engl J Med 1983;308:614.
45. Julian DG. Is the use of beta-blockade contraindicated in the patient with coronary spasm? Circulation 1983;67(Suppl):1.
46. Steinbeck G, Andresen D, Bach P, et al. A comparison of electrophysiologically guided anti-arrhythmic drug therapy with beta-blocker therapy in patients with symptomatic sustained ventricular tachyarrhythmias. N Engl J Med 1992;327:987.
47. Steinbeck G, Andresen D, Bach P, et al. A comparison of electrophysiologically guided antiarrhythmic drug therapy with beta-blocker therapy in patients with symptomatic, sustained ventricular tachyarrhythmias. N Engl J Med 1992;327:987 [erratum: N Engl J Med 1993;328:71].
48. Matterson BJ, Reda DJ, Cushman WC, et al. Single drug therapy for hypertensive men: A comparison of 6 hypertensive agents with placebo. N Engl J Med 1993;328:914.
49. Medical Research Council Working Party. MRC trial of treatment of hypertension in older adults: Principal results. BMJ 1992;304:405.
50. Phillips T, Anlauf M, Distler A, et al. Randomised, double blind, multicentre comparison of hydrochlorothiazide, atenolol, nitrendipine, and enalapril in antihypertensive treatment: Results of the HANE study. BMJ 1997;315:154.
51. Devreux RB. Do antihypertensive drugs differ in their abilities to regress left ventricular hypertrophy? Circulation 1997;95:1983.
52. International Collaborative Study Group. Reduction of infarct size with early use of timolol in acute myocardial infarction. N Engl J Med 1984;310:9.
53. CAPRICORN: The Capricorn Investigators: Effect of carvedilol on outcome after myocardial infarction in patients with left-ventricular dysfunction. Lancet 2001;357:1385.
54. Second Cardiac Insufficiency Bisoprolol Study (CIBIS II). Presented by E. Merck at the 20th Congress of the European Society of Cardiology, August 1998, Vienna, Austria.
55. COPERNICUS: Packer M, Coast JS, Fowler MB, et al. for the Carvedilol Prospective Randomized Cumulative Survival Study Group: Effect of carvedilol on survival in severe chronic heart failure. N Engl J Med 2001;344:1651.
56. MERIT-HF Study Group. Dose of metoprolol CR/XL and clinical outcomes in patients with heart failure. Analysis of the experience in metoprolol CR/XL randomized intervention trial in chronic heart failure (MERIT-HF). J Am Coll Cardiol 2002;40:491–498.
57. Chan AW, Quinn MJ, Bhatt DL, et al. Mortality benefit of beta-blockade after successful elective percutaneous coronary intervention. J Am Coll Cardiol 2002;40:669–675.
58. Wheat MW Jr. Treatment of dissecting aneurysms of the aorta: Current status. Prog Cardiovasc Dis 1973; 16:87.
59. Ponce FE, Williams LC, Webb HM, et al. Propranolol palliation of tetralogy of Fallot: Experience with long-term drug treatment in pediatric patients. Pediatrics 1973;52:100.
60. Brophy CM, Tilson JE, Tilson MD. Propranolol stimulates the crosslinking of matrix components in skin from the aneurysm-prone blotchy mouse. J Surg Res 1989;46:330.
61. Boucek RJ, Gunja-Smith Z, Noble NL, et al. Modulation by propranolol of the lysyl cross-links in aortic elastin and collagen of the aneurysm-prone turkey. Biochem Pharmacol 1983;32:275.
62. Handlin LR, Kindred LH, Beauchamp GD, et al. Reversible left ventricular dysfunction after subarachnoid hemorrhage. Am Heart J 1993;126:235.
63. Mangano DT, Layug EL, Wallace A, et al. Effect of atenolol on mortality and cardiovascular morbidity after non-cardiac surgery. N Engl J Med 1996;335:1713.
64. Theodorakis JM, Kremastinos T, Stephanokis GS, et al. The effectiveness of beta-blockade and its influence on heart rate variability in vasovagal patients. Eur Heart J 1993;14:1499.
65. SOLVD Investigators. Effect of enalapril on mortality and the development of heart failure in asymptomatic patients with reduced left ventricular ejection fractions. N Engl J Med 1992;327:685.
66. Cunnane JG, Blackwood GW. Psychosis with propranolol: Still not recognized? Postgrad Med J 1987; 63:57.
67. Savola J, Vehvilainen O, Vaatainen NJ. Psoriasis as a side effect of beta-blockers. BMJ 1987;295:637.
68. Medical Research Council Working Party on Mild to Moderate Hypertension. Bendrofluazide and propranolol for the treatment of mild hypertension. Lancet 1981;2:359.
69. Hjalmarson A, Herlitz J, Malek I. Effect on mortality of metoprolol in acute myocardial infarction. Lancet 1981;ii:823.

70. Wallin JD, O'Neill WM. Labetalol: Current research and therapeutic status. Arch Intern Med 1983;143: 485.
71. Poldermans D, Boersma E, Bax JJ, et al. The effect of bisoprolol on perioperative mortality and myocardial infarction in high-risk patients undergoing vascular surgery. N Engl J Med 1999;341:1789.
72. GEMINI: Bakris GL, Fonseca V, Katholi RE, et al. Metabolic effects of carvedilol vs metoprolol in patients with type 2 diabetes mellitus and hypertension: a randomized controlled trial. JAMA 2004;292: 2227–2236.
73. Packer M, Bristol MR, Cohn JN, et al. for the US Carvedilol Heart Failure Study Group: The effect of carvedilol on morbidity and mortality in patients with chronic heart failure. N Engl J Med 1996;334:1349.
74. Gorczynski RJ. Basic pharmacology of esmolol. Am J Cardiol 1985;56:3F.
75. Cray RJ, Bateman TM, Czer LS, et al. Esmolol: A new ultrashort-acting beta-adrenergic blocking agent for rapid control of heart rate in post-operative supraventricular tachyarrhythmias. J Am Coll Cardiol 1985;5:1451.
76. Platia EV, Michelson EL, Porterfield JK, et al. Esmolol versus verapamil in the acute treatment of atrial fibrillation or atrial flutter. Am J Cardiol 1989;63:925.
77. Morganroth J, Horowitz LN, Anderson J, et al. Comparative efficacy and tolerance of esmolol to propranolol for control of supraventricular tachyarrhythmia. Am J Cardiol 1985;56:33F.
78. Clark JA, Zimmerman HF, Tanner LA. Labetalol hepatotoxicity. Ann Intern Med 1990;113:210.
79. MERIT-HF Study Group. Effect of metoprolol CR/XL in chronic heart failure: Metoprolol CR/XL Randomized Trial in Congestive Heart Failure (MERIT-HF). Lancet 1999;353:2001.
80. Juul-Möller S, Edvardsson N, Rehnqvist-Ahlberg N. Sotalol versus quinidine for the maintenance of sinus rhythm after direct current conversion of atrial fibrillation. Circulation 1990;82:1932–1939.
81. Neutel JM, Smith DHG, Ram CVS. Application of ambulatory blood pressure monitoring in differentiating between antihypertensive agents. Am J Med 1993;94:181.

SUGGESTED READING

Cominacini L, Fratta Pasini A, Garbin U, et al. Nebivolol and its 4-keto derivative increase nitric oxide in endothelial cells by reducing its oxidative inactivation. J Am Coll Cardiol 2003;42:1838–1844.

GEMIMI: Bakris GL, Fonseca V, Katholi RE, et al. Metabolic effects of carvedilol vs metoprolol in patients with type 2 diabetes mellitus and hypertension: A randomized controlled trial. JAMA 2004;292:2227–2236.

Kokkinos P, Chrysohoou C, Panagiotakos D, et al. Beta-blockade mitigates exercise blood pressure in hypertensive male patients. J Am Coll Cardiol 2006;47:794-798.

Nihat K, Emrullah B, Ibrahim O, et al. Protective effects of carvedilol against anthracycline-induced cardiomyopathy. J Am Coll Cardiol 2006;48:2258–2262.

Remme WJ, Torp-Pedersen C, Cleland JGF, et al. Carvedilol protects better against vascular events than metoprolol in heart failure: results from COMET. J Am Coll Cardiol 2007;49:963–971.

Takemoto Y, Hozumi T, Sugioka K, et al. Beta-blocker therapy induces ventricular resynchronization in dilated cardiomyopathy with narrow QRS complex. J Am Coll Cardiol 2007;49:778–783.

Van Melle JP, Verbeek DE, van den Berg MP, et al. Beta-blockers and depression after myocardial infarction: A multicenter prospective study. J Am Coll Cardiol 2006;48:2209–2214.

Wilkinson IB, McEniery CM, Cockcroft JR. Atenolol and cardiovascular risk: An issue close to the heart. Lancet 2006;367:627–629.

2 Beta-Blocker Controversies

BETA-BLOCKERS ARE NOT A GOOD INITIAL CHOICE FOR HYPERTENSION: TRUE OR FALSE?

A metaanalysis by Lindholm et al. *(1)* concluded that beta-blockers should not remain the first choice in the treatment of primary hypertension. Unfortunately, this analysis included randomized controlled trials (RCTs) with poor methodology (*see* Chapter 9).

- In most of the RCTs analyzed by these investigators, atenolol was the beta-blocker used for comparison. Worldwide, atenolol is the most prescribed beta-blocker (more than 44 million prescriptions annually).
- Their analysis indeed suggests that atenolol does not give hypertensive patients adequate protection against cardiovascular disease (CVD). However, these investigators failed to recognize that beta-blockers possess important and subtle clinical properties. Their analysis does not indicate that other beta-blockers provide the same poor CVD protection as atenolol.

The second edition of Cardiac Drug Therapy *(1988) emphasized that beta-blockers are not all alike:*

- Those with ISA activity (oxprenolol, pindolol) are not cardioprotective; *see* discussion of ISA activity in Chapter 1.
- Propranolol proved cardioprotective in BHAT *(2)*, and in the Medical Researach Council (MRC) trial of treatment of mild hypertension *(3)*, but only in nonsmokers (*see* the last section of Chapter 1, Which Beta-Blocker Is Best for Your Patients?)
- Bucindolol, a newer vasodilatory beta-blocker, surprisingly proved to be of no value for the treatment of heart failure (HF) *(4)*, whereas carvedilol (in COPERNICUS *[5]* and CAPRICORN *[6]*) significantly decreased coronary heart disease (CHD) outcomes.
- Bisoprolol (in CIBIS *[7]*) and metoprolol succinate (in MERIT/HF *[8]*) significantly reduced fatal and nonfatal myocardial infarction (MI) and recurrence of HF.
- In CAPRICORN, carvedilol achieved a 50% reduction in nonfatal MI patients aged mainly >55 yr. There was a 30% reduction in total mortality and nonfatal MI. Carvedilol decreased CHD events in elderly normotensive and hypertensive patients.
- The causation of a fatal or nonfatal MI in patients with CHD is the same in a hypertensive and nonhypertensive individual. Thus calcium antagonist or diuretic therapy used for management of hypertension cannot give more cardioprotection (decrease in fatal and nonfatal MI) than treatment with beta-blockers that are proven in RCTs to prevent outcomes. Experts *(1)* who make claims for calcium antagonists and diuretics based on faulty metaanalyses are misguiding clinicians.
- Newer beta-blockers have other possible benefits. Carvedilol and nebivolol are beta- blockers with direct vasodilating and antioxidant properties. Nebivolol stimulates the endothelial L-arginine/nitric oxide pathway and produces vasodilation; the drug increases nitric oxide (NO) by decreasing its oxidative inactivation *(9)*.

From: *Contemporary Cardiology: Cardiac Drug Therapy, Seventh Edition*
M. Gabriel Khan © Humana Press Inc., Totowa, NJ

- These two beta-blockers should be subjected to long-term outcome trials in the treatment of primary hypertension.
- Atenolol is a hydrophilic beta-blocker that attains low brain concentration. Increased brain concentration and elevation of central vagal tone confers cardiovascular protection *(10)*. Lipid-soluble beta-blockers (bisoprolol, carvedilol, metoprolol, propranolol, and timolol) with high brain concentration block sympathetic discharge in the hypothalamus better than water-soluble agents (atenolol and sotalol) *(10)*.
- Abald et al. *(11)*, in a rabbit model, showed that although metoprolol (lipophilic) and atenolol (hydrophilic) caused equal beta-blockade, only metoprolol caused a reduction in sudden cardiac death. Metoprolol, but not atenolol, caused a significant increase, which indicates an increase in sympathetic tone.
- Importantly, only the lipophilic beta-blockers (carvedilol, bisoprolol, bisoprolol, propranolol, and timolol) have been shown in RCTs to prevent fatal and nonfatal MI and sudden cardiac death. In the timolol infarction RCT, the drug caused a 67% reduction in sudden deaths *(12)*. These agents have been shown to quell early morning catecholamine surge and control early morning and exercise-induced excessive rise in blood pressure better compared with atenolol *(13,14)*.
- Importantly, the duration of action of atenolol varies from 18 to 24 h and fails in some individuals to provide 24 h of CVD protection. The drug leaves an early morning gap, a period crucial for the prevention of fatal MI and sudden cardiac death.
- The observation that atenolol is less effective than other antihypertensives including vasodilatory beta-blockers at lowering aortic pressure despite an equivalent effect on brachial pressure may partly explain the poor cardioprotection. In the Conduit Artery Function Evaluation (CAFE) study *(15)*, brachial and aortic pressures were measured in a subset of 2199 patients from ASCOT *(16)*. Despite virtually identical reductions in brachial pressure, the aortic systolic pressure was 4.3 mmHg lower in the amlodipine/perindopril arm versus those on atenolol/bendroflumethiazide (*see* discussion in Chapter 9, Hypertension Controversies).

It is clear that beta-blockers are not all alike with regard to their salutary effects, and older beta-blocking drugs including atenolol should become obsolete *(17)*. Beta-blockers are CVD protective provided that bisoprolol, carvedilol, or metoprolol are chosen and not atenolol *(18)*.

It is poor logic to accept the conclusions drawn from the Lindholm et al. metaanalysis *(1)*.

- I strongly advise the use of an appropriate beta-blocker (bisoprolol carvedilol, or metoprolol succinate extended release) for the initial management of mild primary hypertension depending on the age and ethnicity of the individual (*see* treatment tables and algorithms in Chapter 9, Hypertension Controversies).

BETA-BLOCKERS ARE NOT RECOMMENDED FOR TREATMENT OF ELDERLY HYPERTENSIVES: TRUE OR FALSE?

In 1998, Messerli et al. *(19)* concluded that this statement is true based on their metaanalysis, which included the poorly run MRC trial in the elderly *(20)*. Evidence is cited in Chapter 9 of this text indicating that the statement is false. The beta-blocker hypertension controversy, including appropriate use in elderly hypertensive patients, is discussed fully in Chapters 8 and 9, and algorithms are provided indicating which initial drug is best depending on the age and ethnicity of the hypertensive patient.

BETA-BLOCKERS CAUSE DIABETES: TRUE OR FALSE?

A small presumed increased risk for the development of type 2 diabetes caused by beta-blocker therapy in hypertensive individuals has become a concern. Insulin secretion is probably partly beta$_2$ mediated.Glucose-sulfonylurea–stimulated insulin secretion is partially inhibited by beta-blockers *(21)*. Clinically, however, no significant worsening of glycemic control is seen when beta-blockers are combined with these agents. Long-term beta-blocker therapy may increase blood glucose concentration by approx 0.2–0.5 mmol/L (approx 3–9 mg/dL), as observed in RCTs with follow-up beyond 5 yr.

In **ASCOT-BPLA** *(16)*, baseline glucose concentration for amlodipine and the atenolol-based regimen was 6.24 versus 6.4 mmol/L. At follow-up 5 yr later, levels for the atenolol regimen were 0.2 mmol/L higher than in the amlodipine group. Without clearly confirming a diabetic state, the investigators proclaimed that beta-blockers caused a 30% increase in diabetes.

- The diagnosis of diabetes mellitus was not confirmed by a 2 h glucose assessment.
- It is surprising that *The Lancet*, a peer-reviewed journal, would print such erroneous conclusions.
- Physicians who incorrectly label individuals as diabetics are in line for medicolegal action.

In **UKPDS** *(22)*, the longest follow-up study in diabetics (9 yr), the studied 1148 hypertensive patients with type 2 diabetes to determine whether tight control of blood pressure with either a beta-blocker or an ACE inhibitor has a specific advantage or disadvantage in preventing the macrovascular and microvascular complications of type 2 diabetes. At 9-yr follow-up, blood pressure lowering with captopril or atenolol was similarly effective in reducing the incidence of major diabetic complications. Glycated hemoglobin concentration was similar in the two groups over the second 4 yr of study (atenolol 8.4% versus captopril 8.3%; *see* Chapters 9 and 22).

Gress et al. conducted a prospective study of 12,550 adults 45–64 yr old who did not have diabetes *(23)*. A health evaluation conducted at baseline included assessment of medication use. The incidence of type 2 diabetes was assessed after 3 and 6 yr by assessment of fasting serum glucose. Individuals with hypertension treated with beta-blockers had a 28% higher risk of subsequent diabetes.

- The diagnosis of diabetes mellitus versus mild glucose intolerance was not clarified. Thus this analysis is flawed.

Padwal and colleagues conducted a systematic review of antihypertensive therapy and the incidence of type 2 diabetes *(24)*. Data from the highest quality studies indicate that diabetes incidence is unchanged or increased by beta-blocker and thiazide diuretics and unchanged or decreased by ACE inhibitors and calcium antagonists.

- The authors concluded that current data are far from conclusive. These investigators warned that poor methodologic quality limits the conclusions that can be drawn from the several nonrandomized studies quoted by many.
- Most important, in the studies analyzed by Padwal et al., the increase in diabetic incidence reported is presumptive because type 2 diabetes was not proved by appropriate diagnostic testing.

In most studies, including **LIFE**, post hoc analysis suggests that increased risk of new-onset diabetes is confined to individuals with an elevated blood glucose at baseline and family predisposition to diabetes *(25)*. This finding strongly suggest that in prediabetics beta-blockers bring to light type 2 diabetes at an earlier point in time but do not cause diabetes in nondiabetic individuals.

STOP-2, a large RCT, showed no difference between ACE inhibitors and beta-blockers in preventing cardiovascular events and no difference in incidence of diabetes *(26)*.

I believe that the diagnosis of diabetes was not correctly established in many of the quoted studies. Clinicians and trialists should ask whether this increased incidence of diabetes is real, or are there other explanations for the observed modest increase in fasting glucose concentrations observed. Murphy et al. completed a 14-yr follow-up in hypertensive patients treated with diuretics that caused a major increase in the incidence of glucose intolerance *(27)*.

- *This effect, however, was promptly reversed in most (60%) of the patients on discontinuation of the diuretic (27).* Thus, these individuals developed benign reversible glucose intolerance, and it is important for clinicians to note that these patients were not classified as diabetics by these investigators. Similar findings have been reported when beta-blocker therapy is discontinued.
- The study of Murphy et al. shows without doubt that diuretics do not cause genuine diabetes mellitus and this information should be made known to trialists and experts in the field who continue to issue misleading medical reports.
- Trialists and those who claim to be experts in the field must be warned not to label individuals as diabetic solely on a fasting glucose level range of 6.4–7.4 mmol/L (115–133 mg/dL) without further diagnostic confirmation in patients treated with a beta-blocker, a diuretic, or a combination of both.
- It remains unclear whether ACE inhibitors reduce diabetic risk or whether long-term treatment with beta-blockers and diuretics increases glucose levels 0.2–0.5 mmol/L (3–9 mg/dL) in normal subjects.
- **In some subjects with prediabetes or a positive family history of type 2 diabetes, beta-blockers and diuretics might bring the diabetic state to light at an earlier point in time, and thus energetic treatment can commence. This presents a reassuring, rather than alarming, scenario.**
- It must be reemphasized that the finding of glucose intolerance does not necessarily mean the diabetic state exists. Beta-blockers do not cause type 2 diabetes, as proclaimed by several trialists and notable clinicians.
- In nondiabetics, beta-blockers may cause mild glucose intolerance that is benign and reversible on discontinuation of these agents.

DO ALL BETA-BLOCKERS CAUSE GLUCOSE INTOLERANCE?

The GEMINI trial *(28)* compared the effects of two different beta-blockers on glycemic control as well as other cardiovascular risk factors in a cohort with glycemic control similar to the UKPDS.

- Carvedilol stabilized HbA_{1c}, improved insulin resistance, and slowed development of microalbuminuria in the presence of renin-angiotensin system (RAS) blockade compared with metoprolol.
- Carvedilol treatment had no effect on HbA_{1c} (mean [SD] change from baseline to end point, 0.02% [0.04%]; 95% CI, –0.06–0.10%; $p = 0.65$), whereas metoprolol increased HbA_{1c} (0.15% [0.04%]; 95% CI, 0.08–0.22%; $p < 0.001$) *(28)*.
- HOMA-IR was reduced by carvedilol and increased with metoprolol, which resulted in a significant improvement from baseline for carvedilol (–9.1%, $p = 0.004$) but not metoprolol which lowers insulin resistance *(28)*, an effect that correlated with HbA_{1c}. This finding sup-

ports the effect of carvedilol on reducing insulin resistance, which has been previously shown by Giugliano et al. in more time-intensive insulin clamp studies *(29)*.

- Treatment with carvedilol was associated with improvement in total cholesterol and a smaller increase in triglyceride levels relative to metoprolol *(28)*.

BETA-BLOCKERS SHOULD NOT BE GIVEN TO PATIENTS DURING THE EARLY HOURS OF ACUTE MI: TRUE OR FALSE?

The results of COMMIT/CCS-2: Clopidogrel and Metoprolol in Myocardial Infarction Trial/Second Chinese Cardiac Study *(30)* may cause changes in the American College of Cardiology/American Heart Association (ACC/AHA) guidelines. In this huge RC, patients received aspirin and were randomized to receive clopidogrel 75 mg/d or placebo; within these two groups, patients were then randomized to metoprolol (*15 mg IV in three equal doses followed by 200 mg/d orally*) or placebo. Patients were randomized within 24 h of suspected acute MI and demonstrating ST elevation or other ischemic abnormality.

- Metoprolol produced a significant 18% RRR in reinfarction (2.0% versus 2.5%; $p = 0.001$) as well as a 17% RRR in ventricular fibrillation (2.5% versus 3.0%; $p = 0.001$); there was no effect on mortality. However, metoprolol significantly increased the relative risk of death from cardiogenic shock, by 29%, with the greatest risk of shock occurring primarily on d 0–1 *(30)*.
- Cardiogenic shock was understandably more evident in patients in Killip class II and III; this adverse effect was largely iatrogenic because the dose of metoprolol was excessive and given to patients in whom these agents are contraindicated.
- Oral beta-blocker therapy is preferred, and IV use is cautioned against, particularly in patients with pulmonary edema or systolic blood pressure (BP) < 100 mmHg. In this study *(30)*, a large dose of metoprolol was given IV to patients with systolic BP < 95 mmHg and in those with Killip class II and III.
- Study co-chair Rory Collins emphasized that it may generally be prudent to wait until a heart attack patient's condition has stabilized before starting beta-blocker therapy."
- The advice should be restated: do not give beta-blockers to patients who are hemodynamically unstable or in whom heart failure is manifest. Most patients with acute MI can be given metoprolol at an appropriate dose within the early hours of onset of acute MI (*see* Chapter 22).

REFERENCES

1. Lindholm LH, Carlberg B, Samuelsson O. Should β blockers remain first choice in the treatment of primary hypertension? A meta-analysis. Lancet 2005;366:1545–1553.
2. β-Blocker Heart Attack Trial Research Group. A randomised trial of propranolol in patients with acute myocardial infarction. I: Mortality results. JAMA 1982;247:1707–1714.
3. Treatment of hypertension: The 1985 results. Lancet 1985;2:645–647.
4. Beta-Blocker Evaluation of Survival Trial Investigators. A trial of the beta-blocker bucindolol in patients with advanced chronic heart failure N Engl J Med 2001;62:1659–1667.
5. Packer M, Fowler MB, Roecker EB, et al. Effect of carvedilol on the morbidity of patients with severe chronic heart failure: results of the Carvedilol Prospective Randomized Cumulative Survival (COPERNICUS) study. Circulation 2002;106:2194–2199.
6. The CAPRICORN Investigators. Effect of carvedilol on outcome after myocardial infarction in patients with left-ventricular dysfunction: The CAPRICORN randomised trial. Lancet 2001;357:1385–1390.
7. CIBIS-II Investigators and Committees. The Cardiac Insufficiency Bisoprolol Study II (CIBIS-II): A randomised trial. Lancet 1999;353:9–13.
8. MERIT-HF Study Group. Effect of metoprolol CR/XL in chronic heart failure: Metoprolol CR/XL Randomised Intervention Trial in Congestive heart failure (MERIT-HF). Lancet 1999;353:2001–2007.

9. Cominacini L, Fratta Pasini A, Garbin U, et al. Nebivolol and its 4-keto derivative increase nitric oxide in endothelial cells by reducing its oxidative inactivation. J Am Coll Cardiol 2003;42:1838–1844.
10. Pitt B The role of beta-adrenergic blocking agents in preventing sudden cardiac death. Circulation 1992; 85(I Suppl):107.
11. Äblad B, Bjurö T, Björkman JA, Edström T, Olsson G. Role of central nervous beta-adrenoceptors in the prevention of ventricular fibrillation through augmentation of cardiac vagal tone. J Am Coll Cardiol 1991; 17(Suppl):165.
12. Norwegian Multicentre Group. Timolol induced reduction in mortality and reinfarction in patients surviving acute myocardial infarction. N Engl J Med 1981;304:801–807.
13. Neutel JM, Smith DHG, Ram CVS. Application of ambulatory blood pressure monitoring in differentiating between antihypertensive agents. Am J Med 1993;94:181.
14. Kokkinos P, Chrysohoou C, Panagiotakos D, et al. Beta-blockade mitigates exercise blood pressure in hypertensive male patients. J Am Coll Cardiol 2006;47:794–798.
15. CAFE investigators for the Anglo-Scandinavian Cardiac Outcomes Trial (ASCOT) investigators. Differential impact of blood pressure-lowering drugs on central aortic pressure and clinical outcomes: Principal results of the Conduit Artery Function Evaluation (CAFE) Study. Circulation 2006;113:1213–1225.
16. Dahlof B, Sever PS, Poulter NR, et al. for the ASCOT investigators. Prevention of cardiovascular events with an antihypertensive regimen of amlodipine adding perindopril as required versus atenolol adding bendroflumethiazide as required, in the Anglo-Scandinavian Cardiac Outcomes Trial-Blood Pressure Lowering Arm (ASCOT-BPLA): A multicentre randomised controlled trial. Lancet 2005;366:895–906.
17. Khan M Gabriel. Hypertension. In: Cardiac Drug Therapy, 6th ed. Philadelphia, WB Saunders, 2003; 46–48.
18. Khan M Gabriel. Which beta blocker to choose. In: Heart Disease Diagnosis and Therapy, a Practical Approach, 2nd ed. Totowa, NJ, Humana Press, 2005, pp. 311–314.
19. Messerli FH, Grossman E, Goldbourt U. Are β-blockers efficacious as first-line therapy for hypertension in the elderly? JAMA 1998;279:1903–1907.
20. MRC Working Party. Medical Research Council Trial of treatment of hypertension in older adults: Principal results. BMJ 1992;304:405–412.
21. Loubatiere A, Mariani MM, Sorel G, et al. The action of beta adrenergic blocking drugs and stimulating agents on insulin secretion. Characteristic of the type of beta receptor. Diabetologica 1971;7:127–132.
22. UK Prospective Diabetes Study Group. Efficacy of atenolol and captopril in reducing risk of macrovascular and microvascular complications in type 2 diabetes: UKPDS. BMJ 1998;317:713–720.
23. Gress TW, Nieto FJ, Shahar E, et al. for The Atherosclerosis Risk in Communities Study: Hypertension and antihypertensive therapy as risk factors for type 2 diabetes mellitus. N Engl J Med 2000;342:905–912.
24. Padwal R, Laupacis A. Antihypertensive therapy and incidence of type 2 diabetes. A systematic review. Diabetes Care 2004;27:247–255.
25. Lindholm LH, Ibsen H, Borch-Johnsen K, et al. Risk of new-onset diabetes in the Losartan Intervention For Endpoint reduction in hypertension study. J Hypertens 2002;20:1879–1886.
26. Hansson L, Lindholm LH, Ekbom T, et al. Randomised trial of old and new antihypertensive drugs in elderly patients: cardiovascular mortality and morbidity. The Swedish Trial in Old Patients with Hypertension-2 study. Lancet 1999;354:1751–1756.
27. Murphy MB, Lewis PJ, Kohner E, Schumer B, Dollery CT. Glucose intolerance in hypertensive patients treated with diuretics: A fourteen-year follow-up. Lancet 1982;2:1293–1295.
28. GEMINI: Bakris GL, Fonseca V, Katholi RE, et al. Metabolic effects of carvedilol vs metoprolol in patients with type 2 diabetes mellitus and hypertension: a randomized controlled trial. JAMA 2004;292: 2227–2236.
29. Giugliano D, Acampora R, Marfella R, et al. Metabolic and cardiovascular effects of carvedilol and atenolol in non-insulin-dependent diabetes mellitus and hypertension: a randomized, controlled trial. Ann Intern Med 1997;126:955–959.
30. COMMIT (Clopidogrel and Metoprolol in Myocardial Infarction Trial) Collaborative Group. Early intravenous then oral metoprolol in 45,852 patients with acute myocardial infarction: Randomised placebo-controlled trial. Lancet 2005;366:1622–1632.

SUGGESTED READING

Remme WJ, Torp-Pedersen C, Cleland JGF, et al. Carvedilol protects better against vascular events than metoprolol in heart failure: results from COMET. J Am Coll Cardiol 2007;49:963–971.

3 Angiotensin-Converting Enzyme Inhibitors and Angiotensin II Receptor Blockers

Angiotensin-converting enzyme (ACE) inhibitors and angiotensin II receptor blockers (ARBs) play a pivotal role in the management of heart failure (HF) and hypertension. These agents are *cardioprotective* and increase survival in patients with

- HF.
- Left ventricular (LV) dysfunction.
- Acute myocardial infarction (MI). The Survival of Myocardial Infarction Long-Term Evaluation (SMILE) study *(1)* showed that zofenopril administered to patients with acute anterior infarction improved survival.
- Hypertension with LV hypertrophy (LVH).
- Hypertension with diabetes and proteinuria.
- A high risk for cardiovascular events, as documented by the Heart Outcomes Prevention Evaluation HOPE study *(2)*.

Tissue angiotensin II production appears to be an important modulator of tissue function and structure. Angiotensin II produced in cardiac myocytes has been shown to play a role in stretch-induced hypertrophy and in the process of myocardial remodeling post infarction *(3)*.

Three classes of ACE inhibitors have been developed. Most ACE inhibitors except captopril and lisinopril possess a carboxylic radical, are transformed in the liver to the active agent, and are thus prodrugs.

Class I: Captopril is not a prodrug; it is the active drug, but with metabolism, the metabolites are also active. Only captopril and zofenopril contain a sulfhydryl (SH) group.
Class II: All other available agents except lisinopril are prodrugs and become active only after hepatic metabolism to the diacid (Table 3-1).
Class III: Lisinopril is not a prodrug and is the only water-soluble agent; it is excreted unchanged by the kidneys. Lipid solubility does not confer clinical benefits beyond those observed with lisinopril.

The pharmacologic features and dosages of ACE inhibitors are given in Tables 3-1 and 3-2 and in Chapter 8.

MECHANISM OF ACTION

Vascular stretch of the renal afferent arteriole and the sodium concentration in the distal tubule, sensed by the macula densa and an interplay of beta-adrenergic receptors,

From: *Contemporary Cardiology: Cardiac Drug Therapy, Seventh Edition*
M. Gabriel Khan © Humana Press Inc., Totowa, NJ

Table 3-1
Pharmacologic Profile and Dosages of ACE Inhibitors

	Benazepril	*Captopril*	*Cilazapril*	*Enalapril*	*Fosinopril*	*Lisinopril*	*Perindopril*	*Quinapril*	*Ramipril*	*Trandolapril*
USA + Canada	Lotensin	Capoten	Inhibace	Vasotec	Monopril	Prinivil,	Aceon Zestril	Accupril	Altace	Mavik
UK	—	Capoten	Vascace	Innovace	Staril	Carace, Zestril	Aceon	Accuprin	Tritace	Gopten/ Odrik
Europe	Cibace	Lopril, Lopirin	Inibace	Xanef, Renitec		Carace, Zestril	Acertil	Accupro	Tritace	Gopten
Prodrug	Yes	No	Yes	Yes	Yes	No	Yes	Yes	Partial	Yes
Action										
Apparent (h)	1	0.5		2–4		2–4			3–6	
Peak effect (h)	2	1–2		4		4–8			3–6	
Duration (h)	12–24	8–12	>24	12–24		24–30			24–48	
Half-life (h)	10–11	2–3	>40	11	>24	13	>24	>24	14–30	24
Metabolism	—	Partly hepatic		Hepatic		None			Partial	
Elimination	Renal	Renal	Renal	Renal	Renal + heptatic	Renal	Renal	Renal	Renal	Renal
SH group	No	Yes	No	No	No	No	No	No	No	No
Tissue specificity	No	No	Yes	No	Yes	No	Yes		Yes	Yes
Equivalent dose	10 mg	100 mg	2.5	20 mg	10	20 mg	3	15	10 mg	2
Initial dose	5–10 mg	6.25 mg	1.5	2.5mg	5	2.5 mg	2	2.5–5	2.5–5	0.5
Total daily dose										
Hypertension	10–20 mg	25–150 mg	1.5–5 mg	5–40 mg	5–40 mg	5–40 mg	2–8 mg	5–40 mg	2.5–15 mg	1–4 mg
Heart failure	—	75–150 mg	—	10–35 mg	—	10–35 mg				—
Dose frequency[a]	1 daily	2–3 daily	1 daily	1–2 daily	1 daily	1 daily	1 daily	1 daily	1 daily	1 daily
Supplied, tabs	5, 10, 20, 40 mg	12.5, 25, 50, 100 mg	1, 2.5, 5 mg	2.5, 5, 10, 20 mg	10, 20 mg	2.5, 5, 10, 20, 40 mg	2, 4 mg	5, 10, 20, 40 mg	1.25, 2.5, 5, 10 mg	0.5, 1, 2 mg

[a]Increase dosing interval with renal failure or in the elderly.

Table 3-2
Profile of Angiotensin II Receptor Blockers

Drug	*Active metabolite*	*Bioavailability (%)*	*Half-life (h)*	*Food effect*	*Dose once daily (mg)*
Candesartan	No	15	9	None	4–16
Irbesartan	No	60–80	11–15	None	150–300
Losartan	Yes	33	6–9	Minimal	50–100
Valsartan	No	25	6	50%	80–160

control the release of renin from the juxtaglomerular cells located in the media of the afferent renal arteriole *(4–7)*.

Stimuli to the release of renin include

- A decrease in renal blood flow (ischemia), hypotension, and reduction of intravascular volume.
- Sodium depletion or sodium diuresis.
- Beta-adrenoceptor activation.

The enzyme renin is a protease that cleaves the leucine 10–valine 11 bond from angiotensinogen to form the decapeptide angiotensin I *(7)*. ACE now cleaves histidine–leucine from angiotensin I, resulting in the formation of angiotensin II, which causes

- Vasoconstriction about 40 times more intense than that caused by norepinephrine. Vasoconstriction occurs predominantly in arterioles and, to a lesser degree, in veins; this action is more pronounced in the skin and kidney, with some sparing of vessels in the brain and muscle *(8)*.
- Renal effects: marked sodium reabsorption occurs in the proximal tubule.
- Adrenal effects: aldosterone release enhances sodium and water reabsorption and potassium excretion in the renal tubule distal to the macula densa. Angiotensin II also promotes release of catecholamines from the adrenal medulla.
- Increased sympathetic outflow and facilitated ganglionic stimulation of the sympathetic nervous system *(7,9)*.
- Modest vagal inhibition, which may explain the lack of tachycardia in response to the marked vasodilator effect of ACE inhibitors.
- Enhanced antidiuretic hormone secretion, resulting in free water gain.

ACE inhibitors are competitive inhibitors of angiotensin-converting enzyme, and therefore they prevent the conversion of angiotensin I to angiotensin II. The consequences of this action are as follows:

- Arteriolar dilation causes a fall in total systemic vascular resistance, blood pressure, and afterload; these three terms are interrelated but are not synonymous *(10)*.
- **Sympathetic activity decreases** because of attenuation of angiotensin-related potentiation of sympathetic activity and release of norepinephrine. The diminished sympathetic activity causes further vasodilation with additional reduction in afterload and some decrease in preload. It is because of this further indirect antisympathetic and vagal effect that heart rate is not increased by ACE inhibitors, as opposed to several other groups of vasodilators.
- Reduction in aldosterone secretion promotes sodium excretion and potassium retention.
- **Vascular oxidative stress is favorably influenced** *(9)* because vascular superoxide is reduced. Thus, ACE inhibitors are believed to have important antioxidant properties superior

to those of vitamin E and other antioxidants. A review by Burnier gives details and relevant references *(10)*. Vascular wall endothelium, smooth muscle, and fibroblasts contain enzyme systems that use nicotinamide adenine dinucleotide and its reduced form (NADH and NADPH) for the production of superoxide anion that is increased in response to angiotensin II. ACE activity has been noted to increase in atheromatous plaques, and inhibition appears to influence inflammatory reaction favorably within the arterial wall. Angiotensin II is a mitogen for vascular smooth muscle cells that can be inhibited. Superoxide is a major source of hydrogen peroxide; thus, smooth muscle cell proliferation may be limited. Also, nitric oxide (NO) activity appears to improve because superoxide reacts with NO *(10)*.

- **Increased free water loss** by blocking of angiotensin-mediated vasopressin release causes free water loss, resulting in some protection from dilutional hyponatremia. This action is important in patients with severe HF.
- **Increased bradykinin-converting enzyme** is the same as kinase II, which causes degradation of bradykinin. *The accumulation of bradykinin stimulates release of vasodilatory NO and prostacyclin that may protect the endothelium and contribute to arterial dilation and to a decrease in peripheral vascular resistance.* Thus, indomethacin and other prostaglandin inhibitors reduce the effectiveness of ACE inhibitors. Captopril has been shown to be uricosuric *(11)*, and it reduces hyperuricemia.
- **Arteriolar hyperplasia is decreased.** ACE inhibitors have been shown to decrease arteriolar hyperplasia caused by hypertension. Therapy with cilazapril for 1 yr appears to correct the structural and functional abnormalities in the resistance arteries of patients with mild essential hypertension.

ACE gene polymorphism contributes to the modulation and adequacy of the neurohormonal response to ACE inhibitor long-term administration in HF *(12)*. Patients with HF with aldosterone escape have been shown to have a higher prevalence of DD genotype compared with patients with normal aldosterone levels *(12)*. The antihypertensive response to ACE inhibition has also been shown in a small series to be more pronounced in subjects with ACE DD genotype than in those with the ACE-11 genotype *(12)*. Genetic screening of large populations of patients, however, remains controversial.

ACE INHIBITORS VERSUS OTHER VASODILATORS

The reversal of iatrogenic hypokalemia caused by ACE inhibition is an important asset in the management of patients with hypertension and HF, who often require diuretic therapy.

The suppression of ADH activity by ACE inhibitors decreases free water gain, which is useful in the management of the hyponatremic patient with HF. This salutary effect is not observed with other vasodilators.

- Both **ACE inhibitors** and calcium antagonists are effective in preventing LVH and also cause it to regress when present, but other vasodilators do not consistently prevent hypertrophy or cause regression. LVH is an independent risk factor for sudden death, and its prevention is therefore an important aspect of pharmacologic therapy. ACE inhibitors are generally well tolerated, with few adverse effects, whereas fewer than 33% of patients tolerate hydralazine or alpha$_1$-blockers after 6 mo of therapy at doses sufficient to achieve goal blood pressure. ACE inhibitors cause marked arteriolar vasodilation and a significant decrease in venous tone, resulting in a decrease in afterload and preload. In contrast with other vasodilators, with the exception of calcium antagonists, they cause afterload reduction, but their administration sets in motion compensatory mechanisms that have several effects tending to counteract their beneficial action.

- **Prazosin** and other alpha$_1$-blockers cause a decrease in afterload and a mild decrease in preload, but they increase heart rate and cardiac ejection velocity, resulting in a deleterious rate of rise of aortic pressure. These agents cause sodium and water retention that necessitates an increase in prazosin dosage and often requires added diuretic therapy. Tachyphylaxis occurs, and clinical trials have proved prazosin to be ineffective for prolonging life in the setting of HF.
- **Hydralazine** has had extensive clinical testing. The Veteran's Administration Heart Failure Trial (VHeFT II) *(12)* showed the drug to be effective in HF when combined with the venodilator effect of nitrates. Hydralazine causes a marked enhancement in heart rate and cardiac ejection velocity. This action is undesirable in patients with ischemic heart disease and limits the usefulness of this agent. Other vasodilators of this class, including alpha$_1$-adrenergic receptor blockers (trimazosin, indoramin, terazosin), cause undesirable effects similar to those of prazosin and hydralazine. Other vasodilators, except for those that have a primary renal and adrenal action, of necessity cause a stimulation of the renin-angiotensin system as well as an adrenal release of catecholamine and sympathetic stimulation to compensate for the arteriolar dilation. These untoward effects, however, allow for the occasional combination of one of the aforementioned vasodilators with an ACE inhibitor.
- **Nitroglycerin** is predominantly a venous dilator and decreases preload. A minimal decrease in afterload occurs with the use of intravenous (IV) nitroglycerin, but not oral nitrates. These agents are useful in the management of chronic HF only when they are added to arteriolar vasodilators.

CLINICAL INDICATIONS

Hypertension

ACE inhibitors and ARBs are indicated for hypertension of all grades. Because these agents do not cause sodium and water retention, they can often be used as monotherapy without a diuretic. This is a major advantage in terms of compliance and avoids the biochemical and lipid derangements produced by diuretics. Also, one-a-day preparations are available. Their low side effect profile, especially with the quality-of-life advantages over some other antihypertensive agents, has resulted in their widespread use.

As outlined earlier, their built-in protection from reflex sympathetic stimulation, resulting in an increase in heart rate and the rate of rise of aortic pressure, is a major advantage over alpha$_1$-adrenergic receptor antagonists (alpha-blockers) and similar vasodilators. ACE inhibitors and ARBs retain potassium and avoid the need for gastric-irritating potassium supplements. These agents have proved to be effective in the prevention of LVH and therefore have the potential to decrease cardiac mortality, because LVH is an independent risk factor for sudden death.

Rebound hypertension observed after withdrawal of clonidine, guanabenz, guanfacine, methyldopa, and, rarely, calcium antagonists and beta-blockers is not a feature of ACE inhibition.

ACE inhibitors are most effective in young patients, aged less than 55 yr, with essential hypertension who usually have increased renin activity. In this subset of patients, ACE inhibitors prescribed as monotherapy are effective in about 50% of cases. In patients with more severe hypertension, ACE inhibitors in combination with diuretics are effective in up to 65%. ACE inhibitors are slightly less effective in reducing blood pressure in nonwhite patients and in the elderly, although studies indicate a sufficiently good response to justify a trial of ACE inhibitors or ARBs as monotherapy in the elderly when other agents are contraindicated or poorly tolerated. The antihypertensive action of ACE inhibitors is multifactorial and partially depends on the renin and sodium status. Thus, it is not surprising that ACE inhibitors have been shown to be effective in elderly patients with low renin status.

ACE inhibitors and ARBs are particularly effective in lowering blood pressure in patients with high renin-angiotensin states, such as

- In combination with moderate to high doses of diuretics for the management of resistant hypertension.
- In malignant hypertension.
- In hypertension resulting from oral contraceptive use.
- In coarctation of the aorta.
- Immediately after dialysis in patients with chronic renal failure, when sodium and volume depletion is associated with enhancement of the renin-angiotensin system and responds to ACE inhibition *(13)*.
- For the management of hypertensive patients with concomitant HF, for which ACE inhibitors are ideal. In this subset of patients, the systolic blood pressure should be maintained at less than 140 mmHg. The use of ACE inhibitors complements therapy with diuretics because diuretic use in this context stimulates the renin-angiotensin system.

ACE inhibitors are highly recommended in the following clinical situations:

- In the hypertensive diabetic patient, ACE inhibitors are first-choice agents because they do not adversely affect glucose metabolism, they have a proven effect in reducing diabetic proteinuria, and there is some evidence suggesting prolongation of nephron life. ACE inhibition enhances insulin-mediated uptake of glucose, and this effect may be important in the management of hypertensives with diabetes.
- These drugs are useful in hypertensive patients with hyperlipidemia because these agents produce no change in lipid parameters. When needed, a combination with a beta-blocking drug may provide cardioprotection.
- Tissue ACE inhibition allows for the use of ACE inhibitors to decrease blood pressure in patients who have undergone nephrectomy.

Although these agents are very effective in patients with renovascular hypertension, they must be used, if at all, with extreme caution because severe renal insufficiency may occur in patients with bilateral renal artery stenosis or stenosis in a solitary kidney. Because ACE inhibitors cause dilation of the efferent arteriole, they may precipitate renal failure or the loss of a kidney.

Heart Failure

ACE inhibitors have provided a major improvement in the management of HF, resulting in both amelioration of symptoms and an increase in survival when they are used in combination with diuretics and digoxin *(14)*. The fall in cardiac output with HF triggers a compensatory response that involves enhancement of the sympathetic nervous system and the renin-angiotensin-aldosterone system. As a result of these adjustments, systemic vascular resistance and afterload are increased inappropriately, with further deterioration in cardiac performance, and a vicious circle ensues (*see* Chapter 12). ACE inhibitors play a vital role in halting the counterproductive pathophysiologic events that tend to perpetuate, rather than correct, cardiac decompensation.

The beneficial effects of diuretics in the management of HF are limited by excessive stimulation of the renin-angiotensin system; the addition of ACE inhibitors results in further amelioration. This improvement is partly the result of reduced arterial and venous tone, but changes in fluid and electrolyte balance are also important.

Stimulation of the sympathetic and the renin-angiotensin-aldosterone system causes intense sodium and water retention in the proximal and distal nephron. Also, an increase in venous tone occurs. Both adjustments result in an increase in filling pressure, which enhances preload. ACE inhibitors partially inhibit sodium and water retention and decrease venous tone, which produces a decrease in preload, an improvement or decrease in symptoms and signs of pulmonary congestion, and an increase in exercise tolerance. The improvement in functional capacity is superior to that observed with hydralazine and is similar to the combination of hydralazine and isosorbide dinitrate.

The Cooperative North Scandinavian Enalapril Survival Study (CONSENSUS) *(15)* indicated an increased survival in New York Heart Association (NYHA) class IV patients treated for over 6 mo with enalapril added to diuretics and digoxin. The 6-mo mortality rate was 26% in patients treated with enalapril, versus 44% in those given diuretic and digoxin alone ($p < 0.001$). Forty-two percent of the group treated with enalapril showed functional class improvement compared with 22% in the control group ($p = 0.001$). In a study of patients with HF with an ejection fraction of less than 35%, enalapril improved survival and decreased the number of hospitalizations for HF *(16)*. The VHeFT II trial, at an average 2.5-yr follow-up, showed a modest improvement in survival, the mortality rate being 33% for enalapril added to diuretics and digoxin, versus 38% in patients given a diuretic and digoxin along with hydralazine and isosorbide dinitrate *(12)*.

It is clear that ACE inhibitors improve survival in certain categories of patients, and benefit is beyond question for patients with NYHA class IV HF *(15)*. There is as yet no convincing evidence that these drugs decrease mortality in patients with NYHA class II HF and, although VHeFT II results suggest some benefit in class II patients, this is not statistically significant (*see* Chapter 12).

In the management of patients with HF, it is of paramount importance to commence with the smallest dose of ACE inhibitor, enalapril 2.5 mg or captopril 6.25 mg once or twice daily, and to titrate the dose slowly over several days, to avoid relative hypovolemia and hypotension, which can worsen cerebral and coronary perfusion. In a randomized study, patients with HF and concomitant angina showed an increase in angina and a reduced exercise tolerance when treated with captopril *(17)*. The deleterious effects were related to the hypotensive effect of captopril. Poor diastolic coronary perfusion to contractile myocardial segments supplied by arteries with significant stenosis may precipitate angina in patients with HF. Caution is therefore especially necessary when ACE inhibitors are combined with calcium antagonists, nitrates, or other agents that may result in the lowering of blood pressure.

Acute Myocardial Infarction

After acute MI, there is stimulation of the renin-angiotensin system resulting in increased myocardial wall stress, as well as cardiac dilation that may ultimately increase morbidity and mortality. The process by which the left ventricle dilates and progressively enlarges after infarction is called ventricular remodeling. After MI, some patients develop an increase in LV size and an increase in end-systolic and end-diastolic volumes. ACE inhibitors cause favorable myocardial remodeling. These agents have been shown to decrease the incidence of HF and the rate of hospitalization in postinfarction patients with ejection fraction < 40 in the Survival and Ventricular Enlargement (SAVE) and Acute Infarction Ramipril Efficacy (AIRE) studies (*see* Chapter 12).

In the SMILE trial *(1)*, patients with anterior MI were treated early with zofenopril regardless of HF. Treatment lasted only 6 wk and resulted in a significant reduction in deaths and HF. After 1 yr, mortality was lower in the treated group than in the placebo group. In the AIRE trial, ramipril administered to patients within 3–10 d of acute MI with transient signs and symptoms of HF caused a significant 27% reduction in the risk of death at 15 mo, a benefit that was maintained for 5 yr.

Renoprotection

Based mainly on retrospective studies, ACE inhibitors were noted to slow the progression of renal disease in nondiabetic patients. In the African American Study of Kidney Disease and Hypertension, an ACE inhibitor was shown to be more effective than a calcium antagonist in retarding the progression of renal disease. ACE inhibitors have been shown in trials to slow progression in patients with type 1 diabetes with microalbuminuria, but they have not been conclusively shown in RCTs to cause renoprotection in patients with type 2 diabetes. A small study of 92 patients comparing enalapril and losartan in hypertensive type 2 diabetes indicated equal protection.

Results of two large randomized controlled trials (RCTs) with ARBs are now available: both losartan *(18)* and irbesartan *(19)* retarded the progression of nephropathy caused by type 2 diabetes independent of reduction in blood pressure. The average blood pressure during the course of the irbesartan trials was 144/83 mmHg with placebo and 143/83 mmHg in the treated group (*see* Chapter 22). ARBs are the first line of treatment for patients with type 2 diabetes with or without hypertension. **Most important, lowering of blood pressure to <130 mmHg, a difficult goal with monotherapy, appears to be nonessential** (see also the blood pressure range and the discussion of the benefit of beta-blockers in the United Kingdom Prospective Diabetes Study Group in Chapter 1).

Coarctation of the Aorta

In this condition, the renin-angiotensin system is especially active, and these agents have a role.

Pulmonary Hypertension

ACE inhibitors may lower pulmonary artery pressure and may increase cardiac output and functional capacity. As with other agents, the improvement is generally not spectacular.

Scleroderma Renal Crisis

This condition is associated with activation of the renin-angiotensin system with rapid progression of renal failure. ACE inhibitor therapy may prevent disease progression and improve survival *(20)*. An interesting case report *(21)* indicates the failure of losartan to control blood pressure caused by scleroderma renal crisis but with excellent control achieved with an ACE inhibitor. Thus, there may be subtle differences between ACE inhibitors and ARBs that may be important in clinical management.

Bartter's Syndrome

Correction of hyperkalemia is achieved.

CONTRAINDICATIONS

- **Renal artery stenosis** in a solitary kidney or significant bilateral renal artery stenosis *(22)*. In patients with tight renal artery stenosis, renal circulation is critically dependent on high levels of angiotensin II. A sharp decrease in angiotensin II concentration causes dilation of the glomerular efferent arteriole, resulting in a marked fall in renal blood flow that may cause the loss of a kidney. This catastrophic event is heralded by a sharp rise in serum creatinine concentration.

- **Significant aortic stenosis** is a contraindication.
- **Hypertrophic and restrictive cardiomyopathy**, **constrictive pericarditis**, and hypertensive hypertrophic "cardiomyopathy" of the elderly with impaired ventricular relaxation *(23)* are contraindications.
- **Severe carotid artery stenosis** is a contraindication.
- **Renal failure**, serum creatinine level greater than 2.3 mg/dL, 203 μmol/L (glomerular filtration rate [GFR] 40 mL/min). Caution is necessary when ACE inhibitors are used in patients with renal failure because worsening of renal failure or hyperkalemia may occur.
- **Angina** complicating HF or hypertension is a contraindication because, in these situations, ACE inhibitors may cause an increase in angina *(17)*.
- **Severe anemia** is a relative contraindication to the use of all vasodilators.
- **Preexisting neutropenia** is a contraindication because of the effect on white blood cell function.
- **Pregnancy and lactation** are contraindications.
- **Immune-related renal disease** or coadministration of agents that alter immune function, immunosuppressives, procainamide, tocainide, probenecid, hydralazine, allopurinol, and perhaps acebutolol and pindolol, which have been reported to cause a lupus-like syndrome, are contraindications.
- **Porphyria** is a contraindication.
- **Uric acid renal calculi** are contraindications because these agents are uricosuric *(11)*.

ADVICE, ADVERSE EFFECTS, AND INTERACTIONS

Hypotension

Symptomatic hypotension is not uncommon in patients with HF who are already being treated with diuretics or in patients with unilateral tight renal artery stenosis with high circulating renin levels.

Renal Failure

Development or worsening of renal failure may result from relative hypotension or in patients with tight renal artery stenosis.

Hyperkalemia

This may be precipitated by an increase in renal failure, by the use of potassium-sparing diuretics or potassium supplements or the use of salt substitutes, and in patients with hyporeninemic hypoaldosteronism.

Cough

A dry, ticklish, irritating, nonproductive cough occurs in up to 20% of patients, but it was observed in 32% in one series and is clearly dose related, occurring with equal frequency with captopril, enalapril, and lisinopril. ACE is the same as kinase II, which degrades bradykinin completely. The accumulation of bradykinin appears to be responsible for the cough. The cough responds to treatment with sulindac or other nonsteroidal anti-inflammatory drugs (NSAIDs). ARBs, however, do not cause cough, and angioedema rarely occurs. This newer class of cardioactive agents is discussed at the end of this chapter.

Loss of Taste Sensation

This side effect is uncommon and can occur with all ACE inhibitors because the effect appears to be related to the binding of zinc by the ACE inhibitor. A metallic or sour taste in the mouth occurs in some patients with most agents. Mouth ulcers are not uncommon.

Angioedema

This rare complication is important because it can be life-threatening, and deaths have occurred *(24,25)*. The occurrence appears to be slightly more common with longer acting ACE inhibitors than with captopril. Bradykinin and kallidin mediate hereditary angioedema. Thus, ACE inhibition results in an accumulation of bradykinin, which can cause angioedema.

Angioedema is usually observed after the very first few doses or within the first month *(24)*, but it can occur after the first dose or after several months of therapy. Cases have been reported within the first year of therapy. Warning signs include localized facial swelling or unilateral facial edema and periorbital edema, which is usually mild and subsides with cessation of drug therapy. Swelling may progress over a few hours to the lips, tongue, and larynx, with obstruction to the airway, which may be resistant to antihistamines and IV epinephrine. The severity of laryngeal edema may render endotracheal intubation impossible *(25,26)*, and it may necessitate emergency tracheostomy. Thus, all patients taking an ACE inhibitor who develop mild facial edema and initially respond to antihistamine should be hospitalized, given epinephrine and antihistamine, and observed in an intensive care setting, because, rarely, a rebound, worsening, life-threatening situation can ensue *(25,26)* and should be prevented. Antihistamines alone may not suffice and, whereas an injection of antihistamine may appear to cause relief over a few hours, severe angioedema may still develop *(25,26)*.

Rash

A pruritic rash may occur in up to 10% of patients, typically maculopapular on the arms and trunk, occasionally involving the face. Pruritus may be severe. An urticarial or erythematous eruption, sometimes associated with eosinophilia, may ensue, and, very rarely, pemphigus and onycholysis have been reported. Captopril and enalapril appear to exhibit the same incidence of rash.

Proteinuria

This occurs in fewer than 1% of captopril-treated patients and mainly in those with underlying renal collagen vascular disease or other immunologic abnormality with a dose of captopril in excess of 150 mg/d. Proteinuria results from stimulation of immune mechanisms and relative hypotension, and it also occurs with other ACE inhibitors.

Neutropenia, Agranulocytosis

This complication is very rare and occurs mainly in patients with collagen vascular disease and other immunologic disturbances. This complication usually manifests within the first 4 mo of therapy and reverses about 3 wk after cessation of ACE inhibitor therapy.

Mild Dyspnea and/or Wheeze

This may develop, particularly in some asthmatic patients, within the first few weeks of ACE inhibitor therapy *(27)*.

Anaphylactoid Reactions

In patients given ACE inhibitors, anaphylactoid reactions may occur during desensitization treatment with bee or wasp venom. Discontinuation of the ACE inhibitor for at least 24 h before treatment is advisable.

Captopril

This drug appears to inhibit the diuretic action of furosemide in ambulatory patients (*see* Chapter 12).

Uncommon Adverse Effects

These include headache, dizziness, fatigue, nausea, diarrhea, impotence, loss of libido, myalgia, muscle cramps, hair loss, hepatitis, cholestatic jaundice, acute pancreatitis, and the occurrence of antinuclear antibodies.

Interactions

Interactions may occur with allopurinol, acebutolol, hydralazine, procainamide, pindolol, tocainide, and immunosuppressives because these drugs alter the immune response. With diuretics, hypotensive effects have been emphasized, and potassium-sparing diuretics or potassium supplements may cause life-threatening hyperkalemia. Lithium levels may increase, and toxicity has been reported.

INDIVIDUAL ACE INHIBITORS

Pharmacologic Profile and Individual Differences

The pharmacologic profiles of the commonly used ACE inhibitors are given in Table 3-1.

Subtle Differences

Short-acting ACE inhibitors such as captopril have obvious advantages in the treatment of hypertensive emergencies because the several hours' delay of peak action of other ACE inhibitors does not allow their use when blood pressure lowering is required urgently. Angioedema appears to be slightly more common with enalapril than is observed with captopril, and the longer-acting ACE inhibitors are not exempt from this life-threatening adverse effect. Quinapril, ramipril, and some other ACE inhibitors inhibit tissue renin production. The renin-angiotensin system not only is confined to blood vessels and the kidney but also exists in the heart, liver, adrenals, brain, pituitary glands, salivary glands, gut, uterus, ovaries, and other tissues. The possible theoretical benefit of inhibiting tissue renin-angiotensin systems, however, has not yet been translated into clearly defined clinical differences among the various ACE inhibitors. Quinapril and ramipril penetrate to myo-cardial ACE binding sites. Myocardial angiotensin has a minimal positive inotropic effect and thus could conceivably be implicated in the development of myocardial hypertrophy. Long-acting preparations with half-lives ranging from 24 to 48 h include cilazapril, perindopril, quinapril, ramipril, spirapril, and zofenopril. Zofenopril is five times more potent than captopril, but it is the only other compound of those mentioned that has an SH group.

Hypotension

Short-acting compounds have an advantage in the initial management of patients with HF. The observation period after the first dose is 1–2 h for captopril, 2–4 h for enalapril, and 2–10 h for longer acting compounds. When hypotension occurs, cessation of the drug leads to quicker recovery with the shorter acting compounds. Also, renal failure may be more protracted with longer-acting agents. The agents that are not prodrugs (Table 3-1) have a rapid onset of action. Lisinopril is not a prodrug, and its action is not affected by concurrent administration of food or liver transformation.

Drug name:	**Captopril**
Trade name:	Capoten
Supplied:	12.5, 25, 50 mg
Dosage:	Hypertension: 12.5–50 mg twice daily, max. 150 mg daily; *see* text for further advice Heart failure: 6.25 mg test dose, 6.25–12.5 mg twice daily; titrate over days to weeks to 25–50 mg twice daily; *see* text for further advice

Dosage (Further Advice)

Heart failure: When feasible, discontinue diuretics for 24 h before the initial dose of captopril 6.25 mg. Lower doses (e.g., 3 mg) have been used in special situations, including HF after MI. Observe the blood pressure every 15 min after dosing for 2 h. If hypotension does not occur, give 6.25 mg twice daily for 1–2 d and then, depending on the urgency of the situation, 12.5 mg twice daily, increasing, if needed, to 25 mg twice daily. Most patients require a dose of 37.5–50 mg daily. Maximum suggested dose is 100 mg daily in two or three divided doses if renal function is normal. If interrupted, diuretics should be recommenced approx 24–36 h after the initial dose of captopril. At times, it is not possible to discontinue diuretics completely, and the dose is halved. Also, nitrates should be withheld, to allow the introduction of captopril without producing hypotension or presyncope.

Hypertension: The initial dose is 12.5 mg on d 1 and then twice daily, increasing over the next days or weeks as needed, to a maintenance dose of 25–50 mg twice daily. The maximum dose is 150 mg daily in two divided doses in patients with normal renal function. In patients with renal dysfunction, the total dose should be decreased and the dosing interval increased. In elderly hypertensive patients and in patients with renal impairment or with concomitant diuretic use, the initial dose should be 6.25 mg.

The action, indications, contraindications, and adverse effects of captopril are given under the general discussion of ACE inhibitors.

Pharmacokinetics

Food has been shown to cause about a 33% reduction in absorption of captopril, so the drug should be given 1 h before meals on an empty stomach. The effect on blood pressure, however, does not appear to be affected by giving the drug with food. About 50% of the absorbed captopril is metabolized by the liver and is eliminated with the active drug by the kidney, with a plasma half-life of approximately 2–3 h. Captopril is 25–30% albumin bound; some binding occurs to endogenous thiol compounds, and the drug does not cross the blood-brain barrier. An apparent action on blood pressure is observed within half an hour of oral ingestion, with a peak effect in 1–2 h and duration of 8–12 h, so in the management of hypertension or HF, twice-daily dosage produces a 24-h therapeutic effect.

Drug name:	**Enalapril**
Trade names:	Vasotec, Innovace (UK)
Supplied:	2.5, 5, 10, 20 mg
Dosage:	Hypertension: 5–20 mg daily, max. 40 mg; *see* text for further advice Heart failure: 2.5 mg test dose, then 10–15 mg once or twice daily, max. 30 mg daily; see text for further advice

Dosage (Further Advice)

Heart failure: The dose of diuretics should be halved or held for 24 h to allow for the introduction of enalapril. This is sometimes not possible, and the initial dose of enalapril must be given under close hospital supervision. The initial dose is 2.5 mg orally; observe under close supervision with blood pressure monitoring for 2–6 h. In the absence of hypotension, give 2.5 mg twice daily for a few days, and reintroduce diuretics as soon as possible to prevent the recurrence or worsening of HF. The dose of enalapril is increased to 5 mg twice daily for several days and, if needed, to 7.5–10 mg twice daily, which is approximately equivalent to 75–100 mg captopril daily; the suggested maximum dose is 30 mg, preferably in two divided doses. Patients with HF often have concomitant renal dysfunction, and the once-daily dosing of enalapril is usually sufficient to produce a salutary response. A twice-daily enalapril dose, however, allows for finer titration and may avoid relative hypotension. The effective median dose in CONSENSUS was 18 mg, and in VHeFT it was 15 mg.

Hypertension: Discontinue diuretics for 2–3 d, and then give 2.5 mg daily, increasing slowly over several weeks to 5–10 mg daily. With more severe hypertension, the starting dose could be 2.5 mg on the first day and then 5 mg daily. If blood pressure control is not achieved with a dose of 10 mg, increase the dose to 10 mg in the morning and 5 mg at night. Failure to control the condition with this dose should prompt the reintroduction of the diuretic. The maximum dose of enalapril should be kept to 30 mg daily, equivalent to 150 mg captopril. A dose of 40 mg is rarely necessary, except with severe or resistant hypertension requiring therapy.

Pharmacokinetics

After oral dosing, about 60% of the drug is absorbed and is not influenced by ingestion of food. Enalapril is inactive and undergoes hepatic hydrolysis to the active enalaprilat. Peak effect of enalaprilat is at about 5 h; after multiple dosing, the plasma half-life is approx 11 h. The peak hypotensive effect is observed from 4 to 6 h after oral dosing, and excretion is virtually all renal. The dose of enalapril may need to be increased in patients with severe liver dysfunction.

The adverse effects and contraindications of enalapril have been given earlier under ACE inhibitors.

Drug name:	**Lisinopril**
Trade names:	Prinivil, Zestril, Carace
Supplied:	2.5, 5, 10, 20 mg
Dosage:	Hypertension: 5–20 mg once daily, max. 40 mg; *see* text for further advice Heart failure: 2.5–5 mg once daily, increasing over weeks to 10–20 mg daily, max. 40 mg daily

Dosage (Further Advice)

As with other ACE inhibitors, it is recommended, if feasible, to discontinue diuretics for at least 2 d before commencing lisinopril and to recommence diuretics a few days to weeks later, if needed. Initially, give 2.5 mg daily, increasing slowly over weeks with evaluation of blood pressure and renal function, to a maintenance dose of 5–20 mg once daily. The maximum suggested dose of lisinopril is 30 mg daily; doses in excess of 20 mg usually do not cause further lowering of blood pressure *(27–29)*. In the Assessment of Treatment with Lisinopril and Survival (ATLAS) trial *(29)*, a daily dose of 30–35 mg versus 2.5–5 mg reportedly caused a significant decrease in hospitalizations, but the decrease was only 14%, with no reduction in total mortality.

Pharmacokinetics

The drug is well absorbed when given orally, and absorption is not influenced by food. Lisinopril is not a prodrug and does not undergo hepatic metabolism. The drug is hydrophilic and is completely eliminated by the kidney with a plasma half-life of 13 h, but the elimination half-life is long, up to 30 h. An apparent action is observed in 2–4 h with peak effect at 4–8 h and duration of action of 24–30 h. Lisinopril is the only water-soluble ACE inhibitor.

Drug name:	**Benazepril**
Trade name:	Lotensin
Supplied:	5, 10, 20, 40 mg
Dosage:	5 mg daily, increasing over weeks to 10–20 mg daily, max. 40 mg

The plasma half-life is about 11 h; the terminal half-life is 21–22 h.

Drug name:	**Cilazapril**
Trade names:	Inhibace, Vascace (UK)
Supplied:	1, 2.5, 5 mg
Dosage:	1–2, 5 mg daily, max. 5 mg

Cilazapril is a prodrug and undergoes hepatic metabolism to the active form cilazaprilat with a terminal half-life that exceeds 40 h.

Drug name:	**Fosinopril**
Trade names:	Monopril, Staril (UK)
Supplied:	10, 20 mg
Dosage:	5–10 mg once daily, increasing gradually to 20 mg daily, max. 40 mg; *see* text for further advice

Dosage (Further Advice)

Avoid taking within 2 h of antacids. Fosinopril undergoes hepatic and renal elimination. More of the drug is removed through the liver with increasing renal failure *(30)*. Fosinopril appears to cause less cough than is observed with other ACE inhibitors. The terminal half-life is approximately 13 h, but inhibition of serum ACE lasts 24 h after a 40-mg dose of the drug.

Drug name:	**Perindopril**
Trade name:	Aceon
Supplied:	2, 4, 8 mg
Dosage:	2 mg daily; maintenance 4 mg, max. 8 mg

The drug is long acting, given once daily, and has tissue specificity, although the exact benefit of this activity is not yet clinically apparent. The terminal half-life is 27–33 h.

Drug name:	**Quinapril**
Trade names:	Accupril, Accupro (UK)
Supplied:	5, 10, 20, 40 mg
Dosage:	2.5–5 mg initially, increasing to 10–40 mg daily, max. 60 mg

Drug name:	**Ramipril**
Trade names:	Altace, Tritace (UK)
Supplied:	1.25, 2.5, 5, 10 mg
Dosage:	1.25–2.5 mg daily, increasing over weeks to 5–10 mg; max. 15 mg once daily or two divided doses

The drug is partially metabolized to the active form, ramiprilat, and is partially a prodrug. Ramiprilat is about 70% and ramipril approximately 50% protein bound. The effective half-life is 14–18 h, but accumulation of the drug occurs resulting in a terminal half-life of up to 110 h. The maximal effect is observed in about 6 h, with duration of action exceeding 24 h. The drug has tissue-specific ACE inhibitor activity.

The HOPE study showed that in a high-risk group of patients (81% ischemic heart disease, 11% stroke, 38% diabetes), 10 mg of ramipril given for a mean of 4.5 yr caused a reduction of 22% in the primary outcome of MI, stroke, or death from cardiovascular diseases *(2)*. In diabetic patients after adjustment for the changes in systolic (2.4 mmHg) blood pressure, ramipril lowered the risk of the combined primary outcome by 25%.

Drug name:	**Spirapril**
Trade names:	Renpress, Sandopril
Supplied:	12.5 mg
Dosage:	6.5–12.5 mg daily, max. 30 mg

The drug is well absorbed when given orally. The onset of action occurs in 1 h after ingestion, with a prolonged duration of action reflecting a half-life of about 72 h. The drug is eliminated by the liver and kidney.

Drug name:	**Trandolapril**
Trade names:	Mavik, Gopten (UK)
Supplied:	0.5, 1, 2 mg
Dosage:	0.5–1 mg daily, max. 4 mg

This agent without SH moiety has a long plasma half-life of 24 h. It is rapidly hydrolyzed to trandolaprilat, the active compound, which has high lipophilicity that enhances tissue penetration *(31)*.

Drug name:	**Zofenopril**
Dosage:	Initially 7.5 mg every 12 h; titrate slowly to 15–30 mg daily

The dose outlined under dosage was administered for 6 wk in the SMILE study *(1)*. Patients with acute anterior infarcts were randomized at a mean of 15 h from the onset of symptoms. Therapy resulted in a significant reduction in the incidence of severe HF and improved survival at 1-yr follow-up. Efficacy was observed mainly in patients with previous infarction. Further clinical trials with ACE inhibitors administered within 6 h of onset of symptoms are required to document the safety and efficacy of very early ACE inhibitor therapy.

ANGIOTENSIN II RECEPTOR BLOCKERS

There are two main types of angiotensin II receptor: AT_1 and AT_2. Most actions of angiotensin II are mediated through the AT_1 receptor. ARBs specifically block the angiotensin II receptor AT_1, and this causes blockade of the renin-angiotensin aldosterone system, although we know that the blockade is not complete. Because angiotensin can be synthesized outside the renin-angiotensin system, angiotensin receptor antagonists could produce more effective control of angiotensin II than ACE inhibitors. The major pathway for angiotensin II production in the heart is not ACE but a serine protease, chymase. Angiotensin I can be converted to angiotensin II by enzymes such as cathepsin, trypsin, and heart chymase, but the exact contribution of these alternative pathways to the generation of angiotensin II is unclear.

Angiotensin II blockade causes an increased flux of superoxide that improves NO bioactivity. Most important, AT_2 receptors are not blocked by ARBs. It appears that AT_2 receptors mediate a physiologic cardioprotective role: production of bradykinin, NO, prostaglandins in the kidney, inhibition of cell growth, promotion of cell differentiation, and apoptosis. *A review by Burnier (10) gives details and relevant references. Their proven beneficial effect in type 2 diabetes (18,19,31)*, in which no proven effect of ACE inhibitors has emerged, will render ARBs a popular choice in diabetics, particularly because of the absence of cough and the virtual absence of angioedema *(32)*. ACE inhibitors need to be tested against ARBs in patients with type 2 diabetes. Of all drug classes, patients are more likely to remain on long-term treatment with ARBs *(33)*. ARBs work selectively at the AT_1 receptor and have no effect at the AT_2 receptor. The most notable advantage of ARBs is that they do not cause cough, a bothersome complication of ACE inhibitors; the rare but serious occurrence of angioedema with ACE inhibitors does not appear to be provoked by ARBs, although a few cases have been reported.

Overall differences between ARBs and ACE inhibitors have not been noted in clinical trials. The Evaluation of Losartan in the Elderly (ELITE) study *(32)* reported nearly equivalent effects for losartan and captopril on the progression of HF, but there was an unexpected reduction in the incidence of sudden death in the losartan group. This study was underpowered and was not confirmed by the better powered ELITE II study *(34)*, which did not show a difference in mortality or in sudden death. *One should be careful, however, before concluding that ARBs are less effective than ACE inhibitors for HF based solely on the results of ELITE II.* The results of CHARM clearly indicated that the ARB candesartion is equal to ACE inhibitor therapy for the management of heart failure (*see* the results of CHARM in Chapter 22).

Drug name:	**Candesartan**
Trade names:	Atacand, Amias (UK)
Supplied:	8, 16, 32 mg; 8, 16 mg; UK 4, 8, 16 mg
Dosage:	Initially 8 mg once daily (4 mg in the elderly or in hepatic/renal impairment), then 8–16 mg; max. 32 mg daily
Half-life:	9 h, 9–12 h in elderly
Excretion:	60% renal; 40% bile

Drug name:	**Irbesartan**
Trade names:	Avapro, Aprovel (UK)
Supplied:	75, 150, 300 mg
Dosage:	150–300 mg once daily (initial dose 75 mg in the elderly)
Half-life:	11–15 h
Excretion:	80% renal; 20% bile

Drug name:	**Losartan**
Trade name:	Cozaar
Supplied:	25, 50 mg
Dosage:	25–50 mg once or twice daily (initially in the elderly and in those with hepatic or renal impairment 25 mg daily); max. 100 mg daily

See Table 3-2 for a comparison of ARBs. *Olmesartan (Benicar)* causes significant reductions in blood pressure at 20–40 mg once daily.

Drug name:	**Valsartan**
Trade name:	Diovan
Supplied:	40, 80 mg
Dosage:	80–160 mg once daily (initial dose in the elderly 40 mg); max. 320 mg

Caution: Neutropenia has been reported in 1.9% of valsartan-treated patients. Increased hepatic enzymes and the rare occurrence of severe hepatic dysfunction with two fatalities have been reported in association with marketed ARBs.

Drug name:	**Telmisartan**
Trade name:	Micardis
Supplied:	40, 80 mg
Dosage:	20–80 mg once daily
Half-life:	24 h
Excretion:	98% in the feces

Drug name:	**Eprosartan**
Trade name:	Teveten
Supplied:	400, 600 mg
Dosage:	300–400 mg twice daily; or 300–800 mg once daily
Half-life:	7 h

REFERENCES

1. Ambrosioni E, Borghi C, Magnani B, et al. for the Survival of Myocardial Infarction Long-term Evaluation (SMILE) Study Investigators. The effect of the angiotensin-converting enzyme inhibitor zofenopril on mortality and morbidity after anterior myocardial infarction. N Engl J Med 1995;332:80.
2. HOPE Investigators. Yusuf S, Sleight P, Pogue J, et al. The Heart Outcomes Prevention Evaluation Investigators. Effects of an angiotensin-converting enzyme inhibitor, ramipril, on death from cardiovascular causes, myocardial infarction, and stroke in high-risk patients. N Engl J Med 2000;342:145.
3. Pfeffer MA, Braunwald E. Ventricular remodelling after myocardial infarction: Experimental observations and clinical implications. Circulation 1990;81:1161.
4. Davis JO, Freeman RH. Mechanisms regulating renin release. Physiol Rev 1976;56:1.
5. Torretti J. Sympathetic control of renin release. Annu Rev Pharmacol Toxicol 1982;22:167.
6. Reid IA. The renin-angiotensin system and body function. Arch Intern Med 1985;145:1475.
7. Ganong WF. The brain renin-angiotensin system. Annu Rev Physiol 1984;46:17.
8. Khan M Gabriel. Heart failure. In: Heart Disease, Diagnosis and Therapy. Totowa, NJ, Humana Press, 2005.
9. Munzel T, Keaney JF. Are ACE inhibitors a "magic bullet" against oxidative stress? Circulation 2001; 104:1571.
10. Burnier M. Angiotensin II type 1 receptor blockers. Circulation 2001;103:904.
11. Leary WP, Reyes AJ. Angiotensin I converting enzyme inhibitors and the renal excretion of urate. Cardiovasc Drugs Ther 1987;1:29.
12. Cicoira M, Zanolla L, Rossi A. Failure of aldosterone suppression despite angiotensin converting enzyme (ACE) inhibitor administration in chronic heart failure is associated with ACE DD genotype. J Am Coll Cardiol 2001;37:1808.
13. Weber KT. Aldosterone and spironolactone in heart failure. N Engl J Med 1999;341:753.
14. Cohn JN, Johnson G, Ziesche S, et al. A comparison of enalapril with hydralazine-isosorbide dinitrate in the treatment of chronic congestive heart failure. N Engl J Med 1991;325:303.
15. CONSENSUS Trial Study Group. Effects of enalapril on mortality in severe congestive heart failure: Results of the Cooperative North Scandinavian Enalapril Survival Study (CONSENSUS). N Engl J Med 1987;316:1429.
16. SOLVD Investigators. Effect of enalapril on survival in patients with reduced left ventricular ejection fractions and congestive heart failure. N Engl J Med 1991;325:293.
17. Cleland JGF, Henderson E, McLenachan J, et al. Effect of captopril, an angiotensin converting enzyme inhibitor, in patients with angina pectoris and heart failure. J Am Coll Cardiol 1991;17:733.
18. RENAAL study investigators. Brenner BM, Cooper ME, Zeeuw D de, et al. Effects of losartan on renal and cardiovascular outcomes in patients with type 2 diabetes and nephropathy. N Engl J Med 2001;345: 861.
19. Parving H-H, Lehnert H, Brochner-Mortensen J, et al. for the Irbesartan in Patients with Type 2 Diabetes and Microalbuminuria Study Group. The effect of irbesartan on the development of diabetic nephropathy in patients with type 2 diabetes. N Engl J Med 2001;345:870.
20. Ferner RE, Simpson JM, Rawlings MD. Effects of intradermal bradykinin after inhibition of angiotensin converting enzyme. BMJ 1987;294:1119.
21. Caskey FJ, Thacker EJ, Johnston PA, et al. Failure of losartan to control blood pressure in scleroderma renal crisis. Lancet 1997;349:620.
22. Hricik DE, Browning PJ, Kopelman R, et al. Captopril-induced functional renal insufficiency in patients with bilateral renal-artery stenoses or renal-artery stenosis in a solitary kidney. N Engl J Med 1983;308: 373.
23. Topol EJ, Thomas A, Fortuin NJ. Hypertensive hypertrophic cardiomyopathy of the elderly. N Engl J Med 1985;312:277.

24. Jett GK. Captopril-induced angioedema. Ann Emerg Med 1984;13:489.
25. Giannoccaro PJ, Wallace GJ, Higginson L, et al. Fatal angioedema associated with enalapril. Can J Cardiol 1989;5:335.
26. Cameron DI. Near fatal angioedema associated with captopril. Can J Cardiol 1990;6:265.
27. Lunde H, Hedner T, Samuelsson O, et al. Dyspnoea, asthma, and bronchospasm in relation to treatment with angiotensin converting enzyme inhibitors. BMJ 1994;308:18.
28. Kochar MS, Bolek G, Kalbfleish JF, et al. A 52 week comparison of lisinopril, hydrochlorothiazide and their combination in hypertension. J Clin Pharmacol 1987;27:373.
29. ATLAS Study Group. Packer M, Poole-Wilson PA, Armstrong PW, et al. Comparative effects of low and high doses of the angiotensin-converting enzyme inhibitor, lisinopril on morbidity and mortality in chronic heart failure. Circulation 1999;100:2312.
30. Hui KK, Duchin KL, Kripalani KJ, et al. Pharmacokinetics of fosinopril in patients with various degrees of renal function. Clin Pharmacol Ther 1991;49:457.
31. Lewis EJ, Hunsicker LG, Clarke WR, et al. for the Collaborative Study Group. Renoprotective effect of the angiotensin receptor antagonist irbesartan in patients with nephropathy due to type 2 diabetes. N Engl J Med 2001;345:851.
32. Khan M Gabriel. Cardiac Drug Therapy, 5th ed. Philadelphia, WB Saunders, 2000, p 53.
33. Bloom BS. Continuation of initial medication after 1 year therapy. Clin Ther 1999;20:671.
34. ELITE II: Pitt B, Poole-Wilson PA, Segal R, et al. Effect of losartan compared with captopril on mortality on patients with symptomatic heart failure: Randomized trial. The Losartan Heart Failure Study. Lancet 2000;255:1582.

SUGGESTED READING

Jhund P, McMurray JV. Does aspirin reduce the benefit of an angiotensin-converting enzyme inhibitor?: Choosing between the Scylla of observational studies and the Charybdis of subgroup analysis. Circulation 2006;113:2566–2568.

Cardinale D, Colombo A, Sandri MT, et al. Prevention of high-dose chemotherapy–induced cardiotoxicity in high-risk patients by angiotensin-converting enzyme inhibition. Circulation 2006;114:2474–2481.

4 ACE Inhibitor Controversies

ACE INHIBITORS VERSUS ARBs: DOES THE CHOICE MATTER?

- Angiotensin-converting enzyme (ACE) inhibitors have been shown in large randomized controlled trials (RCTs) to prevent cardiovascular disease (CVD) outcomes significantly in patients with hypertension and heart failure (HF) and in patients with acute myocardial infarction (MI) with left ventricular (LV) dysfunction. Several recent RCTs including Condesartan in Heart Failure Assessment of Reduction in Mortality and Morbidity (CHARM) *(1)* and Valsartan in Acute Myocardial Infarction Trial (VALIANT) *(2)* have proved the equivalence of ACE inhibitors and angiotensin II receptor blockers (ARBs). Their adverse effects, however, deserve careful scrutiny if we are to give patients medications that have a lower adverse effect profile.
- ACE inhibitors cause cough in more than 15% of treated individuals and, most important, produce a significantly higher incidence of angioedema versus ARBs; this incidence is much higher in patients of African origin. Deaths owing to angioedema have been reported in several hypertension RCTs.

Angioedema: In the well-run large Antihypertensive and Lipid-Lowering Treatment to Prevent Heart Attack Trial (ALLHAT) *(3)*, angioedema occurred in 8 of 15,255 (0.1%), 3 of 9048 (<0.1%), and 38 of 9054 (0.4%) persons in the chlorthalidone, amlodipine, and lisinopril treatment groups, respectively. Significant differences for angioedema were seen for the lisinopril versus chlorthalidone comparison overall ($p < 0.001$):

- In blacks angioedema was seen in 2 of 5369 (<0.1%) for chlorthalidone and 23 of 3210 (0.7%) for lisinopril ($p < 0.001$). Caution is urged in the use of ACE inhibitors in blacks; it is preferable to use an ARB if cost is not a concern.
- In non-blacks (angioedema was seen in 6 of 9886 (0.1%) for chlorthalidone and 15 of 5844 for lisinopril (0.3%; $p = 0.002$).
- The only death from angioedema was in the lisinopril group.

Death should not occur in the treatment of healthy individuals; the patient with mild primary hypertension is invariably healthy and asymptomatic. Importantly, most patients with angioedema caused by an ACE inhibitor require emergency room treatment. Because hypertensive patients are mostly asymptomatic, ARBs offer major advantages over ACE inhibitors with regard to safety profile. The clinician's objective is to produce salutary effects for patients without causing harm.

ACE INHIBITORS/ARBs CAUSE RENOPROTECTION: TRUE OR FALSE?

- It is said by experts and clinical teachers that ACE inhibitors and ARBs have specific renoprotective effects. Guidelines indicate that these are the drugs of choice for the treatment of hypertension in patients with renal disease with or without proteinuria.

From: *Contemporary Cardiology: Cardiac Drug Therapy, Seventh Edition*
M. Gabriel Khan © Humana Press Inc., Totowa, NJ

Casas et al. *(4)* assessed electronic databases for RCTs of antihypertensive drugs and progression of renal disease. Effects on primary discrete end points (doubling of creatinine and end-stage renal disease) and secondary continuous markers of renal outcomes (creatinine, albuminuria, and glomerular filtration rate) were calculated with random-effect models. Comparisons of ACE inhibitors or ARBs with other antihypertensive drugs yielded a relative risk of 0.71 (95% CI 0.49–1.04) for doubling of creatinine and a small benefit in end-stage renal disease (relative risk 0.87, 0.75–0.99). In patients with diabetic nephropathy, no benefit was seen in comparative trials of ACE inhibitors or ARBs on the doubling of creatinine (1.09, 0.55–2.15), end-stage renal disease (0.89, 0.74–1.07), glomerular filtration rate, or creatinine amounts. Placebo-controlled trials of ACE inhibitors or ARBs showed greater benefits than comparative trials on all renal outcomes but were accompanied by substantial reductions in blood pressure in favor of ACE inhibitors or ARBs. These investigators concluded that:

- The benefits of ACE inhibitors or ARBs on renal outcomes in placebo-controlled trials probably result from a blood-pressure-lowering effect *(4)*.

ACE INHIBITORS DECREASE THE INCIDENCE OF DIABETES: TRUE OR FALSE?

In the Losartan Intervention for Endpoint Reduction in Hypertension (**LIFE**) study *(5)*, atenolol was compared with losartan. In a post hoc analysis it is claimed that there was a significant 15% excess of new-onset diabetes over 5 yr, but the absolute rise in glucose was not stated. A large number of patients in the beta-blocker group received diuretics, and the frequency of diuretic use in each study arm was not given. In most studies, including LIFE, post hoc analysis *(6)* suggested that increased risk of new-onset diabetes was confined to individuals with an elevated blood glucose at baseline and family predisposition to diabetes *(6)*.

In the Valsartan Antihypertensive Long-Term Use Evaluation (**VALUE**) trial, new-onset type 2 diabetes was 25% more frequent in the patients on amlodipine than in those on valsartan (13.1% versus 16.4%; $p < 0.0001$) *(7)*. Other RCTs combined ACE inhibitors with diuretics and calcium antagonists, and firm conclusions cannot be ascertained (*see* CONVINCE and PROGRESS trials in Chapters 8 and 9).

ACE inhibitors appear in RCTs to lower the incidence of new diabetes compared with beta-blockers and diuretics, but this effect might be owing to

1. Masking of latent diabetes, a situation that has long-term effects, because treatment of the diabetic process is delayed.
2. Reducing the incidence of benign reversible glucose intolerance (*see* Chapters 8 and 9).

COMBINATION OF ACE INHIBITOR AND ARB PROVEN EFFECTIVE: TRUE OR FALSE?

The search for virtually complete renin-angiotensin-aldosterone system (RAAS) blockade appears to make good sense. The combination of ACE inhibitor and ARB, however, did not result in satisfactory therapeutic goals in the valsartan RCT. Combination therapy did not result in significant reduction in primary outcomes in patients with HF. Most important, the combination of valsartan with a beta-blocker needed for HF treatment increased mortality *(2)*.

In CHARM-Added, after 41 mo of follow-up patients receiving candesartan were 15% less likely to experience the primary end point compared with those given placebo (42% versus 37.9%; $p = 0.0011$). This result occurred regardless of whether or not patients were given a beta-blocker and independent of the dose of ACE inhibitor used *(1)*. Addition of candesartan to an ACE inhibitor led to further clinically important reduction in cardiovascular death and hospitalization for HF, but total mortality was not reduced. Caution is needed when a combination of ACE inhibitor and ARB is administered because hyperkalemia may ensue, especially if renal dysfunction is present, a scenario that is common in the elderly. In CHARM, hyperkalemia occurred in 2.7%, and creatinine increased 3.7% above placebo.

It is preferable to add an aldosterone antagonist to an ACE inhibitor rather than adding an ARB. Caution is needed in HF patients treated with aldosterone antagonists because these agents may cause hyperkalemia, and the addition of an ARB would cause severe hyperkalemia. The strategy of complete RAAS blockade with the combination of ACE inhibitor and ARB remains controversial, particularly when the combination of an ACE inhibitor and an aldosterone antagonist has been proved successful in RCTs (spironolactone in RALES *[8]* and eplerenone in EPHESUS *[9]*.)

ACE INHIBITORS FOR HF WITH PRESERVED SYSTOLIC FUNCTION

ACE inhibitors have been shown conclusively to improve outcomes in patients with MI and HF. However, the evidence for significant benefit in MI patients with preserved LV systolic function is probably not conclusive. Al-Mallah et al. *(10)* analyzed 6 of 61 RCTs that met specified inclusion criteria. There were 16,772 patients randomized to an ACE inhibitor and 16,728 patients randomized to placebo. Treatment was associated with a decrease in cardiovascular mortality (relative risk [RR] 0.83, 95% CI 0.72–0.96; $p = 0.01$), nonfatal MI (RR 0.84, 95% CI 0.75–0.94, $p = 0.003$), all-cause mortality (RR 0.87, 95% CI 0.81–0.94, $p = 0.0003$), and revascularization rates (RR 0.93, 95% CI 0.87–1.00, $p = 0.04$). Treatment of 100 patients for an average duration of 4.4 yr prevents either one death, or one nonfatal MI, or one cardiovascular death. The cumulative evidence provided by this meta-analysis showed a modest favorable effect of ACE inhibitors on the outcome of patients with CHD and preserved LV systolic function *(10)*.

REFERENCES

1. Swedberg K, Granger CB, McMurray JJV, et al. Effects of candesartan in patients with chronic heart failure and reduced left-ventricular systolic function taking angiotensin-converting-enzyme inhibitors: the CHARM-Added trial. Lancet 2003;362:767–771.
2. Pfeffer MA et al. Valsartan, captopril, or both in myocardial infarction complicated by heart failure, left ventricular dysfunction or both. N Engl J Med 2003;349:1893–1906.
3. The ALLHAT Officers and Coordinators for the ALLHAT Collaborative Research Group. Major outcomes in high-risk hypertensive patients randomized to angiotensin-converting enzyme inhibitor or calcium channel blocker vs. diuretic: The Antihypertensive and Lipid-Lowering Treatment to Prevent Heart Attack Trial (ALLHAT). JAMA 2002;288:2981–2997.
4. Casas JP, Chau W, Loukogeorgakis S, et al. Effect of inhibitors of the renin-angiotensin system and other antihypertensive drugs on renal outcomes: Systematic review and meta-analysis. Lancet 2005;366: 2026–2033.
5. Dahlöf B, Devereux RB, Kjeldsen SE, et al. for the LIFE Study Group. Cardiovascular morbidity and mortality in the Losartan Intervention for Endpoint Reduction in Hypertension study (LIFE): A randomised trial against atenolol. Lancet 2002;359:995–1003.

6. Lindholm LH, Ibsen H, Borch-Johnsen K, et al. Risk of new-onset diabetes in the Losartan Intervention for Endpoint Reduction in Hypertension study. J Hypertens 2002;20:1879–1886.
7. Julius S, Kjeldsen SE, Weber M, et al. for the VALUE Trial Group. Outcomes in hypertensive patients at high cardiovascular risk treated with regimes based on valsartan or amlodipine: the VALUE randomised trial. Lancet 2004;363:2002–2031.
8. Pitt B, Zannad F, Remme WJ, et al. for the Randomized Evaluation Study Investigators. The effect of spironolactone on morbidity and mortality in patients with severe heart failure. N Engl J Med 1999;341: 709.
9. Pitt B, Remme W, Zannad F, et al. for the Eplerenone Post-Acute Myocardial Infarction Heart Failure Efficacy and Survival Study Investigators. Eplerenone, a selective aldosterone blocker, in patients with left ventricular dysfunction after myocardial infarction. N Engl J Med 2003;348:1309–1321.
10. Al-Mallah MH, Tleyjeh IM, Abdel-Latif AA, et al. Angiotensin-converting enzyme inhibitors in coronary artery disease and preserved left ventricular systolic function. A systematic review and meta-analysis of randomized controlled trials. J Am Coll Cardiol 2006;47:1576–1583.

SUGGESTED READING

Jhund P, McMurray JJV. Does aspirin reduce the benefit of an angiotensin-converting enzyme inhibitor?: Choosing between the Scylla of observational studies and the Charybdis of subgroup analysis. Circulation 2006;113:2566–2568.

5 Calcium Antagonists (Calcium Channel Blockers)

This chapter emphasizes

- That these excellent blood pressure-lowering agents have been proved in randomized clinical trials (RCTs) to decrease cardiovascular disease (CVD) outcomes in patients with hypertension but carry a significant risk for heart failure (HF) in the elderly and in blacks. This increased incidence of HF appears to be ignored by analysts of RCTs and is discussed in Chapter 8.
- **When to choose a calcium antagonist**.
- **Which one to choose**.

There are important differences among these agents that may affect choice in treating individual patients. Recommendations are given after discussion of the mechanism of action.

MECHANISM OF ACTION

Calcium antagonists act at the plasma membrane to inhibit calcium entry into cells by blocking voltage-dependent calcium channels. Calcium ions play a vital role in the contraction of all types of muscle: cardiac, skeletal, and smooth. **Myoplasmic calcium** depends on calcium entry into the cell. Calcium binds to the regulatory protein troponin, removing the inhibitory action of tropomyosin, and in the presence of adenosine triphosphate allows the interaction between myosin and actin with consequent contraction of the muscle cell. During phase 0 of the cardiac action potential, there is a rapid inward current of sodium through so-called fast channels. During phase 2 (the plateau phase), there is a slow inward current of calcium through channels that are 100 times more selective for calcium than for sodium; these channels have been termed slow calcium channels.

Fleckenstein *(1)* showed that **calcium channels** can be selectively blocked by a class of agents he termed calcium antagonists (also called calcium channel blockers, calcium channel antagonists, and calcium entry blockers).

There are at least two types of calcium channels: L and T. L channels are increased in activity by catecholamines. The calcium antagonists available for clinical use are mainly L channel blockers. A second type of channel, termed the T channel, appears at more negative potentials and seems to play a role in the initial depolarization of the sinoatrial (SA) and atrioventricular (AV) nodal tissue. T channels are also present in vascular smooth muscle cells, Purkinje cells, and neurohormonal secretory cells. Mibefradil was touted as a T channel blocker; it caused bradycardia and has a host of adverse effects and interactions. **The drug has been withdrawn from the market.**

From: *Contemporary Cardiology: Cardiac Drug Therapy, Seventh Edition*
M. Gabriel Khan © Humana Press Inc., Totowa, NJ

Table 5-1
Clinical Classification of Calcium Antagonists

Group	*Characteristics*
I	L channel blockers: no action on SA or AV nodes: no effect Dihydropyridines: amlodipine, felodipine, isradipine, nifedipine, nicardipine, niludipine, nimodipine, nisoldipine, nitrendipine, ryosidine
II	L channel blockers and probably some T channel blockade: additional action on SA and TV nodes: EP effects Phenylalkylamines: verapamil Benzothiazepines: diltiazem
III	Mainly T-type channel blocker: mibefradil (Posicor, withdrawn)

Calcium movement into the cell is mediated by at least seven mechanisms *(2)*. The slow channels represent two of these mechanisms. Two or more types of slow channels exist:

1. **Voltage-dependent** calcium channels are blocked by calcium antagonists.
   - **Nifedipine** is one of the most potent calcium antagonists and appears to act by plugging the calcium channels. It causes dilation of coronary arteries and arterioles and considerable peripheral arteriolar dilation. Nifedipine has a small and usually unimportant negative inotropic effect on the heart.
   - **Verapamil and diltiazem** cause distortion of calcium channels and also cause coronary artery dilation: there are additional effects on the SA and AV nodes; in addition, these drugs have a negative inotropic effect. Peripheral vasodilation is relatively milder than that noted after nifedipine administration.
2. **Receptor-operated** calcium channels are blocked by beta-adrenoceptor blockers. Beta-agonists increase calcium influx through such channels, and this effect is blocked by beta-adrenoceptor blocking agents, which cause the failure of a certain proportion of the calcium channels to open. Beta-adrenergic blockers reduce intracellular levels of cyclic adenosine monophosphate; this, in turn, decreases the number of receptor-operated calcium channels available for calcium influx and thus lowers intracellular calcium and actuates a decrease in heart rate and myocardial contractility. In other words, beta-adrenoceptor blockers have a calcium channel blocking property. In fact, verapamil was first investigated because its action resembled that of the beta-adrenoceptor blocking agents.

   A clinical classification of calcium antagonists is given in Table 5-1.

MAJOR CALCIUM ANTAGONISTS

The dihydropyridines (DHPs), phenylalkylamines, and benzothiazepines have vastly different actions (Table 5-2). Their indications are necessarily different, as well as several of their important adverse effects and cautions. They are interchangeable only in the management of coronary artery spasm. For use in other clinical situations (in angina, in hypertension, or in the elderly), care is necessary in their selection. Only amlodipine and felodipine have proved safe in patients with mild left ventricular (LV) dysfunction. (*See* Table 5-2 for a comparison of cardiac effects and peripheral dilation.)

The DHPs are discussed first because they were used in clinical practice much before the benzothiazepine diltiazem.

Although nifedipine and most DHPs have no serious side effects, they may have a slightly higher incidence of minor side effects compared with verapamil *(4)*. Conversely, verapamil has a lower incidence of minor side effects, but it has the potential to produce more serious side effects including a high incidence of constipation, which is particularly bothersome in the elderly *(12)*. Peripheral edema may occur during nifedipine or DHP therapy in the absence of HF. Edema is believed to result from an increase in capillary permeability. In patients developing bilateral leg edema, symptoms and signs of HF should be sought. All calcium antagonists can produce severe **hypotension**.

Interactions include the following:

- Nifedipine may depress **quinidine** blood levels, and levels may rebound when nifedipine is withdrawn *(13,14)*.
- An interaction has been noted with **prazosin**, and hypotension can be precipitated.
- **Cimetidine and ranitidine** interfere with hepatic metabolism.
- **Phenytoin** blood levels have been noted to increase (*see* Chapter 21).

Drug name:	**Verapamil**
Trade names:	Isoptin SR, Securon SR (UK), Univer, Covera-HS-new 1998*, Chronovera (C)
Supplied:	120, 180, 240 mg; *180, 240 mg
Dosage:	120–240 mg once daily

Verapamil structurally is a phenylalkylamine calcium antagonist and is a derivative of papaverine.

Action

Verapamil is a moderately potent vasodilator. Peripheral vasodilation is much less conspicuous than that seen with nifedipine. Verapamil has a marked negative inotropic effect. The electrophysiologic effects are mild depression of the sinus node function and of conduction through the AV node.

Advice, Adverse Effects, and Interactions

The side effects are illustrated in Table 5-3 and are compared with those of DHPs.

Contraindications include the following:

- **Bradycardia and sinus and AV node disease:** The drug is contraindicated in patients with bradycardia or AV block. Patients with sick sinus syndrome are often very sensitive to verapamil: sinus arrest and asystole unresponsive to atropine have been reported.
- **Heart failure:** The drug is contraindicated in patients with cardiomegaly or LV function, EF < 40%.
- **Acute myocardial infarction:** The manufacturer's warning in North America is that the drug should not be used in this condition. Earlier studies had suggested that verapamil could have salutary effects on jeopardized myocardium after coronary occlusion. It is now fairly clear that verapamil and other calcium antagonists do not salvage myocardium when they are given after arterial occlusion has occurred. *The prediction in the first edition of this book has been borne out by more recent studies. Patients with unstable angina, threatened infarction, or acute infarct appear to have an increased risk of death (15,16)*. No routine role for verapamil in the management of patients with infarction is advised.
- **Hypotension:** Precautions similar to those for DHPs should be taken.
- The drug is contraindicated in patients with **Wolff-Parkinson-White (WPW) syndrome** associated with atrial fibrillation or flutter because ventricular fibrillation can be precipitated

(17). Patients with WPW syndrome and AV nodal reentrant tachycardia may develop atrial fibrillation, so verapamil is best regarded as contraindicated in patients with WPW syndrome (*see* Chapter 14). The dose should be reduced in patients with liver dysfunction and in those treated with cimetidine.

Adverse effects include the following:

- Constipation may be distressing, especially in the elderly.
- Galactorrhea and minor degrees of hepatotoxicity may rarely occur.
- Rare occurrences include hepatotoxicity resulting from a hypersensitivity reaction.
- Respiratory arrest has been reported in a patient with muscular dystrophy *(18)*.

Interactions include the following:

- **Beta-blockers:** Oral administration of verapamil combined with beta-blockers should be used with caution and only in selected patients because the negative inotropic effect of both drugs may precipitate HF. Verapamil should not be given as an intravenous (IV) bolus to patients receiving beta-blockers. It is preferable to give an oral preparation that takes about 2 h to act, especially if the reduction of ventricular rate is not urgent. Interaction of verapamil and timolol eyedrops producing severe bradycardia may occur.
- **Digoxin:** Verapamil should never be given to a digitalized patient when digitalis toxicity is suspected. Serum digoxin levels may be increased 50–70% by verapamil. Verapamil also reduces both the renal and nonrenal elimination of digoxin.
- **Amiodarone:** There have been reports of serious interactions between verapamil and amiodaone, which may also depress the SA and AV nodes. Verapamil is usually avoided in patients taking amiodarone.
- **Tranquilizers:** When verapamil is combined with tranquilizers, the patient should be warned about the possible sedative effect.
- **Oral anticoagulants:** There is some evidence that verapamil increases the effect of oral anticoagulants.
- **Quinidine:** Plasma levels of quinidine may increase during the administration of verapamil. Marked hypotension has been reported when IV verapamil has been given to patients receiving oral quinidine.
- **Disopyramide** and verapamil have added negative inotropic effects that can result in HF.
- **Prazosin** and calcium antagonists have added vasodilator effects, and hypotension may be produced.

Drug name:	**Diltiazem**
Trade names:	Cardizem CD, Tiazac, Adizem-XL (UK), Viazem XL
Supplied:	Cardizem CD 120, 180, 240, 300 mg Tiazac 120, 180, 240, 300, 360 mg Adizem-XL 180, 240, 300 mg
Dosage:	Extended-release 120–300 mg once daily; short-acting formulations not recommended; *see* text

Diltiazem has a structural relationship to benzothiazepine.

Action

Diltiazem causes moderate dilation of arteries. Its dilatory effect is not as powerful as that of nifedipine or other DHPs (*see* Table 5-2). The effect on the SA node is more powerful than that of verapamil, but its action on the AV node is less so. Thus, the drug is not as effective as verapamil in the termination of AV nodal reentrant tachycardia. The modest actions give the drug a balanced profile of action. Diltiazem causes a decrease in the rate pressure product at any given level of exercise. The drug has a mild negative inotropic effect.

Advice, Adverse Effects, and Interactions

The large multicenter study of 1998, including 2466 patients randomized to diltiazem or placebo, showed no decrease in overall mortality and no significant decrease in reinfarction rates in patients with Q-wave versus non-Q-wave infarction *(19). A significant increase in mortality was observed resulting from diltiazem in patients with pulmonary congestion and LV dysfunction, EF < 40%.* The increase in mortality persisted through long-term therapy beyond 1 yr *(20)*. Congestive HF occurred in 39 (12%) patients receiving placebo and in 61 (21%) patients given diltiazem. Diltiazem is currently not approved by the U.S. Food and Drug Administration (FDA) for the management of non-Q-wave infarction, except when angina is a complication.

For several years, the drug was prescribed inappropriately for patients with non-Q-wave infarction. Headaches, dizziness, sedation, rash, edema, and constipation may occur. Reversible acute hepatic injury with extreme increases in the levels of liver enzymes occurs rarely. Occasionally, mild reversible increases in the levels of transaminase can occur. Myopathy with marked increase of creatinine kinase, acute mania with psychosis *(21)*, and acute renal failure *(22)*, precipitated by diltiazem, have been reported.

Contraindications include HF, sick sinus syndrome, second- or third-degree AV block, hypotension, and pregnancy and lactation.

Interactions have been reported, with amiodarone producing sinus arrest and hypotension *(23)*. Also, digoxin levels are increased by about 46% *(24)*. In general, beta-blockers and diltiazem are a relatively safe and effective combination for the management of stable and unstable angina. In rare instances, the addition of diltiazem to a beta-blocker can decrease the pulse rate to low levels, and HF is occasionally precipitated. Interactions occur with cimetidine, cyclosporine, and carbamazepine (*see* Chapter 21).

Drug name:	**Amiodipine**
Trade names:	Norvasc, Istin (UK)
Supplied:	5, 10 mg
Dosage:	2.5 mg daily increasing to 5–7.5 mg; max. 10 mg

Amlodipine has a half-life of 35–50 h, and peak blood levels are reached after 6–12 h. The antihypertensive effect is equal to that of nadolol *(25)*. A 9-mg dose appears to be equal to 320 mg verapamil *(26)*.

Caution: Reduce dosage in the elderly; avoid in LV dysfunction, pregnancy, and lactation.

Drug name:	**Isradipine**
Trade names:	DynaCirc, Prescal (UK)
Supplied:	2.5 mg
Dosage:	2.5 mg twice daily; max. 10 mg

Drug name:	**Felodipine**
Trade names:	Plendil, Renedil
Supplied:	2.5, 5, 10 mg
Dosage:	Hypertension: 2.5–5 mg once daily; max. 10 mg; reduce dosage in the elderly and in hepatic impairment

With isradipine and felodipine, interactions occur with cimetidine, antiepileptic agents, and grapefruit juice. Felodipine (Plendil) was the calcium antagonist used in the Hypertension Optimal Treatment (HOT) study *(27)*. The drug proved remarkably safe and in combination with other agents was effective in decreasing diastolic pressures to the desired goal; it resulted in a significant reduction of fatal and nonfatal strokes.

Drug name:	**Nicardipine**
Trade name:	Cardene
Dosage:	5–30 mg twice daily

Nicardipine has actions, effects, and indications similar to those of nifedipine.

Drug name:	**Nimodipine**
Trade name:	Nimotop
Dosage:	0.35 mg/kg four times hourly; *see* text for further advice

Nimodipine is useful in the management of cerebral arterial spasm after subarachnoid hemorrhage *(28)*.

Dosage (Further Advice)

For patients over 70 kg, use an IV central line, 1 mg/h initially, increasing after 2 h to 2 mg/h, if hypotension does not occur. Halve the dose in patients weighing less than 70 kg. Use the IV route for 5 d and then give orally 60 mg every 4 h starting within 4 d of subarachnoid hemorrhage and for 21 d.

Drug name:	**Nisoldipine**
Trade names:	Sular, Syscor (UK)
Dosage:	10 mg daily; max. 40 mg

Nisoldipine has been observed to cause enhanced platelet aggregation as well as exacerbation of myocardial ischemia on abrupt withdrawal.

Other DHPs include azodipine, diazodipine, flordipine, iodipine, and lacidipine (Motens, UK); the dose is 2–4 mg daily, maximum 6 mg once daily. Also available are mesudipine, niludipine, nilvadipine, nitrendipine, oxodipine, riodipine, ryosidine, and vadipine.

What has been described in the earlier discussion of actions, advice, and adverse effects for nifedipine should apply to the aforementioned drugs, except for their duration of action.

Mibefradil (Posicor), a T channel blocker, has caused severe bradycardia and torsades de pointes; caution was necessary. In addition, rhabdomyolysis occurred when a statin was used in combination. The drug has been withdrawn.

WHEN TO CHOOSE A CALCIUM ANTAGONIST

These cardioactive agents, which were favorites in the 1980s, have fallen from grace. Controversies raged during the early 1990s as to their safety. It became clear that the short-acting rapid-release agents increase cardiovascular mortality in some categories of patients, and their use has been curtailed by cardiologists and virtually all internists in the United States and Canada.

During 1996 and 1997, the extended-release formulations, when indicated, were considered effective and safe by most internists and expert panels, but opinions today vary. The Prospective Randomized Amlodipine Survival Evaluation (PRAISE) study *(29)* indicated that, although amlodipine treatment did not show improvement in total cardiac mortality in patients treated for HF, the drug did not increase total mortality. The drug was considered safe in patients with EF > 30%. The drug, however, caused a significant increase in pulmonary edema in patients with a low EF. Thus, caution is necessary with any DHP in patients with HF. Amlodipine is not approved by the FDA for the treatment of HF. Other calcium antagonists are contraindicated in patients with HF and in patients with LV dysfunction.

The following discussion relates only to extended-release calcium antagonists. Rapid-release formulations are not recommended for clinical use except in special circumstances.

- Although calcium antagonists are excellent antihypertensive agents, effective for all grades of hypertension (grades I–III and emergencies), RCTs have not shown a significant decrease in overall mortality. The Systolic Hypertension in Europe (Syst-Eur) study *(30)* showed a 42% reduction in fatal and nonfatal strokes with the use of nitrendipine; overall mortality and cardiovascular mortality rates, however, were not significantly reduced.
- In patients with coexisting disease, particularly diabetes, patients with ischemic heart disease (IHD), and those with LV dysfunction, caution is required *(29,31–37)*. RCTs in hypertensive patients with diabetes have shown increased mortality and cardiovascular mortality rates with the use of isradipine *(34)* and nisoldipine (Table 5-4) *(35)*. Diabetic patients are at high risk for IHD events.
- The HOT study was reported in 1998 *(27)*.

INDICATIONS FOR CALCIUM ANTAGONISTS

Isolated hypertension without organ damage or coexisting disease is an indication (*see* Chapter 8).

- In older African-American people, an RCT by Matterson and associates *(38)* showed that diltiazem was slightly more effective than hydrochlorothiazide (HCTZ). Thus, in older black patients *with isolated hypertension,* diltiazem or a DHP calcium antagonist is indicated if HCTZ does not achieve goal blood pressure.
- In younger black people, in the study by Matterson and colleagues *(38)*, diltiazem was effective in 64% compared with 47% for atenolol and 40% for HCTZ. Thus, diltiazem or amlodipine should be tried if a small dose of a beta-blocking agent fails to control blood pressure. Failure to reach goal blood pressure should prompt the combination of a DHP and a beta-blocker.
- In older white people with isolated systolic hypertension, diltiazem showed a 64% effectiveness versus 68% for atenolol. Thus, a calcium antagonist is a second- or third-line drug after a trial of a beta-blocker or a diuretic and/or combination.
- Patients with severe, stage II and III, hypertension require the combination of several agents, and calcium antagonists are appropriate, except in patients with LV dysfunction.

Table 5-4
Relative Risk of Cardiovascular Events
or Death for Calcium Antagonists versus Other Agents[a]

Study	*Agents*	*Relative risk*[b]
ABCD *(35)*	Nisoldipine versus enalapril	5.5 (2.1–14.6)
FACET *(36)*	Amlodipine versus fosinopril	2.04 (1.05–3.84)
MIDAS *(34)*	Isradipine versus HCTZ	2.7 (1.07–6.86)

[a]Randomized controlled trials in hypertensives with diabetes or impaired glucose tolerance.

[b]Values in parentheses are 95% confidence intervals.

- In the presence of renal disease or renal failure with or without proteinuria (nondiabetic), if ACE inhibitors are contraindicated or poorly effective, DHPs have a role.

Caution: Calcium antagonists appear to possess diabetogenic effects and are not generally advisable in diabetic patients unless other agents are ineffective or intolerable. RCTs in hypertensive diabetic patients have shown an increase in cardiovascular events (*see* Table 5-4) *(34–37)*, but beneficial effects with beta-blockers or ACE inhibitors. (For the results of NORDIL, INSIGHT, and other trials, *see* Chapter 8.)

Stable Angina

These drugs are considered second-line agents in

- The management of angina added to a beta-blocker or a nitrate (*see* Chapter 1, Table 1-1).
- Silent ischemia: combined with a beta-blocker, they decrease the occurrence of silent ischemia.
- Prinzmetal's variant angina (coronary artery spasm). These agents are useful and are first-line drugs in the management of this category of patients; they may be used in combination with nitrates. This condition is rare, however. Because of the widespread discussion of coronary artery spasm in the 1980s, calcium antagonists became commonly used agents in patients with stable angina. Coronary artery spasm is no longer considered to play an important role in stable or unstable angina; thus, the role of these agents has been downgraded.
- **Caution: DHPs are contraindicated in unstable angina.** Diltiazem is also contraindicated, but diltiazem may be tried if a beta-blocker is contraindicated. These agents are not recommended for acute MI. Diltiazem was thought to be useful following non-Q-wave MI. In a clinical trial, diltiazem decreased early reinfarction rates, but the incorrect use of a one-tailed probability test brought about statistical doubt. Further studies have not confirmed the usefulness of diltiazem in non-Q-wave MI. In addition, the drug increases the incidence of pulmonary edema in patients with acute MI and LV dysfunction *(19)*. Verapamil is contra-indicated in unstable angina or acute MI.
- Supraventricular tachycardia: Verapamil is well known for its excellent effect on AV nodal reentrant tachycardia.
- Diltiazem IV has a role for emergency ventricular rate control of atrial fibrillation.
- Hypertrophic cardiomyopathy: Verapamil is advisable in selected patients when beta-blockers are contraindicated.
- Aortic regurgitation: The unloading effect of nifedipine has been shown to reverse LV dilation and hypertrophy; this therapy may delay the need for valve surgery *(12)*.
- Pulmonary hypertension: Calcium antagonists have shown a variable response in patients with primary pulmonary hypertension. The beneficial effect of nifepidine and verapamil, however, carries a risk of causing HF.
- Raynaud's phenomenon.

The clinical application of calcium antagonists versus beta-blockers is shown in Table 5-5.

WHICH CALCIUM ANTAGONIST TO CHOOSE

- Amlodipine is indicated for isolated systolic hypertension in the elderly if a beta-blocker and diuretic are contraindicated or fail to achieve blood pressure goal. Combination with a beta-blocker is relatively safe, except in patients with EF < 40%. Patients with stable angina with mild LV dysfunction, EF > 40%, may be tried on amlodipine. **The PRAISE study *(29)* indicated that amlodipine is relatively safe in patients with EF > 30%.** *Pulmonary edema was precipitated in some patients with EF < 30%, so caution is required to avoid all calcium antagonists if there is LV dysfunction.*
- RCTs indicate that amlodipine *(29)* and felodipine *(27)* possess the best safety profile among the currently available DHP calcium antagonists.
- Other DHPs (e.g., nifedipine and amlodipine) may be used in combination with a beta-blocker and in other situations in which a beta-blocker is used in combination. The nifedipine combination should not be used in patients with EF < 40%.
- Diltiazem is a mild vasodilator and has gained acceptance for the treatment of both hypertension and stable angina. The drug, however, is not advisable in patients with EF < 40%.
- Verapamil has a role in patients with stable angina when beta-blockers are contraindicated. The drug is a more effective antianginal agent than diltiazem or DHPs. The combination of nitrates often proves effective in patients with class II or III angina. The drug should not be used in patients with EF < 40% or in those with unstable angina.

COMBINATION OF CALCIUM ANTAGONISTS WITH BETA-BLOCKERS, NITRATES, OR DIGOXIN

The combination of **amlodipine and a beta-blocker** has been well established as relatively safe and effective. A small dose of a beta-blocker combined with amlodipine 5–10 mg once daily is an effective and generally safe combination. Caution is necessary, however, because amlodipine or another DHP added to a beta-blocker may precipitate HF in patients with serious impairment of LV contractility.

There is a more serious risk when diltiazem is combined with a beta-blocker. Verapamil carries considerable risk when combined with beta-blockers because HF, severe bradycardia, or AV block may ensue in significant numbers of patients. In a randomized double-blind study, Subramanian and colleagues *(40,41)* have shown the combination of **verapamil with propranolol** to be more **effective** than monotherapy with either drug in the management of severe angina pectoris. Among 40 treated patients, hypotension occurred in four, cardiac failure in three, bradycardia in one, and junctional rhythm in two (i.e., 25% side effects, serious enough to require withdrawal in 15% of the patients). The frequency of similar side effects with the combination of propranolol and nifedipine or another DHP is less than 1%. *Therefore, the combination of verapamil and a beta-blocker in more than minimal doses should be used only in selected patients with angina pectoris unresponsive to or intolerant of beta-blockers plus DHP.* If side effects require the withdrawal of the DHP, then diltiazem may be added to the beta-blocker, provided there are no contraindications to this combination, but it is, as a rule, wise to **reduce the dose** of the beta-blocking agent by half at the time of the change in therapy.

Contraindications to the aforementioned combination are the same as those for the use of beta-blockers or verapamil independently.

Table 5-5
Clinical Applications of Calcium Antagonists versus Beta-Blockers

	Heart failure I–III	*Hypertensive with nephropathy and proteinuria*	*Diabetics with hypertension*	*Diabetics with IHD*	*Lone Systolic hypertension/ elderly*	*Angina*	*Unstable angina*	*Acute MI*	*Post-MI prevention*
Amlodipine	Not FDA approved	Indicated if ACE inhibitor CI	Not advisable	Not advisable	Second-line therapy	Second-line therapy	CI Not FDA approved	Not FDA approved	Not FDA approved
Diltiazem	CI	CI	Not advisable	Not advisable	Second-line therapy	Second-line therapy	CI		
Nifedipine	CI	CI	Not advisable	Not advisable	Second-line therapy		CI	Not FDA approved	
Verapamil	CI	CI	Not advisable	Not advisable	Not advisable	Second-line therapy	CI	Not FDA approved CI	Not FDA approved
Isradipine	CI	CI	Not advisable	Not advisable		Second-line therapy	CI		
Beta-blocker	FDA approved[a]	Second-line therapy	Advisable if not prone to hypoglycemia	Advisable if not prone to hypoglycemia	First-line therapy approved	First-line therapy approved	First-line therapy approved	First-line therapy approved	First-line therapy approved

[a]Carvedilol.

CI, contraindicated; ACE, angiotensin-converting enzyme; IHD, ischemic heart disease; MI, myocardial infarction.

Long-acting oral nitrates (isosorbide dinitrate or mononitrate) added to calcium antagonists may be necessary in patients with Prinzmetal's variant angina who fail to respond to high doses of DHP, diltiazem, or verapamil. There is no need to give a nitrate preparation routinely when using calcium antagonists, but the combination may, of course, be employed when shown to be necessary in the individual patient. Because DHPs cause extensive peripheral arterial dilation, and nitrates cause venous dilation with reduction in preload, there will be an increase in the probability of dizziness and/or light-headedness when the drugs are combined.

Note: Prinzmetal's variant angina often undergoes spontaneous remission, and episodes may recur similar to those of cluster headache. Théroux and colleagues *(42)* suggest that low-risk patients who are free of angina for 1 yr during treatment may be slowly weaned from calcium antagonists.

REFERENCES

1. Fleckenstein A. Specific pharmacology of calcium in myocardium, cardiac pacemakers and vascular smooth muscle. Annu Rev Pharmacol Toxicol 1977;17:149.
2. Braunwald E. Mechanism of action of calcium-channel-blocking agents. N Engl J Med 1982;307:1618.
3. Krikler DM, Harris L, Rowland E. Calcium-channel blockers and beta blockers: Advantages and disadvantages of combination therapy in chronic, stable angina pectoris. Am Heart J 1982;104:702.
4. Terry RW. Nifedipine therapy in angina pectoris: Evaluation of safety and side effects. Am Heart J 1982; 104:681.
5. Lette J, Gagnon RM, Lemire TG, et al. Rebound of vasospastic angina after cessation of long-term treatment with nifedipine. Can Med Assoc J 1984;130:1169.
6. Choong CYP, Roubin GS, Shen WF, et al. Effects of nifedipine on arterial oxygenation at rest and during exercise in patients with stable angina. J Am Coll Cardiol 1986;8:1461.
7. Ballester E, Roca J, Rodriquez-Roisin R, et al. Effect of nifedipine hypoxemia occurring after metacholine challenge in asthma. Thorax 1986;41:468.
8. Diamond JR, Cheung JT, Fang LST. Nifedipine-induced renal dysfunction: Alteration in renal hemodynamics. Am J Med 1984;77:905.
9. Bhatnagar SK, Amin MM, Al-Yusuf AR. Diabetogenic effects of nifedipine. BMJ 1984;289:19.
10. McKenney JM, Goodman RP, Wright JT Jr. Use of antihypertensive agents in patients with glucose intolerance. Clin Pharm 1985;4:649.
11. Steele RM, Schuna AA, Schreiber RT. Calcium antagonist-induced gingival hyperplasia. Ann Intern Med 1994;120:663-664.
12. Khan M Gabriel. Angina. In: Heart Disease, Diagnosis and Therapy. Baltimore, Williams & Wilkins, 1996.
13. Farringer JA, Green JA, O'Rourke, et al. Nifedipine-induced alterations in serum quinidine concentrations. Am Heart J 1984;108:1570.
14. VanLith RM, Appleby DH. Quinidine-nifedipine interaction. Drug Intell Clin Pharm 1985;19:829.
15. Verapamil in acute myocardial infarction: The Danish Study Group on Verapamil in Myocardial Infarction. Eur Heart J 1984;5:516.
16. Scheidt S, Frishman WF, Packer M, et al. Long term effectiveness of verapamil in stable and unstable angina pectoris: One year follow-up of patients treated in placebo-controlled, double-blind randomized clinical trial. Am J Cardiol 1982;50:1185.
17. Gulamhusein S, Ko P, Klein GJ. Ventricular fibrillation following verapamil in the Wolff-Parkinson-White syndrome. Am Heart J 1983;106:145.
18. Zalman F, Perloff TK, Durant NN, et al. Acute respiratory failure following intravenous verapamil in Duchenne's muscular dystrophy. Am Heart J 1983;105:510.
19. Multicenter Diltiazem Postinfarction Trial Research Group. The effect of diltiazem on mortality and reinfarction after myocardial infarction. N Engl J Med 1989;319:385.
20. Goldstein RE, Boccuzzi ST, Cruess D, et al. Diltiazem increases late onset congestive heart failure in postinfarction patients with early reduction in ejection fraction. Circulation 1991;83:52.
21. Palat GK, Hooker EA, Morahed A. Secondary mania associated with diltiazem. Clin Cardiol 1984;7:611.
22. Terwee PM, Rosman JB, Van Der Geest S. Acute renal failure due to diltiazem. Lancet 1984;2:1337.

23. Lee TH, Friedman PL, Goldman L, et al. Sinus arrest and hypotension with combined amiodarone-diltiazem therapy. Am Heart J 1985;109:163.
24. Kuhlmann J. Effects of nifedipine and diltiazem on plasma levels and renal excretions of beta-acetyldigoxin. Clin Pharmacol Ther 1985;37:150.
25. Singh S, Doherty J, Udhop V, et al. Amlodipine versus nadolol in patients with stable angina pectoris. Am Heart J 1989;118:1137.
26. Lorimer AR, Smedsrud T, Walker P, Tyler HM. Comparison of amlodipine and verapamil in the treatment of mild to moderate hypertension. J Cardiovasc Pharmacol 1988;12(Suppl 7):S89.
27. Hansson L, Zanchetti A, Carruthers SG, et al. Effects of intensive blood-pressure lowering and low-dose aspirin in patients with hypertension: Principal results of the Hypertension Optimal Treatment (HOT) randomised trial. Lancet 1998;351:1755.
28. Allen GS, Ahn HS, Preziosi TJ, et al. Cerebral arterial spasm: A controlled trial of nimodipine in patients with subarachnoid hemorrhage. N Engl J Med 1983;308:619.
29. PRAISE: Packer M, O'Connor CM, Ghali JK, et al. Effect of amlodipine on morbidity and mortality in severe chronic heart failure: For the Prospective Randomised Amlodipine Survival Evaluation Study Group. N Engl J Med 1996;335:1107.
30. Staessen JA, Fagard R, Lutgarde T, et al. Randomised double-blind comparison of placebo and active treatment for older patients with isolated systolic hypertension: For the Systolic Hypertension in Europe (Syst-Eur) Trial Investigators. Lancet 1997;350:757.
31. Michels KB, Rosner BA, Manson JE, et al. Prospective study of calcium channel blocker use, cardiovascular disease, and total mortality among hypertensive women: The Nurses' Health Study. Circulation 1998;97:1540.
32. Califf RM, Kramer JM. What have we learned from the calcium channel blocker controversy? Circulation 1998;97:1529.
33. Cutler JA. Calcium-channel blockers for hypertension: Uncertainty continues. N Engl J Med 1998;338: 679.
34. Borhani NO, Mercury M, Borhani PA, et al. Final outcome results of the Multicenter Isradipine Diuretic Atherosclerosis Study (MIDAS): A randomised controlled trial. JAMA 1996;276:785.
35. Estacio RO, Jeffers BW, Hiatt WR, et al. The effect of nisoldipine as compared with enalapril on cardiovascular outcomes in patients with non-insulin dependent diabetes and hypertension. N Engl J Med 1998; 338:645.
36. Tatti P, Pahor M, Byington RP, et al. Results of the Fosinopril Amlodipine Cardiovascular Events Trial (FACET) in hypertensive patients with non-insulin dependent diabetes mellitus (NIDDM). Circulation 1997;96(Suppl I):I-764.
37. Pahor M, Kritchevsky SB, Zuccla G, et al. Diabetes and risk of adverse events with calcium antagonists. Diabetes Care 1998;21:193.
38. Matterson BJ, Reda DJ, Cushman WC, et al. Single-drug therapy for hypertension in men: A comparison of six hypertensive agents with placebo. N Engl J Med 1993;328:914.
39. Khan M Gabriel. Valvular heart disease. In: Heart Disease, Diagnosis and Therapy. Baltimore, Williams & Wilkins, 1996.
40. Subramanian B, Bowles MJ, Davies AB, Raftery EB. Combined therapy with verapamil and propranolol in chronic stable angina. Am J Cardiol 1982;49:125.
41. Subramanian VB. Calcium Antagonists in Chronic Stable Angina Pectoris. Amsterdam, Excerpta Medica/ Elsevier, 1983, p 213.
42. Theroux P, Taeymans Y, Waters DD. Calcium antagonists: Clinical use in the treatment of angina. Drugs 1983;25:178.

6 Calcium Antagonist Controversies

CALCIUM ANTAGONISTS AND HEART FAILURE

Calcium Antagonists Cause an Increased Incidence of Acute MI or HF: True or False?

Calcium antagonists without doubt cause an increased incidence of heart failure (HF) as observed in several well-run randomized controlled trials (RCTs):

- Amlodipine in Antihypertensive and Lipid-Lowering Treatment (ALLHAT): HF 38% versus diuretic *(1)*.
- Nifedipine in Intervention as a Goal in Hypertension Treatment (INSIGHT): HF 46% versus diuretic *(2)*.
- Verapamil in Controlled Onset Verapamil Investigation of Cardiovascular End Points (CONVINCE): HF 30% *(3)*.
- Amlodipine in Prospective Randomized Amlodipine Survival Evaluation (PRAISE) caused significant increased pulmonary edema in patients with left ventricular (LV) dysfunction *(4)*.
- Diltiazem caused a significant increase in HF in a non-Q-wave infarction study *(5)*.

The short-acting preparations of nifedipine and other dihydropyridines have been shown in RCTs to cause an increased incidence of myocardial infarction (MI), and controversies raged during the 1990s. These formulations are no longer used.

- Although the sustained-release formulations have been shown to be much safer than the rapid-acting older preparations, these agents are contraindicated in patients with unstable angina or acute MI. Verapamil is also contraindicated in patients with acute ST-elevation MI (STEMI) and non-STEMI.
- Diltiazem is contraindicated in patients with LV dysfunction but may be used in patients with unstable angina if beta-blockers are contraindicated.

Newer Calcium Antagonists Are Better Than Older Agents: True or False?

Lercanidipine was introduced into the United Kingdom a few years ago and is not available in the United States and Canada. It appeared to have major advantages over amlodipine and older dihydropyridines. Because the drug dilates both afferent and efferent arterioles, the high incidence of peripheral edema caused by older calcium antagonists was reportedly reduced more than 50%. The balanced effect of lercanidipine and manidipine on efferent and afferent arterioles was believed to be important in renoprotection; older calcium antagonists dilate only afferent arterioles.

Lercanidipine is only indicated for hypertension and is contraindicated in patients with LV dysfunction; sick sinus syndrome (if pacemaker not fitted); hepatic impairment; aortic stenosis; unstable angina; uncontrolled HF; within 1 mo of MI; and renal impairment.

From: *Contemporary Cardiology: Cardiac Drug Therapy, Seventh Edition*
M. Gabriel Khan © Humana Press Inc., Totowa, NJ

Adverse effects include: flushing, peripheral edema, palpitations, tachycardia, headache, dizziness, and asthenia; also gastrointestinal disturbances, hypotension, drowsiness, myalgia, polyuria, and rash. Thus, such agents are not more effective and do not possess more safety than older agents. Most important, the combination of lercanidipine and digoxin is potentially hazardous.

ARE CALCIUM ANTAGONISTS USEFUL FOR HYPERTENSIVES WITH CAD?

Calcium antagonists have been used in patients to treat coronary artery disease (CAD) events, particularly stable angina, since about 1981. Their role in patients with unstable angina is limited, and caution is required for acute MI. Post-MI prophylaxis with verapamil has been advocated by few in the field and remains controversial. The author does not recommend verapamil post-MI.

Their use in hypertensive patients with unsuspected or stable CAD has been widespread for more than two decades because they cause more effective and consistent lowering of blood pressure than angiotensin-converting enzyme (ACE) inhibitors/ARBs, beta-blockers, and diuretics.

Their salutary effects on adverse cardiovascular disease (CVD) outcomes appear similar to the other three classes in patients without CAD. The large RCT International Verapamil-Trandolapril (INVEST) trial *(6)* studied hypertensive patients with CAD.

- 22,576 hypertensive CAD patients aged 50 yr or older were randomly assigned to either CAS (verapamil sustained release) or NCAS (atenolol). However, at 24 mo, in the CAS group, 6391 patients (81.5%) were taking verapamil sustained release, 4934 (62.9%) were taking trandolapril, and 3430 (43.7%) were taking hydrochlorothiazide.
- In the NCAS group, 6083 patients (77.5%) were taking atenolol, 4733 (60.3%) were taking hydrochlorothiazide, and 4113 (52.4%) were taking trandolapril.
- **Primary outcomes:** First occurrence of death (all cause), nonfatal MI, or nonfatal stroke; others: cardiovascular death, angina, adverse experiences, hospitalizations, and blood pressure control at 24 mo.
- **Results:** 2269 patients had a primary outcome event with no statistically significant difference between treatment strategies (9.93% in CAS and 10.17% in NCAS; relative risk (RR), 0.98; 95% confidence interval (CI), 0.90–1.06). **It is impossible to draw conclusions about the contribution of any single agent in this complex, open-label study that used blunderbuss drug combinations**.
- The exception was patients with prior HF: those assigned to the NCAS strategy appeared to have fewer events ($p = 0.03$ for interaction). Most important, verapamil, as expected, increased the incidence of HF even when combined with an angiotensin-converting enzyme (ACE) inhibitor and diuretic.

Thus, calcium antagonists are not the drugs of choice to treat hypertensive patients who have significant CAD, particularly those with LV dysfunction.

Principal results of the Controlled Onset Verapamil Investigation of Cardiovascular End Points (CONVINCE) trial *(3)* were as follows:

- Aim: To determine whether initial therapy with controlled-onset extended-release (COER) verapamil is equivalent to a physician's choice of atenolol or hydrochlorothiazide in preventing cardiovascular disease.

- An RCT of 16,602 hypertensive patients who had one or more additional risk factors for CVD was conducted. After a mean of 3 yr of follow-up, the sponsor closed the study before unblinding the results.
- Initially, 8241 participants received 180 mg of COER verapamil, and 8361 received either 50 mg of atenolol or 12.5 mg of hydrochlorothiazide. Other drugs (e.g., a diuretic, beta-blocker, or ACE inhibitor) could be added in specified sequence if needed.
- **Primary outcomes:** First occurrence of stroke, MI, or cardiovascular disease (CVD)-related death.
- **Results:**
  - 364 primary CVD-related events occurred in the COER verapamil group versus 365 in the atenolol or hydrochlorothiazide group (hazard ratio [HR], 1.02; 95% CI, 0.88–1.18; $p = 0.77$).
  - Nonstroke hemorrhage was more common with participants in the COER-verapamil group ($n = 118$) compared with the atenolol or hydrochlorothiazide group ($n = 79$) (HR, 1.54; 95% CI, 1.16–2.04; $p = 0.003$).
  - Most important, verapamil caused a 30% increase in HF.
  - Importantly, more CVD-related events occurred between 6 AM and noon in both the COER verapamil (99/277) and atenolol or hydrochlorothiazide (88/274) groups.

I must emphasize that atenolol often has a less than 22-h duration of action, and studies have shown that it fails to quell early morning catecholamine surge, which is suppressed by other beta-blockers including metoprolol, timolol, bisoprolol, and carvedilol. Because most MIs occur during the hours of 6 AM and 11 AM, caution should be used with administration of poorly cardioprotective verapamil and atenolol.

- **Clinicians should recognize that both verapamil and atenolol are not suitable antihypertensive agents, particularly in patients with CAD; verapamil is potentially harmful in the elderly who are at high risk for HF, and atenolol has only mild cardiovascular protective effects.**

See the discussion of atenolol's poor effectiveness in Chapters 2 and 9, Hypertension Controversies.

REFERENCES

1. The ALLHAT Officers and Coordinators for the ALLHAT Collaborative Research Group. Major outcomes in high-risk hypertensive patients randomized to angiotensin-converting enzyme inhibitor or calcium channel blocker vs. diuretic: The Antihypertensive and Lipid-Lowering Treatment to Prevent Heart Attack Trial (ALLHAT). JAMA 2002;288:2981–2997.
2. Brown MJ, Palmer CR, Castaigne A, et al. Morbidity and mortality in patients randomised to double-blind treatment with a long-acting calcium-channel blocker or diuretic in the International Nifedipine GITS study: Intervention as a Goal in Hypertension Treatment. Lancet 2000;356:366–372.
3. CONVINCE: Black HR, Elliott WJ, Grandits G, et al. for the CONVINCE Research Group. JAMA 2003; 289:2073–2082.
4. Packer M, O'Connor CM, Ghali JK, et al. Effect of amlodipine on morbidity and mortality in severe chronic heart failure: For the Prospective Randomised Amlodipine Survival Evaluation Study Group. N Engl J Med 1996;335:1107.
5. Multicenter Diltiazem Postinfarction Trial Research Group. The effect of diltiazem on mortality and reinfarction after myocardial infarction. N Engl J Med 1989;319:385.
6. INVEST: Pepine CJ, Handberg EM, Rhonda M, et al. for the INVEST Investigators. A calcium antagonist vs a non-calcium antagonist hypertension treatment strategy for patients with coronary artery disease. The International Verapamil-Trandolapril Study (INVEST): A randomized controlled trial. JAMA 2003;290: 2805–2816.

7 Diuretics

Diuretics have appropriately maintained a stable place in the management of hypertension and heart failure (HF) because of their proven efficacy and low cost. The aldosterone antagonists spironolactone and its analog eplerenone are diuretics but have added actions that improve myocardial function and are an important part of our armamentarium for the management of patients with HF.

The generic and trade names of available diuretics are listed in Table 7-1.

INDICATIONS

- Hypertension.
- Management and relief of symptoms of HF: dyspnea, orthopnea, paroxysmal nocturnal dyspnea, and edema.
- **Spironolactone** has been shown to have an important role in the management of class III and IV HF.
- Edema due to renal dysfunction, or ascites due to cirrhosis.
- Edema associated with corticosteroids, estrogen, or vasodilator therapy.

Note: Edema of the legs presumed to be caused by HF, edema resulting from obstruction of venous return, and dependent edema caused by lack of muscle pump action are some of the commonest reasons for diuretic abuse.

Cautions

- **Cardiac tamponade:** When the jugular venous pressure (JVP) is grossly raised (>7 cmH_2O) and the patient is not responding to conventional therapy for HF, before giving diuretics to such patients, consideration should be given to a diagnosis of cardiac tamponade or constrictive pericarditis.
- Obstructive and restrictive **cardiomyopathy**.
- Tight mitral **stenosis** or aortic stenosis.
- **Ascites** with impending hepatic coma.
- **Edema** with acute renal failure.
- **Pulmonary embolism** with shortness of breath: Edema caused by cor pulmonale should not be treated aggressively with diuretics. Correct the hypoxemia, and then try to accomplish a very mild diuresis over several weeks.

Monitor intensive diuretic therapy as follows: If any of the following six-point checklist occurs, discontinue diuretics for 24 h and then recommence at approximately half the dose.

1. Systolic blood pressure is <95 mmHg or orthostatic hypotension is present.
2. More than 2 kg weight loss per day is associated with symptoms (1 kg of water loss = 140–150 mEq (mmol) of Na^+ loss in the presence of normal serum Na^+).

From: *Contemporary Cardiology: Cardiac Drug Therapy, Seventh Edition*
M. Gabriel Khan © Humana Press Inc., Totowa, NJ

Table 7-1
Generic and Trade Names of Diuretics

Generic name	*Trade name*	*Tablets (mg)*	*Usual maintenance (mg daily)*
Group I: Thiazides			
Chlorothiazide	Diuril, Saluric	250, 500	500–1000
Hydrochlorothiazide	HydroDiuril, Hydrosaluric, Esidrix, Esidrex, Oretic, Direma	25, 50, 100	12.5–25
Bendrofluazide	Aprinox, Berkozide, Centyl, Neo-NaClex	2.5, 5	2.5–5
Bendroflumethiazide	Naturetin	2.5, 5, 10	2.5–10
Benzthiazide	Aquatag, Exna, Hydrex	50	50–100
Cyclothiazide	Anhydron	2	2
Hydroflumethiazide	Diucardin, Hydrenox, Saluron	50	50
Chlorthalidone	Hygroton	25, 50, 100	25–50
Methylclothiazide	Enduron, Aquatensen, Diutensen-R	2.5, 5	2.5–5
Polythiazide	Renese, Nephril	1, 2, 4	0.5–4
Trichlormethiazide	Naqua, Metahydrin	2, 4	2–4
Cyclopenthiazide	Navidrex, Navidrix	0.5	0.5–1
Metolazone	Zaroxolyn, Metenix	2.5, 5, 10	2.5–5
Quinethazone	Aquamox, Hydromox	50	50–100
Indapamide	Lozol, Natrilix, Lozide (C)	2.5	2.5
Group II: Loop diuretics			
Furosemide, Frusemide (UK)	Lasix, Dryptal, Frusetic, Frusid	20, 40, 80, 500	40–120
Ethacrynic acid	Edecrin	25, 50	50–150
Bumetanide	Burinex, Bumex	0.5, 1, 5	1–2
Piretanide	Arlix	6 (capsule)	6–12
Torsemide	Demadex	5, 10, 20, 100	5–20
Group III: K^+-sparing diuretics			
Spironolactone	Aldactone	25, 50 (UK), 100	25–100
Triamterene	Dyrenium, Dytac	50, 100	50–100
Amiloride	Midamor	5	5–10
Group IV			
Thiazide + K^+-sparing	Aldactazide, Dyazide, Moduretic, Moduret		
Frusemide + K^+-sparing	Frumil, Frusene, Lasoride		
Group V			
Acetazolamide	Diamox	250	—

3. Electrolytes:
   a. Blood urea: >7.0 mmol/L from baseline.
   b. Serum chloride (Cl^-): <94 mEq (mmol)/L.
   c. Serum sodium (Na^+): <128 mEq (mmol)/L.

d. Serum potassium (K^+): <3 mEq (mmol)/L.
e. CO_2: >32 mEq (mmol)/L.
f. Uric acid: >10 mg/dL (588 mmol/L).
g. JVP is <1 cm if previously raised. The Frank-Starling compensatory mechanism is lost if diuresis is too excessive and filling pressures fall below a critical point, thereby causing cardiac output and tissue perfusion to fall.

4. Arrhythmias develop or worsen.
5. The 24-h urinary Na^+ excretion is >150 mEq (mmol).

For the management of moderate to severe HF with bilateral edema and pulmonary crepitations, the goal should be

6. Weight loss, a little more than 1 kg/d for 3 d, and then 0.5 kg/d for 7 d, with a minimum of 4 kg to a maximum of 10 kg in 10 d.

Note: A 24-h urinary Na^+ excretion < 20 mEq (mmol) indicates inadequate diuretic therapy; 24-h urinary excretion > 100 mEq (mmol), with no weight loss, requires reduction of Na^+ intake. This estimation is, however, seldom required.

THIAZIDES

The thiazide diuretics are discussed in Chapter 8.

LOOP DIURETICS

The rapid onset of action of loop diuretics, together with their potency in the presence of normal and abnormal renal function and their venodilator effect, renders them more effective than thiazides for the management of acute and chronic HF and life-threatening pulmonary edema.

Mechanism of Action

Loop diuretics inhibit the $Na^+/K^+/Cl^-$ transport system of the luminal membrane in the thick ascending loop of Henle, and thus they block Cl^- reabsorption at the site where approximately 40% of filtered Na^+ is normally reabsorbed (Fig. 7-1). Loop diuretics, through their action on Na^+-Cl^- cotransport, inhibit Ca^{2+}, K^+, and Mg^{2+} reabsorption in the loop where some 25% of filtered K^+, 25% of Ca^{2+}, and 65% of Mg^{2+} are normally reabsorbed.

Drug name:	**Furosemide; Frusemide**
Trade name:	Lasix
Supplied:	20, 40, 80, 500 mg
Dosage:	20, 40, or 80 mg each morning until desired effect achieved; maintenance 20–40 mg daily or every second day; *see* text for further advice

Dosage (Further Advice)

Patients with severe HF may require between 80 and 160 mg furosemide daily, rarely 240 mg daily for a few days and then a lower maintenance dose. In such patients, it is preferable to give the total dose of furosemide as **one dose each morning**. If a second dose is necessary, this should be given before 2 PM to avoid bothersome nocturia. Hypokalemia is more common with twice-daily dosage. Also, if the patient was formerly resistant

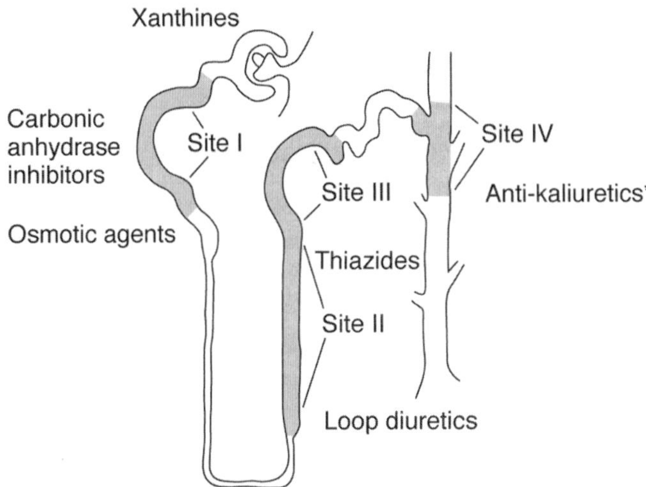

Fig. 7-1. Diagrammatic representation of the nephron showing the four main tubular sites where diuretics interfere with sodium reabsorption. The main action of xanthines on the kidney is on vascular perfusion of the glomerulus, although some effect on sodium reabsorption at site I also is likely. (From Lant A. Diuretic drugs: Progress in clinical pharmacology. Drugs 1985;31(Suppl 4):40.)

to 80 mg, the renal tubule may be resistant to the 80 mg given later in the day. If a dose of furosemide >60 mg per day is predicted to be necessary for several weeks, then it is advisable to add a K^+-sparing diuretic or angiotensin-converting enzyme (ACE) inhibitor. This will increase diuresis by inhibiting aldosterone and at the same time will conserve K^+. **The addition of spironolactone to the HF regimen of ACE inhibitor and furosemide has been shown to improve survival.**

Intravenous (IV) dosage: Ampules are available in 10 mg/mL, 20 mg/2 mL, 40 mg/4 mL, and 250 mg/25 mL. The IV dose is given slowly (20 mg/min), and if renal failure is present, it should not exceed 4 mg/min (to prevent ototoxicity).

Action and Pharmacokinetics

Furosemide inhibits Na^+ and Cl^- reabsorption from the ascending limb of the loop of Henle with, in addition, weak effects in the proximal tubule and the cortical diluting segment. The drug is excreted by the proximal tubule. Because of the site and potency of action, loop diuretics are much more effective than thiazides when the glomerular filtration rate (GFR) is markedly reduced. Loop diuretics remain effective even at GFRs as low as 10 mL/min *(1)*. If a diuretic is required in a patient with a serum creatinine level > 2.3 mg/dL (203 μ/mol/L), it is reasonable to choose furosemide. Furosemide is also used in preference to thiazide as maintenance therapy in patients with moderate to severe or recurrent HF, that is, in patients in whom further episodes may be predicted because of the extent of cardiac disease. IV furosemide has a **venodilator** effect, and, when it is given to patients with pulmonary edema, relief may appear in 5–10 min.

Intravenous Indications

This route is indicated in emergency, life-threatening situations, such as the following:

- Pulmonary edema or interstitial edema resulting from left ventricular failure.
- Severe HF; with poor oral absorption.

Table 7-2
Diuretic-Induced Metabolic Adverse Effects

- Hypokalemia
- Hyponatremia
- Hypochloremic metabolic alkalosis:
  $Cl^- < 94$ mEq (mmol)/L
  $CO_2 > 32$ mEq (mmol)/L
- Azotemia
- Hyperuricemia
- Hypomagnesemia
- Dyslipidemia
- Glucose intolerance
- Nonketotic hyperosmolar coma
- Hypocalcemia (loop diuretics)
- Hypercalcemia (thiazides)
- Hyperkalemia (K^+-sparing diuretics)

- Hypertensive crisis.
- Hypercalcemia and hyperkalemia.

In addition to the mechanism of action of loop diuretics outlined earlier, furosemide causes venodilation. This action involves prostaglandins and can be inhibited by nonsteroidal antiinflammatory drugs (NSAIDs). Furosemide has a half-life of 1.5 h and a duration of action of 4–6 h. Diuresis commences some 15–20 min after IV administration, but relief of shortness of breath may be apparent within 10 min because of an increase in systemic venous capacitance, reduced cardiac preload, and a decrease in left atrial pressure. After oral administration, diuresis peaks in 60–90 min.

Contraindications

- Hepatic failure.
- Hypokalemia or electrolyte depletion, hyponatremia, or hypotension.
- Hypersensitivity to furosemide or sulfonamides.
- In women of child-bearing potential, except in life-threatening situations, in which IV furosemide may be absolutely necessary. Furosemide has caused fetal abnormalities in animal studies.

Warnings

- Commence with a minimum dose of 20–40 mg, especially in the elderly.
- Monitor electrolytes, blood urea, creatinine, complete blood counts, and uric acid, especially when the dose exceeds 60 mg daily.

Adverse Effects

Hypokalemia, dehydration, anemia, leukopenia, thrombocytopenia, rare agranulocytosis, and thrombophlebitis have been noted, but aplastic anemia seems to be more common with thiazides than with furosemide. Hypotension, hyperuricemia and precipitation of gout, hypocalcemia, and precipitation of nonketotic hyperosmolar diabetic coma may occur. Table 7-2 summarizes the metabolic adverse effects.

Drug Interactions

1. Use carefully in the presence of renal dysfunction when combined with **cephalosporin** or **aminoglycoside antibiotics**, because increased nephrotoxicity has been noted.

2. Care should be taken when loop diuretics or thiazides are given to **lithium-treated** patients. The decreased Na^+ reabsorption in the proximal tubules causes an increased reabsorption of lithium and may cause **lithium toxicity** *(2)*. Patients receiving concomitant chloral hydrate may experience hot flushes, sweating, and tachycardia. Prostaglandin inhibitors indomethacin and other NSAIDs antagonize the actions of loop diuretics as well as thiazides *(3)*.
3. The effects of tubocurarine may be increased.

Drug name:	**Ethacrynic acid**
Trade name:	Edecrin
Supplied:	50 mg
Dosage:	Oral dose of 50–150 mg daily or in an emergency IV 50 mg diluted with 50 mL 5% dextrose/water given slowly

This is a potent loop diuretic, similar in action to furosemide. The drug may cause slightly more Cl^- loss than furosemide. Ethacrynic acid has slightly more side effects (although there is less increase in serum uric acid concentration), and it is therefore reserved for patients who are resistant to the effects of furosemide.

Ethacrynic acid is not a sulfonamide and exhibits no cross-sensitivity with the thiazides. Ethacrynic acid is therefore useful in patients allergic to sulfonamides. The anticoagulant effect of warfarin is increased by ethacrynic acid.

Drug name:	**Bumetanide**
Trade names:	Burinex, Bumex
Supplied:	Tablets: 0.5, 1, and 5 mg Ampules: 2, 4, 10 mL; 500 mg/mL
Dosage:	Oral: 0.5–1 mg daily increased if required to 2–4 mg; 5 mg in oliguria IV: 1–3 mg over 1–2 min, repeated after 20 min

Bumetanide is as effective as furosemide, and it has a similar site of action in the medullary diluting segment *(4)*. The drug is excreted along with its metabolites in the urine and is believed to cause less Mg^{2+} loss than furosemide during long-term administration. Bumetanide and furosemide have similar pharmacokinetic characteristics. Bumetanide is more potent than furosemide: 1 mg bumetanide = 40 mg furosemide. The drug is absorbed more rapidly in patients with HF and has a bioavailability twice that of furosemide. Bumetanide is more nephrotoxic but appears to be less ototoxic than furosemide, so it is prudent not to use the drug with aminoglycosides or other potentially nephrotoxic drugs. Indications are as listed for furosemide. The drug is not approved in the United States for hypertension.

Drug name:	**Torsemide; torasemide (UK)**
Trade names:	Demadex, Torem (UK)
Supplied:	Tablets: 5, 10, 20, 100 mg Ampules: 50 mg
Dosage:	Oral: 2.5– 40 mg once daily; HF dose 20–200 mg IV: 5–50 mg

Toresemide given orally achieves high bioavailability, and a 10-mg dose produces diuresis equivalent to 40 mg furosemide *(5)*.

POTASSIUM-SPARING DIURETICS

Mechanism of Action

Increased renin release from the juxtaglomerular cells is caused by several conditions:

- Reduction in renal blood flow from HF, blood loss, hypotension, or ischemia.
- Na^+ diuresis.
- Beta-adrenergic stimulation.

Renin converts liver angiotensinogen to angiotensin I. Angiotensin II and adrenocorticotrophic hormone stimulate adrenal aldosterone production.

The "aldosterone antagonists" are very weak diuretics. Aldosterone handles approximately 2% of filtered Na^+ at the distal tubule, so only a small diuresis is achieved. Diuretics that block aldosterone or act at the same site distal to the macula densa cause a small amount of Na^+ excretion and prevent exchange of K^+. Only spironolactone and potassium canrenoate antagonize aldosterone. Spironolactone interferes with the effect of aldosterone to increase the rate of Na^+-K^+ exchange at the basolateral surface *(6)*. Amiloride and triamterene interact with lumen membrane transporters to prevent urinary Na^+ entry into the cytoplasm *(6)*. They are direct inhibitors of K^+ secretion.

K^+-sparing diuretics play a vital role in conserving K^+ and Mg^{2+} in patients treated with thiazides or loop diuretics. The addition of a K^+-sparing drug to low-dose thiazide therapy results in a reduced risk of cardiac arrest *(7)*.

The four available K^+-sparing diuretics are **amiloride** (Midamor), **spironolactone** (Aldactone), **triamterene** (Dyrenium, Dytac), and **potassium canrenoate** (Spiroctan-M). **These weak diuretics are very important in the following situations:**

1. **Spironolactone** 25 mg added to an ACE inhibitor in patients with HF causes a more complete block of aldosterone production than is achieved with ACE inhibition and reduces mortality and morbidity in these patients. The salutary effects are related not only to Na^+ loss but also to a decrease in cardiac fibrosis, retardation of endothelial dysfunction, and increased nitric oxide production caused by inhibition of aldosterone. Aldosterone, a compensatory "good" hormone, appears to have fibrogenic and other deleterious properties. Tissue collagen turnover and fibrosis appear to be important facets of HF, and spironolactone may attenuate deleterious structural remodeling *(8)*.
2. When added to thiazides or loop diuretics, diuresis is greatly augmented. The serum K^+ often remains within the normal range.
3. Clinical situations in which secondary aldosteronism is involved. The "aldosterone antagonists" are first-line diuretics in conditions associated with **secondary aldosteronism**:
   - Cirrhosis with ascites.
   - Nephrotic syndrome.
   - Chronic **recurrent HF**. (They can be extremely effective and beneficial when added to loop or to thiazide diuretics and ACE inhibitors.)
   - Cyclical edema.
   - Renovascular hypertension.

Spironolactone is also of value in the diagnosis of primary aldosteronism and in treatment of Bartter's syndrome.

The following are suggested **guidelines** for the diuretic management of the patient with marked ascites caused by cirrhosis. Ensure that

- Hepatic encephalopathy is not present.
- The patient can sign his or her name and constructional apraxia is not present.
- The patient can tolerate a 60–80-g protein diet for 1 wk without the precipitation of encephalopathy.
- Jaundice is either not present or not increasing.

If these four assessments are passed for more than 7 d, then commence spironolactone 25–100 mg twice daily. Some 2–8 wk later, if there is no encephalopathy, add 25 mg of hydrochlorothiazide (HCTZ) every second day and then if needed daily, or furosemide 40 mg daily. It may be necessary to wait 2–3 mo to achieve a 75% reduction in the ascites.

Contraindications and Warnings

The following are contraindications and warnings for the use of K^+-sparing diuretics or combinations with thiazides or furosemide:

1. Acute or chronic renal failure. These drugs should be avoided if there is any evidence of renal failure, in particular a serum creatinine level > 1.3 mg/dL (115 μmol/L) in patients aged <70 yr, and > 1.0 mg/dL (88 μmol/L) for those > 70 yr, or urea > 7 mmol/L. These ground rules should be broken only if the patient is under strict observation in hospital and an order is written to discontinue the medications if the serum K^+ level is >5 mEq (mmol)/L.
2. Do not use in conjunction with K^+ supplements or ACE inhibitors or in patients who have metabolic acidosis because these diuretics may themselves increase acidosis by retaining H^+ along with K^+.
3. Do not use triamterene combined with indomethacin or other NSAIDs; acute renal failure may be precipitated *(9,10)*. Triamterene is relatively insoluble and may precipitate as **renal calculi** *(11)*. This agent is contraindicated in patients who have had a renal stone.

Spironolactone is a competitive inhibitor of aldosterone.

Drug name:	**Spironolactone**
Trade names:	Aldactone, Spiroctan (UK)
Dosage:	25–100 mg daily in single or two divided doses

Advantages

- **The drug appears to decrease cardiac fibrosis** *(12)* **and endothelial dysfunction** *(13)* **and to increase nitric oxide bioactivity** (*see* Chapter 12, Management of Heart Failure). These actions appear to explain the beneficial effects of the drug in patients with HF, as shown in the Randomized Aldactone Evaluation Study (RALES) *(12)*.
- Spironolactone is metabolized in the liver, whereas amiloride is excreted by the kidney, so if renal dysfunction supervenes, the risk of hyperkalemia is less with spironolactone.
- Spironolactone does not cause aplastic anemia or have any other serious hematologic effects. Amiloride and triamterene have been associated with aplastic anemia (although rarely).
- The drug does not cause megaloblastic anemia, seen rarely with triamterene.
- Spironolactone has a positive inotropic effect independent of and additive to that of digitalis. Stroke volume is increased.

Table 7-3
Interactions of Spironolactone

- Aspirin antagonizes the diuretic effect of spironolactone
- ACE inhibitors and spironolactone both cause hyperkalemia
- Digoxin levels are increased (laboratory reaction)
- NSAIDs combined with spironolactone may precipitate acute renal failure

Disadvantages

- Gynecomastia. This depends on the dose and its duration. Keep the maintenance dose at less than 50 mg/d. Eplerenone is as effective as spironolactone. Most important, the drug does not cause gynecomastia and will replace spironolactone.
- **Caution:** Potential human metabolic products are carcinogenic in rodents and tumorigenic in rats.

Interactions are summarized in Table 7-3.

Drug name:	**Eplerenone**
Trade name:	Inspra
Dosage:	12.5–25 mg once daily, max. 50 mg daily

Eplerenone is an important addition to our therapeutic armamentarium for the management of HF and hypertension (*see* Chapters 12 and 22).

Combination of a Thiazide or Furosemide and Potassium-Sparing Diuretic

It is now well established that thiazide diuretics cause significant **K^+ loss**, which increases the incidence of arrhythmias, cardiac arrest *(7)*, and cardiac mortality. Conservation or replacement of K^+ is therefore essential and has been proved to decrease the risk of cardiac arrest. K^+-sparing diuretics are useful and can prevent the use of gastric-irritating potassium chloride (KCl) preparations in most patients if these drugs are used with **careful restrictions**.

Dyazide: Tablets (capsules, US) of 50 mg triamterene and 25 mg HCTZ.

Dytide: Tablets of triamterene 50 mg and 25 mg benzthiazide. *Dosage:* one tablet each morning or every second day; for mild to moderate hypertension, a dose of one tablet daily for maintenance; **contraindicated** in patients who have had a **renal stone** *(11)* or renal failure.

Aldactazide: Tablets of 25 mg spironolactone and 25 mg HCTZ.

Aldactide: Tablets of 25 mg spironolactone and 25 mg hydroflumethiazide; tablets of 50 mg spironolactone and 50 mg hydroflumethiazide.

Moduretic (Moduret): Tablets of 50 mg HCTZ and 5 mg amiloride hydrochloride; Moduret 25 or nonproprietary in the United Kingdom, co-amilozide = HCTZ 25 mg, amiloride 2.5 mg; *Dosage:* 1 tablet each morning; **not advisable to use more than 1 tablet daily**.

Maxzide: Tablets of 75 mg triamterene and 50 mg of HCTZ. *Dosage:* half to 1 tablet each morning.

Frumil (Lasoride): Tablets of 40 mg frusemide and 5 mg amiloride, given 1 to 2 tablets daily.

Frusene: Tablets of 40 mg frusemide and 50 mg triamterene.

Warnings

- K^+-sparing diuretics must not be given concomitantly with K^+ supplements or ACE inhibitors except under strict supervision; severe hyperkalemia may result.
- Elderly diabetic patients may develop hyporeninemic hypoaldosteronism and may therefore retain K^+ despite a normal serum creatinine level.
- If the patient develops gynecomastia during spironolactone therapy, then triamterene or amiloride can replace the spironolactone because these two agents do not cause gynecomastia. They are devoid of the hormonal effects of spironolactone. Triamterene, however, is slightly insoluble and can precipitate as renal calculi.
- K^+-sparing diuretics may rarely produce mild metabolic acidosis.

OTHER DIURETICS

Drug name:	**Metolazone**
Trade names:	Zaroxolyn, Metenix (UK)
Supplied:	2.5, 5, 10 mg
Dosage:	2.5–5 mg once daily; rarely 10 mg

Metolazone has a prolonged action of up to 24 h. The drug acts in both the proximal convoluted tubule and the distal nephron, similar to thiazide. Both thiazides and metolazone have secondary effects in the proximal tubule that are not usually manifest because the proximally rejected ions are ordinarily reabsorbed in the loop. **Thus, combinations of metolazone and loop diuretics are very effective in the management of intractable HF.** Sequential nephron blockade is a proven concept.

Thiazides become ineffective when the GFR falls to <30 mL/min, whereas loop diuretics and metolazone retain effectiveness. **The combination of metolazone and a loop diuretic is very potent** and useful, but K^+ loss is often pronounced.

Drug name:	**Acetazolamide**
Trade name:	Diamox
Supplied:	250 mg
Dosage:	250 mg three times daily, max. 4 d; treatment can be repeated once or twice in a month.

This drug is a carbonic anhydrase inhibitor. It causes excretion of HCO_3^-, retention of Cl^-, and, consequently, metabolic acidosis and hyperchloremia. Acetazolamide is a very weak diuretic, and the action is lost after 4 d. It is of importance only in the management of hypochloremic metabolic alkalosis in the presence of a normal serum K^+ level *(15)*. The typical case is one of refractory HF in a patient taking furosemide and K^+-sparing diuretics. The electrolyte picture shows $Cl^- < 92$ mEq (mmol)/L, CO_2 >30 mEq (mmol)/L, and K^+ 3.5–5 mEq (mmol)/L. In such cases, acetazolamide, added to the spironolactone with the furosemide dose discontinued or halved, results in continued diuresis and correction of the normokalemic hypochloremic metabolic alkalosis.

Acetazolamide is contraindicated in patients with renal failure, renal calculi, metabolic acidosis, and severe cirrhosis.

Table 7-4
K⁺-Enriched Foods

Food	*Amount*	*K^+ (mEq)*
Orange juice	Half cup	6
Milk (skim-powdered)	Half cup	27
Milk (whole-powdered)	Half cup	20
Melon (honeydew)	Quarter	13
Banana	One	10
Tomato	One	6
Celery	One	5
Spinach	Half cup	8
Potato (baked)	Half	13
Beans	Half cup	10
Strawberries	Half cup	3
Meats, shellfish, and avocado	All contain increased K^+	

POTASSIUM CHLORIDE SUPPLEMENTS

To physicians caring for cardiac and hypertensive patients, diuretics are the commonest cause of hypokalemia. The incidence of hypokalemia is about 5–30% with HCTZ and 5–20% with loop diuretics, but as high as 50–100% with chlorthalidone *(16)*. The author concurs with these observations and ceased to use chlorthalidone in 1974. Nephrologists may use the drug successfully in patients with mild renal impairment because K^+ is usually retained in that situation. Thus, the nephrologist may recommend this drug, inappropriately, for general use.

Mild hypokalemia of 3–3.5 mEq (mmol)/L is of concern and must be corrected if the patient is taking digoxin or has arrhythmias, cardiac disease, or weakness. If metabolic acidosis is present, a serum K^+ level < 3.5 mEq (mmol)/L constitutes a definite total body K^+ deficit. Minor decreases in serum K^+ concentration to 3 mEq (mmol)/L may be corrected in most patients by asking them to ingest foods that are rich in K^+ (Table 7-4).

It is a relatively useless exercise to tell the patient to take an extra glass of orange juice, as is commonly done (6 oz = 8.4 mEq K^+). Note that salt substitutes, such as Co-salt, Nosalt, and other brands, also aid in increasing serum K^+ levels. However, salt substitutes contain KCl and may therefore cause gastric irritation in some patients.

It is important **not** to give KCl mixtures along with K^+-sparing diuretics or an ACE inhibitor and then continue with enriched diets and salt substitutes without knowledge of renal function, because this occasionally causes hyperkalemia.

Patients taking thiazide diuretics should be allowed to continue for at least 1–2 mo and the electrolytes reassessed. Depending on the dose, hypokalemia occurs in 30–50% of patients. If, however, patients are instructed to follow a diet containing K^+-rich foods, such as those outlined in Table 7-4, the incidence of hypokalemia can be reduced. Patients showing even mild hypokalemia should be given KCl supplements or preferably taken off thiazides and given a thiazide K^+-sparing diuretic.

As an alternative, patients may be started on Moduretic or Dyazide or Frumil if renal function is normal.

If the serum K^+ concentration is <2.5 mEq (mmol)/L, IV K^+ is given. In the range of 2.5–3.5 mEq (mmol)/L, oral K^+ is usually sufficient, but it must always be in the form of Cl^- except in renal tubular acidosis, in which citrates and bicarbonates can be used.

Diuretics cause significant hypokalemia, but only rarely do they cause a significant fall in total body K^+. Compare extracellular 65 mEq (mmol) with 4000 mEq (mmol) intracellular total K^+. Thus, the importance of determining the **serum K^+** level is emphasized, because it is abnormalities at this level that dictate alterations of the K^+ gradient across the myocardial cell membrane and that can result in severe electrical changes and cardiac arrhythmias. **Fluctuations** of the serum K^+ concentration are often exaggerated by **acidosis**, causing hyperkalemia, and by **alkalosis**, causing hypokalemia. It is necessary to watch for the occurrence of the two conditions because they can be altered within minutes (e.g., metabolic acidosis during seizures, diabetic ketoacidosis, cardiac arrest, or respirator hyperventilation causing respiratory alkalosis and perhaps triggering ventricular tachycardia or ventricular fibrillation). A low serum K^+ level **reduces ventricular fibrillation threshold** and therefore increases the potential for sudden death *(17)*.

Note:

1. Hypokalemia produced by catecholamines is mediated by $beta_2$-adrenoceptors *(18)*. The increase in catecholamines that occurs during acute myocardial infarction can cause a significant decrease in serum K^+ concentration. Catecholamine-induced hypokalemia may be prevented by $beta_2$-blockade.
2. The $beta_2$-stimulants salbutamol, terbutaline, and pirbuterol may precipitate hypokalemia that is transient but perhaps important.

Potassium Chloride

1. **Mixtures:** Patients dislike the taste of these costly mixtures. A dose of 20 mEq (mmol)/L is given twice daily, and it is usually adequate, along with a K^+-rich diet. Patients in whom the serum K^+ level consistently falls to <3 mEq (mmol)/L, despite this regimen, and who are taking necessary doses of diuretics may require as much as 40 mEq KCl three times daily. It is preferable in these patients to add a K^+-retaining diuretic rather than using KCl.
2. The **effervescent** potassium preparations contain very little KCl and are not recommended.
3. KCl **tablets**, **capsules**, or **slow-release wax matrix** are not completely satisfactory because there is a significant incidence of ulceration of the gastrointestinal tract, including perforations *(19)*. Controlled-release preparations, K-Dur 20 (US) and K-Contin (UK), are safer than wax matrix KCl. Nonwax matrix preparations include Micro-K and K-Dur 20. The dispersion and slow-release characteristics of these preparations are believed to minimize contact between erosive K^+ and the mucosal lining, but caution is required *(20)*.

Diuretic-K^+ combinations are not recommended.

Salt Substitutes

The patient who has edema, HF, or hypertension must be on a restricted-Na^+ diet. There is a definite case, therefore, for salt substitutes in which K^+ takes the place of Na^+. There are many such products on the market—Nosalt, Cosalt, Morton's salt substitute, and Featherweight-K all have a reasonable taste. It is important, however, to recognize that the occasional patient may develop gastric discomfort. Thiazide and loop diuretics cause K^+ and Mg^{2+} losses. Some patients with severe K^+ deficiency may require supplemental **Mg^{2+}** to achieve correction of the K^+ and Mg^{2+} deficiency. The Mg^{2+} deficiency often continues undetected. Importantly, K^+-sparing diuretics are also Mg^{2+} sparing.

Intravenous Potassium Chloride

Care should be taken with IV KCl (Table 7-5) because death from **iatrogenic hyperkalemia** is not uncommon.

Table 7-5
Potassium Supplements[a]

	Ingredients	K^+ *mEq (mmol)*	Cl^- *mEq (mmol)*
Liquids			
Kay Ciel; Kay-Cee-L 1 mmol/mL	KCl	20	20
Potassium chloride 10%	KCl	20	20
K-Lor (paquettes)	KCl	20	20
K-Lyte Cl	KCl	25	25
Kaochlor 10% (or sugar free)	KCl	20	20
Klorvess 10%	KCl	20	20
Kolyum	KCl	20	3[b]
Kaon Elixir	K gluconate	20	—[b]
Kaon Cl 20%	KCl	40	40
K-Lyte (effervescent)	KH_2CO_3	25	—[b]
Potassium triplex	not KCl	15	—[b]
Potassium sandoz	KCl	12	8[b]
Rum K	KCl	20	20
Tables/capsules: slow release			
K-Long	KCl	6[b]	6
Kalium durules	KCl	10[b]	10
Kaon	K gluconate	5[b]	—[b]
Leo K	KCl	8	8[b]
Nu-K	K	8	8[b]
Sando K	K	12	8[b]
Slow-K	KCl	8[b]	8[b]
K-Dur 20	KCl	20	20
Micro-K	KCl	8	8
Micro-K-10	KCl	10	10

[a]Dosage: usual range 20–60 mEq (mmol) K^+ daily.
[b]Not recommended because of low K^+ or Cl^- content.

- Use IV KCl only when necessary, that is, when $K^+ < 2.5$ mEq (mmol)/L.
- Ensure an adequate urine output and that renal failure is absent.
- Do not give along with K^+-sparing diuretics, captopril, or enalapril.
- Correct metabolic acidosis or alkalosis.

Note:

1. In the presence of **metabolic alkalosis** with a pH > 7.5 and CO_2 > 30 mEq (mmol)/L, smaller amounts of KCL are required.
2. **Metabolic acidosis**, with a pH < 7.3 and serum K^+ level < 3 mEq (mmol)/L, means a major K^+ deficit and therefore the need for correction over several days.

Dilute KCl as much as possible: 40–60 mEq (mmol)/L. In noncardiac patients, dilute KCl in **normal saline**, especially if severe hypokalemia is present. In life-threatening situations, dilute in saline for all patients.

Dilute in dextrose:

- If aggressive therapy is not required and there is a need to limit Na+ load, as in the presence of HF or poor cardiac contractility in patients with recurrent or past HF.
- If on the first day of therapy the KCl was diluted in saline.

Observations and Warnings

- The container must not usually contain >40 mEq (mmol) KCl.
- The rate should not exceed 10 mEq (mmol)/h, except in severe hypokalemia <2.5 mEq (mmol)/L or when symptoms or arrhythmias are present.
- If the rate must exceed 10 mEq (mmol)/h, an electrocardiographic monitor is necessary with observations every 15 min. The maximum rate of 30 mEq (mmol)/h is rarely necessary.

NEW CONCEPTS

- The loop diuretic **torsemide** (torasemide, UK) is completely absorbed and appears to have higher reliability and predictability compared with furosemide. The variability of absorption is 9 for torsemide and 30 for furosemide.
- Torsemide has been shown in a small study to cause a dramatic decrease in hospitalization and reduced mortality in patients with class III and IV HF compared with furosemide *(5)*. The simple expedient of the choice of a diuretic can result in a decrease in hospitalization for HF of >33%.
- Food further reduces absorption of furosemide, and not many physicians recognize that this well-known drug must be taken on an empty stomach.

Aldosterone antagonists hold the key. The therapeutic value of aldosterone antagonists must not be underestimated in the management of HF of all grades. The drug should not be reserved for class IV HF.

- A therapeutic dose of loop diuretic must reach the kidney site of action. A small dose of a poorly absorbed drug has no effect; a large dose loses effect later and also stimulates the renin-angiotensin aldosterone system that causes Na^+ and water retention, hence the not surprising proven value of **spironolactone** (Aldactone) in the RALES study *(12)* in patients with class III and IV HF, in whom this agent is strongly recommended.
- In more than 55% of patients admitted with CHF, the precipitating factor is Na^+ and water retention. Consequently, we must focus on a better choice of loop diuretic and insist on combination with an aldosterone antagonist in virtually all patients admitted for HF.
- Patients with Class II–III HF can benefit from a smaller maintenance dose of loop diuretic: 20 mg furosemide (instead of 40–60 mg) plus spironolactone 25–50 mg or eplerenone 25 mg daily, with monitoring of serum potassium.
- Importantly, aldosterone antagonists are administered not only for the enhancement of diuresis but also because of their beneficial actions on cardiac myocytes. Spironolactone blockade of aldosterone actions appears to decrease cardiac fibrosis *(12)* and endothelial dysfunction *(13)* and to increase nitric oxide bioactivity.
- Aldosterone blockade prevents ventricular remodeling and collagen formation in patients with left ventricular (LV) dysfunction after acute myocardial infarction (MI) *(21)*.
- These agents favorably modify myocardial collagen and the development of fibrosis and may thus improve cardiac performance, ameliorating the disease process. Loop diuretics do not possess such salutary effects (*see* earlier discussion under Loop Diuretics). In addition, spironolactone appears to have a positive inotropic effect independent of and additive to digitalis; stroke volume is increased. Further studies and randomized controlled trials are in progress.
- Because ACE inhibitors only partially block aldosterone activity, and aldosterone causes myocardial and other deleterious effects in patients with HF, the use of aldosterone antagonists or receptor blockers constitutes a major addition to our effective armamentarium. In the RALES study *(14)*, there was a 30% reduction in the rate of death **and a similar reduction in sudden deaths and** hospitalizations among class III and IV patients with HF

who were treated with spironolactone 25 mg in combination with an ACE inhibitor loop diuretic, compared with patients who received placebo. Baseline serum creatinine was <2.5 mg/dL (221 μmol/L); severe hyperkalemia occurred in 2% of patients. Importantly, 75% of patients received digoxin. Only 11% received a beta-blocker. *See* cautions given earlier for use in patients with GFR < 50 mL/min.

- The derivative compound of spironolactone, eplerenone (Inspra), does not cause gynecomastia and impotence. In the Eplerenone Post-Acute Myocardial Infarction Heart Failure Efficacy and Survival Study (EPHESUS) *(22)*, the drug reduced adverse outcomes in patients with acute MI and LV dysfunction. This agent binds more specifically to the aldosterone receptor and does not bind as avidly to the androgen receptor. It blocks the mineralocorticoid receptor and not glucocorticoid, progesterone, or androgen receptors *(23)*.
- In EPHESUS, patients 3–14 d post acute MI were randomly assigned to eplerenone (25 mg daily titrated to a maximum of 50 mg (3313 patients) or placebo (3319 patients) in addition to optimal medical therapy *(22)*.
  - The primary end points were death from any cause and death from cardiovascular causes or hospitalization for HF acute MI. At 16-mo follow-up, there were 478 deaths in the eplerenone group and 554 deaths in the placebo group (relative risk [RR], 0.85; 95% confidence interval [CI], 0.75–0.96; $p = 0.008$).
  - Cardiovascular deaths were: 407 in the eplerenone group and 483 in the placebo group; (RR, 0.83; 95% CI, 0.72–0.94; $p = 0.005$) *(22)*.
  - The cardiovascular mortality reduction observed was caused mainly by a 21% reduction in the rate of sudden death from cardiac causes. A significant reduction in the rate of hospitalization for cardiovascular events was caused by a 15% reduction in the risk of hospitalization for HF and a 23% reduction in the number of episodes of hospitalization for HF *(22)*.
  - The risk of serious hyperkalemia was significantly increased in patients with significant renal dysfunction: creatinine clearance at baseline < 50 mL/min *(22)*.
- Eplerenone reduces coronary vascular inflammation and the risk of subsequent development of interstitial fibrosis in animal models of myocardial disease *(24,25)*. Eplerenone also reduces oxidative stress, improves endothelial dysfunction *(26,27)*, attenuates platelet aggregation *(4)*, decreases activation of matrix metalloproteinases, and improves ventricular remodeling *(28)*. In addition, aldosterone blockade decreases sympathetic drive in rats through direct actions in the brain *(29)*, improves norepinephrine uptake in patients with HF *(30)*, and improves heart-rate variability *(31)*—all factors known to have important effects on the risk of sudden death from cardiac causes.

Francis and colleagues *(32)* emphasized the following:

- In animal studies, excessive aldosterone has been associated with collagen deposition, myocardial fibrosis, and myocardial remodeling *(33)*.
- Blocking the synthesis or function of aldosterone has also been demonstrated to improve diastolic dysfunction in hypertensive patients with diastolic heart failure *(34)* and to improve endothelial function in patients with asymptomatic LV dysfunction or mild HF *(35)*.
- Most important, in EPHESUS, eplerenone was beneficial in patients who were receiving optimal therapy including an ACE inhibitor or an ARB, a beta-blocker, aspirin, a lipid-lowering agent, and coronary reperfusion therapy *(22)*. In RALES, only 11% of patients received a beta-blocker *(14)*.

REFERENCES

1. Maclean D, Tudhope GR. Modern diuretic treatment. BMJ 1983;286:1419.
2. Kerry RJ, Ludlow JM, Owen G. Diuretics are dangerous with lithium. BMJ 1980;281:371.

3. Yeung Laiwah AC, Mactier RA. Antagonistic effect of non-steroidal anti-inflammatory drugs on frusemide-induced diuresis in cardiac failure. BMJ 1981;283:714.
4. Puschett JB. Renal effects of bumetanide. J Clin Pharmacol 1981;21:575.
5. Sherman LG, Liang C, Baumgardner S, et al. Piretanide, a potent diuretic with potassium-sparing properties, for the treatment of congestive heart failure. Clin Pharmacol Ther 1986;40:587.
6. Narins RG (ed). Maxwell & Kleeman's Clinical Disorders of Fluid and Electrolyte Metabolism, 5th ed. New York, McGraw-Hill, 1994.
7. Siscovick DS, Raghunathan TE, Psaty BM. Diuretic therapy for hypertension and the risk of primary cardiac arrest. N Engl J Med 1994;330:1852.
8. Webert KT. Aldosterone in congestive heart failure. N Engl J Med 2001;345:1689.
9. Favre L, Glasson P, Vallotton MB. Reversible acute renal failure from combined triamterene and indomethacin: A study in healthy subjects. Ann Intern Med 1982;96:317.
10. Weinberg MS, Quigg RJ, Salant DJ, et al. Anuric renal failure precipitated by indomethacin and triamterene. Nephron 1985;40:216.
11. Ettinger B, Oldroyd NO, Sorgel F. Triamterene nephrolithiasis. JAMA 1980;244:2443.
12. Weber KT. Aldosterone and spironolactone in heart failure. N Engl J Med 1999;341:753.
13. Farquharson CAJ, Struthers AD. Spironolactone increases nitric oxide bioactivity, improves endothelial vasodilator dysfunction, and suppresses vascular angiotensin I/angiotensin II conversion in patients with chronic heart failure. Circulation 2000;101:594.
14. RALES: Pitt B, Zannad F, Remme WJ, et al. for the Randomized Aldactone Evaluation Study investigators. The effect of spironolactone on morbidity in patients with severe heart failure. N Engl J Med 1999;341:709.
15. Khan M Gabriel. Treatment of refractory congestive heart failure and normokalemic hypochloremic alkalosis with acetazolamide and spironolactone. Can Med Assoc J 1980;123:883.
16. Whelton A. An overview of national patterns and preferences in diuretic selection. Am J Cardiol 1986; 57:2A.
17. Hohnloser SH, Verrier RL, Lown B, et al. Effect of hypokalemia on susceptibility to ventricular fibrillation in the human and ischemic canine heart. Am Heart J 1986;112:32.
18. Clausen T. Adrenergic control of Na^+-K^+-homoeostasis. Acta Med Scand 1983;Suppl 672:111.
19. Farquharson-Roberts MA, Giddings AEB, Nunn AJ. Perforation of small bowel due to slow release potassium chloride (Slow-K). BMJ 1975;3:206.
20. Mahon FG, Ryan JR, Akdamar K, et al. Upper gastrointestinal lesions after potassium chloride supplements: A controlled clinical trial. Lancet 1982;2:1059.
21. Rodríguez JA, Godoy I, Castro P, et al. Ramipril vs. espironolactona en el remodelamiento ventricular izquierdo post-infarto: randomizado y dobleciego. Rev Med Chile 1997;125:643-652.
22. EPHESUS: Pitt B, Remme W, Zannad F, et al. for the Eplerenone Post-Acute Myocardial Infarction Heart Failure Efficacy and Survival Study Investigators. Eplerenone, a selective aldosterone blocker, in patients with left ventricular dysfunction after myocardial infarction. N Engl J Med 2003;348:1309–1321.
23. de Gasparo M, Joss U, Ramjoue HP, et al. Three new epoxy-spirolactone derivatives: Characterization in vivo and in vitro. J Pharmacol Exp Ther 1987;240:650–656.
24. Rocha R, Rudolph AE, Frierdich GE, et al. Aldosterone induces a vascular inflammatory phenotype in the rat heart. Am J Physiol Heart Circ Physiol 2002;283:H1802–H1810.
25. Sun Y, Zhang J, Lu L, Chen SS, Quinn MT, Weber KT. Aldosterone-induced inflammation in the rat heart: role of oxidative stress. Am J Pathol 2002;161:1773–1781.
26. Struthers AD, MacDonald TM. Review of aldosterone- and angiotensin II-induced target organ damage and prevention. Cardiovasc Res 2004;61:663–670.
27. Rajagopalan S, Duquaine D, King S, Pitt B, Patel P. Mineralocorticoid receptor antagonism in experimental atherosclerosis. Circulation 2002;105:2212–2216.
28. Suzuki G, Morita H, Mishima T, et al. Effects of long-term monotherapy with eplerenone, a novel aldosterone blocker, on progression of left ventricular dysfunction and remodeling in dogs with heart failure. Circulation 2002;106:2967–2972.
29. Zhang ZH, Francis J, Weiss RM, Felder RB. The renin-angiotensin-aldosterone system excites hypothalamic paraventricular nucleus neurons in heart failure. Am J Physiol Heart Circ Physiol 2002;283:H423–H433.
30. Barr CS, Lang CC, Hanson J, Arnott M, Kennedy N, Struthers AD. Effects of adding spironolactone to an angiotensin-converting enzyme inhibitor in chronic congestive heart failure secondary to coronary artery disease. Am J Cardiol 1995;76:1259–1265.

31. Korkmaz ME, Muderrisoglu H, Ulucam M, Ozin B. Effects of spironolactone on heart rate variability and left ventricular systolic function in severe ischemic heart failure. Am J Cardiol 2000;86:649–653.
32. Francis GS, Tang WHW. Should we consider aldosterone as the primary screening target for preventing cardiovascular events? J Am Coll Cardiol 2005;45:1249–1250.
33. Struthers AD, MacDonald TM. Review of aldosterone- and angiotensin II-induced target organ damage and prevention. Cardiovasc Res 2004;61:663–670.
34. Mottram PM, Haluska B, Leano R, Cowley D, Stowasser M, Marwick TH. Effect of aldosterone antagonism on myocardial dysfunction in hypertensive patients with diastolic heart failure. Circulation 2004; 110:558–565.
35. Macdonald JE, Kennedy N, Struthers AD. Effects of spironolactone on endothelial function, vascular angiotensin converting enzyme activity, and other prognostic markers in patients with mild heart failure already taking optimal treatment. Heart 2004;90:765–770.

SUGGESTED READING

Bauersachs J, Heck M, Fraccarollo D, et al. Addition of spironolactone to angiotensin-converting enzyme inhibition in heart failure improves endothelial vasomotor dysfunction: Role of vascular superoxide anion formation and endothelial nitric oxide synthase expression. J Am Coll Cardiol 2002;39:351–358.

Beygui F, Collet J-P, Benoliel J-J, et al. High plasma aldosterone levels on admission are associated with death in patients presenting with acute ST-elevation myocardial infarction. Circulation 2006;114:2604–2610.

Calhoun DA. Aldosterone and cardiovascular disease: smoke and fire. Circulation 2006;114:2572–2574.

Francis GS, Tang WHW. Should we consider aldosterone as the primary screening target for preventing cardiovascular events? J Am Coll Cardiol 2005;45:1249–1250.

Jaffe IZ, Mendelsohn ME. Angiotensin II and aldosterone regulate gene transcription via functional mineralocortocoid receptors in human coronary artery smooth muscle cells. Circ Res 2005;96:643–650.

Macdonald JE, Kennedy N, Struthers AD. Effects of spironolactone on endothelial function, vascular angiotensin converting enzyme activity, and other prognostic markers in patients with mild heart failure already taking optimal treatment. Heart 2004;90:765–770.

Mottram PM, Haluska B, Leano R, Cowley D, Stowasser M, Marwick TH. Effect of aldosterone antagonism on myocardial dysfunction in hypertensive patients with diastolic heart failure. Circulation 2004;110: 558–565.

Pitt GS, Pitt B. Aldosterone, ion channels, and sudden death: another piece of the circle? Am J Physiol 2006; 290:H2176–H2177.

8 Hypertension

RELEVANT KEY ISSUES

There are more than one billion individuals with hypertension worldwide, and only four classes of antihypertensive agents are available.

- More than 60 million Americans, 20% of the population, have hypertension that requires drug therapy. At age 65–75, however, more than 60% of individuals have hypertension. The incidence is higher in blacks. The prevalence of hypertension in industrialized countries in general is similar to that in the white population of the United States. Hypertension is the most common indication both for visits to physicians and for the use of prescription drugs in the United States.
- **Most important, we only have four groups of drugs (diuretics, beta-blockers, angiotensin-converting enzyme (ACE) inhibitors, or angiotensin 11 receptor blockers (ARBs) and calcium antagonists) to treat this most common condition** that leads to devastating events, particularly death and disability. I have purposely left out centrally acting agents (methyldopa and clonidine) and alpha-blockers because their use is limited to a few selected individuals.
- At the onset of my discussions, I must emphasize that ACE I/ARBs are excellent, well-tested, but mild antihypertensive agents, and that calcium antagonists are the most powerful of the four antihypertensive agents available for management of moderate and severe hypertension. We would be lost if these agents were not part of our antihypertensive armamentarium.
- ACE inhibitors and the identically acting ARBs are a major advance but represent a single class of agent.
- Calcium antagonists are not superior, however, to the two older classes of agents, beta-blockers and diuretics, when used as monotherapy to treat mild hypertension.
- *Alpha-blockers cause heart failure (HF) and are not recommended agents (1,2); they do not enter the equation, as discussed below.*
- *This is an appalling situation* because, in clinical practice, patients who cannot tolerate one or two of the four types of agents are frequently encountered, and many patients require two agents to attain adequate control.
- **Thus, drug choice is limited. This situation will change only if pharmaceutical companies and experts who formulate hypertension therapeutic guidelines will admit that after more than 50 yr of research and numerous randomized clinical trials (RCTs), we only have four classes of agents.** The recognition of the truth should promote more intensive research to discover new groups of agents to add to our present armamentarium of four groups.
- **In addition, the organizers of RCTs must provide sound methodology, which has been lacking in many such trials (see the later criticisms of RCTs).**
- For example, the beta-blocker atenolol is the main beta-blocker that has been compared with other agents. However, the non-lipid-soluble atenolol may not be as cardioprotective

From: *Contemporary Cardiology: Cardiac Drug Therapy, Seventh Edition*
M. Gabriel Khan © Humana Press Inc., Totowa, NJ

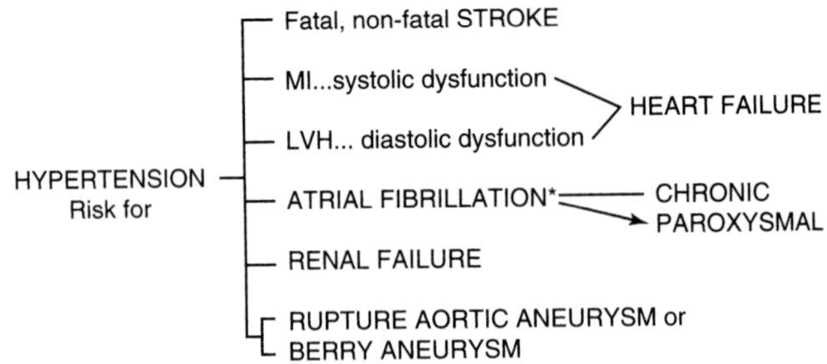

Fig. 8-1. Common detrimental effects of hypertension. *, not well appreciated: epidemic of atrial fibrillation with its management problems.

as metoprolol, timolol, carvedilol, bisoprolol, or propranolol, the only beta-blockers shown in RCTs to be cardioprotective *(1)*. *Beta-blockers have subtle and important* differences *(1)* (*see* Chapters 1, 2, and 9).

Consider the following:

- Hypertension is the leading cause of cardiovascular disease (CVD) morbidity and mortality.
- The prevalence of left ventricular hypertrophy (LVH) as a function of blood pressure (BP) have been proved. The incidence of myocardial infarction (MI) in Framingham subjects with hypertension shows a stepwise increase in risk as BP rises. In more than 40% of patients with acute MI, an antecedent history of hypertension is obtained. MI is a critical factor in the development of heart failure (HF).
- Renal failure caused by renal diseases is often nonpreventable, but that caused by hypertension is. The risk of renal failure is increased in patients with diabetes and in blacks.

Most physicians are cognizant of the aforementioned statements, but few are aware of the following distressing facts:

- Studies indicate that about 66% of elderly patients with HF had antecedent hypertension. The bulk of HF is related to hypertension and MI. The message is that effective hypertension control is the single greatest means to prevent diastolic and systolic HF (Fig. 8-1). *Importantly, diastolic HF has no effective therapy, and prevention is the key* (*see* Chapters 12 and 13).
- Hypertension is the most common underlying cause of atrial fibrillation, which is the most common sustained arrhythmia encountered in the office and emergency room.
- In North America, <33% of hypertensive patients have their BP controlled to goal.
- Drug therapy guidelines as recommended by the Joint National Committee (JNC) *(3)* and the World Health Organization-International Society of Hypertension (WHO-ISH) during 1990 to 2001 were meritorious but were subject to serious criticisms regarding their initial choice of agents. Also, their recommendations for patients with coexisting diseases required revision based on the results of the RCTs, as discussed later. Their newer guidelines are faulty (*see* later discussion).

This chapter discusses antihypertensive agents and emphasizes

- Which drugs are best for the management of mild hypertension in younger and older white and black patients. BP reductions caused by antihypertensive agents differ in different ethnic groups and in younger and older patients.
- Which drugs are best for patients with major risk factors, target organ damage, and coexisting disease: ischemic heart disease (IHD), diabetes, and hyperlipidemia. These three conditions markedly increase the risk of cardiovascular death. The risk of cardiovascular morbidity

Table 8-1
Major Risk Factors, Target Organ Damage, and Coexisting Disease

Major risk factor	*Target organ damage*	*Coexisting disease*
Smoking	Heart failure	Diabetes
Age	LV dysfunction	Hyperlipidemia
Men > 45 yr	LV hypertrophy	IHD
Women > 55 yr	Retinopathy	Angina
Family history of IHD or stroke	Renal insufficiency	Silent ischemia
Men < 55 yr		MI
Women < 65 yr		Previous CABG
		LV dysfunction
		Stroke or TIA
		Nephropathy
		Peripheral vascular disease

IHD, ischemic heart disease; LV, left ventricular; MI, myocardial infaraction; TIA, transient ischemic attack.

and mortality is determined not only by the BP but also by the presence or absence of these coexisting diseases, target organ damage, and risk factors (Table 8-1). **Thus, risk stratification is necessary for the formulation of appropriate antihypertensive therapy.**

- The author criticizes some important aspects of the JNC and British recommendations. Practitioners should be aware that committee recommendations are not always completely accurate. The results of RCTs indicate that the JNC and WHO guidelines for the management of patients with isolated systolic hypertension and hypertension with coexisting diabetes, IHD, and dyslipidemia are not logical.
- Answers to the calcium antagonist controversy. Are these drugs potentially dangerous? When are they considered appropriate agents for the treatment of hypertension?
- A new look at drugs for hypertensive emergencies.

DEFINITIONS

- The JNC has reclassified BP into three stages; stage 4 has been deleted (Table 8-2). When systolic BP and diastolic pressures fall into different categories, the higher category should be selected to classify the patient's BP status.
- Except when the initial BP reading corresponds to stage 3, the diagnosis of hypertension grading is based on an average of two or more readings taken at each of two or more visits during the next 1–8 wk, after the initial reading.
- In addition to classifying stages of hypertension on the basis of BP readings (*see* Table 8-2), it is generally accepted that systolic hypertension is as important as diastolic hypertension.
- The results of the Hypertension Optimal Treatment (HOT) trial *(2)* indicate that, in patients with diastolic BP mean 105 mmHg, it is safe to decrease the diastolic BP to <90 mmHg; further lowering to <85 mmHg did not result in a significant decrease in mortality or event rates but was not harmful. In diabetic patients, a decrease in diastolic BP to ≤80 mmHg resulted in a 51% reduction in major cardiovascular events compared with target group ≤90 mmHg.
- Stage 1 (mild) hypertension is common worldwide and affects more than 60 million Americans, with approximately 2 million new cases diagnosed annually.
- **Isolated systolic hypertension in older patients:** Approximately 64% of Americans over the age of 65 yr are hypertensive. Isolated systolic hypertension is defined as systolic BP > 140 mmHg, diastolic BP < 90 mmHg present in the absence of target organ damage and coexisting disease (*see* Table 8-1). Isolated systolic hypertension in individuals aged over 65 yr is a major cause of stroke, left ventricular failure (LVF), and mortality from IHD.

Table 8-2
Classification and Management of Blood Pressure for Adults[a]

				Initial drug therapy	
BP classification	*SBP[a] mmHg*	*DBP[a] mmHg*	*Life style modification*	*Without compelling indication*	*With compelling indication*
Normal	<120	and <80	Encourage		
Prehypertension	120–139	or 80–89	Yes	No antihypertensive drug indicated	Drug(s) for compelling indications[b]
Stage 1 Hypertension	140–159	or 90–99	Yes	Thiazide-type diuretics for most; may consider ACE I, ARB, BB, CCB, or combination	Drug(s) for the compelling indications[b] Other antihypertensive drugs (diuretics, ACE I, ARB, BB, CCB as needed)
Stage 2 Hypertension	≥160	or ≥100	Yes	Two-drug combination for most[c] (usually thiazide-type diuretic and ACE I or ARB or BB or CCB)	

DBP diasolic blood pressure; SBP, systolic blood pressure.

Drug abbreviations: ACE I, angiotensin converting enzyme inhibitor; ARB, angiotensin receptor blocker; BB, beta-blocker, CCB, calcium channel blocker.

[a]Treatment determined by highest BP category.

[b]Treat patients with chronic kidney disease or diabetes to BP goal of <130/80 mmHg.

[c]Initial combined therapy should be used cautiously in those at risk for orthostatic hypotension.

Modified from Seventh Report of the Joint National Committee on Prevention, Detection, Evaluation and Treatment of High Blood Pressure (NIH Publication No. 03-5233, May 2003).

- The prevalence of high BP in African Americans is among the highest in the world, and organ damage occurs earlier in these patients than in whites.
- In approximately 95% of individuals, hypertension exists without a known cause and is termed **primary (essential) hypertension**. In the remaining 5%, hypertension is secondary to known causes (Table 8-3).
- Proper technique for BP measurement is essential for adequate diagnosis and patient care.

NONDRUG THERAPY

Nondrug therapy should be tried rigorously before drug therapy in all patients with mild hypertension. Nondrug therapy—low-sodium diet, weight reduction, cessation of smoking, reduction in alcohol intake, removal of stress and/or learning to deal with stress, relaxation, exercises, and a potassium-enriched diet—may result in adequate control of hypertension in up to 40% of patients with stage 1 or isolated systolic hypertension in the elderly. In addition, low saturated fat intake is often necessary because of coexisting hyperlipidemia, which increases risk.

Table 8-3
Causes of Secondary Hypertension

Cause	%
Renal parenchymal disease	3
Renal vascular disease	1
Cushing's syndrome	0.1
Pheochromocytoma	0.1
Primary hyperaldosteronism	0.1
Coarctation of the aorta	0.1
Estrogens	0.4
Alcohol	0.2 or more

LABORATORY WORK-UP

- Complete blood count and platelets.
- Electrolytes, blood urea, creatinine, estimated GFR, and uric acid.
- Urinalysis.
- Serum cholesterol and high-density and low-density lipoprotein (HDL and LDL) cholesterol.
- Chest radiography and electrocardiography.
- Urinary and plasma metanephrine and normetanephrine if pheochromocytoma is suspected.

WHICH DRUGS TO CHOOSE

- The physician should strive for monotherapy in the treatment of mild primary hypertension whenever possible. If the choice of initial agent is based on age and ethnicity, about 45% of patients attain goal BP with monotherapy.
- The combination, however, of two agents at low dose may achieve the therapeutic goal with less potential for adverse effects.
- It is advisable to give a trial of individual agents before using combinations of drugs or fixed-dose combinations.
- The patient should have a thorough understanding of the problems associated with drug therapy to facilitate acceptance and compliance during medication changes.
- It is important for the physician to consider the efficacy and the pharmacologic and adverse effects of the antihypertensive agent to be chosen, as well as the cost to the patient and the ability of the drug to prolong life.

Recommendations for Patients Without Coexisting Disease

Mild Primary Hypertension in Younger Patients

There is abundant evidence from RCTs that whites and African Americans differ in their response to antihypertensive agents; see Fig. 8-2.

Recommendations for White Patients Younger than Age 65

It may appear old-fashioned to recommend beta-blockers and diuretics as first-line agents in the new millennium, but the scientific evidence gleaned from RCTs *(5)* reemphasizes their efficacy, safety, and costs (Figs. 8-2 to 8-5).

- A metaanalysis by Staessen et al. 2001 *(5)* and ALLHAT *(2)* indicates that new drugs are not more effective, they do not have more beneficial effects, and, importantly, calcium antagonists significantly increase the risk of HF (Fig. 8-4).

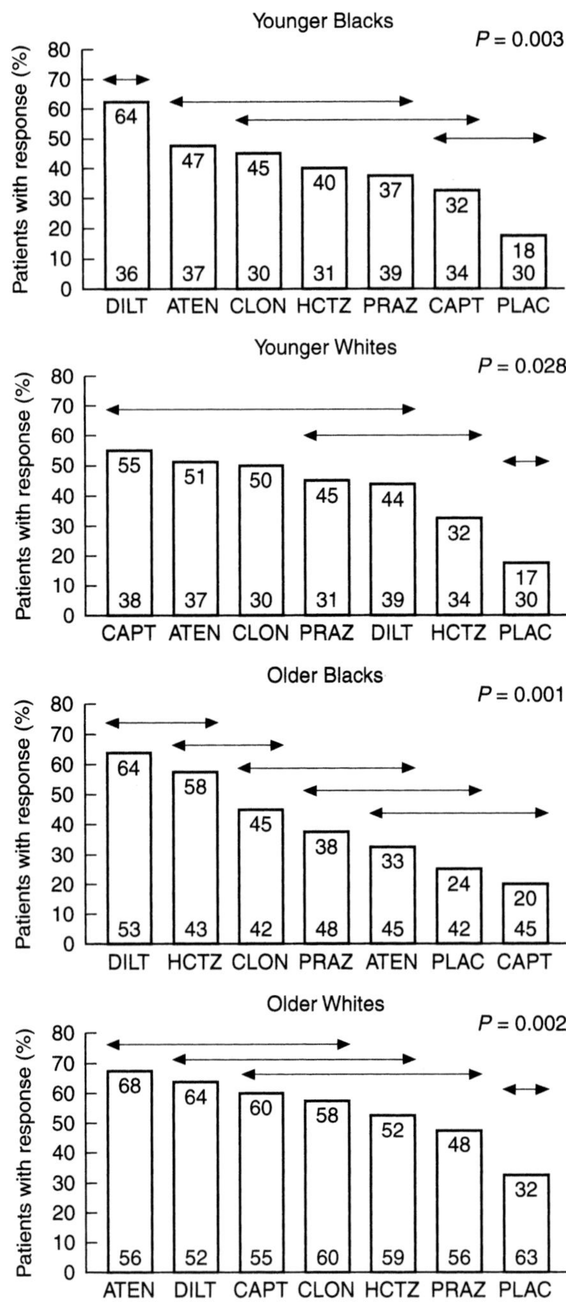

Fig. 8-2. Younger black patients, younger white patients, older black patients, and older white patients with responses in each of the study groups. The *arrows* group the drugs whose effects do not differ from each other by more than 15%. (From Materson BJ, Reda DJ, Cushman WC, et al. Single-drug therapy for hypertension in men: A comparison of six antihypertensive agents with placebo. N Engl J Med 1993;28:919; *see* Table 9-3 for corrected values.)

- Alpha-blockers increase the risk of HF *(2)* and have deleterious effects on the cardiovascular system. Thus, they have little or no role in the management of hypertension as emphasized in the second edition of this book in 1998. A warning was issued by the American College of Cardiology following the ALLHAT *(2)* findings in 2000.

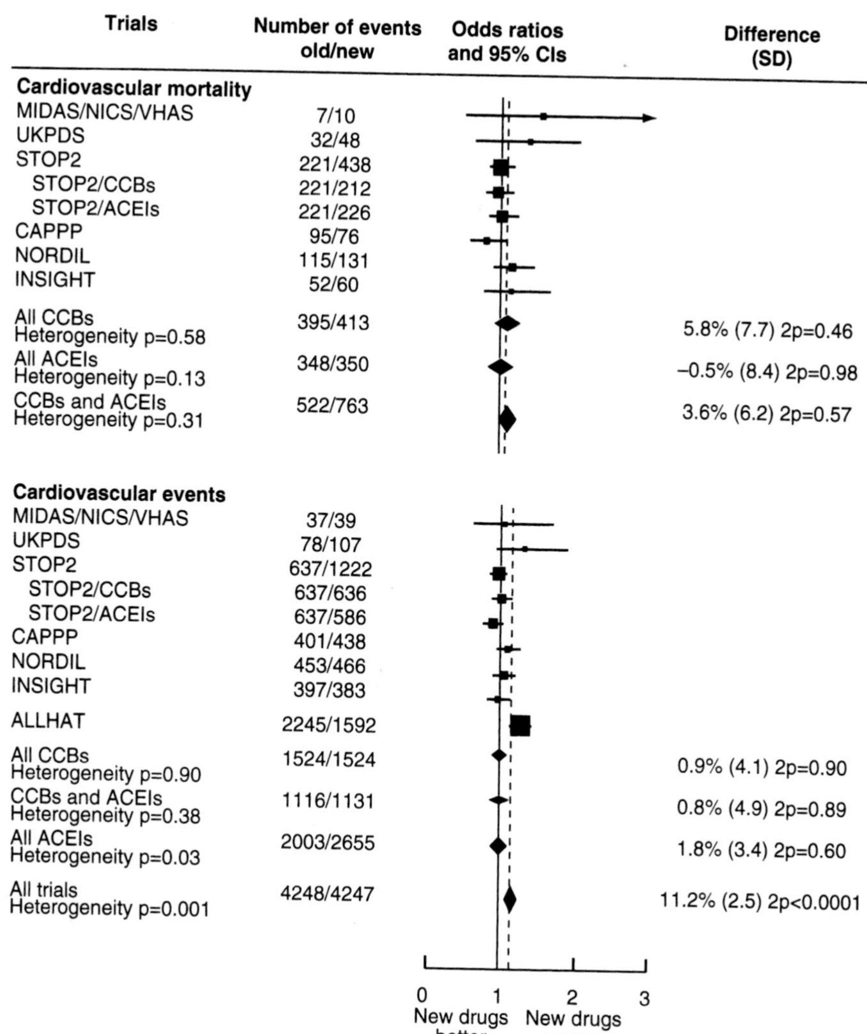

Trials
Number of events old/new
Odds ratios and 95% CIs
Difference (SD)
Cardiovascular mortality
MIDAS/NICS/VHAS 7/10
UKPDS 32/48
STOP2 221/438
STOP2/CCBs 221/212
STOP2/ACEIs 221/226
CAPPP 95/76
NORDIL 115/131
INSIGHT 52/60
All CCBs Heterogeneity p=0.58 395/413 5.8% (7.7) 2p=0.46
All ACEIs Heterogeneity p=0.13 348/350 −0.5% (8.4) 2p=0.98
CCBs and ACEIs Heterogeneity p=0.31 522/763 3.6% (6.2) 2p=0.57
Cardiovascular events
MIDAS/NICS/VHAS 37/39
UKPDS 78/107
STOP2 637/1222
STOP2/CCBs 637/636
STOP2/ACEIs 637/586
CAPPP 401/438
NORDIL 453/466
INSIGHT 397/383
ALLHAT 2245/1592
All CCBs Heterogeneity p=0.90 1524/1524 0.9% (4.1) 2p=0.90
CCBs and ACEIs Heterogeneity p=0.38 1116/1131 0.8% (4.9) 2p=0.89
All ACEIs Heterogeneity p=0.03 2003/2655 1.8% (3.4) 2p=0.60
All trials Heterogeneity p=0.001 4248/4247 11.2% (2.5) 2p<0.0001
0 1 2 3
New drugs better
New drugs worse

Fig. 8-3. Effects of antihypertensive treatment on cardiovascular mortality and all cardiovascular events in trials comparing old with new drugs. (Redrawn from Staessen JA, Wang Ji-Guang, Thijs L. Cardiovascular protection and blood pressure reduction: A meta-analysis. Lancet 2001;358:1307, with permission.)

- An RCT by Materson and colleagues *(6)* and the HANE Study *(7)* both indicate that beta-blockers are effective in younger whites (Fig. 8-2).
- ACE inhibitors are more effective than diuretics in younger whites. Recommendations are given in Table 8-4.

Recommendations for Younger Black Patients. Calcium antagonists are the most effective agents, followed by beta-blockers; *the latter may be tried first because these agents are safe and inexpensive and are particularly useful in patients with diabetes* (*see* the United Kingdom Prospective Diabetes Study Group [UKPDS] discussion in Chapters 2 and 22).

Mild Primary Hypertension in Older Patients

Recommendations for White Patients Older than Age 65. There is no sound evidence to support the WHO, JNC, and other national committees' choice of calcium antagonists

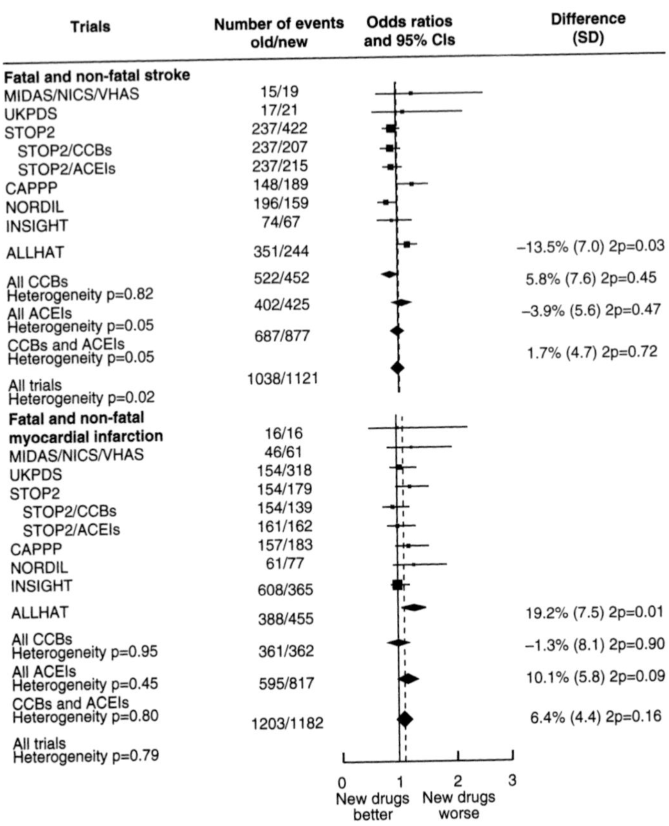

Trials
Number of events old/new
Odds ratios and 95% CIs
Difference (SD)
Fatal and non-fatal stroke
MIDAS/NICS/VHAS 15/19
UKPDS 17/21
STOP2 237/422
STOP2/CCBs 237/207
STOP2/ACEIs 237/215
CAPPP 148/189
NORDIL 196/159
INSIGHT 74/67
ALLHAT 351/244 −13.5% (7.0) 2p=0.03
All CCBs Heterogeneity p=0.82 522/452 5.8% (7.6) 2p=0.45
All ACEIs Heterogeneity p=0.05 402/425 −3.9% (5.6) 2p=0.47
CCBs and ACEIs Heterogeneity p=0.05 687/877 1.7% (4.7) 2p=0.72
All trials Heterogeneity p=0.02 1038/1121
Fatal and non-fatal myocardial infarction
MIDAS/NICS/VHAS 16/16
UKPDS 46/61
STOP2 154/318
STOP2/CCBs 154/179
STOP2/ACEIs 154/139
CAPPP 161/162
NORDIL 157/183
INSIGHT 61/77
ALLHAT 608/365 19.2% (7.5) 2p=0.01
All CCBs Heterogeneity p=0.95 388/455 −1.3% (8.1) 2p=0.90
All ACEIs Heterogeneity p=0.45 361/362 10.1% (5.8) 2p=0.09
CCBs and ACEIs Heterogeneity p=0.80 595/817 6.4% (4.4) 2p=0.16
All trials Heterogeneity p=0.79 1203/1182
0 1 2 3
New drugs better
New drugs worse

Fig. 8-4. Effects of antihypertensive treatment on fatal and nonfatal stroke and myocardial infarction in trials comparing old with new drugs. (Redrawn from Staessen JA, Wang Ji-Guang, Thijs L. Cardiovascular protection and blood pressure reduction: A meta-analysis. Lancet 2001;358:1307, with permission.)

for the management of isolated hypertension in elderly whites. Beta-blockers are as effective *(6,7)* and are safer and much less expensive. Beta-blockers are safe in patients aged 65–79 yr; and the safety and ability of these drugs to prevent HF and death have been endorsed in two RCTs: CAPRICORN *(8)* and COPERNICUS *(9)*.

In the excellent meta-analysis by Staessen and associates *(5)*, (Figs. 8-2 and 8-3), the authors concluded: "All antihypertensive drugs have similar long-term efficacy and safety," but *in the same article indicated that new drugs significantly increased the risk of HF*. HF is a common cause of morbidity, hospitalization, and death; effective control of hypertension is necessary to stem the epidemic of HF. In the Intervention as a Goal in Hypertension Treatment (INSIGHT) study *(10)*, among primary end points HF and MI were statistically more frequent in the Adalat XL group. In the Prospective Randomized Amlodipine Survival Evaluation (PRAISE) study *(11)*, pulmonary edema was more frequent in the amlodipine-treated group. In a non-Q-wave MI study *(12)*, diltiazem increased the risk of HF. These findings are not surprising because calcium antagonists possess significant negative inotropic effects. Elderly hypertensive patients are at a higher risk of HF and MI than younger patients; thus, although calcium antagonists are highly effective antihypertensives in the elderly, *beta-blockers, diuretics, and ACE inhibitors are*

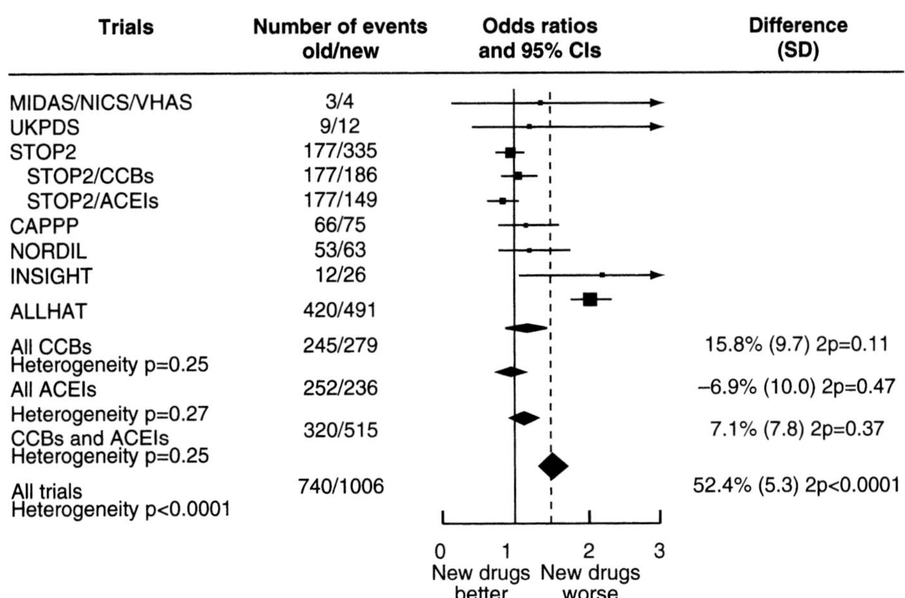

Fig. 8-5. Effects of antihypertensive treatment on fatal and nonfatal congestive heart failure in trials comparing old with new drugs. (Redrawn from Staessen JA, Wang Ji-Guang, Thijs L. Cardiovascular protection and blood pressure reduction: A meta-analysis. Lancet 2001;358:1305, with permission.)

preferred because these drugs have proved useful in the prevention and management of HF. The combination of ACE inhibitor and beta-blocker is not considered complementary, because these drugs do not enhance antihypertensive effects. However, they are both cardioprotective and deserve a trial.

- The JNC advises a diuretic, as preferred, based on the results of the Systolic Hypertension in Elderly Programs (SHEP) study *(4)*.
- In the SHEP study, atenolol was the second agent used, after a diuretic. After 5 yr of follow-up, IHD was reduced by 25%, with a major reduction in stroke. The Swedish Trial in Old Patients with Hypertension (STOP) *(5)* in the elderly showed a significant reduction in mortality and strokes as a result of beta-blocker therapy.
- A calcium antagonist, long-acting dihydropyridine (DHP), is recommended by the JNC as an alternative to diuretics based on the results of the Systolic Hypertension in Europe (Syst-Eur) trial *(6)*: nitrendipine, a long-acting DHP, was combined when required with diuretic or enalapril. The treated group showed a 42% reduced occurrence of all strokes; total mortality and cardiovascular mortality rates were not significantly reduced ($p = 0.07$; $p = 0.22$). The trial was not done solely with nitrendipine; follow-up was not sufficiently long to determine the absolute safety of DHPs in the elderly, who may have undetected IHD and are at high risk of HF and IHD events.

Recommendations for Elderly Black Patients. A diuretic and calcium antagonist have been shown to have better antihypertensive effects than beta-blockers and ACE inhibitors and are recommended. However, caution is required in patients with ejection fraction < 45% because the risk of HF may increase with long-term calcium antagonist therapy. Thus, *a diuretic is the first choice in elderly patients of African origin.*

The following RCTs are relevant to decision-making strategies in the elderly 65–80 yr old. Few patients over age 80 were included in RCTs to enable us to draw conclusions; a

Table 8-4
Choice of Drug for the Treatment of Mild Primary Hypertension Based on Age and Ethnicity*

White patients *younger than age 65*

1. Beta-blocker: bisoprolol, carvedilol, or metoprolol (Toprol XL) preferred over other beta-blockers: monotherapy success in ~65% in this age and ethnic category: *Warning:* avoid atenolol
2. ACE inhibitor: monotherapy success in ~62%; often requires combination with diuretic to achieve goal BP[a]
3. Diuretic: monotherapy success in ~32%
4. Beta-blocker or ACE I/ARB + diuretic
5. Calcium antagonist: success in ~58%

Black patients *younger than age 65*

1. Calcium antagonist: monotherapy success in ~70%
2. Beta-blocker (bisoprolol, carvedilol, metoprolol extended release [Toprol XL]): success in ~51%; avoid atenolol
3. Calcium antagonist + beta-blocker success in >90% (avoid verapamil)[b]
4. Diuretic: success in ~48%

White patients *older than age 65*

1. Diuretic: monotherapy success in ~68% (first choice because of safety)
2. Beta-blocker: carvedilol, bisoprolol, metoprolol extended release; avoid atenolol; success expected in ~72%; second choice because safer than calcium antagonists in the elderly[c]
3. ACE inhibitor: success in ~62%[a]
4. Calcium antagonist (avoid verapamil): success in ~72%

Black patients *older than age* 65

1. Diuretic: success in ~64%; preferred over calcium antagonist heart failure risk[c]
2. Calcium antagonist (avoid verapamil): success in ~85%
3. Diuretic + calcium antagonist

*Approximations from Materson et al. *(62)*; *see* Table 9-3. ACE I/ARB and beta-blockers: low efficacy in blacks; ARB preferred over ACE I in view of angioedema risk.

[a]PROGRESS only 42% goal BP achieved in mixed population *(9)*.

[b]Severe bradycardia risk.

[c]*See* Table 9-2; HF risk.

subgroup metaanalysis of RCTs in patients over age 80 indicated no treatment benefit for cardiovascular death and a nonsignificant relative excess of death from all causes. The calcium antagonist isradipine *(7)* caused an increase in cardiovascular events compared with hydrochlorothiazide (HCTZ), particularly in patients with diabetes. An RCT with nisoldipine *(8)* in patients with hypertension and non-insulin-dependent diabetes was terminated early because nisoldipine-treated patients had a higher risk of fatal and nonfatal acute MI than observed in the enalapril group: 25/235 versus 5/235 ($p < 0.001$). These results indicate that sustained-release calcium antagonists may increase the risk of cardiac mortality in patients who are at risk of IHD events, particularly in those with diabetes, dyslipidemia, and coexisting IHD and in the elderly with silent ischemia or undetected IHD. Long-term RCTs are necessary before DHPs may be considered safe alternatives to diuretics and beta-blockers.

Beta-blockers: The Swedish STOP 2 study *(13)* in the elderly showed a significant reduction in mortality and strokes as a result of beta-blocker therapy. Newer agents were not superior to beta-blockers or diuretics. *The beta-blockers used were atenolol and the noncardioprotective pindolol.*

Table 8-5
Reasons for Poor Drug Control of Blood Pressure

- Poor compliance
  Inconvenient drug dosing, e.g., b.i.d. or t.i.d.
  Inability to purchase drug (financial)
  Adverse effect of drug
- Related to drug
  Inappropriate drug selection or drug combination
  Interactions with NSAIDs, nasal decongestants, cocaine
- Volume overload
  Diuretic required
  ↑Na^+ intake
  Renal failure
- Weight gain
- Alcohol intake >4 oz/d
- Renovascular hypertension
- Other causes of secondary hypertension
- Cuff size
- White coat syndrome
- Pseudohypertension

Some RCTs used propranolol, a beta-blocker influenced unfavorably by cigarette smoking. Smoking interferes with hepatic metabolism of propranolol and decreases blood levels of this agent *(14)*. In the Beta-Blocker Heart Attack Trial (BHAT), propranolol failed to prevent fatal and nonfatal MI in smokers *(15)*.

Propranolol and oxprenolol lose their effects in smokers; metoprolol and timolol *(16)* have been shown to prevent fatal MI, nonfatal MI, and sudden cardiac death in smokers and nonsmokers.

In addition, the physician must be aware of the reasons for poor drug control of BP in the treated patient (Table 8-5).

RCTs of **ACE inhibitors** have not shown these drugs to be superior to beta-blockers or diuretics *(17)*. Importantly, *RCTs have indicated that ACE inhibitors rarely achieve goal BP without the addition of a diuretic. In the large PROGRESS trial (18), only 42% achieved goal BP; 58% required addition of diuretics.*

ARBs are as effective as ACE inhibitors; the absence of cough and angioedema and the better patient tolerance are advantages; angioedema is common in blacks treated with ACE inhibitors, and if costs are not a concern ARBs are preferred.

Therapy for Patients with Coexisting Diseases

In the presence of coexisting disease and target organ damage with comorbid conditions (*see* Table 8-1), agents are recommended as follows:

- *Angina, after MI, or suspected IHD:* Beta-blockers are strongly recommended. The JNC also recommends calcium antagonists, but the author qualifies this with the following statement: use diltiazem sustained-release preparation (e.g., Cardizem CD) or amlodipine if beta-blockers are contraindicated. Other DHPs are advisable only if a beta-blocker is being used in combination. A DHP used without a beta-blocker may increase mortality if unstable angina or acute MI supervenes.
- Atrial fibrillation or other arrhythmias: Beta-blockers and ACE inhibitors are strongly advisable. Hypertension is the leading cause of atrial fibrillation and HF (*see* Fig. 8-1).

Table 8-6
Rationale for Not Recommending $Alpha_1$-Blockers

- They cause an increase in cardiac ejection velocity, ↑ in heart rate. This action results in:
  ↑ in cardiac work and myocardial oxygen requirement
  Damage to arteries at branching points: may cause rupture of aneurysms. These agents are contraindicated in patients with CHD and aneurysms.
- They cause an ↑ in circulating norepinephrine and activate the renin-angiotensin system, causing:
  Na^+ and water retention.
  ↑ Risk for HF
  Their use often requires addition of a diuretic
- They may cause retrograde ejaculation
- They do not prevent or cause regression of left ventricular hypertrophy

From Khan M Gabriel. Cardiac Drug Therapy, 4th ed. London, WB Saunders, 1995.

- Aortic and other aneurysms: Beta-blockers are strongly indicated because they decrease ejection velocity and shearing stress in arteries; thus, they may provide some protection from rupture or further expansion of the aneurysm *(19)*.
- Diabetes type 2 without proteinuria: The JNC recommends diuretics *(20)*. In the Antihypertensive and Lipid-Lowering Treatment to Prevent Heart Attack Trial (ALLHAT) *(21)*, diuretics were as effective as ACE inhibitors and calcium antagonists in decreasing CVD outcome.
- Diabetic patients have a high incidence of MI and cardiac death; thus, both ACE inhibitors and beta-blockers are strongly recommended. The UKPDS study *(22)* showed beta-blocker therapy to be as effective as captopril in reducing the risk of macrovascular and microvascular complications in type 2 diabetes *(16)*. Importantly, glycemic control was not different between groups (*see* the UKPDS discussion in Chapter 1).
- Stroke or transient ischemic attack: BP must be cautiously reduced, if at all, in the acute stage. A beta-blocker or diuretic or combination is advisable. An RCT of perindopril 18 among 6105 patients with previous stroke or transient ischemic attack showed no reduction in the risk of cardiovascular events or stroke, but the combination with indapamide significantly reduced adverse events. In the large Captopril Prevention Project (CAPP) study of captopril versus diuretic and beta-blocker *(23)*, fatal and **nonfatal stroke was increased in the captopril group ($p = 0.044$)**, with no significant differences in other events. In addition, some captopril-treated patients required addition of diuretic to achieve goal BP.
- Dyslipidemia: During the years 1988 to 2001 prior to the results of ALLHAT, which indicated that the alpha-blocker doxazosin caused a high incidence of HF *(2)*, the JNC recommended alpha-blockers with no alternatives. Many internists agreed and promoted this fallacy.
- Alpha-blockers may increase cardiovascular mortality and have not been shown to prevent or reduce LVH. Alpha-blockers were recommended by the JNC because these agents do not unfavorably alter lipid levels, but alpha-blockers have undesirable cardiovascular effects and have not been shown to prolong life (Table 8-6). Patients with dyslipidemia are at high risk of IHD events. Because beta-blockers are strongly recommended by the JNC for patients at high risk of IHD events, these agents are the logical choice. *See* Chapter 1 for a discussion of the effects of beta-blockers on lipids. If beta-blockers are contraindicated, an ACE inhibitor and low-dose diuretic are advisable.
- Congestive heart failure (CHF) classes I–II and III: Diuretics plus ACE inhibitor plus a beta-blocker. In this subset, beta-blockers have been shown in RCTs to prolong life and to reduce the risk of hospitalization *(8,9)*. Thus, beta-blockers are strongly indicated for patients with LV dysfunction, ejection fraction 25–45%.

- Preoperative hypertension: Beta-blockers are recommended by the JNC. Atenolol *(24)* and bisoprolol have proved successful in RCTs.
- Renal insufficiency, except renovascular hypertension, creatinine clearance < 265 μmol/L, 3 mg/dL: ACE inhibitor plus loop diuretic is indicated, but a beta-blocker and/or calcium antagonist may be necessary to achieve goal BP; see later discussion of **metolazone**.
- LVH: Beta-blockers and/or ACE inhibitors are preferred. Avoid alpha-blockers. Calcium antagonists and alpha-blockers have not been shown to reduce LV mass consistently *(25,26)*.
- Liver disease: Avoid methyldopa and labetalol; the latter may cause hepatic necrosis *(27)*.
- Severe depression: Diuretics or ACE inhibitors are recommended; a calcium antagonist may be used in the absence of diabetes. Beta-blockers may increase depression, but this effect is rare and does not contraindicate the use of beta-blocker therapy if needed. Reserpine, methyldopa, clonidine, and other central alpha-agonists are contraindicated.
- Stasis edema or varicose veins with edema: Avoid calcium antagonists, particularly the DHPs.
- Renal vascular hypertension: Avoid ACE inhibitors and ARBs.
- Gastroreflux syndrome: Avoid calcium antagonists because they may increase reflux.
- Gout: Avoid diuretics.
- Sensitivity to sulfonamides: Avoid all diuretics except ethacrynic acid and amiloride.
- Severe peripheral vascular disease: Avoid beta-blockers; these agents are not contraindicated in patients with mild or stable peripheral vascular disease because these patients often have coexisting IHD, and beta-blockers may ameliorate symptoms and prolong life in this subset.
- Renal calculi: Avoid triamterene because this agent may precipitate calculi (*see* Chapter 7).
- Prostatism: An alpha-blocker has a role except when IHD or HF is present.
- Migraine: A nonselective beta-blocker is the most logical agent because vasoconstriction may relieve symptoms.
- Osteoporosis: Thiazides have been shown to increase bone mass *(28–30)*.
- Mitral valve prolapse: Beta-blockers are the obvious choice.
- Hyperthyroidism: Beta-blockers are recommended for the management of arrhythmias; propranolol is the most effective.
- Cyclosporine-induced hypertension: Calcium antagonists are of value.
- Pregnancy: Avoid ACE inhibitors and ARBs. Methyldopa, atenolol, or propranolol may be indicated at certain periods. For preeclampsia, a diuretic should be avoided. For eclampsia, hydralazine or labetalol is recommended (*see* Chapter 20).
- Subarachnoid hemorrhage: Nimodipine or a beta-blocking agent such as labetalol should suffice.
- Silent myocardial ischemia is commoner than nonsilent ischemia (angina): Beta-blockers are strongly indicated.

BETA-BLOCKERS

A beta-blocker is strongly recommended for the management of

- All hypertensive patients, white or black, aged < 70 yr with no coexisting disease (*see* Table 8-6).

Dosage

The dosage of beta-blockers is given in Table 8-7. In the elderly, it is preferable to start with smaller doses, for example, bisoprolol 5 mg, metoprolol succinate extended release (Toprol XL) 50 mg, carvedilol 12.5–25 mg, or timolol 5 mg daily. It is not advisable to use a dose higher than that given in Table 8-7. If BP goal is not attained, a low-dose diuretic should be added or the beta-blocker should be discontinued and the patient commenced on a diuretic or other agent.

Table 8-7
Doses[a] of Beta-Blockers

Drug	Before addition of diuretics (mg daily)	With diuretics (mg)
Acebututolol	300–400	400
Atenolol	50–100	25–50
Bisoprolol[b]	5–10	5–10[b]
Carvedilol	12.5–50	12.5–50
Metoprolol	100–300	100–200
Nadolol	40–80	20–80
Propranolol LA	120–240	120–160
Timolol	10–20	5–15

[a]Probable cardioprotective dose.

[b]Ziac: 5, 7.5, 10 mg bisoprolol with 6.25 mg HCTZ. (Atenolol is not recommended by the author.)

Action of Beta-Blockers

Beta-blockers lower BP by

- Decreasing cardiac output.
- Inhibiting the release of renin, thus decreasing angiotensin and aldosterone (*see* Chapter 1).
- Decreasing central vasomotor activity.
- Releasing norepinephrine from sympathetic neurons.

For other actions and salutary effects of beta-blockers, *see* Chapter 1.

Individual Beta-Blockers

Drug name:	**Metoprolol succinate**
Trade name:	Toprol XL
Supplied:	50, 100, 200 mg
Dosage:	50–200 mg once daily

Drug name:	**Metoprolol tartrate**
Trade names:	Betaloc, Lopressor
Supplied:	50, 100, 200 mg
Dosage:	50–100 mg twice daily

Toprol XL has a 24-h duration of action. A combination of Toprol XL and low-dose HCTZ 6.25 mg should be appropriate for the control of more than 80% of patients with stage 1 isolated hypertension. *Metoprolol tartrate* is given 50–100 mg twice daily.

Drug name:	**Atenolol**
Trade names:	Tenormin, Totamol
Supplied:	25, 50, 100 mg
Dosage:	the drug *is not recomended by the author; see* Chapter 9

Drug name:	**Bisoprolol**
Trade names:	Zebeta, Monocor, Emcor
Supplied:	5, 10 mg
Dosage:	5–10 mg once daily (rarely 15 mg) once daily

Ziac is a combination of bisoprolol 2.5-, 5-, and 10-mg tablets with HCTZ 6.25 mg. This combination showed response rates of up to 84% in two well-controlled RCTs. Ziac has been approved by the U.S. Food and Drug Administration (FDA) as initial therapy; Monozide 10 = bisoprolol 10 mg, HCTZ 6.25 mg, in the United Kingdom.

Drug name:	**Carvedilol**
Trade names:	Coreg, Eucardic
Dosage:	12.5–25 mg twice daily

DIURETICS

The Systolic Hypertension in the Elderly Program (SHEP) *(4)*, in which a diuretic was used in patients aged 65–85 yr, showed a 36% reduction in the risk of stroke ($p = 0.0003$), a 27% decrease in IHD event rates, and a 54% decrease in the risk of LVF. In the SHEP trial, a low-dose diuretic was used as initial therapy, and a beta-blocker was added if necessary. There is no question about the efficacy of diuretics in patients with mild to moderate hypertension, and, when they are combined with other antihypertensive agents, they can be used in all types and degrees of hypertension.

Recommendations for the use of diuretics are as follows:

- Low-dose diuretic therapy is strongly recommended as first-line therapy in older patients (age > 70 yr) of any ethnic group *(3,20)*.
- If the diuretic was not the first-choice agent, it is logical to add a diuretic if goal BP has not been achieved.
- Diuretics are highly recommended in patients with coexisting disease (*see* Fig. 8-6) for special situations, in particular in combination with ACE inhibitors for HF. Renal failure with increased volume overload is a common cause of resistant hypertension that requires the addition of a diuretic to enhance the efficacy of other agents.
- **Metolazone is a thiazide diuretic that has a unique property of retaining effectiveness when other thiazides become ineffective in patients with renal failure GFR < 30 mL/min. Dosage 2.5 to 7.5 mg daily.**

Drug name:	**Hydrochlorothiazide**
Trade names:	HydroDIURIL, Esidrex, Hydro-Saluric
Supplied:	25, 50 mg
Dosage:	12.5–25 mg each morning; max. 50 mg daily

The 50-mg dose was necessary to achieve control of BP in one study *(31)*, and it was commonly used from 1965 to 1985.

Action

The exact mechanism of action and antihypertensive effect are unknown, and the effect is believed to be related to decrease in vascular volume, negative sodium (Na^+) balance, and arteriolar dilation, causing a decrease in total peripheral resistance.

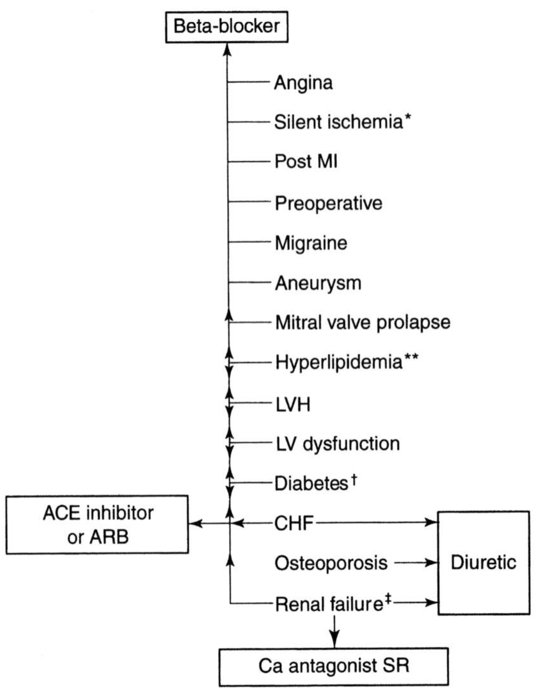

*More common than angina in men >50 yr.
**Statin and beta-blocker or ACE inhibitor, not alpha-blocker.
†Not prone to hypoglycemia.
‡Not renovascular.

Fig. 8-6. Choice of antihypertensive agent in patients with coexisting diseases.

Advice, Adverse Effects, and Interactions

Contraindications

- Hypersensitivity to thiazides or sulfonamides.
- Anuria or severe renal failure.
- Pregnancy and breastfeeding (*see* Chapter 20).
- Concomitant lithium therapy.

Adverse Effects

These include the following:

1. Dehydration and electrolyte imbalance are the most common adverse effects. The dose is too large if signs of dehydration or orthostatic hypotension develop, or if the patient has increased urea > 10.0 mmol/L or an increase of 7.0 mmol/L from baseline, chlorides < 94 mEq (mmol)/L, total carbon dioxide > 32 mEq (mmol)/L, and uric acid > 7 mg/dL (420 μmol/L).
2. Hypokalemia occurs in a significant number of patients receiving thiazides and contributes to increased risk of cardiac arrest *(32)*. Chlorthalidone causes a greater loss of potassium (K^+) than for equivalent doses of HCTZ. The incidence of hypokalemia can be decreased by the use of low-dose thiazide regimens with K^+-sparing diuretics. It is advisable to use the following:
   a. A thiazide-K^+-sparing diuretic, such as amiloride with HCTZ (Moduretic, Moduret), if renal function is normal: for patients aged < 75 yr, serum creatinine level < 1.3 mg/dL (115 μmol/L); for patients aged > 75 yr, serum creatinine level < 1.0 mg/dL (88 μmol/L).

b. If mild renal dysfunction exists, hyperkalemia may occur with the use of K^+-sparing diuretics; therefore, a plain thiazide is recommended without potassium supplements.

3. If the physician does not wish to use the combination of amiloride and HCTZ (Moduretic) or the combination of triamterene and HCTZ (Dyazide) when the serum creatinine concentration is normal, a thiazide can be used and the K^+ rechecked in months to evaluate whether the patient is a K^+ retainer or has a tendency to lose K^+. If the serum K^+ level is less than 3.5 mEq (mmol)/L, the deficiency should be corrected with potassium chloride (KC1) and the thiazide replaced with the combination of amiloride and HCTZ (Moduretic). The possibility of alternate-day therapy may be considered because the antihypertensive effect is significant and the risk of electrolyte imbalance is greatly reduced.
4. Gastrointestinal effects include anorexia, gastric irritation, intrahepatic cholestatic jaundice, and pancreatitis.
5. Central nervous system effects include dizziness, vertigo, paresthesia, and headache.
6. Hematology and blood disturbances include leukopenia, rare agranulocytosis, thrombocytopenia, aplastic anemia and hemolytic anemia; increased serum cholesterol, decreased HDL cholesterol, and increased blood viscosity.
7. Cardiovascular effects include orthostatic hypotension, low cardiac output, and arrhythmias from hypokalemia, especially if the patient is taking digitalis.
8. Hepatic coma may be precipitated, so do not use in patients with impending hepatic coma or moderate to severe hepatic dysfunction.
9. In diabetes, insulin requirement may be increased; latent diabetes may become manifest; rarely, hyperosmolar, nonketotic hyperglycemic diabetic coma may be precipitated. If the patient has ever had this condition, avoid all diuretics.
10. For use in pregnant or nursing mothers, thiazides cross the placental barrier, appear in breast milk, and can cause fetal or neonatal jaundice, thrombocytopenia, decreased vascular volume and placental perfusion, and acute pancreatitis.
11. Precipitation of gout and hyperuricemia is a well-known complication of all diuretics. If gout or hyperuricemia occurs, this is treated in the usual fashion, and the diuretic is discontinued. There is no reason to add allopurinol to the regimen to prevent further episodes of gout. This is commonly done and adds to polypharmacy and expense.
12. Thiazides decrease calcium (Ca^{2+}) excretion, but hypercalcemia rarely occurs.
13. Acute allergic interstitial pneumonitis *(33,34)* is an extremely rare, but life-threatening, complication.
14. Drug interactions with lithium, steroids, and oral anticoagulants have been reported.

Drug name:	**Bendrofluazide**
Trade names:	UK Aprinox, Berkozide, Centyl, Neo-Naclex, Urizide
Supplied:	2.5, 5 mg
Dosage:	2.5–5 mg daily

Advice and Adverse Effects

Recommendations are the same as for HCTZ.

Drug name:	**Triamterene and Hydrochlorothiazide**
Trade name:	Dyazide
Supplied:	Tablets containing 50 mg triamterene and 25 mg hydrochlorothiazide
Dosage:	1 tablet each morning

Advice and Adverse Effects

Contraindications are the same as those outlined for HCTZ; special note should be made of the following:

1. Triamterene is a K^+-sparing diuretic and is contraindicated in patients with past or present renal dysfunction or renal calculi (*see* Chapter 7).
2. The use of Dyazide (triamterene and HCTZ) is not recommended if the serum creatinine level is > 1.3 mg/dL (115 μmol/L) in patients aged < 70 yr. For patients > 70 yr of age, the lower creatinine value of not more than 1.0 mg/dL (88 μmol/L) should be used to prevent hyperkalemia. Do not use along with KC1, ACE inhibitor, or any other K^+-sparing regimen. Do not use with indomethacin: renal failure may be precipitated.

Drug name:	**Hydrochlorothiazide and Amiloride**
Trade names:	Moduretic, Moduret (C)
Supplied:	Tablets containing 50 mg hydrochlorothiazide and 5 mg amiloride
Dosage:	Half a tablet daily; *see* text for further advice

Dosage (Further Advice)

The manufacturer indicates up to four tablets daily. The physician must insist on a lower dose of diuretics. *A more appropriate combination, co-amilozide, available in the United Kingdom and Europe, contains amiloride 2.5 mg, HCTZ 25 mg.*

Advice and Adverse Effects

Do not use along with potassium supplements. *See* Chapter 7 for amiloride, Aldactazide, eplerenone, spironolactone, and triamterene.

Drug name:	**Furosemide; Frusemide**
Trade name:	Lasix
Supplied:	Tablets: 20, 40, 80, 500 mg Injectable: 20 mg in 2-mL ampule; 100 mg in 10-mL ampule

Advice and Adverse Effects

Furosemide is less effective than thiazides in mild to moderate hypertension, and therefore it is not advisable to use this drug unless the patient has significant renal dysfunction, such as a creatinine level > 2.3 mg/dL (203 μmol/L). Because furosemide inhibits the reabsorption of a very high percentage of filtered sodium, it is more effective than thiazides in patients with reduced glomerular filtration rate (GFR). As with thiazides, the combination with a K^+-sparing diuretic has proved to be useful in causing further diuresis and in reducing K^+ loss.

Ziac (US) or Monocor (UK) is a combination of bisoprolol 2.5, 5, and 10 mg with 6.25 mg HCTZ. This is an appropriate combination of a diuretic and a beta-blocker. BP is lowered to goal levels in about 80% of patients. This combination-type therapy with Ziac has shown consistently low discontinuation rates because of adverse effects, compared with enalapril.

Drug name:	**Eplerenone**
Trade name:	Inspra
Dosage:	25 mg once daily, max. 50 mg

ACE INHIBITORS AND ANGIOTENSIN II RECEPTOR BLOCKERS

ACE inhibitors and ARBs play a major role in the management of hypertension, particularly in patients with target organ damage and coexisting diseases (*see* Table 8-1). The major advantage of ARBs over ACE inhibitors is the absence of cough and very rare occurrence of angioedema; these agents are as effective as ACE inhibitors for the control of hypertension and HF. The failure of losartan, however, to control BP in scleroderma renal crisis with responsiveness to lisinopril has been reported *(35)*.

- In patients with target organ damage and coexisting conditions and special situations (*see* Table 8-6), particularly HF, LVH, diabetes with proteinuria, and selected cases of nephropathy (excluding renovascular hypertension), these agents are indicated. They are, however, not superior to other agents in diabetic patients, as is often claimed (*see* Chapter 9, Hypertension Controversies).

Action

ACE inhibitors prevent the conversion of angiotensin I to angiotensin II; ARBs block the effects of angiotensin II on blood vessel walls and do not interfere with the breakdown of bradykinin. These actions of ACE inhibitors and ARBs result in

- Arteriolar dilation, which causes a fall in total systemic vascular resistance.
- Attenuation of angiotensin potentiation of sympathetic activity and release of norepinephrine. The diminished sympathetic activity causes vasodilation, reduction in afterload, and some decrease in preload. Also, heart rate is not increased by these agents, as opposed to other vasodilators.
- Reduction in aldosterone secretion. The latter action promotes Na^+ excretion and K^+ retention.
- Blocking of angiotensin-mediated vasopressin release, which appears to be important in HF.
- Converting enzyme (the same as kinase II), which causes degradation of bradykinin. The accumulation of bradykinin stimulates release of vasodilator prostaglandins that contribute to the decrease in peripheral vascular resistance. Thus, indomethacin and other prostaglandin inhibitors reduce the effectiveness of ACE inhibitors.

Advice, Adverse Effects, and Interactions

ACE inhibitors retain K^+, so these drugs should not be given with potassium supplements or K^+-sparing diuretics, Aldactazide (spironolactone and HCTZ), Dyazide (triamterene and HCTZ), Maxzide (triamterene and HCTZ), or Moduretic (Moduret) (amiloride and HCTZ). Hyperkalemia may also occur with renal failure. Cough occurs in up to 20% of patients; angioedema is discussed in Chapter 3. Captopril causes proteinuria in about 1% of patients; this finding has occurred mainly in patients with preexisting renal disease who are taking doses of captopril in excess of 150 mg daily. Proteinuria caused by diabetes is not a contraindication because the drug has been shown to diminish proteinuria in some diabetic patients *(36,37)*. Adverse reactions reportedly include severe pruritus and rash in 10% and loss of taste in 7% of patients *(38)*, as well as mouth ulcers, neurologic dysfunction, and gastrointestinal disturbances. Occasionally, tachycardia, increased angina, and precipitation of MI may occur. Neutropenia and agranulocytosis are rare and occur mainly in patients with serious intercurrent illness, particularly immunologic disturbances, and in those with an altered immune response, in particular collagen vascular disease. Precipitation of renal failure in patients with tight renal artery stenosis has been reported *(39,40)*. Uncommon side effects include fatigue, Raynaud's phenomenon, cough and/or wheeze, myalgia, muscle cramps, hair loss, angioedema of the face, mouth, or larynx, impotence or decreased libido, pemphigus, hepatitis, and the occurrence of anti-nuclear antibodies.

Contraindications

The use of ACE inhibitors and ARBs should be avoided in the following clinical situations:

- Hypotension: systolic pressures < 95 mmHg.
- Moderate or severe aortic stenosis.
- Severe renal failure; serum creatinine level > 2.3 mg/dL, 203 μmol/L. If the use of an ACE inhibitor is necessary, alter the dose and dosing interval.
- Hyperkalemia or concomitant use of K^+-sparing diuretics or potassium supplements.
- Tight renal artery stenosis or stenosis in a solitary kidney.
- Immune problems, in particular collagen vascular disease and autoimmune disease; ACE inhibitors are necessary. Discontinue the following drugs, which alter immune response: steroids, procainamide, hydralazine, probenecid, tocainide, allopurinol, acebutolol, pindolol, and others.
- Patients known to have neutropenia or thrombocytopenia.
- Severe carotid artery stenosis.
- Restrictive, obstructive, or hypertrophic cardiomyopathies, constrictive pericarditis, cardiac tamponade, and hypertensive hypertrophic cardiomyopathy of the elderly with impaired ventricular relaxation *(41)*.
- Pregnancy and breastfeeding.
- **Women aged < 45 yr who may wish to become pregnant; these drugs should be avoided.**
- Chlorpromazine therapy because severe hypotension may occur.
- Uric acid renal calculi: Captopril increases uric acid excretion. The drug has been proposed as strongly indicated in hypertensive patients with gout or hyperuricemia *(42)*. However, excretion of increased uric acid may predispose to accretion of renal calculi. Further, the usual measures of alkalinizing the urine are not acceptable in hypertensive or cardiac patients; probenecid interacts with captopril and so may allopurinol.

Drug name:	**Captopril**
Trade name:	Capoten
Supplied:	12.5, 25, 50 mg
Dosage:	Hypertension: 12.5 mg twice daily for a few days and then three times daily for about 1 wk, and then 25 mg three times daily; max. 75–100 mg daily; *see* text for further advice

Dosage (Further Advice)

The 75-mg dose appears to be as effective as higher doses. Do not exceed 150 mg daily. A twice-daily maintenance dose is effective for hypertension. If the BP is not excessively high (systolic > 180 mmHg, diastolic > 100 mmHg), it is advisable to discontinue diuretics 24–48 h before commencing the ACE inhibitor and to restart them a few days to weeks later, depending on BP response.

In renal failure, increase the dose interval depending on creatinine clearance (GFR) (*see* Appendix II):

GFR 75–35 mL/min dose every 12–24 h
GFR 34–20 mL/min dose every 24–48 h
GFR 9–6 mL/min dose every 48–72 h

Table 8-8
ACE Inhibitors

Drug	*Trade name*	*Dosage (mg)*[a]	*Max/d (mg)*
Benazepril	Lotensin	5–30	30
Captopril	Capoten	25–100 (2)	100
Cilazapril	Inhibace, Vascase	1–5	5
Enalapril	Vasotec, Innovace	5–20 (1–2)	30
Fosinopril	Monopril	10–30 (1–2)	30
Lisinopril	Prinivil, Zestril	5–30 (1)	30
Moexipril	Perdix	7.5–15 (2)	15
Perindopril	Coversyl	2–8	8
Quinapril	Accupri, Accupro	5–40 (1–2)	40
Ramipril	Altace, Tritace	1.25–15 (1)	15
Trandolapril	Mavik, Gopten	1–4(1)	4

[a]*See* text: suggested maximum is slightly lower than manufacturer's maximum. (1), once daily; (2), two divided doses.

Table 8-9
Angiotensin II Receptor Blockers

Drug	*Trade name*	*Dosage (mg)*[a]	*Max/d (mg)*[a]
Candesartan	Atacand, Amias	4–10	32
Losartan	Cozaar	25–100 (1, 2)	100
Valsartan	Diovan	80–160 (1)	160
Irbesartan	Avapro, Aprovel	75–225 (1)	300
Telmisartan	Micardis	20–80 (1)	80
Eprosartan	Teveten	300–400 (2)	800

[a]*See* text: suggested maximum is slightly lower than manufacturer's maximum. (1), once daily; (2), two divided doses. Halve the initial dose in elderly patients and in the presence of hepatic or renal impairment.

Drug name:	**Enalapril**
Trade names:	Vasotec, Innovace (UK)
Supplied:	2.5, 5, 10, 20 mg
Dosage:	Hypertension: 2.5 mg once daily for 1–2 d, and then 5 mg increasing over weeks or months to 10–20 mg; max. 30 mg (rarely 40 mg); *see* text for further advice

Dosage (Further Advice)

Occasionally, the daily dose must be given in two divided doses to achieve 24-h control of BP. The usual recommended initial dose in patients not taking a diuretic is 5 mg once daily, except in the elderly or in those with renal impairment, and in suspected high renin states as seen with renal artery stenosis, prior diuretic use, and low-sodium diets. Here 2.5 mg is advisable. Note that the serum creatinine level may be normal in patients aged > 70 yr with renal impairment, and caution with dosage is necessary.

The dosages of ACE inhibitors and ARBs are given in Tables 8-8 and 8-9, respectively. The maximum doses given in these tables are approximately 20% lower than those stated by the manufacturer. The author does not recommend the use of the manufacturer's maximum for BP control. The goal BP should be achieved with approximately 75% of the maximum dose; if this is not achieved, the drug should be combined with a small dose of another agent.

For other ACE inhibitors, the action, pharmacokinetics, and adverse effects of ACE inhibitors, and ARBs, *see* Chapter 2.

ACE Inhibitor-Diuretic Combination

Capozide: 15–30 mg contains 15 mg captopril with 30 mg HCTZ for twice-daily dosage. These preparations carry the disadvantages of fixed combinations.

Vaseretic: 10–25 mg contains enalapril 10 mg with HCTZ 25 mg and is effective when given once daily. The combinations are not recommended if there is moderate renal impairment: serum creatinine level > 2.3 mg/dL, 203 μmol/L.

Hyzaar: This is a combination of losartan 50 mg and HCTZ 12.5 mg. This agent should not be prescribed as initial therapy but only after a trial of a diuretic or ACE inhibitor independently. This drug is contraindicated in patients with renal vascular hypertension.

CALCIUM ANTAGONISTS (EXTENDED RELEASE)

Calcium antagonists are recommended by the JNC for the following situations:

- In older African Americans or if diuretics are contraindicated or cause adverse effects (*see* Table 8-4).
- In younger African Americans if beta-blockers are contraindicated or not well tolerated.
- In older white patients with isolated systolic hypertension if beta-blockers or diuretics are contraindicated or cause adverse effects *(6)* provided that left ventricular function is normal.
- As second-line therapy in combination with beta-blockers or other agents in patients with angina or renal dysfunction.

The calcium antagonists are used with caution in the following situations:

- Patients with IHD, with silent ischemia, and after MI: diltiazem is indicated if beta-blockers are contraindicated. DHPs may be used in this subset of patients if a beta-blocker is being used concomitantly.
- Patients with hypertension and diabetes: RCTs have shown an increase in mortality in patients treated with extended-release calcium antagonists. The isradipine and nisoldipine studies *(7,8)* confirm an increased risk of IHD events caused by calcium antagonists in diabetic patients. ACE inhibitors and beta-blockers are preferred.
- Patients with HF, LV dysfunction, or ejection fraction < 45%.

Drug name:	**Amlodipine**
Trade names:	Norvasc, Istin (UK)
Supplied:	Tablets 5, 10 mg
Dosage:	5 mg, max. 10 mg once daily; initial 2.5 mg in the elderly

Drug name:	**Nifedipine**
Trade names:	Procardia XL, Adalat CC, Adalat LA (UK), Adalat XL (C)
Dosage:	30 mg daily increasing to 60 mg, max. 60 mg

DHPs cause a significant increase in sodium excretion, and a diuretic may not be necessary or may not lower BP further.

The rapid-release capsule of nifedipine is no longer recommended. The extended-release preparation has been used worldwide since the 1980s. The drug has a role in renovascular hypertension and in the perioperative management of pheochromocytoma *(43)*. Nifedipine and other DHPs may cause rebound hypertension. A case of an increase from 170/100 to 300/200 mmHg has been reported on sudden cessation of nifedipine therapy *(44)*. The INSIGHT trial *(10)* showed nifedipine equivalent to diuretic in preventing stroke, but it increased the risk of HF significantly.

Drug name:	**Diltiazem extended release**
Trade names:	Cardizem CD, Tiazac, Adizem-XL (UK), Viazem XL
Supplied:	Cardizem CD, Tiazac: 120, 180, 240, 300 mg
Dosage:	120 mg increasing to 240 mg daily, max. 300 mg

Diltiazem is a weak vasodilator, 50% less potent than DHPs. Caution is needed when this drug is combined with a beta-blocker because bradycardia or LVF may ensue. Interactions occur with digoxin and amiodarone. *A diltiazem-lithium interaction causing psychosis has been reported (45).* The NORDIL trial *(46)* indicated that diltiazem was as safe as a beta-blocker or diuretic, but there was a small increase in the combined end point of MI and HF.

Drug name:	**Verapamil extended release**
Trade names:	Covera-HS*, Chronovera*, Isoptin SR, Securon SR (UK)
Supplied:	120, 180, 240 mg
Dosage:	120 mg once daily, max. 240 mg. *180–240 mg daily; reduce the dose in liver disease, renal failure, or the elderly

Caution: Short-acting formulations are not recommended, Verapamil should not be used in patients with cardiomegaly or LV dysfunction. Also avoid in HF, conduction defects, and sick sinus syndrome. Constipation and bradycardia are limiting considerations, particularly in patients aged > 70 yr. Combination with a *beta-blocker is contraindicated.*

Drug name:	**Felodipine**
Trade names:	Plendil, Renedil
Supplied:	Extended-release tablets: 2.5, 5, 10 mg
Dosage:	2.5–10 mg once daily

Other calcium antagonists are discussed in Chapter 5.

CENTRALLY ACTING DRUGS

Drug name:	**Clonodine**
Trade name:	Catapres
Supplied:	0.1, 0.3 mg
Dosage:	0.1 mg at bedtime; increase to twice daily with a larger dose at night; maintenance 0.2–0.8 mg

Caution: Clonidine is contraindicated in patients with depression. Rebound hypertension can pose a major problem. **Newer agents have rendered centrally acting drugs obsolete.**

Drug name:	**Methyldopa**
Trade name:	Aldomet
Supplied:	125, 250, 500 mg
Dosage:	250 mg twice daily, increasing over days to weeks to 250 mg three times daily; max. 500 mg two or three times daily

Caution: This drug should be avoided in patients with active liver disease, depression, or pheochromocytoma. Hemolytic anemia is a well-known complication, and myocarditis causing death has been reported *(47)*. The drug has a role mainly in pregnancy (*see* Chapter 20) and in special situations as combination therapy when other agents have failed or are contraindicated.

ALPHA$_1$-BLOCKERS

The ACC has issued a caution regarding the use of alpha-blockers. The *author issued a caution in the second edition of this book in 1988.*

Drug name:	**Prazosin**
Trade names:	Minipress, Hypovase (UK)
Supplied:	1, 2, 5 mg
Dosage:	0.5 mg test dose, then 1–2 mg twice daily, max. 10 mg daily; *see* text

Dosage

Withhold diuretics for 24 h. For mild hypertension, start a 0.5-mg test dose at bedtime. If no syncope or other adverse effects occur 24 h later, use 1 mg twice daily. If a dose > 6 mg is used, a beta-blocker and diuretic are usually necessary.

Caution: Rare syncopal reactions after the first dose has been documented. Postural hypotension, dizziness, tachycardia, and palpitations with rare precipitation of angina have been documented. The drug is not recommended by the author.

Prazosin may cause

- Increase in heart rate.
- Increase in pulsative force and cardiac peak ejection velocity.
- Increase in circulating norepinephrine levels.
- Activation of the renin-angiotensin system.

Dosaxozin prazosin, terazosin, hydralazine, and vasodilators of this class do not significantly prevent or reduce LVH and have some nonbeneficial effects on the cardiovascular system (*see* Table 8-8).

Drug name:	**Terazosin**
Trade name:	Hytrin
Supplied:	1, 2, 5, 10 mg
Dosage:	Discontinue diuretics and give a daily 1-mg dose at bedtime, increasing if needed to 2 mg in a few weeks; maintenance 2–5 mg daily

The main advantage over prazosin is a half-life three to four times greater, which allows for once-daily dosing. The agent is widely used in men with benign prostatic hypertrophy. Caution is required in combination with calcium antagonists.

Drug name:	**Phentolamine**
Trade name:	Rogitine
Supplied:	10 mg/dL; as 1- or 5-mL ampules
Dosage:	IV: 10–20 μg/kg/min; average 5–10-mg dose IV repeated as necessary Infusion: 5–60 mg over 10–30 min at rate of 0.1–2 mg/min

Phentolamine and phenoxybenzamine block alpha$_1$-receptors and especially alpha$_2$-receptors. The drug is very expensive; action is rapid and lasts only minutes. Thus, nitroprusside is preferred for control of most hypertensive crises including pheochromocytoma.

Drug name:	**Phenoxybenzamine**
Supplied:	10-mg capsules
Dosage:	Pheochromocytoma: 10 mg every 12 h, increasing the dose every 2 days by 10 mg daily; usual dosage 1–2 mg/kg daily in divided doses; saline may be needed to prevent postural hypotension

The drug is given for 1–2 wk before surgical removal of pheochromocytoma. Postoperative hypotension may be avoided by discontinuing the drug several days before operation and limited use in selected patients. Beta-blockers may be added after 1 wk of alpha-blockade, but only if it is necessary to treat catecholamine-induced arrhythmias.

Contraindications

HF is a contraindication.

HYPERTENSIVE CRISIS

Hypertensive crisis is usually subclassified into either **hypertensive emergency or urgency**.

- *Hypertensive emergency* is defined as a severe sudden elevation in BP, generally diastolic > 120–130 mmHg; some clinicians add: and/or systolic BP > 220 mmHg. The systolic pressures should reflect a knowledge of previous BPs, such as a rise within days from 160–170 to >220 mmHg systolic; the rate of rise of BP in relation to previous BP is more important than the absolute BP. Most important, the sudden excessive elevation in BP should be associated with **acute** organ damage or dysfunction, which confers an immediate threat to the integrity of the cardiovascular system and to life.

In aortic dissection or acute pulmonary edema, a BP of 200/110 mmHg must be reduced. Conditions associated with emergencies are given in Table 8-10.

Emergencies require reduction in BP within minutes by intravenous (IV) therapy. The emergencies and the drugs of choice are given in Table 8-11; because these are rare occurrences and memory may elude the reader, I have provided a second approach (Table 8-12) that gives the drugs and their indications.

For hypertensive emergencies, the goal is to produce an immediate but modest reduction in BP. The objective, in most patients, is to achieve no greater than a 20% reduction from baseline of the mean arterial pressure or to reduce the diastolic BP to 110 mmHg

Table 8-10
Types of Hypertensive Emergencies

- Accelerated malignant hypertension[a]
- Acute coronary insufficiency
- Acute pulmonary edema (LVF)
- Acute renal dysfunction
- Aortic dissection
- Catecholamine crisis
- Eclampsia
- Hypertensive encephalopathy
- Subarachnoid hemorrhage
- Perioperative hypertension

[a]Severe elevation of blood pressure with papilledema and/or microangiopathic hemolytic anemia, or encephalopathy, or renal dysfunction.

Table 8-11
Hypertensive Emergencies and IV Drug of Choice as Listed

Emergency	*Drug choice*	*Caution or comment*
Accelerated malignant hypertension	Labetalol	Asthma
	Fenoldopam	Asthma, glaucoma, IHD
	Enalaprilat	Renal artery stenosis
	Urapidil (Europe)	
Acute coronary syndrome	Nitroglycerin + morphine + metoprolol	
Aortic dissection	Nitroprusside + beta-blocker	Hepatic and renal failure
	Labetalol	May not be effective if on alpha- or beta-blocker
Catecholamine crisis	Nitroprusside + beta-blocker	
	Labetalol + nitroglycerin if cocaine	
Eclampsia	Hydralazine	+$MgSO_4$ for seizures
	Labetalol, Urapidil	
LVF with acute pulmonary edema	Nitroglycerin + furosemide + morphine	
	Urapidil	
	Enalaprilat	Renal artery stenosis; crash hypotension
Perioperative or post-operative	Labetalol or nitroprusside	Clipping aneurysms, neurosurgical or ear surgery
	Fenoldopam	
	Nitroglycerin	Coronary bypass surgery
Renal dysfunction	Fenoldopam	
	Labetalol, calcium antagonist	

and no less than 100 mmHg over a period of several minutes to several hours depending on the clinical situation. The BP is maintained at this level for a further 12–24 h, at which time oral therapy should be instituted and a decision made as to the necessity for further lowering of BP. These guidelines do not apply in patients with aortic dissection, in whom

Table 8-12
Drugs and Indications for Hypertensive Emergencies

Drug	*Indication*
Labetalol	Accelerated malignant hypertension, aortic dissection, hypertensive encephalopathy, eclampsia, catecholamine excess, renal dysfunction, perioperative use
Nitroglycerin	Acute coronary syndrome, LVF, perioperative use, e.g., coronary artery bypass
Fenoldopam	Malignant hypertension, renal dysfunction, hypertensive encephalopathy
Nitroprusside	Aortic dissection[a]
Enalaprilat	LVF (but may cause crash hypotension)
Urapidil (Europe)	Malignant hypertension, hypertensive encephalopathy LVF, eclampsia
Hydralazine	Eclampsia
Nicardipine	Renal failure, malignant hypertension
Nimodipine	Subarachnoid hemorrhage
Esmolol	Aortic dissection with nitroprusside

[a]Newer drugs have displaced nitroprusside because of an arterial line is needed, fear of cyanide and thyocyanate, the need to shield the infusion and the patient, and the risk of coronary steal.

BP must be reduced to a much lower level along with the use of a beta-blocking agent to decrease the rate of rise of aortic pressure *(19)*.

Caution is necessary: nitroprusside and labetalol have caused precipitous reductions in BP in some patients, resulting in cerebral and myocardial ischemia and/or MI. A titrated reduction in BP with one of the agents listed in Table 8-12 is superior and safer than the widespread use of sublingual nifedipine, which has resulted in cerebral and myocardial ischemia and/or MI *(41,42)*. Sublingual nifedipine is not approved by the FDA in the United States. In countries where sublingual or oral rapid-release nifedipine 5–10 mg is still used, caution is necessary to avoid the medication in patients who are suspected of having myocardial ischemia, MI, or cerebral ischemia.

Hypertensive urgencies refer to other situations in which it is advisable to reduce markedly elevated BP within a day or two, rather than within minutes using oral drugs. These situations include

- Upper level of stage 3 hypertension: BP commonly systolic > 220 mmHg, diastolic > 120 mmHg; decrease to 180/100 mmHg.
- Presence of papilledema but without acute deterioration of specific organ systems.
- Progressive but not acute target organ damage, as outlined earlier for hypertensive emergencies.
- Rebound hypertension, for example, after withdrawal of methyldopa, clonidine, or DHPs. If stroke, decrease only to 180/105 mmHg.
- Refractory hypertension: patients in this category, with diastolic BP > 120 mmHg and no acute complications, should be tried first on oral antihypertensive therapy and sedation plus furosemide 40–80 mg IV initially; this is especially necessary if the history suggests that volume expansion is present; with renal failure, volume overload is usually present.

Drug name:	**Sodium nitroprusside**
Trade name:	Nipride
Dosage:	*See* text

Dosage

IV administration is given by infusion pump only. Take care to avoid extravasation. Wrap the infusion bottle in aluminum foil or other opaque material to protect it from light. The prepared solution must be used within 4 h.

One vial (50 mg) sodium nitroprusside in 500 mL 5% dextrose = 100 μg/mL.

Dose/kg	μg/kg/min	mL/kg/min
Average	3	0.03
Range	0.25–10	0.005–0.08
Dose for a 60-kg patient	mg/60 kg/min	mL/60 kg/min
Average	180	1.8
Range	30–300	0.30–3.0

Start the infusion at the lower dose range (0.5 μg/kg/min) and adjust in increments of 0.2 μg/kg/min, usually every 5 min until the desired BP reduction is obtained. The average dose is 3 μg/kg/min (range, 0.5–8 μg/kg/min). An alternative dosing schedule using less volume is given in Table 11-5.

Oral antihypertensive agents should be started immediately so that the patient can be weaned from nitroprusside as quickly as possible.

Action and Metabolism

Nitroprusside is a potent, rapidly acting, IV antihypertensive agent. The hypotensive effects are caused by peripheral vasodilation and reduction in peripheral resistance as a result of a direct action on vascular smooth muscle, partly through nitric oxide. There is also venous pooling. Because of vasodilation, variable reflex tachycardia occurs. There is a slight decrease in stroke volume and cardiac output. Myocardial oxygen consumption is reduced. The drug's effect on BP is almost immediate (within 0.5–2 min) and usually ends when the IV infusion has stopped. The brief duration of drug action is the result of its rapid biotransformation to thiocyanate. The ferrous ion in nitroprusside reacts with the sulfhydryl groups of red blood cells to produce cyanide ion, which is further reduced to thiocyanate in the liver, which, in turn, is excreted by the kidney.

Advice, Adverse Effects, and Interactions

Contraindications

- Hepatic failure.
- Compensatory hypertension, such as arteriovenous shunt or coarctation of the aorta; corrected hypovolemia or severe anemia.
- Abnormalities of cyanide metabolism: Leber's optic atrophy and tobacco amblyopia.
- Malnutrition, vitamin B_{12} deficiency, and hypothyroidism.
- Severe renal failure and inadequate cerebral circulation; caution is necessary in these patients.
- Pregnancy.
- Raised intracranial pressure.

Fatalities have resulted from cyanide poisoning. In the presence of liver disease, cyanide levels increase with evidence of metabolic acidosis, so it is necessary to measure cyanide levels. If kidney disease exists, thiocyanate levels must be monitored, especially if treatment is to be extended for more than 2 d. Acceleration of infusion from an accident or faulty equipment and failure to monitor the BP accurately have all been associated with hypotension and shock. Retrosternal chest pain and palpitations may also be experienced.

Methemoglobinemia has been reported. Hydroxocobalamin decreases cyanide levels and may be useful to increase the margin of safety. Rebound hypertension can be a problem.

Management of Adverse Effects

Amyl nitrite inhalations and IV sodium thiosulfate are used to treat acute cyanide poisoning. Nitrites form methemoglobin, which combines with cyanide ions to form relatively nontoxic cyanomethemoglobin.

Drug name:	**Fenoldopam**
Trade name:	Corlopam
Dosage:	IV infusion: initial 0.1 μg/kg/min, titrate 0.05 to 0.1 μg/kg/min at intervals of 15 min to 1–1.6 μg/kg/min (*see Suggested Readings*)

Action

Onset of action is within 5 min, and duration of action is 30 min, Unlike dopamine, fenoldopam (Corlopam) does not have alpha- or beta-adrenergic agonist activity. Fenoldopam is a peripherally acting selective D_1-receptor antagonist. The agent causes peripheral arterial dilation, and, importantly, significant renal, mesenteric, and coronary vasodilation occurs.

Advantages over nitroprusside include the absence of significant rebound hypertension and an increase in renal blood flow and lack of coronary steal and thiocyanate and cyanide intoxication. Unlike other dopaminergic agonists, fenoldopam does not cross the blood-brain barrier.

Caution: Fenoldopam contains sodium metabisulfite ME and may cause allergic-type reactions and may precipitate asthmatic episodes in sensitive asthmatic patients. *Avoid in glaucoma; the drug increases intraocular pressure. Also, avoid in patients with IHD because the drug may cause significant tachycardia that can worsen acute coronary syndrome,* and the tachycardia must not be treated with a beta-blocker. This drug is approved for short-term use, <48 h.

Drug name:	**Labetalol**
Trade names:	Normodyne, Trandate
Supplied:	Ampules: 20 mL, 5 mg/mL
Dosage:	20–80-mg bolus every 10–15 min; IV infusion: 0.5–2 mg/min

Dosage (Further Advice)

IV infusion of 20–160 mg/h (2 mg/min) under close and continuous supervision is given slowly to obtain the desired BP reduction. The onset of action is 5–10 min, and the duration is 3–6 h. The patient must be recumbent throughout the infusion and for at least 4 h afterward. The hypotensive effect may last 1–8 h after cessation of the infusion. Thus, labetalol is not as predictable as nitroprusside. Alternatively, bolus injections are used, starting with a 20-mg dose and gradually increasing the dosage every 10 min to a maximum of 80 mg.

Labetalol is a very useful drug for the management of hypertensive emergencies *(49)*. The drug is especially useful for crises associated with dissecting aneurysm, renal failure, hypertensive encephalopathy, eclampsia, and clonidine withdrawal, as well as in malignant hypertension and in some patients with pheochromocytoma. It is useful perioperatively and postoperatively, such as during neurosurgery for clipping aneurysms and in ear surgery.

Adverse effects include bronchospasm, nausea, vomiting, orthostatic hypotension, and, rarely, hepatic necrosis.

Drug name:	**Hydralazine**
Trade name:	Apresoline
Dosage:	10–20 mg; *see* text

Dosage

Hydralazine intramuscularly, but preferably by IV infusion, is indicated for hypertensive emergencies, particularly if the condition is associated with renal failure or preeclampsia. The recommended test dose is 10 mg followed in 30 min by an IV infusion of 10–20 mg/h, depending on the response. A maintenance dose of 5–10 mg/h is recommended with continuous monitoring of heart rate and BP. Oral hydralazine is commenced within 24 h, 100–200 mg daily. If there is no contraindication to beta-blockers, propranolol is given IV 1–4 mg and then orally 120–240 mg daily in addition (or the equivalent dose of another beta-blocker). Furosemide 40 mg IV followed by oral HCTZ or furosemide greatly improves the control of BP.

Hydralazine is contraindicated in patients with IHD and aneurysms, in particular dissecting aneurysm, because the drug increases cardiac ejection velocity and the rate of rise of aortic pressure.

Other agents have relegated the use of hydralazine to a role in patients with renal failure and eclampsia.

Drug name:	**Diazoxide**
Trade names:	Hyperstat, Eudemine (UK)
Dosage:	50–150 mg IV bolus injected undiluted and within 30 s directly into a peripheral vein; *see* text for further advice

Diazoxide has a small role in the management of hypertensive emergency associated with severe renal dysfunction if infusion pumps and intensive monitoring are unavailable to allow the use of agents listed in Table 8-8. The agents listed in Table 8-8 have rendered diazoxide *obsolete* for hypertensive emergencies.

Drug name:	**Urapidil (Europe)**
Dosage:	12.5-mg bolus followed by infusion of 5–40 mg/h

Urapadil, an alpha-blocker with serotonin-agonist activity, has a role in selected patients with hypertensive emergencies. The dose is 12.5–25 mg by IV bolus and then infusion at 5–40 mg/h. The drug does not increase heart rate significantly.

The time to onset of action is 3–5 min, and the duration of action is 4–6 h; adverse effects include hypotension, headache, and dizziness. The drug is a useful addition to therapy for accelerated malignant hypertension, hypertensive encephalopathy, and eclampsia, and, unlike fenoldopam and nitroprusside, it does not cause tachycardia or coronary steal and thus may be useful for LVF.

Other Agents

Nimodipine is indicated for hypertensive emergencies associated with subarachnoid hemorrhage.

Enalaprilat is advocated by some for LVF but must be avoided in acute MI, ischemia, renal vascular hypertension, and pregnancy. The drug's onset of action is 20 min and duration is 6 h. The drug may cause a precipitous fall in BP; nitrogycerin IV is preferred for the management of LVF; the addition of IV furosemide and sedation provide salutary effects.

REFERENCES

1. Khan M Gabriel. Hypertension. In: Cardiac Drug Therapy, London, WB Saunders, 1988.
2. The ALLHAT Officers and Coordinators for the ALLHAT Collaborative Research Group. Major cardiovascular events in hypertensive patients randomized to doxazosin vs chlorthalidone: The Antihypertensive and Lipid-Lowering Treatment to Prevent Heart Attack Trial (ALLHAT). JAMA 2000;283:1967–1975.
3. Sixth Report of the Joint National Committee on Prevention, Detection, Evaluation and Treatment of High Blood Pressure. Arch Intern Med 1997;157:2413.
4. SHEP Cooperative Study Group. Prevention of stroke by antihypertensive drug treatment in older persons with isolated systolic hypertension: Final results of the Systolic Hypertension in Elderly Programs (SHEP). JAMA 1991;265:3255.
5. Staessen JA, Wang Ji-Guang, Thijs L. Cardiovascular protection and blood pressure reduction: A meta-analysis. Lancet 2001;358:1305.
6. Materson BJ, Reda DJ, Cushman WC, et al. Single-drug therapy for hypertension in men: A comparison of six antihypertensive agents with placebo. N Engl J Med 1993;328:914.
7. HANE: Philipp T, Anlauf M, Distler A, et al. on behalf of the HANE trial research group: Randomised double blind, multicentre comparison of hydrochlorothiazide, atenolol, nitrendipine, and enalapril in antihypertensive treatment: Results of the HANE study. BMJ 1997;315:154.
8. CAPRICORN Investigators. Effect of carvedilol on outcome after myocardial infarction in patients with left-ventricular dysfunction: The CAPRICORN randomized trial. Lancet 2001;357:1385.
9. COPERNICUS: Packer M, Coats JS. Fowler MB, et al. for the Carvedilol Prospective Randomized Cumulative Survival (COPERNICUS) Study Group: Effect of carvedilol on survival in severe chronic heart failure. N Engl J Med 2001;344;l651.
10. INSIGHT: Brown MJ, Christopher RP, Castaigne A. Morbidity and mortality in patients randomized to double blind treatment with a long acting calcium channel blocker or diuretic in the international nifedipine GITS study: Intervention as a Goal in Hypertension Treatment (INSIGHT). Lancet 2000;356:366.
11. PRAISE: Packer M, O'Connor CM, Ghali JK, et al. for the Prospective Randomized Amlodipine Survival Evaluation (PRAISE): Effect of amlodipine on morbidity and mortality in severe chronic heart failure. N Engl J Med 1996;335:1107.
12. Multicenter Diltiazem Postinfarction Trial Research Group. The effect of diltiazem on mortality and reinfarction after myocardial infarction. N Engl J Med 1988;319:385.
13. Dahlof B, Lindholm LH, Hansson L, et al. Morbidity and mortality in the Swedish Trial in Old Patients with hypertension (STOP hypertension). Lancet 1991;338:1281.
14. Materson BJ, Reda D, Freiss ED, Henderson WG. Cigarette smoking interferes with treatment of hypertension. Arch Intern Med 1988;148:2116.
15. BHAT: β-Blocker Heart Attack Trial Research Group. A randomised trial of propranolol in patients with acute myocardial infarction, I: mortality results. JAMA 1982;247:1707–1714.
16. Norwegian Multicentre Study Group. Timolol-induced reduction in mortality in reinfarction in patients surviving acute myocardial infarction. N Engl J Med 1981;304:801.
17. Casas JP, Chau W, Loukogeorgakis S, et al. Effect of inhibitors of the renin-angiotensin system and other antihypertensive drugs on renal outcomes: Systematic review and meta-analysis. Lancet 2005;366: 2026–2033.
18. PROGRESS Collaborative Group. Randomized trial of a perindopril-based blood pressure lowering regimen among, individuals with previous stroke or transient ischaemic attack. Lancet 2001;358:1033.
19. Khan M Gabriel. Aortic dissection. In: Heart Disease Diagnosis and Therapy, a Practical Approach, 2nd ed. Totowa, NJ, Humana Press, 2005, p. 369.
20. The Seventh Report of the Joint National Committee on prevention, detection, evaluation, and treatment of high blood pressure. JAMA 2003;289:2560–2572.

21. The ALLHAT Officers and Coordinators for the ALLHAT Collaborative Research Group. Major outcomes in high-risk hypertensive patients randomized to angiotensin-converting enzyme inhibitor or calcium channel blocker vs. diuretic: The Antihypertensive and Lipid-Lowering Treatment to Prevent Heart Attack Trial (ALLHAT). JAMA 2002;288:2981–2997.
22. UKPDS: UK Prospective Diabetes Study Group. Efficacy of atenolol and captopril in reducing risk of macrovascular and microvascular complications in type 2 diabetes. BMJ 1998;317:713.
23. Hansson L, Lindholm LH, Niskanen L, et al. Effect of angiotensin-converting-enzyme inhibition compared with conventional therapy on cardiovascular morbidity and mortality in hypertension: The Captopril Prevention Project. Lancet 1999;353:611–616.
24. Mangano DT, Layug EL, Wallace A, et al. Effect of atenolol on mortality and cardiovascular morbidity after non-cardiac surgery. N Engl J Med 1996;335:1713.
25. Devereux RB. Do antihypertensive drugs differ in their ability to regress left ventricular hypertrophy? Circulation 1985;95:1983.
26. Dunn FG, Venture HO, Messerli FH, et al. Time course of regression of left ventricular hypertrophy in hypertensive patients treated with atenolol. Circulation 1987;76:243.
27. Clark JA, Zimmerman HF, Tanner LA. Labetalol hepatotoxicity. Ann Intern Med 1990;113:210.
28. Felson DT, Sloutskis D, Anderson J, et al. Thiaxide diuretics and the risk of hip fracture. JAMA 1991; 265:370.
29. LaCroix AZ, Wienpahl J, White LR, et al. Thiazide diuretic agents and the incidence of hip fracture. N Engl J Med 1990;322:288.
30. Ray WA, Griffin Downey W. Long-term use of thiazide diuretics and risk of hip fracture. Lancet 1989;1: 687.
31. Magee PF, Freis ED. Is low-dose hydrochlorothiazide effective? Hypertension 1986;8:III35.
32. Siscovick DS, Raghanathan TE, Psaty BM, et al. Diuretic therapy for hypertension and the risk of primary cardiac arrest. N Engl J Med 1994;330:1852.
33. Biron P, Dessureault J, Napke E. Acute allergic interstitial pneumonitis induced by hydrochlorothiazide. Can Med Assoc J 1991;145:28.
34. Hoegholm A, Rasmussen SW, Kristensen KS. Pulmonary oedema with shock induced by hydrochlorothiazide: A rare side effect mimicking myocardial infarction. Br Heart J 1990;63:186.
35. Caskey FJ, Thacker EJ, Johnston PA, et al. Failure of losartan to control blood pressure in scleroderma renal crisis. Lancet 1997;349:620.
36. Hommel E, Parving Hans H, Mathiesen E, et al. Effect of captopril on kidney function in insulin-dependent diabetic patients with nephropathy. BMJ 1986;293:467.
37. Taguma Y, Kitamoro Y, Futaki G, et al. Effect of captopril on heavy proteinuria in azotemic diabetics. N Engl J Med 1985;313:1617.
38. Jenkins AC, Dreslinski GR, Tadros SS, et al. Captopril in hypertension: Seven years later. J Cardiovasc Pharmacol 1985;7:596.
39. Hricik DE, Browning PJ, Kopelman R, et al: Captopril-induced functional renal insufficiency in patients with bilateral renal-artery stenoses or renal-artery stenosis in a solitary kidney. N Engl J Med 1983;308: 373.
40. Greminger P, Vetter H, Steurer T, et al. Captopril and kidney function in renovascular and essential hypertension. Nephron 1986;4(Suppl 1):91.
41. Topol EJ, Thomas AT, Fortuin NJ. Hypertensive hypertrophic cardiomyopathy of the elderly. N Engl J Med 1985;312:277.
42. Leary WP, Reyes AJ. Angiotensin I converting enzyme inhibitors and the renal excretion of urate. Cardiovasc Drugs Ther 1987;1:29.
43. Chimori K, Miyazaki S, Nakajima T, et al. Preoperative management of pheochromocytoma with the calcium antagonist nifedipine. Clin Ther 1985;7:372.
44. Bursztyn M, Tordjman K, Grossman E, et al. Hypertensive crisis associated with nifedipine withdrawal. Arch Intern Med 1986;146:397.
45. Binder EF, Cayabyab L, Ritchie DJ, et al. Diltiazem-induced psychosis and a possible diltiazem-lithium interaction. Arch Intern Med 1991;151:373.
46. NORDIL: Hansson L, Hedner T, Lund-Johansen P, et al. Randomized trial of effects of calcium antagonists compared with diuretics and beta-blockers on cardiovascular morbidity and mortality in hypertension: The Nordic Diltiazem study. Lancet 2000;356:359.
47. Seeverens H, de Bruin CD, Jordans JGM. Myocarditis and methyldopa. Acta Med Scand 1982;211–233.
48. Wright JT Jr, Wilson DJ, Goodman RP, et al. Labetalol fay continuous infusion in severe hypertension. J Clin Hypertens 1986;2:39.

49. Murphy MB, Murray C, Shorten G. Fenoldopam: A selective peripheral dopamine-receptor agonist for the treatment of severe hypertension: Review article. N Engl J Med 2001;345:1548.

SUGGESTED READING

Brook RD. How to achieve control in managing hypertension. J Am Coll Cardiol Curr Rev May/June:35, 2002.

ALLHAT: Davis BR, Piller LB, Cutler JA, et al. for the Antihypertensive and Lipid-Lowering Treatment to Prevent Heart Attack Trial (ALLHAT) Collaborative Research Group. Role of diuretics in the prevention of heart failure: The Antihypertensive and Lipid-Lowering Treatment to Prevent Heart Attack Trial. Circulation 2006;113:2201–2210.

Grossman E, Messerli FH. The management of hypertensive crisis. Am Coll Cardiol Curr J Rev Jan/Feb, 1999.

Gueffier F, Bulpitt C, Biossel JP, et al. for the INDIANA GROUP. Antihypertensive drugs in very old people: A subgroup meta-analysis of randomized controlled trials. Lancet 1999;353:793.

Materson BJ, Reda DJ. Correction: single-drug therapy for hypertension in men. N Engl J Med 1994;330: 1689.

Messerli FH, Re RN. Do we need yet another blocker of the renin-angiotensin system? J Am Coll Cardiol 2007;49:1164–1165.

Murphy MB, Murray C, Shorten G. Fenoldopam—a selective peripheral dopamine-receptor agonist for the treatment of severe hypertension: Review article. N Engl J Med 2001;345:1548.

Oh Byung-Hee, Mitchell J, Herron JR, et al. Aliskiren, an oral renin inhibitor, provides dose-dependent efficacy and sustained 24-h blood pressure control in patients with hypertension. J Am Coll Cardiol 2007;49: 1157–1163.

Rahman M, Pressel S, Davis BR, et al. for the ALLHAT Collaborative Research Group. Cardiovascular outcomes in high-risk hypertensive patients stratified by baseline glomerular filtration rate. Ann Inter Med 2006;144:172–180.

Yusuf S. Preventing vascular events due to elevated blood pressure. Circulation 2006;113:2166–2168.

9 Hypertension Controversies

BETA-BLOCKERS SHOULD NOT REMAIN FIRST CHOICE IN THE TREATMENT OF PRIMARY HYPERTENSION: TRUE OR FALSE?

This statement is printed on the front cover of *The Lancet* of October 29, 2005. It is surprising that this peer-reviewed journal would print such a misleading statement.

- The quote was based on a metaanalysis by Lindholm et al., who concluded that beta-blockers should not remain first choice in the treatment of primary hypertension and should not be used as reference drugs in future randomized controlled trials (RCTs) of hypertension *(1)*. Unfortunately, many experts in the field have endorsed the conclusions of this faulty meta-analysis.

Beta-blockers have been used for more than 35 yr for the treatment of hypertension. The controversy regarding their continued use is of paramount importance, particularly because there are more than 1 billion hypertensive individuals who require treatment, and only four classes of antihypertensive agents are available: beta-blockers, diuretics, calcium antagonists, and angiotensin-converting enzyme (ACE) inhibitors or angiotensin receptor blockers (ARBs). The two other drug classes (alpha blockers [doxazosin] and centrally acting agents [methyldopa, clonidine]) have been rendered relatively obsolete for the management of primary hypertension (*see* later discussion and alpha-blocker section in Chapter 8). Methyl dopa remains useful mainly for hypertension in pregnancy.

- In 14 studies analyzed by Lindholm et al., atenolol was the beta-blocker used; in four trials, mixtures of atenolol, metoprolol, and pindolol were used (*see* Table 9-1).
- **In a *Lancet* letter, Cruickshank stated that by lumping together all randomized hypertension trials involving beta-blockers, Lars Lindholm and colleagues have arrived at misleading conclusions *(2)*, and I concur with this statement.**

This discussion reviews trials selected by Lindholm and colleagues and emphasizes that the metaanalysis suggests that atenolol is not an effective choice for the management of hypertension but does not indicate that other beta-blockers are ineffective in decreasing cardiovascular disease (CVD) morbidity and mortality associated with hypertension.

- The reasons for the ineffectiveness of atenolol and the subtle differences that prevail among the available beta-blocking drugs are discussed.
- In addition, in the RCTs analyzed, atenolol monotherapy, or calcium antagonist, ACE inhibitor monotherapy was the therapy in <45% of treated individuals. Comparisons of subgroups are fraught with danger.

Trials selected for metaanalysis by Lindholm et al. include the following:

From: *Contemporary Cardiology: Cardiac Drug Therapy, Seventh Edition*
M. Gabriel Khan © Humana Press Inc., Totowa, NJ

Table 9-1
Clinical Trials Assessed in the Metaanalysis by Lindholm et al. *(1)* and Relevant Effects

Trial	*No. of patients (yr of follow-up)*	*Total mortality*	*Stroke*	*Myocardial infarction*
MRC 1985 *(8)*	8700			
Propranolol[a]				
vs placebo		120 vs 253	42 vs 109	103 vs 234
		RR 0.93	RR 0.76	RR 0.87
vs diuretic		120 vs 128	42 vs 18	103 vs 119
		RR 0.91	RR 2.28	RR 0.84
MRC[b] 1992 *(12)*	4396			
Atenolol vs diuretic	(5.8)	—[c]	—[c]	—[c]
IPPSH *(3)*	6357	108 vs 114	45 vs 46	96 vs 104
Oxprenolol[d] vs placebo	(4)	RR 0.94	RR 0.97	RR 0.92
Berglund *(4)*	106	5 vs 4	—	—
Propranolol vs diuretic	(10)	NS		
Yurenev *(5)*	304	1 vs 7	6 vs 11	7 vs 6
Propranolol vs non-beta-blocker	(4)	RR 0.15	RR 0.56	RR 1.2
Dutch TIA *(6)*	1473	64 vs 58	52 vs 62	45 vs 40
Atenolol vs placebo	(2.6)	RR 1.12	RR 0.85	RR 1.14
UKPDS *(41)*	758	59 vs 75	17 vs 21	46 vs 61
Atenolol vs captopril	(9)[d]	RR 0.88	RR 0.90	RR 0.84[e]
LIFE *(43)*	9193	431 vs 383	309 vs 232	188 vs 198
Atenolol vs losartan	(4.8)	RR 1.13	RR 1.34	RR 0.95
ASCOT-BPLA *(25)*	19,257	820 vs 738	422 vs 327	444 vs 390
Atenolol + diuretic	(5.7)	RR 1.11	RR 1.29	RR 1.1[f]
Amlodipine + perindopril				
STOP-2 *(7)*	6614	369 vs 742	237 vs 422	154 vs 318
Atenolol		RR 0.99	RR 1.12	RR 0.96
Pindolol[d]				
Metoprolol	2213			
vs ACE inhibitor	(5)			
or	2205			
calcium antagonist	2196			
NORDIL *(46)*	10,881	228 vs 221	196 vs 159	157 vs 183
Any beta-blocker vs diltiazem	(4.5)	RR 0.98	RR 1.22	RR 0.85[e]
CONVINCE *(14)*	16,476	319 vs 337	118 vs 133	166 vs 133
Atenolol vs verapamil	(3)	RR 0.93	NS	RR 1.23[g]
Not assessed by Lindholm et al.				
CAPP *(47)*	10,985	82 vs 95	193 vs 149	163 vs 164
Captopril vs atenolol or metoprolol	(6)	NS	RR 1.25[h]	NS

Abbreviations: ACE, angiotensin-converting enzyme; NS, not significant; RR, relative risk.
[a]Not effective in smokers; *see* text.
[b]Poorly run RCT; 25% lost to follow-up; *see* text.
[c]The only long-term RCT in diabetics, high-risk patients; beta-blocker = to captopril.
[d]Has intrinsic sympathomimetic activity (ISA): destroys cardioprotection.
[e]Marked significant reduction in fatal and nonfatal myocardial infarction (MI) in high-risk diabetic patients compared with captopril; surely a diuretic cannot outperform a beta-blocker in preventing coronary heart disease (CHD) events in any group of patients; trials that indicate this superior effect of diuretics are obscure: only observed in the poorly run MRC trials. In NORDIL, beta-blocker better than diltiazem for CHD events.
[f]Primary end point.
[g]Verapamil caused a 30% increase in congestive heart failure.
[h]Captopril caused a 29.5% increase in fatal and nonfatal strokes vs beta-blocker; the opposite effect occurred in LIFE.

1. The International Prospective Primary Prevention Study in Hypertension (IPPSH): Oxprenolol was used *(3)*. The drug has intrinsic sympathomimetic activity (ISA), which renders it noncardioprotective; thus all beta-blockers cannot be blamed for a poor choice of oxprenolol. Worldwide, this drug is used rarely if at all.
2. Berglund et al. *(4)*, Yurenev et al. *(5)*, and TEST *(6)*: These investigators studied only 106, 304, and 720 patients, respectively. Should clinicians accept this type of metaanalysis of apples and oranges?
3. The Swedish Trial of Old Patients-2 (STOP-2) *(7)*: In 6614 elderly hypertensive patients, a diuretic or beta-blocker (atenolol, metoprolol, and pindolol, an ISA beta-blocker) or both were compared with newer drugs: ACE inhibitors (enalapril, lisinopril) or calcium antagonists (felodipine or isradipine). The findings at 6 yr were as follows: old and newer antihypertensive drugs were similar in prevention of cardiovascular mortality or events At the final visit, only 61–66% of patients were still taking the agents allocated to them and this was not a comparative beta-blocker trial.
4. Medical Research Council (MRC) 1985 trial *(8)*: For mild hypertension, propranolol was the beta-blocker used compared with diuretic therapy. Propranolol, but not diuretics, reduced the risk of myocardial infarction by 13%, which increased to a significant 18% when silent infarctions were included. In a subsequent subanalysis compared with placebo, the reduction in nonsmokers was 33%. Nonsmokers given propranolol showed a trend toward reduction in coronary events and significant decrease in strokes; the diuretic bendrofluazide showed a reduction in strokes but not in coronary events. A *Lancet* editorial considered the possibility that beta-blockers were preferable in nonsmoking men *(9)*. The expert author of the editorial did not know that the cardioprotective effects of beta-blockers other than propranolol are not decreased by cigarette smoking.

   Cigarette smoke increases the rate of metabolic degradation of propranolol, and a decrease in plasma propranolol levels has been shown in smokers; timolol, a partially metabolized drug has been shown to be effective in reducing deaths *(10)* in smokers and nonsmokers. **The second edition of *Cardiac Drug Therapy* (1988) emphasized that "beta-blockers are not all alike" *(11)*.**
5. MRC trial in the elderly (1992) *(12)*: The beta-blocker used was atenolol.
   - This beta-blocker appears to be a favorite of trialists who failed to recognize the subtle clinical differences that exist among the available beta-blocking drugs *(11)*.
   - The MRC investigators confirmed that 25% of patients were lost to follow-up and more than half the patients were not taking the therapy assigned by the end of the study *(12)*.
   - There was no difference in total mortality between atenolol and diuretic therapy, but, surprisingly, diuretics reduced coronary heart disease (CHD) events, and atenolol did not.
   - **This obscure and misleading finding nevertheless led Messerli et al. *(13)* to publish an article in the *Journal of the American Medical Association* entitled "Are β-Blockers Efficacious as First-Line Therapy for Hypertension in the Elderly?"**
   - These analysts concluded that beta-blockers should not be first-line therapy for elderly hypertensives.
   - **Unfortunately, this faulty expert opinion of Messerli and colleagues has gained access to notable textbooks and journals.**
6. The Controlled Onset Verapamil Investigation of Cardiovascular End Points (CONVINCE) *(14)*: 8241 hypertensive patients received 180 mg of verapamil, and 8361 received either 50 mg of atenolol or 12.5 mg of hydrochlorothiazide. The findings at 3 yr were as follows: "There were 364 primary CVD-related events that occurred in the verapamil group versus 365 in the atenolol or hydrochlorothiazide group (hazard ratio [HR], 1.02; 95% confidence interval [CI], 0.88–1.18; $p = 0.77$)." Importantly, more cardiovascular disease (CVD)-related events occurred between 6 AM and noon in both the verapamil (99/277) and atenolol

or hydrochlorothiazide (88/274) groups. It must be emphasized that atenolol does not provide a full 24-h action and fails to quell early morning catecholamine surge *(15)*. It is not surprising, therefore, that the drug is only partially CVD protective.

Reasons for the Poor Cardiovascular Protective Effects of Atenolol

- Atenolol is a hydrophilic beta-blocker that attains low brain concentration. Lipid-soluble beta-blocking agents with high brain concentration block sympathetic discharge in the hypothalamus better than water-soluble agents and are more effective in the prevention of cardiac deaths *(16)*.
- In a rabbit model, Äblad et al. *(17)* showed that although metoprolol (lipophilic) and atenolol (hydrophilic) caused equal beta-blockade, only metoprolol caused a reduction in cardiac death. Metoprolol, but not atenolol, caused a significant increase in RR interval variation, and thus a favorable alteration in sympathetic tone.
- Importantly, only the lipophilic beta-blockers (carvedilol, bisoprolol, propranolol, and timolol) have been shown in RCTs to prevent fatal and nonfatal myocardial infarction (MI) and sudden cardiac death *(10,18–20)*.
- **Atenolol's poor brain concentration, its less than 24-h duration of action, and failure to quell early morning catecholamine surge account for the drug's weak CVD risk protection.**
- **Other beta-blockers have been shown to control early morning and exercise-induced excessive rise in blood pressure better compared with atenolol and other antihypertensive agents *(15,21)*.**

Recent investigations indicate that atenolol is less effective than other antihypertensive agents at lowering aortic pressure despite an equivalent effect on brachial pressure, an observation that may partly explain poor CVD risk protection *(22,23)*.

- In the Conduit Artery Function Evaluation (CAFÉ) study *(24)*, brachial and aortic pressures were measured in a subset of 2199 patients from the Anglo-Scandinavian Cardiac Outcomes Trial (ASCOT) *(25,25a)*. Despite virtually identical reductions in brachial pressure, the aortic systolic pressure was 4.3 mmHg lower in the amlodipine/perindopril arm versus those on atenolol.
- In patients with renal failure, aortic pressure appears to be an independent predictor of outcome *(26)*.
- Wilkinson et al. *(27)* indicate that, unlike brachial pressure, aortic pressure is influenced by pressure waves that are reflected back toward the heart from branch points throughout the arterial tree. Atenolol tends to increase the effect of these reflected waves because of a reduction in heart rate, thus attenuating the fall in aortic but not brachial pressure *(23,27)*.
- **Kelly et al. *(28)* have shown, however, that vasodilating beta-blockers reduce wave reflection and are more effective in lowering aortic pressure than atenolol. Wilkinson pointed out that we should not extrapolate the results of CAFÉ to all beta-blockers *(29)*. I concur with Wilkinson, and I have emphasized that "sufficient attention has not been paid by the medical profession and researchers regarding the subtle differences that exist amongst the available beta-blocking drugs"; beta-blockers have subtle clinical differences *(30)*.**

Newer beta-blockers (carvedilol and nebivolol) are unlike atenolol and propranolol, both of which have pharmacodynamic concerns. In the Carvedilol Postinfarct Survival Controlled Evaluation (CAPRICORN) *(18)*, carvedilol achieved a 50% reduction in nonfatal MI in patients mainly above the age of 55 yr. There was a 30% reduction in total mortality and nonfatal MI. Carvedilol decreases CHD events in elderly normotensive and hypertensive patients. Newer beta-blockers have other possible benefits.

- Carvedilol and nebivolol are beta-blockers with direct vasodilating and antioxidant properties. Cominacini et al. *(31)* studied the vasodilator mechanisms of nebivolol, a highly selective $alpha_1$-receptor antagonist with antioxidant properties. This agent stimulates the endothelial L-arginine/nitric oxide pathway, and increases nitric oxide (NO) by decreasing its oxidative inactivation, thus causing vasodilation *(31)*. Nevertheless, bucindolol, a newer beta-blocker, unlike carvedilol, bisoprolol, and metoprolol failed to decrease heart failure deaths in a RCT, which had to be halted *(32)*.
- Carvedilol and nebivolol have not been subjected to long-term outcome trials in the treatment of uncomplicated hypertension. Trialists must consider the subtle differences that exist among the available beta-blocking drugs *(30)*.

Conclusions

- Clinicians are presented with the aforementioned facts and can draw their own conclusions.
- The present author, Cruickshank *(2)*, and others strongly believe that by lumping together all randomized hypertension trials involving beta-blockers, in which mainly atenolol was administered, Lindholm et al. have arrived at misleading conclusions *(2)*.
- Beta-blockers, particularly bisoprolol, carvedilol, and metoprolol succinate (extended release), should remain first choice along with diuretics in the treatment of primary hypertension.
- It is now important for the physician to select an appropriate beta-blocker with the understanding that all beta-blockers are not alike *(11,30)*.

DIABETIC RISK WITH BETA-BLOCKERS AND DIURETICS

An Increased Risk: True or False?

An important area of concern is a so-called increased incidence of diabetes caused by beta-blockers and diuretics. The poor CVD outcomes in diabetic patients behoove us to be cautious in recommending agents that might increase the incidence of diabetes.

I have cited evidence from clinical trials to indicate that the increased incidence of type 2 diabetes mellitus reported in RCTs is unproved and is partly false.

Physicians worldwide are perplexed by these controversies, which affect their management of patients.

Physicians worldwide have become concerned with the increased incidence of type 2 diabetes reported in many countries. It is well established that diabetics have the same CVD risk as do patients with established CVD. Diabetes increases the risk of coronary artery disease (CAD) twofold in men and fourfold in women *(33,34)*. Thus the effects of any drug that increases the incidence of type 2 diabetes, should raise an alarm, and the implications of this finding should be taken seriously *(35)*. Beta-blockers and diuretics have recently fallen into this arena. A proclaimed small increased risk for the development of type 2 diabetes caused by beta-blocker and diuretic therapy in hypertensive individuals has become a concern. Clinicians should ask whether this incidence is real, or are there other explanations for the observed modest increase in fasting glucose concentrations observed in a few patients on long-term treatment with these agents.

Other explanations include:

- Incorrect diagnosis of type 2 diabetes mellitus. In virtually all clinical trials (randomized and nonrandomized), a definition of diabetes was an increase in glucose levels > 126 mg/

dL (7 mmol/L). This was the criterion used in ALLHAT, the largest RCT. I must emphasize that a fasting glucose of 7–7.9 mmol/L, even if repeated twice, should qualify as glucose intolerance and is not diagnostic of diabetes mellitus in patients administered a beta-blocking drug and/or a diuretic. The guidelines should be rewritten by clinicians who understand the pathophysiology of diabetes mellitus.

- Mild reversible glucose intolerance is not necessarily diabetes mellitus. When diuretics and or beta-blocker therapy is discontinued, mild glucose intolerance reverts to normal in virtually all patients who are not genuinely diabetics, but glucose levels remain elevated in patients who are prediabetics (*see* further discussion under the Murphy et al. RCT in Diabetes Incidence in Clinical Studies just below).
- **Patients treated with diuretics and/or beta-blockers should take legal action against physicians who unjustifiably label them diabetics without proper documentation of the diagnosis.**

In the ASCOT-Blood Pressure Lowering Arm (BPLA), in which amlodipine was compared with atenolol, the mean change in glucose levels attributed to atenolol therapy from baseline to final visit was 0.2 mmol/L. Nevertheless, the trialists proclaimed a 30% increase incidence of diabetes based on this modest appearance of glucose intolerance *(25)*.

- Most important, Poulter et al. *(25a)*, for the ASCOT investigators in a reanalysis of the trial results, state that "adjustment for the accumulated mean values of blood glucose had little or no appreciable effect on the HRs of either of the end points."
- Unmasking of latent diabetes by raising glucose levels in prediabetic patients and benign reversible glucose elevations can occur in some individuals treated with diuretics and/or beta-blockers. **ACE inhibitors appear in RCTs to lower the incidence of new diabetes compared with beta-blockers, calcium antagonists, and diuretics, but this effect might be due to masking of latent diabetes, a situation that has long-term concerns, because treatment of the diabetic process is delayed.**

Long-term beta-blocker therapy may increase blood glucose concentration by 0.2 to a maximum of 1.0 mmol/L, as observed in RCTs with follow-up beyond 5 yr.

- **Clinicians should be aware, however, that beta-blockers and diuretics do not destroy islet cells or severely impair insulin secretion. They may have a modest effect on insulin resistance in predisposed individuals, and in prediabetics the diabetic state may be brought to light at an earlier point in time that presents a reassuring, rather than alarming, scenarios. Thus treatment for type 2 diabetes may begin earlier in the course of the true disease process.**
- **Insulin secretion is partly beta-2 mediated, and glucose-sulfonyl-urea-stimulated insulin secretion is partially inhibited by beta-blockers *(36)*. Clinically, however, there is no significant worsening of glycemic control when beta-blockers are combined with these agents.**

Diabetes Incidence in Clinical Studies

1. **In 1982 Murphy et al. reported on the results of a 14-yr follow-up in hypertensive patients treated with a diuretic that showed a major increase in the incidence of glucose intolerance *(37)*. *This effect was promptly reversed on discontinuation of the diuretic in more than 60% of individuals (37)*. It must be emphasized that based solely on the finding of glucose intolerance, the learned physicians *(37)* did not classify these individuals as diabetics. Thus, current trialists and experts in the field should avoid putting a label of diabetes mellitus on individuals who might have reversible benign**

glucose intolerance, as did the subjects studied by Murphy and colleagues. Similar findings have been reported when beta-blocker therapy is discontinued.

2. Padwal and colleagues conducted a systematic review of antihypertensive therapy and the incidence of type 2 diabetes *(38)*. Their findings were as follows:
   - Data from the highest quality studies indicate that diabetes incidence is unchanged or increased by beta-blocker and thiazide diuretics and unchanged or decreased by ACE inhibitors and calcium antagonists.
   - The authors concluded that current data are far from conclusive.
   - These investigators warned that poor methodologic quality limits the conclusions that can be drawn from the several nonrandomized studies quoted by many *(38)*.
   - Most important, in the studies analyzed by Padwal et al., the increase in diabetic incidence reported is presumptive because type 2 diabetes was not proved by appropriate diagnostic testing. These analysts admitted that the data are far from conclusive *(38)*.

   A similar metaanalysis was done by Mason et al. *(39)*. These investigators analyzed the following studies, which were not designed to test the hypothesis that diuretics and beta-blockers cause an increased incidence of diabetes: ALLHAT, Captopril Prevention Project (CAPP), Interventions as a Goal in Hypertensive Treatment (INSIGHT), International Verapamil-Trandolapril Trial (INVEST), Losartan Intervention for Endpoint Reduction in Hypertension (LIFE), Nordic Diltiazem (NORDIL), and STOP- H2. The findings were as follows:
   - "The results *suggest* [italics added] that routine combined use of thiazide with a beta-blocker increases the risk of developing new-onset diabetes *(39)*.
   - Mason and colleagues, however, emphasized: "We have conducted a secondary analysis of trials that include subgroups of patients randomly assigned, *thus our analysis is potentially vulnerable to confounding and reporting bias*" *(39)*. Even so, the Mason et al. metaanalysis is quoted by experts as factual data attesting to an increased incidence of diabetes. These studies are criticized later in our discussion.
3. ASCOT-BPLA *(25a)* randomized 19,257 patients with hypertension aged 40–79 yr, assigned either amlodipine 5–10 mg adding perindopril 4–8 mg as required (amlodipine-based regimen; $n = 9639$) or atenolol 50–100 mg adding bendroflumethiazide 1.25–25 mg and potassium as required (atenolol-based regimen; $n = 9618$). The primary end point was nonfatal MI and fatal CHD. At 5.5-yr follow-up, although these data were not significant, compared with the atenolol-based regimen, fewer individuals on the amlodipine-based regimen had a primary end point (429 versus 474; unadjusted HR 0.90, 95% CI 0.79–1.02, $p = 0.1052$).
   - The primary end point of fatal and nonfatal MI was nonsignificantly lowered by 10% in patients allocated the amlodipine-based regimen compared with those allocated the atenolol diuretic-based regimen ($p = 0.12$); Nonetheless, the investigators state that the amlodipine/ACE inhibitor regimen is preferred *(25)*.
   - The guidelines of the British Hypertension Society emphasized the seriousness of drug-induced diabetes and indicated that the "ASCOT Trial will provide much-needed randomized controlled evidence as to whether these concerns are valid" *(35)*. Of the tertiary end points, the incidence of developing diabetes was stated to be 30% less on the amlodipine-based regimen (567 versus 799; HR 0.70; 95% CI 0.63–0.78, $p < 0.0001$). However, this assumption is based on the observation that at the final visit glucose was significantly lower (mean difference 0.20 mmol/L; $p < 0.0001$) in the amlodipine/perindopril arm versus the atenolol/diuretic-based regimen.
   - Baseline glucose concentration for amlodipine and the atenolol-based regimen was 6.24 versus 6.24 mmol/L.

- The mean change in glucose levels attributed to atenolol therapy from baseline to final visit was only 0.2 mmol/L *(25a)*.
- Thus these trialists do not provide a clearly defined diabetic state.

It should be reiterated that Poulter et al. *(25a)*, for the ASCOT Investigators in a reanalysis of the trial results, state that "adjustment for the accumulated mean values of blood glucose had little or no appreciable effect on the HRs of either of the end points."

4. In ALLHAT, 36% of the patients studied had diabetes; they were followed for over 4.9 yr *(40)*.
   - For this important diabetic population, ALLHAT showed that lisinopril or amlodipine appeared to have no special advantage for most CVD and renal outcomes when compared with chlorthalidone *(40)*.
   - Lisinopril was inferior for several CVD outcomes compared with chlorthalidone, which was superior to amlodipine for heart failure (HF) outcomes in both diabetic and nondiabetic individuals *(40)*.
   - The incidence of diabetes (fasting serum glucose ≥ 126 mg/dL [7.0 mmol/L]) at 4 yr was chlorthalidone 11.6%, amlodipine 9.8%, and lisinopril 8.1%. Unfortunately, the diagnosis of new diabetes was based only on a glucose concentration > 7.0 mmol/L. Importantly, for individuals who had a baseline glucose estimation, only 38% had a peak measurement at 4 yr *(40)*.
5. In the UK Prospective Diabetes Study Group (UKPDS) *(41)*, the trialists studied 1148 hypertensive patients with type 2 diabetes to determine whether tight control of blood pressure with either a beta-blocker or an ACE inhibitor had a specific advantage or disadvantage in preventing the macrovascular and microvascular complications of type 2 diabetes.
   - At the end of the lengthy 9-yr follow-up, blood pressure lowering with captopril or atenolol was similarly effective in reducing the incidence of major diabetic complications *(41)*.
   - Glycated hemoglobin concentration was similar in the two groups over the second 4 yr of study (atenolol 8.4% versus captopril 8.3%) *(41)*.
   - **Most important, in this *long-term study* there was no difference in results for the primary end point (any diabetes-related end point) between the two groups, captopril versus atenolol, at 9 yr despite induced mild increases in HbA_{1c}. Beta-blocker therapy significantly reduced all-cause mortality and risk for MI, stroke, peripheral vascular disease, and microvascular disease. Atenolol was not inferior compared with captopril *(41)*.**
6. Gress et al. conducted a prospective study of 12,550 adults 45–64 yr old who did not have diabetes *(42)*. A health evaluation conducted at baseline included assessment of medication use. The incidence of type 2 diabetes was assessed after 3 and 6 yr by assessment of fasting serum glucose *(42)*.
   - Hypertensive individuals treated with thiazide diuretics were not at greater risk for the subsequent development of diabetes than individuals on nondrug therapy *(42)*.
   - Individuals with hypertension treated with beta-blockers had a 28% higher risk of subsequent diabetes (HR, 1.28; 95% CI, 1.04–1.57) *(42)*. The individuals with fasting glucose > 126 mg/dL were not necessarily genuine type 2 diabetics.
7. In the LIFE trial *(43)*, atenolol was compared with losartan. In a *post hoc* analysis it is claimed that there was a significant 15% excess of new-onset diabetes over 5 yr.
   - However, the absolute rise in glucose was not stated. A large number of patients in the beta-blocker group received diuretics, and the frequency of diuretic use in each study arm was not given.
   - In most studies, including LIFE, *post hoc* analysis suggested that increased risk of new-onset diabetes was confined to individuals with an elevated blood glucose at baseline and family predisposition to diabetes *(44)*.

8. In the VALUE trial, new-onset type 2 diabetes was 25% more frequent in the patients on amlodipine than in those on valsartan (13.1% versus 16.4%; $p < 0.0001$) *(45)*.
9. STOP-2 was a large RCT of 6614 patients aged 70–84 yr randomized to a beta-blocker group (mixed beta-blockers) or hydrochlorothiazide or newer drugs (enalapril or lisinopril, felodipine or isradipine) *(7)*. At 5-yr follow-up, there were no differences in the prevention of cardiovascular mortality or major events.
   - There was no increase in diabetes caused by beta blockers, diuretics, or their combination.
10. The CAPP trial *(46)* assessed captopril versus diuretic and beta-blocker (atenolol or metoprolol) in 10,985 patients, with an average follow-up 6.1 yr.
    - There was no difference in total mortality or fatal and nonfatal MI.
    - However, fatal and nonfatal stroke was more common with captopril (189), versus 148 for the diuretic beta-blocker arm ($p = 0.044$) *(46)*.
    - The opposite finding occurred in LIFE *(42)*. **Importantly**, the relative proportions of patients on beta-blocker and diuretic therapy were not given.
11. Elliott and colleagues *(47)* performed a network metaanalysis to determine the incidence of diabetes in RCTs of antihypertensive drugs and concluded that "the association of antihypertensive drugs with incident diabetes is therefore lowest for ARB and ACE inhibitors followed by calcium antagonists and placebo, beta-blockers, and diuretics in rank order. Although Elliott et al. and experts in the field have accepted the misleading accounts of trialists who claimed to have observed an increase in diabetes risk.
12. The GEMINI trial *(48)* compared the effects of two different beta-blockers on glycemic control as well as other CVD risk factors in a cohort with glycemic control similar to the UKPDS *(41)*.
    - Carvedilol significantly stabilized HbA_{1c}, improved insulin resistance, and slowed development of microalbuminuria in the presence of renin-angiotensin system (RAS) blockade with ACE inhibition or ARB compared with metoprolol. The mean difference between carvedilol and metoprolol with respect to the change in HbA_{1c} from baseline was 0.12% (SD, 0.04%; 95% CI, –0.20% to –0.03%; $p = 0.006$).
    - Carvedilol treatment had no effect on HbA_{1c} (mean (SD) change from baseline to end point, 0.02% [0.04%]; 95% CI, –0.06% to 0.10%; $p = 0.65$), whereas metoprolol increased HbA_{1c} (0.15% [0.04%]; 95% CI, 0.08–0.22%; $p < 0.001$).
    - Using the HOMA-IR model, these investigators demonstrated a reduction in insulin resistance with carvedilol compared with metoprolol, an effect that correlated with HbA_{1c} *(49)*.
    - Participants who were normotensive showed a reduction in progression to microalbuminuria with carvedilol, as well as a reduction in existing microalbuminuria.
    - Metoprolol failed to decrease microalbuminuria. A similar finding was observed in the African-American Study of Kidney Disease trial with long-acting metoprolol *(50)*. This result may be related to an improvement in insulin resistance, as noted by differences in the HOMA-IR index or an effect on oxidant stress, as described in other studies with carvedilol *(51,52)*.
    - Treatment with carvedilol was associated with improvement in total cholesterol; metoprolol increased triglycerides (13%; $p < 0.001$), whereas carvedilol had no effect. Significant weight gain was observed in the metoprolol group (mean [SD], 1.2 [0.2] kg for metoprolol, $p < 0.001$ versus 0.2 [0.2] kg for carvedilol; $p = 0.36$).

Conclusions

The aforementioned discussion indicates that:

- In individuals not in a prediabetic state, beta-blockers and/or diuretics do not cause genuine diabetes mellitus.

Table 9-2
Antihypertensive Agents and Risk for Heart Failure

Drugs	*Trial*	*Risk for heart failure*
Doxazosin	ALLHAT *(40)*	82% versus diuretic
Amlodipine	ALLHAT	32% versus diuretic
Lisinopril	ALLHAT	19% versus diuretic
Nifedipine	INSIGHT *(54)*	46% versus diuretic
Carvedilol	CAPRICORN *(18)*	Significantly decreased risk

- In individuals with a family history of diabetes or in those with borderline elevation of blood glucose (6.5–7 mmol/L) prior to therapy with diuretics and/or beta-blockers, these agents do not cause diabetes, but the diabetic state may be brought to light earlier than if treatment with ACE inhibitors/ARB or calcium antagonists is used. Thus, aggressive diabetic management can be commenced earlier in time, a scenario that is reassuring rather than alarming. The diuretic/beta-blocker combination should not be blamed for causing diabetes in these individuals. Most reassuring, the combination therapy can be continued, as indicated by ALLHAT *(39,40)* and UKPDS *(40)*, which some criticize because of the small number of patients studied.

In patients not suspected of being prediabetic and with normal blood glucose, long-term therapy with either a beta-blocker or a diuretic or their combination might cause a mild elevation of blood glucose, and this clinical state should be labeled

- **Benign reversible glucose intolerance** and should not be classified as diabetes mellitus. In virtually all such individuals, the mild elevation in glucose levels observed should return to normal levels on cessation of therapy with these agents. There remains little doubt that long-term treatment of patients (non-prediabetics and prediabetics) with diuretics and beta-blockers increases the incidence of glucose intolerance, but this metabolic defect is reversible in about 60% of individuals on cessation of therapy *(37)*; the remaining about 40% should prove to have diabetes mellitus.
- Evidence from clinical trials and our internal medicine knowledge base allow me to indicate to students and colleagues that the increased incidence of type 2 diabetes mellitus reportedly caused by beta-blockers and diuretics is unproven and false.
- *Medicolegal action might arise and involve physicians and trialists who label such patients as diabetics without appropriate confirmation of the diagnosis.*
- Carefully planned RCTs are needed to test reported findings, but the diagnosis criteria for new-onset diabetes mellitus would need to be redefined for patients given beta-blockers and diuretics in planned RCTs.
- In these planned RCTs, the diagnosis of diabetes mellitus and **benign reversible glucose intolerance** must be carefully differentiated by tests other than a fasting blood glucose > 7.0 mmol/L (126 mg/dL).

HYPERTENSIVE AGENTS INCREASE HEART FAILURE RISK: TRUE OR FALSE?

Beta-blockers and diuretics are effective treatment for heart failure and in hypertensive individuals do not cause an increased risk for HF, but alpha-blockers, including dozaxosin, and calcium antagonists have been shown to cause a significant increase in HF in hypertensive patients in long-term studies *(40,40b)* (*see* Table 9-2).

1. In ALLHAT, a significant 82% higher rate for HF was observed for the alpha-blocker doxazosin *(39)*. "HF risk was doubled (4-yr rates, 8.13% versus 4.45%; RR, 2.04; 95% CI, 1.79–2.32; $p < 0.001$)." I cautioned that the use of alpha-blockers should be curtailed in the second edition of this book (1988) as well as the fourth edition (1995) *(53)*.
2. In the INSIGHT trial, a 46% higher rate of HF was observed with calcium antagonist therapy versus older drug regimens (Table 9-2).
   - There was no difference in RR for dihydropyridines compared with diltiazem and verapamil *(55,56)*.
   - Most important, for amlodipine versus chlorthalidone, secondary outcomes were similar except for a higher 6-yr rate of HF with amlodipine (10.2% versus 7.7%; RR, 1.38; 95% CI, 1.25–1.52).
   - The amlodipine group had a 32% higher risk of HF ($p < 0.001$), with a 6-yr absolute risk difference of 2.5% and a 35% higher risk of hospitalization for fatal HF ($p < 0.001$). Elderly blacks had the highest increase in HF. ACE inhibitor and lisinopril caused a 19% higher risk of HF ($p < 0.001$).

There is no doubt that calcium antagonists cause very effective lowering of blood pressure. They, however, do cause a significant increased incidence of HF, particularly in the elderly and in blacks compared with diuretics and/or beta-blockers, and some caution is required.

IS ANGIOEDEMA A SIGNIFICANT RISK WITH ACE INHIBITORS?

In ALLHAT, angioedema occurred in 8 of 15, 255 (0.1%), 3 of 9048 (<0.1%), and 38 of 9054 (0.4%) persons in the chlorthalidone, amlodipine, and lisinopril treatment groups, respectively *(39)*. Significant differences were seen for the lisinopril versus chlorthalidone comparison overall: ($p < 0.001$) in blacks (2 of 5369 [<0.1%] for chlorthalidone, 23 of 3210 [0.7%] for lisinopril) and in nonblacks (6 of 9886 [0.1%] for chlorthalidone and 15 of 5844 for lisinopril [0.3%]; $p = 0.002$).

- The only death from angioedema was in the lisinopril group.
- Death should not occur in the treatment of healthy individuals; the patient with mild primary hypertension is invariably healthy and asymptomatic.
- Most patients with angioedema caused by an ACE inhibitor require emergency room treatment.
- Angioedema is more common in blacks treated with ACE inhibitors compared with whites. Caution is required with the use of ACE inhibitors in blacks; it is preferable to use an ARB.

AGE AND ETHNICITY HOLD THE KEY FOR DRUG CHOICE

The choice of initial drug in patients without compelling reasons should be based on:

- Age younger or older than 60 yr.
- Ethnicity *(57)*: nonblack or black patients.

It is well established that >60% of hypertensive individuals require more than one drug to attain goal blood pressures. However, monotherapy is worth the effort because in patients with mild primary hypertension (stage I–II), if clinicians use the age and ethnicity formula monotherapy is expected to obtain blood pressure (BP) goal in about 50%.

The Joint National Committee (JNC) V11 advises that initial drug choices for patients without compelling indications are

- Thiazide-type diuretics for monotherapy.
- One may consider an ACE inhibitor or an ARB, a beta-blocker, or a combination *(58)*.

- The advice to begin with a diuretic in most is logical and sound advice based on the results of numerous well-run RCTs including the hallmark ALLHAT.
- Diuretics, however, are not very effective blood pressure-lowering agents in younger whites *(59–61)*.
- ALLHAT *(40)* and SHEP *(62)* gave conclusive proof as to the salutary CVD effects of diuretics versus newer agents in their study of patients with mean ages of 67 and 72 yr, respectively.
- The JNC V11 recommendation to initiate therapy with an ACE inhibitor or ARB *(58)* without regard for age or ethnicity is not sound advice.
- ACE inhibitors or ARBs are as effective as beta-blockers in reducing CVD outcomes in nonblack individuals younger than age 60 yr, and either agent may be chosen depending on the patient's characteristics.
- ACE inhibitors or ARBs, however, are not superior to beta-blocker therapy if atenolol is excluded.

The Perindopril Protection Against Recurrent Stroke Study (PROGRESS) was a large, well-run RCT of 6105 individuals with hypertension and previous stroke or transient ischemic attack *(63)*. The ACE inhibitor perindopril attained blood pressure goal in only about 42% of trial patients, and no discernible reduction in the primary outcome, reduction in the risk of stroke, was observed.

- Reduction in CVD events was observed only with the combination of captopril and diuretic. In CAPP, fatal and nonfatal stroke was more common with the ACE inhibitor captopril (189 versus 148) for the beta-blocker atenolol or metoprolol and diuretic therapy ($p = 0.044$) *(47)*.

Casas et al. conducted a systematic review and metaanalysis on the effect of inhibitors of the RAS and other antihypertensive drugs on renal outcomes *(64)*. These investigators concluded that the benefits of ACE inhibitors or ARBs on renal outcomes in placebo-controlled trials probably result mainly from a blood pressure-lowering effect.

- In patients with diabetes, additional renoprotective actions of these agents beyond lowering blood pressure remain unproven, and there is uncertainty about the greater renoprotection seen in nondiabetic renal disease *(64)*.

The British guidelines use age < or > 55 yr and ethnicity *(35)*; this provides logical advice based on the renin hypothesis. However, their recommendation to use a calcium antagonist in the elderly black or nonblack individual should be reexamined because these agents increase HF risk, particularly so in black hypertensive individuals (*see* Table 9-1).

The following are suggested drug choices based on age and ethnicity:

1. **Nonblack individuals < age 60 yr:**
   - A hallmark randomized parallel group study in 1292 men by Materson et al. compared younger black patients, younger white patients, older black patients, and older white patients treated with a diuretic, a beta-blocker, an ACE inhibitor, or a calcium antagonist. The study indicated that in younger white patients a beta-blocker or ACE inhibitor had equal BP-lowering effects and were superior to diuretic or calcium antagonist therapy *(59)* (*see* Fig. 8-2).
   - **Deary et al. completed a double-blind placebo-controlled crossover comparison of five antihypertensive drugs (amlodipine, doxazosin, lisinopril, bisoprolol. and bendrofluazide) and placebo in 34 young nonblack hypertensives and showed that bendrofluazide performed significantly worse ($p = 0.0016$) and a beta-blocker, bisoprolol, significantly better ($p = 0.004$) *(60)*.**

Table 9-3
Corrected Values for Figs. 2 and 3 of Materson et al. See also Fig. 8-2

	*Study Agent (percentage of patients with treatment success)**						
	Diltiazem	*Clonidine*	*Atenolol*	*Hydrochlorothiazide*	*Prazosin*	*Captopril*	*Placebo*
Figure 2†	72.4 A	62.4 AB	59.6 AB	54.8 B	53.7 B	50.0 B	31.0 C
Figure 3‡							
Younger blacks	70.3	47.5	51.4	47.9	41.9	43.2	22.7
Younger whites	57.5	68.8	64.9	32.4	54.5	61.5	25.8
Older blacks	84.9	57.8	44.7	63.6	49.0	33.3	27.3
Older whites	71.7	73.3	72.4	68.3	69.0	61.8	37.5

*Treatment was considered successful if the diastolic blood pressure was less than 90 mmHg at the end of the titration period and less than 95 mmHg at the end of 1 yr of maintenance therapy.

†Agents that do not share a letter differ significantly ($p < 0.05$) in the percentage for treatment success, e.g., the value for diltiazem differs significantly from that for hydrochlorothiazide or that for placebe. Agents that share a letter do not differ significantly from each other in the percentage with treatment success.

‡A difference between agents of more than 15% was considered clinically important.

With permission: Materson BJ, Reda DJ. Correction: single-drug therapy for hypertension in men. N Engl J Med 1994;330:1689.

- **Dickerson et al. undertook a crossover rotation of the four main classes of antihypertensive drugs in 40 untreated young white hypertensive patients < age 55 yr to assess the response rate with monotherapy achieved by a systematic rotation *(61)*; 36 patients completed all four cycles. Success of monotherapy was achieved (*p* = 0.0001); in half the patients, BP on the best treatment was 135/85 mmHg or less. The responses to the ACE inhibitor or beta-blocker pair were, on average, at least 50% higher than those to the calcium antagonist/diuretic pair (Table 9-3).**
- **Both studies agree with findings of Materson et al. that in younger white patients a beta-blocker or ACE inhibitor are equally effective as monotherapy in approx 45% of nonblack patients with mild primary hypertension.**

Based on the results of these studies, the initial drug for nonblack individuals younger than 60 years

- Should be an appropriate beta-blocker (carvedilol, bisoprolol, or metoprolol succinate extended release) or an ACE inhibitor or ARB (*see* Fig. 9-1 and Table 9-3).

An ACE inhibitor or ARB are appropriate second choices for initial therapy, but physicians may appropriately choose these agents as first line. ACE inhibitors are effective first-line agents in younger nonblack patients; they attain goal BP in about 42% of patients.

2. **Younger black individual < age 60 yr (*see* Fig. 9-2):**
   - The Materson et al. study indicated that calcium antagonists were most effective followed by beta-blockers, and then diuretics and a poor response to ACE inhibitors (*see* Table 9-3).
   - Also, ACE inhibitors cause a higher risk for angioedema in blacks versus white patients. Several studies have documented a lower efficacy of ACE inhibitors in blacks versus nonblack patients. In two RCTs, greater differences were observed in black versus nonblack patients for combined CVD along with a similar trend for HF and lesser BP reduction *(65,66)*.

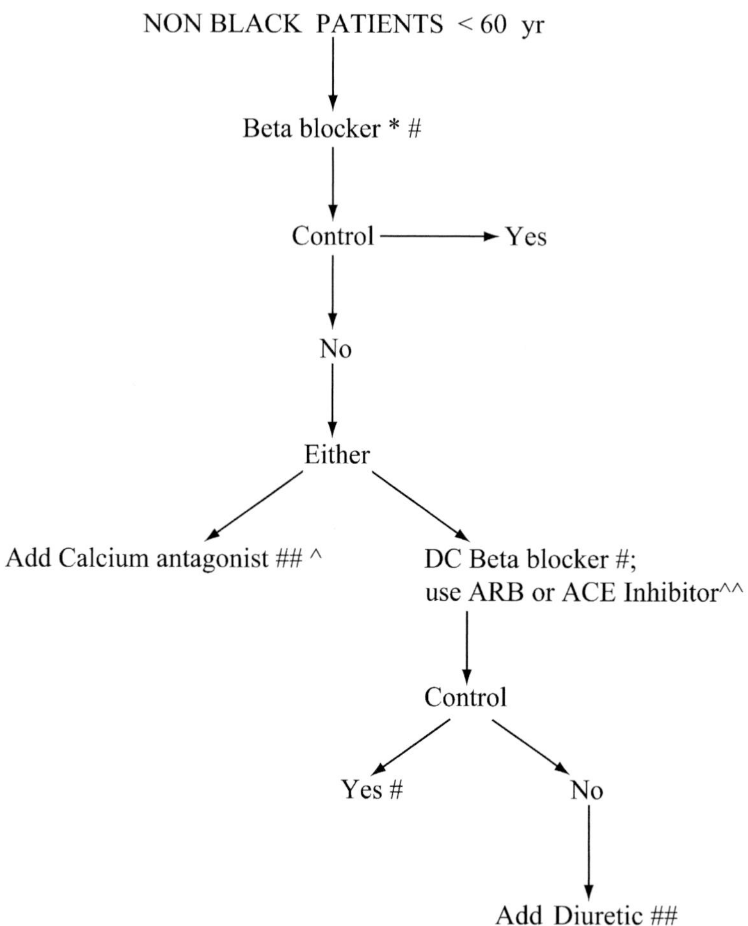

*Carvedilol or bisoprolol. If family history of diabetes or glucose at upper limit of normal exists and beta-blocker is chosen, use carvedilol and avoid combination with diuretic; atenolol is not recommended.

#Monotherapy is worth trying but with drug choice based on age < 60 yr and ethnicity; *see* text.

##Combination attains goal blood pressure with low doses of each drug, thus less adverse effects.

^A high dose of diltiazem is usually required and with a beta-blocker may cause bothersome bradycardia; best to add amlodipine and avoid verapamil.

^^In ALLHAT, the only death from angioedema was in the lisinopril group. A death in asymptomatic individuals is not justifiable. Angioedema, a rare but potentially serious adverse effect of ACE inhibitor use, occurred four times more frequently in participants randomized to lisinopril than in those randomized to chlorthalidone. An ARB is preferred.

Fig. 9-1. Initial drug choice for primary hypertension in nonblack patients < 60 yr old without compelling indications for individual drug classes. ACE, angiotensin-converting enzyme; ARB, angiotensin receptor blocker; DC, discontinue.

3. **Older nonblack individuals > age 60 yr (*see* Fig. 9-3):**
   - The initial agent advised is a diuretic.
   - If goal BP readings are not achieved, the diuretic should be discontinued and a beta-blocker given, preferably carvedilol or bisoprolol.
   - The beta-blockers carvedilol, bisoprolol, and metoprolol are as effective as diuretics in achieving goal BP and in reducing CVD outcomes in the elderly nonblack patient. In

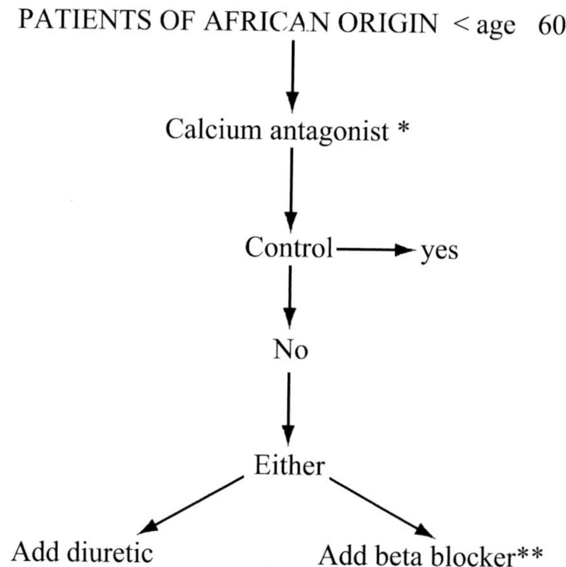

*Good response to monotherapy with these agents.
**To amlodipine, not to verapamil or diltiazem.
The Materson et al. RCT studied younger blacks' response to calcium antagonist and beta-blocker; the latter proved successful, and goal was reached in approx 47% versus diuretics in 40%, diltiazem approx 64%.

Fig. 9-2. Initial drug choice for primary hypertension in black patients < 60 yr old without compelling indications for individual drug classes.

the Materson et al. study, BP goal was achieved by 68%, 64%, and 52% in older white patients treated with beta-blocker, diltiazem, and diuretic, respectively. However, in the MRC trial of hypertension in elderly white patients *(12)*, surprisingly, a reduction in CHD events was attained by diuretic therapy but not with atenolol. In this trial more than 25% of patients were lost to follow-up, and 63% of patients in the atenolol group were either lost to follow-up or withdrawn for various reasons. This obscure trial finding nevertheless led Messerli and colleagues to state incorrectly that diuretics and not beta-blockers are the treatment of choice in elderly hypertensives *(13)*. Unfortunately, their advice was published in most textbooks and journals. A rebuttal with which I concur was made by Kendall et al. *(67)* and others *(68)* regarding the recommendation for treatment with beta-blockers in elderly hypertensives.

- Beta-blockers with proven cardioprotective properties, particularly carvedilol *(18)*, bisoprolol *(19)*, and metoprolol *(69)* have been shown to prevent fatal and nonfatal MI in the elderly with CHD with or without coexisting hypertension. Diuretics do not have a basis for a protective role in atheroma rupture and thus are not expected to prevent the occurrence of fatal and nonfatal MI.
- The meta analysis by Messerli et al. *(13)*, is as misleading as is that of Lindholm et al. *(1)*. In both analyses, atenolol was the principal beta-blocker used. The notion, therefore, that diuretics prevent CHD events in elderly hypertensives and beta-blockers do not should be abandoned.

Failure to achieve target BP should result in a combination of diuretic and beta-blocker, each at small doses (*see* Fig. 9-3).

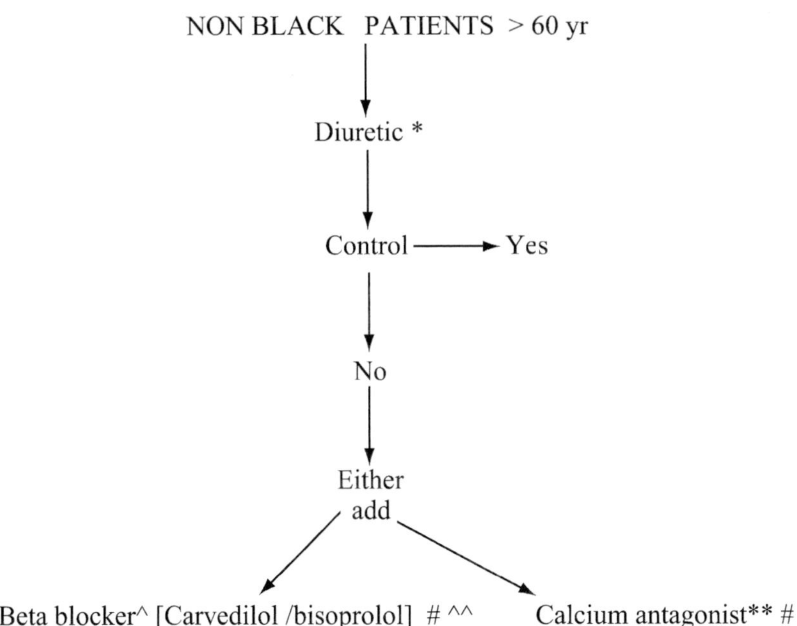

*Chlorthalidone, 25 mg; hydrochlorothiazide 12.5–25 mg; bendrofluazide 2.5–5 mg.

^In ALLHAT, chlorthalidone + add-on beta-blocker in patients with mean age 67 yr achieved goal blood pressure and decreased coronary heart disease events.

#Low-dose combination achieves goal with fewer adverse effects.

^^If family history of diabetes exists, watch for glucose intolerance; *see* text.

Use amlodipine or diltiazem, not verapamil: **caution—increases risk for heart failure in elderly who may have undetected left ventricular (LV) dysfunction. *See* Table 9-2.

....If LV dysfunction is suspected, use angiotensin receptor blocker (ARB) or angiotensin-converting enzyme (ACE) inhibitor instead of calcium antagonist.

Fig. 9-3. Initial drug choice for primary hypertension in nonblack patients > 60 yr old without compelling indications for individual drug classes.

- Diltiazem or amlodipine should be tried next at a low dose plus low-dose diuretic; a low-dose combination decreases risk for HF. The British guideline recommends either a calcium antagonist or a diuretic. Caution is necessary because HF has reached epidemic proportions in the elderly population. Calcium antagonists are effective in achieving goal blood pressure in the elderly, but they carry a substantial risk for HF. In ALLHAT, participants were older than age 55 yr (mean age 67 yr), and amlodipine caused a 32% increased risk for HF *(40)*. Other RCTs have documented that calcium antagonists including the dihydropyridines verapamil and diltiazem increase the risk of HF in the elderly (*see* Table 9-2).

4. **Black patients > age 60 yr (*see* Fig. 9-4):**
   - A diuretic is the drug of choice, as indicated in the Materson et al. study and proved in ALLHAT, in which CVD outcomes were significantly reduced by diuretics, with calcium antagonists showing no advantages.
   - A calcium antagonist may be considered as second line therapy in patients in whom diuretics cause adverse effects and there is no suspicion of left ventricular dysfunction (*see* Fig. 9-4).
   - Calcium antagonists are effective antihypertensive agents equal to diuretics in elderly blacks; 64% and 58% have been shown to achieve goal BP with diltiazem and diuretic

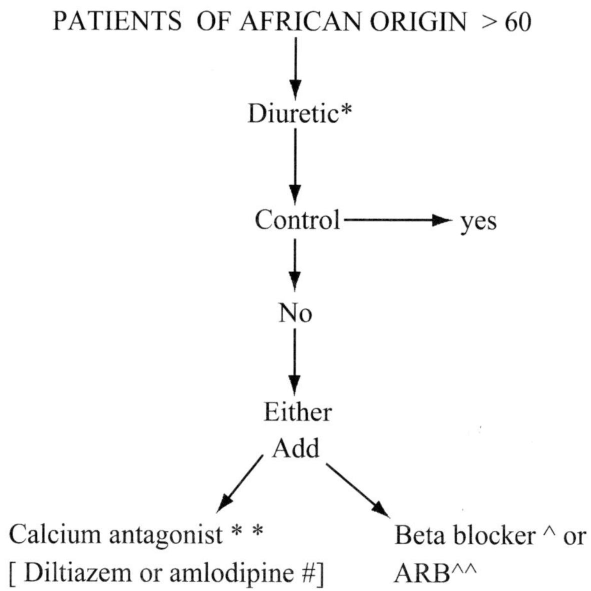

*Chlorthalidone successful in ALLHAT *(40)*.

Caution: elderly blacks have a high incidence of heart failure (HF). Calcium antagonists, although effective in achieving goal blood pressure (BP) carry a substantial risk: amlodipine had a 38% risk of HF in ALLHAT. The risk with nifedipine is higher and even higher for verapamil. Diltiazem carries about the same risk as dihydropyridines, but high dosage of the drug is required because it is a weaker vasodilator. Bothersome edema occurs in about 25% of patients treated with dihydropyridines.

#Low-dose combination achieves goal BP with reduced adverse effects.

^Bisoprolol, but preferably carvedilol or an ARB, if patient is diabetic or prediabetic.

^^ARB instead of ACE inhibitors, which have a higher incidence of angioedema in blacks.

Fig. 9-4. Initial drug choice for primary hypertension in black patients > 60 yr old without compelling indications for individual drug classes. ARB, angiotensin receptor blocker.

therapy, respectively *(59)*. However, an increased risk for HF was observed for verapamil in the CONVINCE study *(14)*, for amlodipine in ALLHAT *(40)*, and for the dihydropyridines in other RCTs. This risk is higher in patients older than age 60 yr than in younger individuals.

RECOMMENDATIONS FOR FUTURE RANDOMIZED TRIALS

The National Heart, Lung, and Blood Institute (NHLBI) working group is planning a study that would define the step-2 drug that should be added to a thiazide-type diuretic *(70)*. Choices for comparison include beta-blockers, calcium antagonists, ARBs, ACE inhibitors, and aldosterone receptor antagonists *(70)*.

- It is reassuring that the NHLBI trialists agree that significant differences in outcomes can be produced by varying the type of beta-blocker and dosing regimen and that significant reductions in CHD events were observed with carvedilol in CAPRICORN *(18)* and COPERNICUS *(71)*, with bisoprolol in CIBIS *(19)*, and with metoprolol in MERIT/HF *(69)*, but a negative result emerged with bucindolol *(32)*.
- The combination of an appropriate beta-blocker (bisoprolol, carvedilol, metoprolol succinate extended release [Toprol XL]), nebivolol, or timolol and the aldosterone antagonist eplerenone deserves study.

REFERENCES

1. Lindholm LH, Carlberg B, Samuelsson O. Should β blockers remain first choice in the treatment of primary hypertension? A meta-analysis. Lancet 2005;366:1545–1553.
2. Cruickshank JM. β blockers for the treatment of primary hypertension. Lancet 2006;367:209.
3. The IPPPSH Collaborative Group. Cardiovascular risk and risk factors in a randomised trial of treatment based on the beta-blocker oxprenolol. The International Prospective Primary Prevention Study in Hypertension (IPPPSH). J Hypertens 1985;3:379–392.
4. Berglund G, Andersin O, Widgren B. Low-dose antihypertensive treatment with a thiazide diuretic is not diabetogenic. Acta Med Scand 1986;220:419–424.
5. Yurenev AP, Dyakonova HG, Novikov ID, et al. Management of essential hypertension in patients with different degrees of left ventricular hypertrophy. Multicenter trial. Am J Hypertens 1992;(6 Pt 2): 182S–189S.
6. The Dutch TIA Trial Study Group. Trial of secondary prevention with atenolol after transient ischemic attack or nondisabling ischemic stroke. Stroke 1993;24:543–548.
7. Hansson L, Lindholm LH, Ekbom T, et al. Randomised trial of old and new antihypertensive drugs in elderly patients: Cardiovascular mortality and morbidity, the Swedish Trial in Old Patients with Hypertension-2 study. Lancet 1999;354:1751–1756.
8. MRC Working Party. MRC trial of treatment of mild hypertension: Principal results. BMJ 1985;291: 97–104.
9. Treatment of hypertension: The 1985 results. Lancet 1985;2:645.
10. Norwegian Multicentre Group. Timolol induced reduction in mortality and reinfarction in patients surviving acute myocardial infarction. N Engl J Med 1981;304:801–807.
11. Khan M Gabriel. Hypertension. In: Cardiac Drug Therapy, 2nd ed. Philadelphia, WB Saunders, 1988, p. 62.
12. MRC Working Party. Medical Research Council Trial of treatment of hypertension in older adults: Principal results. BMJ 1992;304:405–412.
13. Messerli FH, Grossman E, Goldbourt U. Are β-blockers efficacious as first-line therapy for hypertension in the elderly? JAMA 1998;279:1903–1907.
14. CONVINCE: Black HR, Elliott WJ, Grandits G, et al. for the CONVINCE Research Group. Principal results of the Controlled Onset Verapamil Investigation of Cardiovascular End Points (CONVINCE) trial. JAMA 2003;289:2073–2082.
15. Neutel JM, Smith DHG, Ram CVS. Application of ambulatory blood pressure monitoring in differentiating between antihypertensive agents. Am J Med 1993;94:181,
16. Pitt B. The role of beta-adrenergic blocking agents in preventing sudden cardiac death. Circulation 1992; 85(I Suppl):107.
17. Äblad B, Bjurö T, Björkman JA, Edström T, Olsson G. Role of central nervous beta-adrenoceptors in the prevention of ventricular fibrillation through augmentation of cardiac vagal tone. J Am Coll Cardiol 1991;17(Suppl):165.
18. The CAPRICORN Investigators. Effect of carvedilol on outcome after myocardial infarction in patients with left-ventricular dysfunction: The CAPRICORN randomised trial. Lancet 2001;357:1385–1390.
19. CIBIS-II Investigators and Committees. The Cardiac Insufficiency Bisoprolol Study II (CIBIS-II): A randomised trial. Lancet 1999;353:9–13.
20. BHAT: β-Blocker Heart Attack Trial Research Group. A randomised trial of propranolol in patients with acute myocardial infarction. I: Mortality results. JAMA 1982;247:1707–1714.
21. Kokkinos P, Chrysohoou C, Panagiotakos D, et al. Beta-blockade mitigates exercise blood pressure in hypertensive male patients. J Am Coll Cardiol 2006;47:794–798.
22. Morgan T, Lauri J, Anderson A. Effect of different antihypertensive drug classes on central aortic pressure. Am J Hypertens 2004;17:118–123.
23. Dhakam Z, McEniery CM, Cockcroft JR, et al. Atenolol and eprosartan: differential effects on central blood pressure and aortic pulse wave velocity. Am J Hypertens 2006;19:214–219.
24. CAFE investigators for the Anglo-Scandinavian Cardiac Outcomes Trial (ASCOT) investigators. Differential impact of blood pressure-lowering drugs on central aortic pressure and clinical outcomes: Principal results of the Conduit Artery Function Evaluation (CAFE) Study. Circulation 2006;113:1213–1225.
25. ASCOT: Dahlof B, Sever PS, Poulter NR, et al. for the ASCOT investigators. Prevention of cardiovascular events with an antihypertensive regimen of amlodipine adding perindopril as required versus atenolol adding bendroflumethiazide as required, in the Anglo-Scandinavian Cardiac Outcomes Trial-Blood

Pressure Lowering Arm (ASCOT-BPLA): A multicentre randomised controlled trial. Lancet 2005;366: 895–906.

25a. Poulter NR, Wedel H, Dahlöf B, for the ASCOT investigators. Role of blood pressure and other variables in the differential cardiovascular event rates noted in the Anglo-Scandinavian Cardiac Outcomes Trial-Blood Pressure Lowering Arm (ASCOT-BPLA). Lancet 2005;366:907–913.

26. Safar ME, Blacher J, Pannier B, et al. Central pulse pressure and mortality in end-stage renal disease. Hypertension 2002;39:735–738.
27. Wilkinson IB, MacCallum H, Flint L, et al. The influence of heart rate on augmentation index and central arterial pressure in humans. J Physiol 2000;525:263–270.
28. Kelly R, Daley J, Avolio A, O'Rourke M. Arterial dilation and reduced wave reflection: Benefit of dilevalol in hypertension. Hypertension 1989;14:14–21.
29. Wilkinson IB, McEniery CM, Cockcroft JR. Atenolol and cardiovascular risk: An issue close to the heart. Lancet 2006;367:627–629.
30. Khan M Gabriel. Which beta blocker to choose. In: Heart Disease Diagnosis and Therapy, a Practical Approach, 2nd ed. Totowa, NJ, Humana Press, 2005, p. 55.
31. Cominacini L, Fratta Pasini A, Garbin U, et al. Nebivolol and its 4-keto derivative increase nitric oxide in endothelial cells by reducing its oxidative inactivation. J Am Coll Cardiol 2003;42:1838–1844.
32. Beta-blocker Evaluation of Survival Trial Investigators. A trial of the beta-blocker bucindolol in patients with advanced chronic heart failure. N Engl J Med 2001;362:1659– 1667.
33. HOT: Hansson L, et al. for the HOT Study Group. Effects of intensive blood pressure lowering and low-dose aspirin in patients with hypertension: Principal results of the Hypertension Optimal Treatment (HOT) trial. Lancet 1998;351:1755–1762.
34. Zanchetti A, et al. Effects of individual risk factors on the incidence of cardiovascular events in the treated hypertensive patients in the Hypertension Optimal Treatment study. J Hypertens 2001;19:1149–1159.
35. Williams B, Poulter NR, Brown MJ, et al. Guidelines for management of hypertension: Report of the fourth working party of the British Hypertension Society, 2004-BHS IV. J Hum Hypertens 2004;18: 139–185.
36. Loubatiere A, Mariani MM, Sorel G, et al. The action of beta adrenergic blocking drugs and stimulating agents on insulin secretion. Characteristic of the type of beta receptor. Diabetologica 1971;7:127–132.
37. Murphy MB, Lewis PJ, Kohner E, Schumer B, Dollery CT. Glucose intolerance in hypertensive patients treated with diuretics: A fourteen-year follow-up. Lancet 1982;2:1293–1295.
38. Padwal R, Laupacis A. Antihypertensive therapy and incidence of type 2 diabetes. A systematic review. Diabetes Care 2004;27:247–255.
39. Mason JM, Dickinson HO, Nicolson DJ, et al. The diabetiogenic potential of thiazide-type diuretic and a beta blocker combinations in patients with hypertension. J Hypertens 2005;23:1777–1781.
40. The ALLHAT Officers and Coordinators for the ALLHAT Collaborative Research Group. Major outcomes in high-risk hypertensive patients randomized to angiotensin-converting enzyme inhibitor or calcium channel blocker vs. diuretic: The Antihypertensive and Lipid-Lowering Treatment to Prevent Heart Attack Trial (ALLHAT). JAMA 2002;288:2981–2997.
41. UKPDS: UK Prospective Diabetes Study Group. Efficacy of atenolol and captopril in reducing risk of macrovascular and microvascular complications in type 2 diabetes: UKPDS. BMJ 1998;317:713–720.
42. Gress TW, Nieto FJ, Shahar E, et al. for The Atherosclerosis Risk in Communities Study. Hypertension and antihypertensive therapy as risk factors for type 2 diabetes mellitus. N Engl J Med 2000;342:905–912.
43. LIFE: Dahlöf B, Devereux RB, Kjeldsen SE, et al. for the LIFE Study Group. Cardiovascular morbidity and mortality in the Losartan Intervention for Endpoint Reduction in Hypertension Study (LIFE): A randomised trial against atenolol. Lancet 2002;359:995–1003.
44. Lindholm LH, Ibsen H, Borch-Johnsen K, et al. Risk of new-onset diabetes in the Losartan Intervention for Endpoint Reduction in Hypertension Study. J Hypertens 2002;20:1879–1886.
45. Julius S, Kjeldsen SE, Weber M, et al. for the VALUE trial group. Outcomes in hypertensive patients at high cardiovascular risk treated with regimes based on valsartan or amlodipine: The VALUE randomised trial. Lancet 2004;363:2002–2031.
46. Hansson L, Lindholm LH, Niskanen L, et al. Effect of angiotensin-converting-enzyme inhibition compared with conventional therapy on cardiovascular morbidity and mortality in hypertension: The Captopril Prevention Project (CAPPP). Lancet 1999;353:611–616.
47. Elliott WJ, Meyer PM. Incident diabetes in clinical trials of antihypertensive drugs: a network meta-analysis. The Lancet 2007;369:201–207.

48. GEMINI: Bakris GL, Fonseca V, Katholi RE, et al. Metabolic effects of carvedilol vs metoprolol in patients with type 2 diabetes mellitus and hypertension: A randomized controlled trial. JAMA 2004;292: 2227–2236.
49. Khaw KT, Wareham N, Luben R, et al. Glycated haemoglobin, diabetes, and mortality in men in Norfolk cohort of European Prospective Investigation of Cancer and Nutrition (EPIC-Norfolk). BMJ 2001;322: 15–18.
50. Wright JT, Bakris G, Greene T, et al. for the African American Study of Kidney Disease and Hypertension Study Group. Effect of blood pressure lowering and antihypertensive drug class on progression of hypertensive kidney disease: Results from the AASK Trial. JAMA 2002;288:2421–2431.
51. Yasunari K, Maeda K, Nakamura M, Yoshikawa J. Carvedilol inhibits pressure-induced increase in oxidative stress in coronary smooth muscle cells. Hypertens Res 2002;25:419–425.
52. Yasunari K, Maeda K, Nakamura M, Watanabe T, Yoshikawa J, Asada A. Effects of carvedilol on oxidative stress in polymorphonuclear and mononuclear cells in patients with essential hypertension. Am J Med. 2004;116:460–465.
53. Khan M Gabriel. Alpha-1 adrenergic blockers. In: Cardiac Drug Therapy, 4th ed. Philadelphia, WB Saunders, 1995, p. 103.
54. INSIGHT: Brown MJ, Palmer CR, Castaigne A, et al. Morbidity and mortality in patients randomised to double-blind treatment with a long-acting calcium-channel blocker or diuretic in the International Nifedipine GITS study: Intervention as a Goal in Hypertension Treatment (INSIGHT). Lancet 2000;356: 366–372.
55. Neal B, MacMahon S, Chapman N. Effects of ACE inhibitors, calcium antagonists, and other blood-pressure-lowering drugs: results of prospectively designed overviews of randomised trials: Blood Pressure Lowering Treatment Trialists' Collaboration. Lancet 2000;356:1955–1964.
56. Pahor M, Psaty BM, Alderman MH, et al. Health outcomes associated with calcium antagonists compared with other first-line antihypertensive therapies: A meta-analysis of randomised controlled trials. Lancet 2000;356:1949–1954.
57. Khan M Gabriel. Recommendations for hypertension in young and older patients. In: Cardiac Drug Therapy, 6th ed. Philadelphia, WB Saunders, 2003, pp. 134–143.
58. The Seventh Report of the Joint National Committee on Prevention, Detection, Evaluation, and Treatment of High Blood Pressure. JAMA 2003;289:2560–2572.
59. Materson BJ, Reda DJ, Cushman WC, et al. Single-drug therapy for hypertension in men. A comparison of six antihypertensive agents with placebo: The Department of Veterans Affairs Cooperative Study Group on Antihypertensive Agents. N Engl J Med 1993;328:914–921.
59a. Materson BJ, Reda DJ. Correction: single-drug therapy for hypertension in men. N Engl J Med 1994; 330:1689.
60. Deary A, Schumann AL, Murfet H. Double-blind placebo-controlled crossover comparison of five classes of antihypertensive drugs J Hypertens 2002;20:771–777.
61. Dickerson JEC, Hingorani AD, Ashby MJ, et al. Randomisation of antihypertensive treatment by crossover rotation of four major classes. Lancet 1999;353:2008–2013.
62. SHEP Cooperative Research Group. Prevention of stroke by antihypertensive drug treatment in older persons with isolated systolic hypertension: Final results of the Systolic Hypertension in the Elderly Program (SHEP). JAMA 1991;265:3255–3264.
63. PROGRESS Collaborative Group. Randomized trial of a perindopril-based blood pressure lowering regimen among, individuals with previous stroke or transient ischaemic attack. Lancet 2001;358:1033–1041.
64. Casas JP, Chau W, Loukogeorgakis S, et al. Effect of inhibitors of the renin-angiotensin system and other antihypertensive drugs on renal outcomes: Systematic review and meta-analysis. Lancet 2005;366:2026–2033.
65. Saunders E, Weir MR, Kong BW, et al. A comparison of the efficacy and safety of a beta-blocker, a calcium channel blocker, and a converting enzyme inhibitor in hypertensive blacks. Arch Intern Med 1990; 150:1707–1713.
66. Cushman WC, Reda DJ, Perry HM, et al. Regional and racial differences in response to antihypertensive medication use in a randomized controlled trial of men with hypertension in the United States. Arch Intern Med 2000;160:825–831.
67. Kendall MJ, Cohen JD. β-Blockers as first-line agents for hypertension in the elderly. JAMA 1999;281: 131–133.
68. Khan M Gabriel. Hypertension trials. In: Cardiac Drug Therapy, 6th ed. Philadelphia, WB Saunders, 2003, p. 505.

69. MERIT-HF Study Group. Effect of metoprolol CR/XL in chronic heart failure: Metoprolol CR/XL Randomised Intervention Trial in Congestive heart failure (MERIT-HF). Lancet 1999;353:2001–2007.
70. The National Heart, Lung and Blood Pressure Institute Working Group on Future Directions in Hypertension Treatment Trials. Major clinical trials of hypertension. What should be done next? Hypertension 2005;46:1–6.
71. COPERNICUS: Packer M, Fowler MB, Roecker EB, et al. Effect of carvedilol on the morbidity of patients with severe chronic heart failure: Results of the Carvedilol Prospective Randomized Cumulative Survival (COPERNICUS) study. Circulation 2002;106:2194–2199.

SUGGESTED READING

Materson BJ, Reda DJ. Correction: single-drug therapy for hypertension in men. N Engl J Med 1994;330: 1689.

Messerli FH, Re RN. Do we need yet another blocker of the renin-angiotensin system? J Am Coll Cardiol 2007;49:1164–1165.

Oh Byung-Hee, Mitchell J, Herron JR, et al. Aliskiren, an oral renin inhibitor, provides dose-dependent efficacy and sustained 24-h blood pressure control in patients with hypertension. J Am Coll Cardiol 2007;49: 1157–1163.

10 Management of Angina

SALIENT CLINICAL FEATURES

Angina is a pain in the chest or adjacent areas caused by severe, but temporary, lack of blood (ischemia) to a segment of heart muscle, hence the term *myocardial ischemia.* For stable angina, the most important feature is the causation of pain by a particular exertional activity and relief within minutes of cessation of the precipitating activity.

Angina may be classified as

- Stable angina.
- Unstable angina.
- Variant angina (Prinzmetal's), coronary artery spasm (CAS).

The pain of angina must be differentiated from commonly occurring

- Gastroesophageal reflux and motility disorders.
- Musculoskeletal disorders, particularly costochondritis that causes tenderness without swelling of the second to fourth left costochondral junctions and may occur concomitantly with coronary artery disease.

It is necessary to document the presence or absence of diabetes and cigarette smoking, which markedly increases risk, and asthma, which contraindicates the use of beta-blocking drugs.

Physical examination should exclude secondary factors that may precipitate angina:

- Anemia and hypertension.
- Aortic stenosis, severe valvular disease, and hypertrophic cardiomyopathy.
- Arrhythmias.

Relevant baseline investigations include resting and stress electrocardiogram (ECG), total cholesterol, high-density lipoprotein (HDL) cholesterol, low-density lipoprotein (LDL) cholesterol, and triglycerides, as well as hemoglobin, glucose serum creatinine, and estimated glomerular filtration rate (GFR).

Pathophysiologic Implications

Three determinants play major roles in the pathogenesis of myocardial ischemia to cause stable or unstable angina:

- Atheromatous lesions are mainly concentric with stable angina and eccentric with unstable angina and cause >70% coronary stenosis.
- Myocardial oxygen demand is increased.
- Catecholamines are released in response to exertional and emotional stress or other activity. Catecholamines cause an increase in heart rate, velocity, and force of myocardial contraction

From: *Contemporary Cardiology: Cardiac Drug Therapy, Seventh Edition*
M. Gabriel Khan

Table 10-1
Beta-Blocker: First-Line Oral Drug Treatment in Angina Pectoris

Effect on	*Beta-blocker*	*Calcium antagonist*	*Oral nitrate*
Heart rate	↓	↑↓	—
Drastolic filling of coronary arteries	↑	—	—
Blood pressure	↓↓	↓↓	—
Rate pressure product (RPP)	↓	—[a]	—
Relief of angina	Yes	Yes	Variable
Blood flow (subendocardial ischemic area)[b]	↑	↓	Variable
First-line treatment for angina pectoris	Yes	No	No
Prevention of recurrent ventricular fibrillation	Proven	No	No
Prevention of cardiac death	Proven	No	No
Prevention of pain from coronary artery spasm	No	Yes	Variable
Prevention of death in patient with coronary artery spasm	No	No	No

[a]RPP variable decrease on exercise, but not significant at rest or on maximal exercise.
[b]Distal to organic obstruction.
↓, decrease; ↑, increase; —, no significant change.

that increase oxygen demand and ischemia. Increased heart rate decreases the diastolic interval during which coronary artery perfusion occurs. Ischemia further stimulates catecholamine release, thereby perpetuating the vicious circle.

Catecholamine release initiates and perpetuates a dynamic process. Thus, beta-blocking agents play a key role in the management of patients with myocardial ischemia manifested by anginal pain or silent ischemia. The pathophysiology of unstable angina is more complex and is dealt with later in this chapter.

TREATMENT OF STABLE ANGINA

It is crucial to control known risk factors for coronary artery disease strictly:

- Cigarette smoking must be curtailed; weight and stress must be addressed.
- Hypertension must be controlled with an appropriate drug; goal blood pressure (BP): systolic < 135 mmHg.
- Hyperlipidemia must be brought to goal levels: LDL < 2.5 mmol/L (100 mg/dL) and for high-risk patients < 60 mg/dL (1.6 mmol/L); HDL > 1.0 mmol/L (39 mg/dL).
- Diabetes must be treated aggressively.

Beta-Adrenoceptor Blocking Agents

All cardiologists now agree that beta-blockers are standard first-line therapy for stable and unstable angina. **In the first edition of this book in 1984**, I constructed a table that compared beta-blockers, nitrates, and calcium antagonists and indicated the rationale for beta-blockers as first-line treatment; this table has remained unaltered (Table 10-1).

Many patients with left ventricular (LV) dysfunction and borderline and class II–III heart failure (HF) were deprived of beta-blocker therapy from 1970 to 1999. These drugs were believed to be contraindicated in HF. However, beta-blockers continue to surprise us *(1)*. Randomized controlled trials (RCTs) have proved solidly that these drugs decrease mortality and morbidity in patients with all grades of HF (*see* Chapter 12), and at present they are strongly recommended in patients with angina and HF or LV dysfunction. Calcium antagonists and nitrates cannot reduce mortality or morbidity in these patients and are relegated to second-line therapy. **Therefore, virtually all patients with angina should receive a beta-blocker, preferably bisoprolol, metoprolol, or carvedilol, at a cardioprotective dosage** (*see* the later discussion of cardioprotective dose).

These 3 of the 12 available beta-blockers are chosen because they have been shown to decrease mortality in patients with coronary heart disease (*see* Chapter 1). *Atenolol, a water-soluble drug, is frequently used worldwide for angina and hypertension. The water-soluble, non-lipid-soluble beta-blockers atenolol and nadolol have not been shown in RCTs to decrease mortality in patients after myocardial infarction (MI) (2).*

- **It is important to reemphasize that only the cardioselective, lipid-soluble beta-blockers metoprolol, timolol *(3)*, and propranolol (in nonsmokers) and, recently, carvedilol *(4)* have been shown in RCTs to decrease mortality in post-MI patients.** *Beta-blockers have important subtle clinical differences (2).*
- **It remains probable that beta 1 and beta 2 effects are needed to render further cardioprotection** (*see* Chapter 1).

Beta-blockers significantly reduce the number of episodes of angina in more than 75% of patients. Beta-blockers may prevent up to 25% of deaths in patients with angina *(3)*, but reduction in mortality has not been documented in RCTs of patients with angina. Only a few small trials have been conducted, and with poor methodology. With the current use of aspirin, statins, and angiotensin-converting enzyme (ACE) inhibitors as routine therapy in patients with angina, it will take a huge number (>7000) of patients to mount a sound RCT, and such a trial is not planned. Patients receiving a beta-blocking agent have the advantage of pretreatment before a subsequent severe ischemic episode *(3,4)*.

Atenolol has been shown to reduce the number of ischemic episodes on Holter monitoring *(5)*. In a study by Laukkanen and associates *(6)*, silent ischemia detected on exercise test in middle-aged men with coronary risk factors but no prior coronary heart disease was associated with increased coronary events and mortality. The study provides strong support of silent ischemia as a marker of adverse outcome in presumably healthy middle-aged men with one or more risk factors *(7)*.

Observations have established that silent ischemia is common and is easily provoked by daily stressful activities *(8,9)*. Patients with angina may have more silent than painful episodes *(10,11)*. Beta-blockers, nitrates, and calcium antagonists have been shown to abolish silent ischemic episodes *(12)*, but beta-adrenergic blockers are superior. Atenolol and bisoprolol are more effective than nifedipine, especially in reducing the morning surge of silent ischemia *(13,14)*. Suggested steps in how to treat chronic stable angina pectoris are outlined in Figure 10-1.

The salutary effects of beta-adrenoceptor blockade are illustrated in Figure 1-1. These beneficial effects in myocardial ischemia result from

- A decrease in myocardial oxygen demand as a result of a decrease in heart rate.
- A decrease in the velocity and force of myocardial contraction.
- A fall in cardiac output and blood pressure; thus the rate pressure product (heart rate × systolic blood pressure) is reduced.
- Improvement in blood supply caused by a decrease in heart rate, which lengthens the diastolic interval. Because the coronary arteries fill during diastole, coronary perfusion improves.
- Blocking of exercise-induced catecholamine vasoconstriction at sites of coronary stenosis where atheroma could impair the relaxing effects of the endothelium.

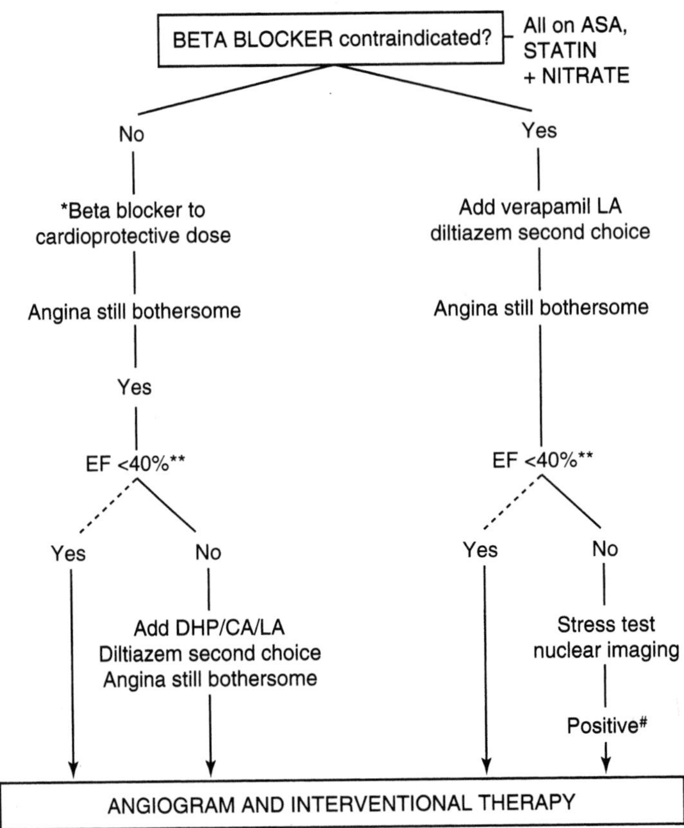

*Preferably carvedilol or metoprolol; *see* text.

**LV dysfunction, diabetes, hypertension, prior MI, silent ischemia, asthma that precludes beta-blockers increase the rationale for more urgent coronary angiograms.

DPH/CA, dihydropyridine calcium antagonist (only if a beta-blocker is combined with EF > 40%); ASA, acetylsalicylic acid; EF, ejection fraction; LA, long acting.

Fig. 10-1. Algorithm for the treatment of stable angina.

- A shift of blood from the epicardium to the subendocardial ischemic area (*see* Table 10-1).
- Decreased conduction through the atrioventricular (AV) node resulting in slowing of the ventricular response in atrial fibrillation or other supraventricular arrhythmias that may occur in patients with myocardial ischemia.
- Decrease in phase four diastolic depolarization producing suppression of ventricular arrhythmias, especially those induced by catecholamines and/or ischemia.
- Increase in ventricular fibrillation (VF) threshold reduces the incidence of VF and sudden deaths that could, at some stage, occur in patients with angina (*see* Chapter 1 for other mechanisms).

Cardioprotection and Dosage of Beta-Blocker

Table 1-4 gives dosages of beta-blockers. The dose of **metoprolol** is 100–300 mg, that of **propranolol** in nonsmokers is 160–240 mg, and that of **timolol** is 10–20 mg daily *(3,4)*, because these doses have been shown to be effective in preventing sudden death and decreasing total cardiac deaths in well-designed clinical trials *(3,15)*, albeit in patients after MI. The salutary effect of smaller doses is unknown, and larger doses are likely to be nonprotective (*see* Chapter 1) *(3)*.

The dose of beta-blocker is kept within the cardioprotective range, to maintain a resting heart rate of 52–60 beats/min bearing in mind that no patient should be allowed to have significant adverse effects from medication. If side effects occur, the dose is reduced, and a nitrate or calcium antagonist is added. If the maximum cardioprotective dose is used and angina is not controlled, the dose of beta-blocker can be increased, but adverse effects may limit the increase. Some patients do better on an average dose of beta-blocker plus a nitrate or calcium antagonist. Trial and error are necessary in many patients. *See* Chapter 1 for the choice of a beta-blocker.

Contraindications to Beta-Blockers

Contraindications to the use of a beta-blocking drug are

- Asthma.
- Severe chronic obstructive pulmonary disease.
- Severe HF (decompensated class IV). These agents have been approved for cautious use in patients with compensated class IV HF.
- Bradyarrhythmias (second- or third-degree AV block).
- Brittle insulin-dependent diabetes and patients prone to hypoglycemia. Beta-blockers are strongly indicated, however, in other diabetic patients because these patients are at high risk of coronary events, and calcium antagonists have been shown in an RCT to increase mortality (*see the discussion of the United Kingdom Prospective Diabetes Study Group in Chapter 1*).

An algorithm for the management of stable angina is depicted in Figure 10-1.

Calcium Antagonists

These agents are used as second-line therapy when beta-blockers are genuinely contraindicated. Several trials have shown that verapamil is as effective as beta-blockers in the control of angina, but this agent does not prolong life. Verapamil is a more effective antianginal agent than diltiazem or dihydropyridines (DHPs) and is considered a first choice, but the drug must be used with caution and must not be combined with a beta-blocker.

Contraindications to the use of verapamil and diltiazem include

- HF, suspected LV dysfunction, and ejection fraction (EF) < 40%, because verapamil has a strongly negative inotropic action and diltiazem is moderately so *(3)*.
- Sinus or AV node disease.
- Bradycardia.

Amlodipine (Norvasc) has a less negative inotropic effect than other DHPs, but in the Prospective Randomized Amlodipene Survival Evaluation (PRAISE) study *(16)*, although amlodipine use was generally safe in patients with HF, it caused an increased incidence of pulmonary edema in patients with EF < 30%. The drug is not recommended if the EF is <35% and should not be combined with a beta-blocker if the EF is <40%.

Combination of Beta-Blockers and Calcium Antagonists

Amlodipine has minimal negative inotropic effects and can be combined with a beta-blocker in patients with EF > 35%. Although beta-blockers may be used in patients with EF < 30%, the combination of a beta-blocker with diltiazem or dihydropyridine should be avoided in patients with EF < 40%.

Verapamil *(17,18)* and, to a lesser extent, **diltiazem** *(18)*, when added to a beta-blocker, may cause conduction disturbances or HF, and the verapamil combination is considered unsafe. The hemodynamic, electrophysiologic, and pharmacokinetic effects, adverse effects, and relative effectiveness of calcium antagonists are given in Tables 5-2 and 5-3 and are discussed in Chapter 5.

Nitrates

Drug name:	**Nitroglycerin: glyceryl trinitrate**
Supplied:	Sublingual nitroglycerin: 0.15, 0.3, 0.6 mg Sublingual glyceryl trinitrate: 300, 500, 600 mg (UK) Spray (Nitrolingual): 0.4-mg metered dose, 200 doses/vial
Dosage:	*See* text

Dosage

Start with 0.15 or 0.3 mg as a test dose with the patient sitting. The drug will not be as effective if the patient is lying down; if the patient is standing, dizziness or presyncope may occur. Thereafter, prescribe 0.3 μg nitroglycerin or 300 μg glyceryl trinitrate. If the systolic blood pressure in routine follow-up is more than 130 mmHg, then it is safe to give 0.4 mg.

The patient must be instructed that nitroglycerin tablets are to be kept in their dark, light-protected bottles; they may be rendered useless after 6 mo, or even earlier, if they are not protected from light. Patients should be advised to have at least two bottles available. These two bottles must contain approx 1 mo supply and no cotton wool, to ensure rapid availability in emergencies. At the end of each month, the containers should be emptied and the supply replenished from a third stock bottle. Patients may take one tablet before precipitating activities. If pain occurs and is not relieved by two tablets, the patient should immediately go to an emergency department. A third tablet can be taken before leaving for the hospital.

Oral Nitroglycerin Tablets

For Nitrong SR 2.6 mg, the dosage is 1 tablet at 7 AM and 2 PM daily. This will allow a 12-h nitrate-free interval to maintain the efficacy of the drug. The maximum dose 6.25 mg tab may cause bothersome headaches. Table 10-2 gives some of the available nitrate preparations.

Action

Nitrates bind to "nitrate receptors" in the vascular smooth muscle wall that activate guanylate cyclase and thereby stimulate the generation of cyclic guanosine monophosphate, which causes relaxation of vascular smooth muscle and thus dilation of veins and, to a lesser extent, arteries. The reason that venous dilation is greater than arterial is unknown. The result is marked dilation of the venous bed and therefore reduction in preload and a minimal decrease in afterload. A modest variable dilation of coronary arteries occurs. Nitrates have a direct effect on the compliance of the left ventricle and cause a downward shift in pressure-volume relationship.

The nonmononitrates are rapidly metabolized in the liver. The large first-pass inactivation of orally administered nitrates causes poor bioavailability to vascular receptors. Transdermal, buccal mononitrates or intravenous (IV) preparations partially overcome this problem.

Table 10-2
Nitrates

Generic	*Trade name or available as*[a]	*Supplied and dosage*[b]
Sublingual		
Nitroglycerin	Nitroglycerin	0.15, 0.3, 0.4, 0.6 mg (USA)
	Nitrostat	0.3, 0.6 mg (C)[c]
	Nitrostabiin	600 μg (C)
	Nitrolingual spray	Metered dose of 0.4 mg
Glyceryl trinitrate (UK)	Giyceryl trinitrate (GTN)	300, 500, 600 μg
	Coro-nitro spray	400 μg/metered dose
	Nitrolingual spray oral	400 μg/metered dose
Nitroglycerin oral tablets	Nitrong SR	2.6 mg (USA, C)
	Nitrostat SR, Nitrobid	7 AM, 2 PM
Buccal tablets	Nitrogard (USA)	1, 2, 3 mg
	Susadrin (USA)	1, 2, 3 mg
	Nitrogard SR (C)	1, 2, 3 mg
	Suscard (UK)	1, 2, 3, 5 mg
Isosorbide dinitrate oral, tablets	Isosorbide dinitrate	10, 20, 30, 40 mg (USA)
		10, 20, 30 mg (UK)
		10, 30 mg (C)
	Isordil	10, 20, 30, 40 mg (USA)
		10, 30 mg (UK)
		10, 30 mg (C)
	Cedocard 10, Cedocard 20	10, 20 mg (UK)
	Cedocard Retard	20 mg
	Isordil Tembids	40 mg capsules
	Sorbitrate	10, 20 mg (USA, UK)
Isosorbide mononitrate	Isosorbide mononitrate	20 mg
	Elantan 20	20 mg
	Elantan 40	40 mg
	Ismo	20 mg b.i.d., 7 h apart
	Imdur	60–120 mg once daily

[a]Several other trade names are available.
[b]For dosage *see* text.
[c]C, Canada.

Cutaneous Nitroglycerins

Long-acting or slow-release cutaneous nitroglycerin preparations are available.

Transderm-Nitro: 0.2, 0.4, 0.6 mg released/h
Nitro-Dur II: 0.2, 0.4, 0.6 mg released/h

The advantage of a cutaneous preparation is that the active drug reaches the target organs before it is inactivated by the liver. A therapeutic effect can be anticipated in 30–60 min and will last 4–6 h with the paste and about 20 h with long-acting preparations. Transdermal preparations should not be applied to the distal parts of the extremities or to the precordium where defibrillator paddles or chest leads may be placed. (Rare explosive events have been reported when contact was made with defibrillator paddles.) Cutaneous preparations are useful during dental work or minor or major surgery in patients with ischemic heart disease or hypertension. It is important, however, to ensure that such patients have tried the preparation and that the systolic blood pressure does not fall to <110 mmHg, because premedication and anesthetics can cause a further decrease in blood pressure. An attempt should be made by the physician to restrict the continuous use of transdermal preparations to up to 3 d and then 12 h daily allowing at least a 10-h nitrate-free interval. The patient should be weaned from the drug slowly, to avoid rebound.

Nitrate Tolerance

- It is well established that nitrate tolerance commonly occurs after several weeks of continuous nitrate use. Continuous infusion of nitroglycerin can result in tolerance within 24 h *(19,20)*.
- All long-acting nitrate preparations—transdermal, isosorbide dinitrate (ISDN) regular strength, or sustained-release isosorbide-5-mononitrate (ISDN 5. MN)—have shown complete attenuation of antianginal effects after 1–2 wk of continuous daily use *(21)*.
- A nitrate-free interval limits the development of nitrate tolerance. When 20 mg ISDN was given at 8 AM and 1 PM for 8 d, leaving a nitrate-free interval during the night, no alteration of the antiischemic effect of the drug occurred *(22)*. However, 15 d of continuous therapy with long-acting ISDN caused a 35–60% alteration of both ST segment and the EF response to exercise *(23)*. The vasodilator effect of transdermal nitroglycerin in HF is maintained with intermittent treatment, whereas tolerance develops with continuous therapy *(24)*.
- Veins and arteries are important sites of nitrate biotransformation. Organic nitrates are converted by intracellular sulfhydryl (SH) groups to nitric oxide and sulfhydryl-containing compounds. Vascular tolerance to nitrates is believed to result from a relative depletion of SH groups in vascular smooth muscle cells. A nitrate-free interval is necessary to allow intracellular generation of an adequate supply of SH groups and to restore vascular responsiveness.
- A nitrate-free interval of 10–12 h is necessary to prevent nitrate tolerance. Suggested steps include the following: ISDN 15–40 mg given at 7 AM, 12 noon, and 5 PM daily, or sustained-release one tablet 8 AM daily; Nitrong SR 7 AM and 2 PM daily; Ismo 20 mg twice daily 7 h apart; Imdur 30–120 mg once daily. Transdermal preparations should be used for about 12 h daily.

Drug name:	**Isosorbide dinitrate**
Trade names:	Coronex, Isordil, Iso-Bid, Sorbitrate (UK)
Supplied:	Isordil: 5-, 10-, 20-, and 30-mg tablets; 40-mg capsules; 10 mL ampules for IV use (1 mg/mL)
Dosage:	30 mg 7 AM, 1 PM daily; *see* text

Dosage

IV: 2–7 mg/h, polyethylene apparatus.

Sublingual: 5 mg before activities known to precipitate angina. Do not use the sublingual preparation instead of nitroglycerin for the relief of pain because the onset of action is delayed for 3–5 min.

Oral: 10–30 mg three times daily; if possible ½–1 h before meals or on an empty stomach. Maintenance: 30 mg at 7 and 11 AM and 4 PM; allow a 12-h nitrate-free interval to prevent tolerance. The 10-mg dose is ineffective.

Drug name:	**Isosorbide mononitrate**
Trade names:	Imdur, Elantan, Ismo (UK)
Dosage:	Initial 30 mg, then 60–120 mg once each AM; max. 240 mg if tolerated
Dosage advice:	Halve the dose for 1 wk if headache occurs with oral nitrate

The 5-mononitrate of isosorbide achieves consistent plasma nitrate levels, but tolerance quickly develops. The drug does not undergo hepatic degradation. It is excreted by the kidneys, unchanged and partially as an inactive compound. Activity lasts for 12 h and thus nitrate tolerance is avoided.

Caution: Gradually discontinue long-term nitrate therapy to avoid the rare occurrence of rebound increase in angina. Cover the nitrate-free interval with a beta-blocker or, if these drugs are contraindicated, administer a calcium antagonist.

Intravenous Nitroglycerin

IV nitroglycerin is of proven value in the management of unstable angina. Onset of action is within 1.5 min, with a duration of about 9 min.

- Low doses predominantly dilate the venous capacitance vessels and therefore decrease preload. The drug reduces LV dimensions and LV wall tension, thereby reducing myocardial oxygen consumption. The drug can also cause an increased myocardial oxygen consumption because of a reflex increase in the heart rate.
- Higher doses cause systemic arteriolar dilation and reduction in afterload.
- In rare instances when the patient does not respond and seems to be doing worse, the physician should entertain the possibility that the nitroglycerin has caused a shunting of blood from the ischemic to the nonischemic zone.

Indications

These include

- Refractory or unstable angina, chest pain, or acute coronary insufficiency. In this setting, continuous IV nitroglycerin is necessary without consideration of tolerance. The dose is titrated to control pain but with careful monitoring of BP.
- CAS.
- Pulmonary edema resulting from LV failure.
- Intraoperative arterial hypertension, especially during cardiac surgery (not routine), and in patients with Prinzmetal's angina and organic obstruction who are undergoing bypass surgery.
- To reduce the size of MI (not proved to be effective). A modest decrease in mortality rate was observed in one study of patients with acute MI.

Contraindications to Intravenous Nitrate or High-Dose Therapy

- Hypovolemia.
- Increased intracranial pressure.
- Cardiac tamponade and constrictive pericarditis.
- Obstructive cardiomyopathy, severe aortic stenosis, or mitral stenosis.
- Right ventricular infarction. (Decrease in preload may cause clinical and hemodynamic deterioration in categories 3, 4, and 5.)
- Glaucoma: closed-angle glaucoma or severe uncontrolled glaucoma.

Warnings

- IV nitroglycerin is a potent vasodilator, and hemodynamic monitoring is usually necessary.
  - The systolic blood pressure should not drop by >20 mmHg; reduce the dose if the systolic blood pressure is <100 mmHg.
  - A diastolic blood pressure of >60 mmHg is necessary for adequate coronary artery perfusion.

Table 10-3
Nitroglycerin Infusion Pump Chart
(50 mg in 500 mL 5% dextrose/water = 100 μg/mL)[a]

Dose (μg/min)	*Infusion rate (mL/h)*
5	3
10	6
15	9
20	12
25	15
30	18
35	21
40	24
45	27
50	30
60	36
70	42
80	48
90	54
100	60
120	72
140	84
160	96
200	120
250	150

[a]Increase by 5 μg/min every 5 min until relief of chest pain; decrease rate if systolic blood pressure < 100 mmHg or falls to 20 mmHg below the baseline, or diastolic blood pressure < 65 mmHg.

  - The pulmonary wedge pressure should be maintained at 15–18 mmHg in patients with acute MI.
- As much as 80% of the nitroglycerin may bind to the polyvinyl chloride infusion set. If such an apparatus is used, the infusion should be slowed down after 2 h because the binding sites in the tubing become saturated. Special polyethylene tubing sets should therefore be used.
- Use an infusion pump to ensure titrated dose response (Table 10-3). IMED infusion pumps are not compatible with the new non-polyvinyl chloride administration sets; however, new pump systems are being developed.
- Wean the patient from the drug slowly.
- Methemoglobinemia may occur after extended, continuous, high doses at levels greater than 7 μg/kg/min; cyanosis with normal arterial blood gases and methemoglobin levels > 1.5 g/dL confirm the diagnosis. Hypoxemia may result from increased venous admixture.
- Interactions with heparin or tissue plasminogen activator may occur.

Aspirin

All patients with stable angina should be administered a chewable or plain aspirin, enteric coated, 75–325 mg daily *(24)*. Aspirin is a potent antiplatelet agent and has been shown to improve survival and to prevent infarction in patients with unstable angina or after MI. A 75-mg dose has been shown to be effective and causes less gastrointestinal bleeding than the commonly prescribed 325-mg dose. An 81-mg enteric-coated aspirin tablet is available.

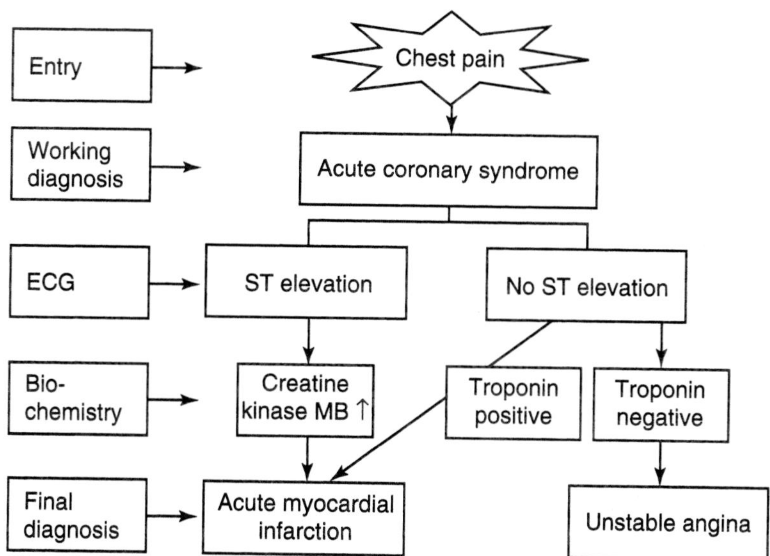

Fig. 10-2. Acute coronary syndrome terminology. (From Hamm CW, Bertrand M, Braunwald E. Acute coronary syndrome without ST elevation: Implementation of new guidelines. Lancet 2001; 358:1534; with permission.

Aspirin inhibits cyclooxygenase and the subsequent suppression of thromboxane A_2, the key moderator of irreversible platelet aggregation. A prospective study *(24)* of 2035 patients with stable angina showed that 75 mg aspirin added to sotalol produced a 34% decrease in primary outcome events of MI and sudden death ($p = 0.003$).

If aspirin use is contraindicated, clopidogrel is advisable. **Clopidogrel** has been shown to have favorable effects on cardiovascular events, equal to those of aspirin, but 75–160 mg coated aspirin is safer.

MANAGEMENT OF UNSTABLE ANGINA

More than half a million individuals are discharged from hospitals in the United States with a proven diagnosis of unstable angina.

Figure 10-2 gives acute coronary syndrome terminology. The pathophysiology of unstable angina has been clarified. In most cases, plaques are asymmetric, with irregular borders and a narrow neck. Rupture of the plaque with overlying thrombus is a common finding on angioscopy *(25)*. In addition, an inflammatory process, probably activated by microorganisms such as *Chlamydia pneumoniae,* appears to play a role in atheroma and plaque formation. There is a strong association between C-reactive protein (CRP) and coronary events. Lipid-rich plaques have a predilection for rupture. Silent ischemia is frequently observed in patients with unstable angina, and the prognosis seems to be worse in this subset *(26,27)*.

- The **order sheet** should indicate the **diagnosis**, rule out acute MI, and have the following suggested orders:

Investigations

- Serial ECGs.
- Troponin T or troponin I, 6- and 12-h to exclude non-ST elevation MI (NSTEMI) assist with risk stratification; measurement of creatine kinase, myocardial bound (CK-MB) isoenzyme levels, every 6 h for 24 h.

Table 10-4
Likelihood of Significant CAD in Patients with Symptoms Suggesting Unstable Angina

High likelihood (e.g., 0.85–0.99)	*Intermediate likelihood (e.g., 0.15–0.84)*	*Low likelihood (e.g., 0.01–0.14)*
Any of the following features:	Absence of high likelihood features and any of the following:	Absence of high or intermediate likelihood features, but may have:
• History of prior MI or sudden death or other known history of CAD	• Definite angina: Men < 60 yr or Women < 70 yr of age	• Chest-pain classified as probably not angina
• Definite angina: Men ≥ 60 or Women ≥ 70 yr of age	• Probable angina: Men ≥ 60 or Women ≥ 70 yr of age	• One risk factor other than diabetes
• Transient hemodynamic or ECG changes during pain	• Chest pain probably not angina and two or three risk factors other than diabetes[a]	• T-wave flattening or inversion < 1 mm in leads with dominant R-waves
• Variant angina (pain with reversible ST-segment elevation)	• Extracardiac vascular disease	• Normal ECG
• ST-segment elevation or depression ≥ 1 mm	• ST-segment depression 0.05–1 mm	
• Marked symmetrical T-wave inversion ≥ 1 mm in multiple precordial leads	• T-wave inversion ≥ 1 mm in leads with dominant R-waves	

[a]Coronary artery disease risk factors include diabetes, smoking, hypertension, and elevated cholesterol.
From Cannon CP. Management of Acute Coronary Syndromes, 2nd ed. Humana Press, Tototwa, NJ, p. 185; with permission.

- Chest radiography.
- Serum cholesterol, HDL, LDL cholesterol, triglycerides.
- Hb for anemia is relevant to angina occurrence.
- Creatinine clearance (eGFR) for adjustment of drug doses particularly low-molecular-weight heparin (LMWH) in patients older than age 70.

Diagnosis and Risk Stratification

Unstable angina, unlike NSTEMI, is a heterogeneous entity and exhibits marked variations in risk for coronary events such that patients admitted with a diagnosis of unstable angina may have no significant or mild coronary artery disease (CAD), and in others severe disease is present. Table 10-4 indicates the likelihood of significant CAD in patients with symptoms suggestive of unstable angina, and Table 10-5 gives the probable short-term risk of death or nonfatal MI.

Medications

- Relief of pain: give **morphine sulfate 2–5 mg IV** and every 30 min if required, to a maximum dose of 15 mg/h for 3 h. (Caution should be exercised in patients with severe pulmonary disease.) If morphine is still required after 3–4 h, this indicates that there may be progression of ischemia, which will require an increase in beta-blockers, IV nitroglycerin, or earlier coronary arteriography.

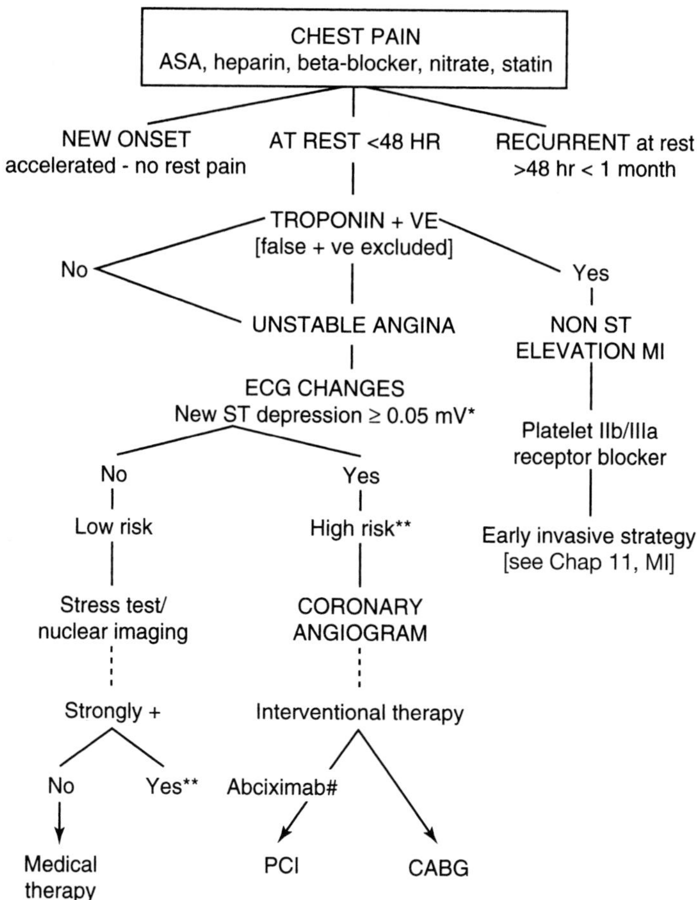

*European Society of Cardiology uses ≥0.1 mV, 1 mm.

**Diabetes, post MI 2 wk, old MI, HF or EF < 40%, hypertension, chronic ASA use increase the rationale for more urgent coronary angiograms.

#Eptifibatide also approved. Platelet IIb/IIIa receptor blocker use varies with the institution.

Fig. 10-3. Management of unstable angina.

- Sedative: give oxazepam 15 mg (or equivalent) at bedtime.
- A stool softener is prescribed.

Specific Cardiac Medications

Figure 10-3 gives an algorithm for the management of unstable angina.

1. **IV nitrates** (if unavailable, use transdermal nitrate plus oral nitrates in high doses). Reduce the dose if the systolic blood pressure is <100 mmHg. A nitrate-free interval may place the patient at risk. It is advisable to continue IV nitroglycerin and titrate the dose upward to pain relief. Failure to gain complete pain relief with IV nitroglycerin, a beta-blocker, and diltiazem, if there is no contraindication to the last combination, should prompt consideration of coronary angiography and interventional therapy.
2. **Must add unless contraindicated: beta-blocker** in sufficient doses (e.g., metoprolol 50–100 mg every 8 h). Hold the dose if the systolic blood pressure is <95 mmHg or the heart rate is <45 per min **or give** IV beta-blockers for one or two doses followed by oral doses (*see* Chapter 1 for doses).

If pain is not completely controlled, add

3. Calcium antagonist: preferably **amlodipine** 5 mg, if no contraindication to combination with beta-blocker (LV dysfunction, EF < 35%, systolic BP < 120 mmHg). Monitor the BP carefully, because calcium antagonists may cause severe hypotension, especially if used concomitantly with IV nitroglycerin, and diltiazem may cause severe bradycardia or sinus arrest in patients with sick sinus syndrome, and a combination with a beta-blocker may be hazardous.
4. Diltiazem plus nitrates should be started at the time of admission if:
   - Beta-blockers are contraindicated, in the following situation:
     - CAS is strongly suspected: the patient gives a clear history of chronic resting angina; or transient ST segment elevation is present during pain. Severe obstructive atherosclerotic coronary artery disease is very common, whereas CAS in its pure form is very rare. Thus, in patients with new-onset resting angina not proved to result from CAS, beta-blocker therapy is strongly indicated.

Newer Antianginal Agents

Ranolazine and nicorandil are discussed in the Controversies section at the end of this chapter.

Aspirin

A timely Veterans Administration Study using 324 mg aspirin in patients with unstable angina resulted in a 50% reduction in mortality rate and nonfatal MIs *(28)*. In another randomized study, aspirin was shown to reduce the cardiac mortality rate by 50% in patients with unstable angina *(29)*. A Swedish study using 75 mg aspirin in patients with stable angina showed a 34% reduction in MI and death.

All patients should receive aspirin 160–325 mg daily if there is no contraindication. Aspirin should be avoided in patients with variant angina because the drug may precipitate episodes of angina.

Clopidogrel

Clopidogrel 600 mg loading dose is given in some hospitals on presentation as soon as the diagnosis of probable NSTEMI/unstable angina is made and is given at the same time as chewable aspirin 75–100 mg. In other hospitals clopidogrel is given 600 mg <2 h before percutaneous coronary intervention (PCI). (*See* Chapters 11, 19, and 22 for further discussion regarding clopidogrel administration.)

Heparin

Paul Wood has observed that heparin reduces the incidence of MI in patients with acute coronary insufficiency; Telford and Wilson *(30)* showed heparin to be effective in the intermediate coronary syndrome. In most patients with unstable angina, a combination of nitrates with a beta-blocker and/or calcium antagonist with aspirin or heparin is advisable *(2,31)*. Heparin is often used in place of aspirin or added to aspirin *(32)*. The study by Theroux and colleagues *(32)* showed no significant differences among the three treatment arms with respect to fatal or nonfatal infarction. A clinical study by Holdright and associates *(33)* showed that combined therapy with heparin and aspirin compared with aspirin alone made no difference in the development of MI, death, or transient myocardial ischemia. A further study by Theroux and colleagues *(34)* showed heparin to be superior to aspirin in preventing infarction during the acute phase of unstable angina; MI occurred in 0.8% of heparin-treated patients and in 3.7% of aspirin-treated patients ($F < 0.05$).

Low-Molecular-Weight Heparin

Several RCTs have shown that LMWH is as effective as standard heparin and is easier to administer. The need for measurement of the prothrombin time is not required, and the incidence of thrombocytopenia appears to be lower. Because this agent can be used at home, it has the potential for cost savings.

The Enoxparin in Unstable Angina and Non Q Wave Myocardial Infarction (ESSENCE) study *(35)* randomized 3171 patients with unstable angina or non-Q-wave MI. Patients received IV dose-adjusted regular heparin plus aspirin 100-160 mg or subcutaneous enoxaparin 1 mg/kg 12 hourly plus aspirin. At 14 d, the risk of death, MI, or recurrent angina was significantly lower in patients assigned to enoxaparin than in those receiving regular heparin (16.6% versus 19.8%; $p = 0.019$). This improvement in events was maintained at 30 d. The 30-d incidence of major bleeding complications was 7% in the regular heparin group and 6.5% in the enoxaparin group. (*See* Chapters 11 and 22 for results of recent RCTS and comparison with fondaparinux.)

Dosage: Enoxaparin: 1 mg/kg every 12 h subcutaneously.

- Patients 75 yr and older should receive 0.75 mg/kg once daily dosing with a caution to assess creatinine clearance; if the estimated GFR is < 50 mL/min, the dose should be given once daily and avoided if estimated GFR is <30 mL/min.
- Patients with estimated GFR 30–40 mL/h should receive half the standard dose given above once daily. LMWH is not advisable if the GFR is <30 mL/min.
- Patients should not be switched from LMWH to UF heparin or vice versa.

Statins

- It is imperative to maintain the LDL cholesterol level at <60 mg/dL (1.6 mmol/L) in patients with unstable angina.
- A level of 60 mg (1.6 mmol/L) or less is now preferred (*see* ASTEROID trial in Chapter 22).

Thus, the use of a high-dose statin (e.g., atorvastatin 60–80 mg or rosuvastatin 20–40 mg daily) should be commenced in most patients during the hospital stay with monitoring of lipid levels in the subsequent weeks. Simvastatin and pravastatin have been shown in several RCTs to cause a decrease in cardiac mortality, a reduction in nonfatal and fatal MI, and angiographic regression of atheroma in patients with ischemic heart disease. Some of the salutary effects of statin therapy may result from modification of endothelial cell dysfunction; this modification occurs within days of therapy. Statins decrease elevated CRP levels, with reduction of CAD. Thus, it is advisable to initiate potent statin therapy when the patient is admitted for acute coronary syndrome (ACS) (*see* the RCT, PROVE IT-TIMI in Chapter 22).

Platelet Glycoprotein IIb/IIIa Receptor Blockers

Several RCTs have studied glycoprotein IIb/IIIa receptor blockers in unstable angina. Abciximab (ReoPro) has proved to be effective in clinical trials. The drug is indicated in patients undergoing coronary angioplasty and in those with unstable angina not responding to conventional medical therapy when angioplasty is planned within 24 h (*see* below).

Tirofiban (Aggrastat) plus aspirin was compared in a clinical study with aspirin plus heparin in patients with unstable angina *(36)*; at 30 d, the frequency of the composite end point with addition of readmission for unstable angina was similar in the two groups: 15.9% in the tirofiban group versus 17.1% in the heparin group ($p = 0.34$). A study of 1915 patients randomly assigned in a double-blind manner to receive tirofiban, heparin, or tirofiban plus heparin was stopped prematurely for the group receiving tirofiban alone because of excess mortality at 7 d *(37)*. There were fewer events at 7 d among patients who received tirofiban plus heparin and aspirin than in those who received heparin and aspirin (4.9% versus 17.9%, $p = 0.004$). The incidence at 30 d was 18.5% versus 22.3% ($p = 0.03$), and at 6 mo it was 27.7% versus 32.1% ($p = 0.02$). The incidence of death or MI at 6 mo was 12.3% in the tirofiban plus heparin and aspirin group compared with 15.3% of the heparin-aspirin group ($p = 0.06$). The results were not significant at 6 mo. Although platelet glycoprotein IIb/IIIa receptor blockers are expensive, the cost effectiveness of **abciximab** (ReoPro) and eptifibatide (Integrilin) in reducing mortality during PCI is favorable.

These agents are strongly recommended in patients at high risk of periprocedural complications, particularly, diabetes. Interventional therapy is necessary in virtually all patients at high risk. Abciximab is effective given as a bolus 10–60 min before the procedure; a pretreatment regimen offers no clear advantages, but the 12-h postprocedural infusion is necessary for a significant prevention of events. The European/Australasian Stroke Prevention in Reversible Ischemia Trial (ESPIRIT) trial results indicate that eptifibatide administered to patients undergoing nonurgent percutaneous transluminal coronary angioplasty (PTCA) with stent caused a **40% reduction in death or MI at 48 h after the procedure**.

Eptifibatide, lamifiban, and tirofiban have been tested in randomized trials with mixed results. Some trials have not shown beneficial effects, and caution is required: Integrilin to Minimize Platelet Aggregation and Coronary Thrombosis (IMPACT) II, eptifibatide ($p = 0.063$ and 0.220); Randomized Efficacy Study of Tirofiban for Outcomes and Restenosis (RESTORE), tirofiban ($p = 0.052$). In the Platelet IIb/IIIa Underpinning the Receptor for Suppression of Unstable Ischemia Trial (PURSUIT), eptifibatide-treated patients who underwent PCI within 72 h showed benefit ($p = 0.01$), **but no benefit at 30 d in those without PCI (*p* = NS)**. Lamifiban (Platelet IIb/IIIa Antagonist for the Reduction of Acute Coronary Syndrome Events in a Global Organization Network [PARAGON]) showed no significant effect on the incidence of death or MI at 30 d (*see* Chapters 11, 19, and 22 for TACTICS and other RCTs).

Antiinflammatory and Antiinfective Therapy

The atheromatous plaque, whatever the causative factor, is exceedingly inflammatory in unstable angina, and reactivation of the process and plaque rupture may trigger new thrombus.

There is a large body of evidence indicating a role for *Helicobacter pylori* and *C. pneumoniae.* Mounting evidence exists implicating *C. pneumoniae.* Particularly high titers of antibodies have been observed in patients with unstable angina, as well as the presence of elementary bodies, DNA, and antigens in the atherosclerotic arterial wall *(38)*.

In a study of 200 patients with unstable angina and non-Q-wave MI, treatment with roxithromycin administered for 30 d reduced the 6-mo mortality rate from MI from 4% to 0%, and the rate of death, MI, or recurrent ischemia from 9% to 2% *(39)*. A larger secondary prevention trial using azithromycin for 6 mo showed no benefit.

Cannon and colleagues enrolled 4162 patients who had had an coronary syndrome event within the prior 10 d and assessed the efficacy of gatifloxacin, a bactericidal antibiotic known to be effective against *C. pneumoniae,* in a double-blind RCT trial *(40)*. Patients were given 400 mg of gatifloxacin daily during an initial 2-wk course of therapy that began 2 wk after randomization, followed by a 10-d course every month for the duration of the trial (mean duration, 2 yr), or placebo.

The primary end point was a composite of death from all causes, MI, documented unstable angina requiring rehospitalization, revascularization, and stroke.

The rates of primary end-point events at 2 yr were 23.7% in the gatifloxacin group and 25.1% in the placebo group (hazard ratio, 0.95; 95% confidence interval, 0.84–1.08; $p = 0.41$). No benefit was observed in subjects with elevated titers to *C. pneumoniae* or CRP *(40)*.

Importantly, the inflammation observed in atheromatous plaques is probably a nonspecific inflammatory response to endothelial injury. This process, which occurs within the media, is nature's modulation, designed to protect and stabilize the injured area of the arterial wall *(41)*.

VARIANT ANGINA (PRINZMETAL'S)

Clues to Diagnosis

- Pain usually occurs at rest (often during sleep between midnight and 8 AM).
- The ECG shows ST-segment elevation during pain.
- Patients have a poor response to beta-blockers alone or a worsening of pain.
- CAS can be provoked by the use of IV ergonovine (with IV nitroglycerin drip on standby; nifedipine may be necessary to reverse spasm, which should be precipitated only in the cardiac laboratory). The test is not necessary, however, to initiate therapy.
- A few patients have ST-segment depression, and it is impossible to separate them from patients with angina from ischemic heart disease with fixed obstruction, except by a history of variable threshold or by an ergonovine test.
- Variable threshold angina may exist.

A subset of patients with variant angina may have significant obstructive coronary artery disease with spasm at the site of the plaque (Prinzmetal's) and may demonstrate any or all of the aforementioned features.

Investigations

Coronary arteriography should be considered in all patients.

Treatment

- Patients should stop smoking.
- Nitroglycerin tablets are taken sublingually.
- Among calcium antagonists, DHPs, verapamil, and diltiazem are equally effective *(41)*.
- It may be necessary to combine both a calcium antagonist and ISDN or isosorbide 5-mononitrate. Occasionally, the patient may respond to nitrates only, but at high doses.
- Beta-blockers provide no benefit, but combined with nitrates they are not as harmful as some would have us believe. Importantly, a review of all trials using beta-blocker monotherapy for CAS indicates neither benefit nor exacerbation *(42)*. Chronic resting angina is usually the result of CAS. New-onset resting angina must be considered as unstable angina, and in this large subset of patients, beta-blocker therapy *(42)* combined with nitrates remains routine *(42)*.
- Avoid aspirin because the drug can precipitate spasm in patients with variant angina *(43)*.

Unfortunately, patients with variant angina, even when the syndrome is completely controlled by calcium antagonists, have died or have had MIs *(42)*. Although calcium antagonists are efficient in controlling the pain of variant angina, **they do not prevent death**. Nitrates are much less effective and also do not appear to improve survival. Cardiac surgery is indicated in patients with significant atheromatous coronary artery obstruction.

Interventional Therapy

1. Seven RCTs of coronary artery bypass grafting (CABG) versus medical therapy were conducted during the 1970s and 1980s. CABG significantly decreased mortality at 5 and 7 yr. However, medical therapy did not include optimal treatment with beta-blockers, aspirin, statins to maintain LDL < 2 mmol/L (<79 mg/dL) *(44)*, and ramipril, the last agent proved in the Heart Outcomes Prevention Evaluation (HOPE) trial *(45)*.
2. Medical therapy versus PCI was assessed by the Randomized Intervention Treatment of Angina (RITA)-2 *(46)* and showed no difference in death and MI. In the small Atorvastatin Versus Revascularization Treatment (AVERT) trial *(44)*, stents were used in 30% of lesions, and aggressive medical therapy with atorvastatin maintained LDL < 77 mg/dL. The ischemic event rate was **13% versus 21%** in the PCI-treated group.
3. CABG versus PTCA in patients with multivessel disease and **normal LV function** was assessed in seven RCTs including the Arterial Revascularization Therapies (ARTS) study *(47)*, which showed no significant difference in mortality or MI. These were relatively low-risk patients, however, with normal LV function and mainly two-vessel disease (68% in ARTS), The ARTS study *(47)* compared stents with CABG; 16.8% of the stent group required a second revascularization, with a 73.8% event-free survival, 79% angina-free survival, and 21% free of anginal medication, versus, 3.5%, 87.8%, 90%, and 41.5%, respectively.

Diabetes: Niles and colleagues *(48)* analyzed a large regional contemporary database of patients with diabetes; 736 had PCI and 5030 had CABG. The 5-yr mortality was significantly increased after initial PCI, and this finding supports the conclusion in the Bypass Angioplasty Revascularization Investigation (BARI) trial *(49)*. Spencer King's editorial *(50)* reads: "Overall, the vote is in, and the winner has been declared. Surgery with at least one **internal mammary artery graft** [emphasis added] is superior to angioplasty in diabetics with multivessel disease" and normal EF (52%). Diabetics, if selected for PCI, should have normal LV function, two-vessel disease, absence of proximal left anterior descending (LAD) coronary artery disease, and suitable lesions from a technical standpoint.

CABG is recommended for patients with

- Triple-vessel disease, most patients with left main coronary artery, and particularly if LV dysfunction is present.
- Diabetes with two-vessel disease with a proximal LAD coronary artery suitable for internal mammary grafting (*see* earlier).
- Diabetes with lesions and LV dysfunction.
- PCI is recommended for patients with single-vessel and two-vessel disease, selected three-vessel disease, normal LV function, and suitable anatomy for the procedure. Diabetic patients with normal LV function who have single- and two-vessel disease in the absence of proximal LAD coronary artery disease may be suitable and selected on an individual basis.

Stable angina: Coronary angiograms with a view to revascularization are indicated in patients with the following: bothersome symptoms affecting lifestyle; ischemia despite optimization of medical therapy with a beta-blocker, nitrate, long-acting DHP (e.g., amlodipine), and statin to goal LDL < 2 mmol/L (80 mg/dL), and ACE inhibitor; patients with high-risk noninvasive test results and left ventricular dysfunction: EF 25–35%.

Unstable angina: Coronary angiograms are needed in patients at high risk (*see* Tables 10-5 and 10-6).

Table 10-5
Short-Term Risk of Death or Nonfatal MI in Patients with Unstable Angina

High risk	*Intermediate risk*	*Low risk*
At least one of the following features must be present:	No high risk feature, but must have any of the following:	No high or intermediate risk feature, but may have any of the following features:
• Prolonged ongoing (>20 min) rest pain	• Prolonged (>20 min) rest angina, now resolved, with moderate or high likelihood of CAD	• Increased angina frequency, severity, or duration
• Pulmonary edema, most likely related to ischemia	• Rest angina (>20 min or relieved with rest or sublingual nitroglycerin)	• Angina provided at a lower threshold
• Angina at rest with dynamic ST-segment changes ≥ 1 mm	• Noctural angina	• New-onset angina with onset 2 wk to 2 mo prior to presentation
• Angina with new or worsening MR murmur	• Angina with dynamic T-wave changes	• Normal or unchanged ECG
• Angina with S3 or new and/or worsening rates	• New-onset CCSC III or IV angina in the past 2 wk with moderate or high likelihood of CAD	
• Angina with hypotension	• Pathologic Q waves or resting ST-segment depression ≤ 1 mm in multiple lead groups (anterior, inferior, lateral)	
	• Age > 65 yr	

Abbreviations: CAD, coronary artery disease; CCSC, Canadian Cardiovascular Society class; MI, myocardial infarction; MR, mitral regurgitation.

From Cannon CP. Management of Acute Coronary Syndromes, 2nd ed. Humana Press, Tototwa, NJ, p. 186; with permission.

In TACTICS-TIMI 18 trial *(51)*, early invasive strategy was beneficial only in patients with elevated troponin T levels (i.e., NSTEMI) and not in unstable angina patients with no elevation of troponins (*see* TACTICS in Chapter 22). The Clopidogrel in Unstable Angina to Prevent Recurrent Events (CURE) study *(52)* suggests that **clopidogrel** plus aspirin has beneficial effects in patients with non-ST elevation acute coronary syndrome, but the benefit was small and was partially offset by an increased risk of bleeding necessitating transfusion (6 of every 1000 treated). **Caution** is also required because the drug can rarely cause thrombotic thrombocytopenic purpura and neutropenia. The 8-mo benefits in patients after PCI resulted in a 31% reduction in cardiovascular death or MI in the PCI-CURE study *(53)* (*see* Chapter 22 for the ACUITY trial).

CONTROVERSIES

1. **Does Clopidogrel plus Aspirin Have Any Value?**
   The CHARISMA trial *(54)* randomized 15,603 patients with either clinically evident CVD or multiple risk factors to receive clopidogrel (75 mg/d) plus low-dose aspirin (75–162 mg/d) or placebo plus low-dose aspirin. At 28 months clopidogrel plus aspirin was

Table 10-6
High-Risk Findings on Noninvasive Stress Testing

Exercise Electrocardiography
- 2.0-mm or greater ST segment depression
- 1.0-mm or greater ST segment depression in stage I
- ST segment depression or longer than 5 min during the recovery period
- Achievement of a workload of less than 4 METs or a low exercise maximal heart rate
- Abnormal blood pressure response
- Ventricular tachyarrhythmias

Myocardial Perfusion Imaging
- Multiple perfusion defects (total plus reversible defects) in more than one vascular supply region (e.g., defects in coronary supply regions of the left anterior descending and left circumflex vessels)
- Large and severe perfusion defects (high semiquantitative defect score)
- Increased lung thallium-201 uptake reflecting execise-induced left ventricular dysfunction
- Postexercise transient left ventricular cavity dilation
- Left ventricular dysfunction on gated single-photon emission computed tomography

Stress Echocardiography
- Multiple reversible wall motion abnormalities
- Severity and extent of these abnormalities (high-global wall motion score)
- Severe reversible cavity dilation
- Left ventricular systolic dysfunction at rest

METs, metabolic equivalents of task.
Adapted from Braunwald E. Heart Disease, 6th ed. Philadelphia, WB Saunders, 2001.

not significantly more effective than aspirin alone in reducing CVD outcomes. However, it is established that after PCI and stenting clopidogrel plus aspirin significantly reduces CVD outcomes and clopidogrel should not be discontinued prematurely.

2. **Are Newer Agents More Useful than Beta-Blockers?**

Ranolazine is a new second-line antianginal agent. The drug acts as a selective inhibitor of the late sodium current, which acts to reduce intracellular calcium in myocytes, thereby reducing the tension or stiffness of the myocardium that occurs during ischemia or HF. The drug may be combined with beta-blockers and ACE inhibitors because the drug does not cause a reduction in heart rate or BP and has no significant effects on myocardial contractility.

In small RCTs the drug reportedly reduced the number of anginal attacks per week and caused a modest improvement in treadmill exercise duration.

- Large-scale RCTs are required to establish this agent as an effective and safe antianginal agent. The drug, causes
- A prolongation of the QT interval, and syncope has been reported.
- Significant interaction occurs with potent CYP3A inhibitors including the antianginal agent diltiazem.

Nicorandil is a nicotinamide nitrate that acts as a potassium channel activator but also has a nitrate-like action. The drug reportedly causes modest dilation of large coronary arteries and reduces preload and afterload. *Indications:* prophylaxis and treatment of angina. The drug is used sparingly in the United Kingdom but extensively in Japan.

The drug has shown low efficacy in small RCTs and is not used in the United States and Canada. Avoid in patients with hypovolemia; low systolic blood pressure, cardiogenic shock; acute pulmonary edema; and acute MI with acute LV failure and low filling pressures. There are several drawbacks: oral ulceration, myalgia, and rash; at high dosage, reduction in blood pressure and/or increase in heart rate; angioedema, hepatic dysfunction, and anal ulceration; headache, flushing; nausea, vomiting, dizziness, weakness also reported.

It seems unlikely that nicorandil or **ranolazine** would fill a role for the effective management of stable angina; use in unstable angina remains controversial.

REFERENCES

1. Cruickshank JM. Beta-blockers continue to surprise us. Eur Heart J 2000;21:354.
2. Khan M Gabriel. Angina. In: Heart Disease, Diagnosis and Therapy. Totowa, NJ, Humana Press, 2005.
3. Norwegian MultiCenter Study Group. Timolol-induced reduction in mortality and reinfarction in patients surviving acute myocardial infarction. N Engl J Med 1981;304:801.
4. CAPRICORN investigators. Effect of carvedilol on outcome after myocardial infarction in patients with LV dysfunction. Lancet 2001;357:1385.
5. Pepine CJ, Cohn PF, Deedwania PC, et al. Effect of treatment on outcome in mildly symptomatic patients with ischemia during daily life: The Atenolol Silent Ischemia Study (ASSIST). Circulation 1994; 90:762.
6. Laukkanen JA, Kurl S, Lakka TA, et al. Exercise induced silent myocardial ischemia and coronary morbidity and mortality in middle aged men. J Am Coll Cardiol 200138:72.
7. Deedwania PC. Silent ischemia predicts poor outcome in high risk healthy men. J Am Coll Cardiol 2001; 38:80.
8. Deanfield JE, Selwyn AP, Chierchia S, et al. Myocardial ischaemia during daily life in patients with stable angina: Its relation to symptoms and heart rate changes. Lancet 1983;2:753.
9. Deanfield JE, Shea M, Kensett M, et al. Silent myocardial ischemia due to mental stress. Lancet 1984;2: 1001.
10. Deanfield JE. Holter monitoring in assessment of angina pectoris. Am J Cardiol 1987;59:18C.
11. Cohn PF. Total ischemic burden: Pathophysiology and prognosis. Am J Cardiol 1987;59:3C.
12. Pepine CT, Hill JA. Management of the total ischemic burden in angina pectoris. Am J Cardiol 1987; 59:7C.
13. Prakash C, Deedwania, Carlsajal EV, et al. Anti-ischemic effects of atenolol and nifedipine in patients with coronary artery disease and ambulatory silent ischemia. J Am Coll Cardiol 1991;17:963.
14. von Arnim T, for the TIBBS investigators. Medical treatment to reduce total ischemic burden: Total Ischemic Burden Bisoprolol Study (TIBBS), a multicenter trial comparing bisoprolol and nifedipine. J Am Coll Cardiol 1995;25:231.
15. Furberg CD, Friedwald WT, Eberlain KA (eds). Proceedings of the workshop on implications on recent beta-blocker trials for post-myocardial infarction patients. Circulation 1983;67(Suppl III):1.
16. PRAISE: Packer M, O'Connor CM, Ghoul JK, et al. for the Prospective Randomized Amlodipine Survival Evaluation study group. Effect of amlodipine on morbidity and mortality in severe chronic heart failure. N Engl J Med 1196;335:1107.
17. Subramanian B, Bowles MJ, Davies AB, et al. Combined therapy with verapamil and propranolol in chronic stable angina. Am J Cardiol 1982;49:125.
18. O'Hara MJ, Khurmi NS, Bowles MJ, et al. Diltiazem and propranolol combination for the treatment of chronic stable angina pectoris. Clin Cardiol 1987;10:115.
19. Elkayam U. Tolerance to organic nitrates: Evidence, mechanisms, clinical relevance and strategies for prevention. Ann Intern Med 1991;114:667.
20. Packer M, Le WH, Kessler P, et al. Induction of nitrate tolerance in heart failure by continuous infusion of nitroglycerin and reversal of tolerance by *N*-acetylcysteine, a sulfhydryl donor (abstract). J Am Coll Cardiol 1986;7:27A.
21. Abrams J. Interval therapy to avoid nitrate tolerance: Paradise regained. Am J Cardiol 198964:931.
22. Rudolph W. Tolerance development during isosorbide dinitrate treatment: Can it be circumvented? Z Kardiol 1983;72:195.
23. Sharpe N, Coxon R, Webster M, et al. Hemodynamic effects of intermittent transdermal nitroglycerin in chronic congestive heart failure. Am J Cardiol 1987;59:895.
24. Juul Moller S, Edvardsson N, Jhnmatz B, et al. Double blind trial of aspirin in primary prevention of myocardial infarction in patients with stable angina pectoris. Lancet 1992;340:1421.

25. Hamm CW, Bertrand M, Braunwald E. Acute coronary syndrome without ST elevation: Implementation of new guidelines. Lancet 2001;358:1533.
26. Gottlieb SO, Weisfeldt ML, Ouyang P, et al. Silent ischemia as a marker for early unfavorable outcomes in patients with unstable angina. N Engl J Med 1986;314:1214.
27. Nademanee K, Intarachot V, Josephson MA, et al. Prognostic significance of silent myocardial ischemia in patients with unstable angina. J Am Coll Cardiol 1987;10:1.
28. Lewis HD, Davis JW, Archibald DG, et al. Protective effects of aspirin against acute myocardial infarction and death in men with unstable angina: Results of a Veterans Administration Cooperative Study. N Engl J Med 1983;309:396.
29. Cairns JA, Gent M, Singer J, et al. Aspirin, sulfinpyrazone or both in unstable angina. N Engl J Med 1985; 313:1369.
30. Telford A, Wilson C. Trial of heparin versus atenolol in prevention of myocardial infarction in the intermediate coronary syndrome. Lancet 1981;1:1225.
31. RISC group. Risk of myocardial infarction and death during treatment with low dose aspirin and intravenous heparin in men with unstable coronary artery disease. Lancet 1990;336:827.
32. Théroux P, Ouimet H, McCans J. Aspirin, heparin or both to treat unstable angina. N Engl J Med 1988; 319:1105.
33. Holdright D, Patel D, Cunningham D, et al. Comparison of the effect of heparin and aspirin versus aspirin alone on transient myocardial ischemia and in-hospital prognosis in patients with unstable angina. J Am Cardiol 1994;24:39.
34. Théroux P, Waters D, Qiu S, et al. Aspirin versus heparin to prevent myocardial infarction during the acute phase of unstable angina. Circulation 1993;88:2045.
35. Cohen M, Demers C, Gurfinkel EP, et al. A comparison of low-molecular-weight heparin wïth unfractionated heparin for unstable coronary artery disease. N Engl J Med 1997;337:447.
36. Platelet Receptor Inhibitor Ischemic Syndrome Management (PRISM) study investigators: A comparison of aspirin plus tirofiban with aspirin plus heparin for unstable angina. N Engl J Med 1998;338:1498.
37. PRISM-PLUS: Platelet Receptor Inhibitor in Ischemic Syndrome Management in Patients Limited by Unstable Signs and Symptoms (PRISM-PLUS) study investigators. Inhibition of the platelet glycoprotein IIb/IIIa receptor with tirofiban in unstable angina and non-Q wave myocardial infarction. N Engl J Med 1998;338:1488.
38. Muhlestin JB, Hammond EH, Carlsquist JF, et al. Increased incidence of *Chlamydia* species within the coronary arteries of patients with symptomatic atherosclerotic versus other forms of cardiovascular disease. J Am Coll Cardiol 1996;27:1555.
39. Gurfinkel E, Bozavich G, Daroca A, et al. for the ROXIS Study Group. Randomized trial of roxithromycin in non-Q wave coronary syndromes: ROXIS pilot study. Lancet 1997;350:404.
40. Cannon CP, Braunwald E, McCabe CH, et al. for the Pravastatin or Atorvastatin Evaluation and Infection Therapy-Thrombolysis in Myocardial Infarction 22 Investigators. Antibiotic treatment of *Chlamydia pneumoniae* after acute coronary syndrome. N Engl J Med 2005;352:1646–1654.
41. Khan M Gabriel. Atherosclerosis. In: Encyclopedia of Heart Diseases. San Diego, Academic Press, 2006, p. 121.
42. Feldman RL. A review of medical therapy for coronary artery spasm. Circulation 1987;75(Suppl V):V-96.
43. Miwa K. Kambara H, Kawai C. Effect of aspirin in large doses on attacks of variant angina. Am Heart J 1983;105:351.
44. Pitt B, Waters D, Brown WV, et al. for the Atorvastatin Versus Revascularization Treatment investigators. Aggressive lipid lowering therapy compared with angioplasty in stable coronary artery disease. N Engl J Med 1999;341:70–76.
45. HOPE Investigators. Yusuf S, Sleigh P, Pogue J, et al. Effects of an angiotensin-converting enzyme inhibitor, ramipril, on death from cardiovascular causes, myocardial infarction, and stroke in high-risk patients. The Heart Outcomes Prevention Evaluation Investigators. N Engl J Med 2000;342:145–153.
46. RITA-2 Trial Participants. Coronary angioplasty versus medical therapy for angina: The second Randomized Intervention Treatment of Angina (RITA-2 Trial). Lancet 1997;350:461–468.
47. ARTS: Serruys PW, Unger F, Sousa JE, et al. for the Arterial Revascularization Therapies study group. Comparison of coronary artery bypass surgery and stenting for the treatment of multivessel disease. N Engl J Med 2001;1344:1117–1124.
48. Niles NW, McGrath PD, Malenka D, et al. for the northern New England Cardiovascular Disease Study group. Survival of patients with diabetes and multivessel coronary artery disease after surgical or percutaneous coronary revaacularization: Results of a large regional prospective study. J Am Coll Cardiol 2001; 37:1008–1015.

49. BARI Investigators. Seven-year outcome in the Bypass Angioplasty Revascularization Investigation (BARI) by treatment and diabetic status. J Am Coll Cardiol 2000;35:1122–1129.
50. King SB. Coronary artery bypass graft or percutaneous coronary interventions in patients with diabetes: another nail in the coffin or "too close to call"? J Am Coll Cardiol 2001;37:1016–1018.
51. TACTICS: Cannon CP, Weintraub WS, Demopoulos LA, et al. for the Thrombolysis in Myocardial Infarction 18 investigators. Comparison of early and conservative strategies in patients with unstable coronary syndromes treated with the glycoprotein llb/lla inhibitor tirofiban. N Engl J Med 2001;344: 1879–1887.
52. CURE: The Clopidogrel in Unstable Angina to Prevent Recurrent Events Trial Investigators. Effects of clopidogrel in addition to aspirin in patients with acute coronary syndromes without ST-segment elevation. N Engl J Med 2001;345:494–502.
53. PCI/CURE: Mehta SR, Yusuf S, Peters RJ, et al. for the clopidogrel in unstable angina to prevent recurrent events trial. Effects of pretreatment with clopidogrel and aspirin followed by long-term therapy inpatients undergoing percutaneous coronary intervention. Lancet 2001358:527–533.
54. CHARISMA: Bhatt DL, Fox KAA, Hacke W, for the CHARISMA Investigators: Clopidogrel and aspirin versus aspirin alone for the prevention of atherothrombotic events. N Engl J Med 2006;354:1706–1717.

SUGGESTED READING

Cairns JA. Ranolazine: Augmenting the antianginal armamentarium. J Am Coll Cardiol 2006;48:576–578.

Jespersen CM, Als-Nielsen B, Damgaard M, et al. CLARICOR Trial Group. Randomised placebo controlled multicentre trial to assess short term clarithromycin for patients with stable coronary heart disease: CLARICOR trial. BMJ 2006;332:22–27.

Smith SC Jr, Feldman TE, Hirshfeld JW Jr, et al. ACC/AHA/SCAI 2005 guideline update for percutaneous coronary intervention: A report of the American College of Cardiology/American Heart Association Task Force on Practice Guidelines (ACC/AHA/SCAI Writing Committee to Update the 2001 Guidelines for Percutaneous Coronary Intervention). J Am Coll Cardiol 2006;47:e1–121.

Stone PH, Gratsiansky NA, Blokhin A, for the ERICA Investigators. Antianginal efficacy of ranolazine when added to treatment with amlodipine: the ERICA (Efficacy of Ranolazine in Chronic Angina) trial. J Am Coll Cardiol 2006;48:566–575.

11 Management of Acute Myocardial Infarction

DIAGNOSIS

Acute coronary syndrome (ACS) embraces ST-segment-elevation myocardial infarction (STEMI) and non-ST-elevation MI (NSTEMI)-ACS *(1)*. The terms Q-wave and non-Q-wave MI are no longer used. Patients presenting with NSTEMI-ACS symptoms without biochemical markers of acute myocardial infarction (AMI) (particularly elevated troponin) are regarded as having unstable angina (Fig. 11-1).

- Troponin levels and creatine kinase, myocardial bound (CK-MB) have no role in the diagnosis of STEMI prior to the institution of thrombolytic therapy or percutaneous coronary intervention (PCI).

  Troponin levels are useful in differentiating NSTEMI from unstable angina.

- Astute observation of the electrocardiographic (ECG) changes of STEMI remain crucial for diagnosis and must be mastered.
- Patients with symptoms of STEMI (chest discomfort with or without radiation to the arms, neck, jaw, epigastrium, or back; shortness of breath; weakness; diaphoresis; nausea; lightheadedness) should be transported to the hospital by ambulance rather than by relatives. If nitroglycerin is available, one tablet or two puffs sublingual should be used and two chewable aspirins are taken while awaiting the ambulance.
- Nitrates should not be used by patients who have received a phosphodiesterase inhibitor for erectile dysfunction within the last 24 h (48 h for tadalafil).

Thuresson and colleagues point out that the typical **symptom onset of AMI is observed in less than 50% of patients with STEMI; only one in five fulfill all the criteria usually associated with an acute MI** *(2)*.

- **Symptoms of AMI in women may differ from those in men but not markedly. Most important, women more frequently report pain/discomfort in the neck or jaw and back, as well as nausea and vomiting; they score their pain/discomfort slightly higher than men *(2)*.**

An **acute MI remains a fatal event in >33% of patients. Approximately 50% of deaths occur within 1 h of onset of symptoms**, mainly because of ventricular fibrillation (VF). The incidence of AMI is similar in Europe; unfortunately, the incidence is increasing in Asia and Latin America.

GENOMICS

Topol *(3)* emphasized that although more than 50 million American adults have some atheromatous coronary artery disease (CAD), only a small fraction will ever

From: *Contemporary Cardiology: Cardiac Drug Therapy, Seventh Edition*
M. Gabriel Khan © Humana Press Inc., Totowa, NJ

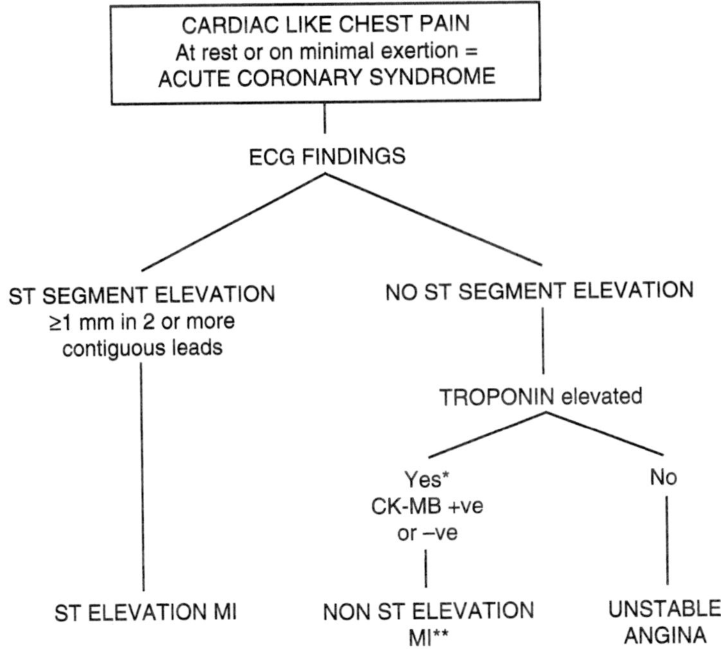

*Exclude false +ve. If troponins unavailable, creatine kinase, myocardial bound (CK-MB) + ve also confirms diagnosis; CK-MB –ve with the associated ECG changes = unstable angina high risk.

**ACC/AHA guideline: associated with ST depression ≥ 0.05 mV, 0.5 mm. European Society of Cardiology ≥ 0.1 mV, 1 mm.

Fig. 11-1. Diagnosis of ST segment elevation MI (STEMI) and non-ST segment elevation MI (NSTEMI) Acute coronary syndrome.

develop erosion, fissuring, or plaque rupture that culminates in AMI. In the United States, the number of hospitalizations for ACS in 2002 was 1,673,000; of these, approx 1 million had an AMI; STEMIs occurred in **approx 500,000 *(4)*; approx 500,000 are diagnosed with NSTEMI and unstable angina, approx 33% of the total.**

Willett *(5)* estimated that more than 80% of CAD may be accountable for by lifestyle issues: weight, diet, exercise, and control of risk factors such as blood pressure and smoking. Nevertheless the evidence for heritability of AMI is striking, with a positive family history being one of the most important risk factors for this complex trait *(6)*. Genetic studies indicate that the heritability of AMI is much more impressive than that of atherosclerotic CAD *(5,6)*, which in the majority remains stable and without plaque erosion or rupture.

RELEVANT KEY STRATEGIES

This chapter outlines the standard therapies for patients with AMI and emphasizes the importance of the early use of

- Aspirin and clopidogrel.
- Beta-blockers (metoprolol or carvedilol) used mainly orally.
- PCI, which if readily available is the first choice for reperfusion (*see* Fig. 11-2).
- Angiotensin-converting enzyme (ACE) inhibitors.
- Statins.
- Thrombolytic therapy when PCI is not readily available.

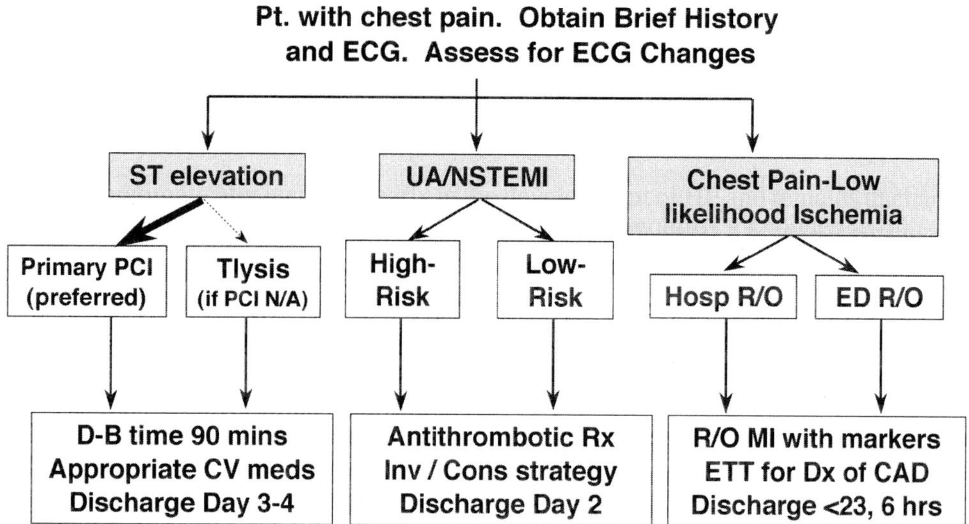

Fig. 11-2. Critical pathways for acute coronary syndromes at Brigham and Women's Hospital. (From Cannon CP. Coronary Syndromes, 2nd ed. Totowa, NJ, Humana Press, 2003, p. 749.)

These six agents have proved in several randomized controlled trials (RCTs) to decrease the incidence of cardiac events and mortality, but they are underused; their administration is often delayed unjustifiably.

AMI is usually caused by occlusion of a coronary artery by thrombosis *(8)* overlying a fissured or ruptured atheromatous plaque. The contents of a ruptured plaque are highly thrombogenic, and exposed collagen provokes platelet aggregation. Thus, the efficacy of aspirin should not be underestimated. Aspirin (160–325 mg) administered at the onset of symptoms markedly improves survival. In the Second International Study of Infarct Survival (ISIS-2), aspirin caused a 32% reduction in the 35-d vascular mortality rate *(9)*. Thus, all patients with known coronary heart disease must be strongly advised to chew and swallow this life-saving agent if chest discomfort exceeds 10 min or if chest pain is not relieved by nitroglycerin (glyceryl trinitrate).

- **Patients and the public must be informed that the use of 160–325 mg chewable aspirin (two 75–80-, or 81-mg soft chewable tablets tablets (not enteric coated) taken at the onset of a heart attack can cause a 25% decrease in the incidence of heart attack or death.** Aspirin should be taken once the decision has been made to proceed to the nearest emergency room. Individuals over age 35 (the MI age) should be warned that soft chewable aspirin acts rapidly and prevents fatal and nonfatal MI, but that nitroglycerin does neither. Nitroglycerin is effective mainly for coronary artery spasm, which is indeed a rare cause of acute MI.
- **In the United Kingdom advice for aspirin** is as follows: chewed or dispersed in water at a dose of 150–300 mg. If aspirin is given before arrival at hospital, a note saying that it has been given should be sent with the patient.
- Patients may be motivated to use this strategy if they are informed that **aspirin is more important than the use of nitroglycerin** because nitroglycerin may relieve pain of mild angina but does not prevent a heart attack or save lives. If chewable aspirin has not been used, then the dose should be given immediately on arrival at an emergency room.

Aspirin does not block catecholamine-induced platelet aggregation and does not decrease the incidence of sudden cardiac death or the occurrence of early-morning AMI. Beta-

Table 11-1
Thrombolytic Therapy: Timing of Admission and Survival

Time from onset of symptoms	*Lives saved per 1000 treated*
Within 1 h	65
2–3 h	27
4–6 h	25
7–12 h	8

blocking agents are successful here. The combination of aspirin and beta-blockers is life-saving and has proved to be effective.

- The thrombogenic properties of atherosclerotic plaques cannot all be nullified by aspirin or heparin, and clopidogrel has found a niche. New agents are being sought in clinical trials. Fondaparinux and bivalirudin are promising agents *(10)* (*see* Chapter 22).

After occlusion of the artery, myocardial cell death begins in about 20 min, and the area of myocardium supplied by the occluded artery usually becomes necrotic over 4–6 h. PCI completed within 90 min or thrombolytic agents given within the first hour of onset of symptoms markedly improve survival and morbidity. Although improvement in survival has been shown in clinical trials to occur with thrombolytic therapy given up to 6 h after the onset of symptoms, the gain is greatest within the first 2 h and then falls off dramatically after the fourth hour. Thrombolytic therapy administered at the earliest moment (<2 h) is of the utmost importance. Although clinical trials have indicated improved survival in patients treated between 6 and 12 h, the salvage is small (Table 11-1).

The delay in the emergency room from the arrival of the patient to the administration of thrombolytic therapy varies from 30 to 90 min. The door-to-needle time is stated to vary widely among hospitals. *A delay beyond 15 min is inexcusable (1).* Delays may result from duplication of assessments by different teams of clinicians. Thrombolytic therapy should be administered in the emergency room. The emergency room physician and assistants should have the training and authority necessary to administer a thrombolytic agent.

Extensive public education is essential. This is especially important in patients with known CAD. The patient and relatives must be aware of the early symptoms and signs of AMI. The patient may therefore quickly summon transport by a mobile emergency service that should be equipped with semiautomated defibrillators and provide the use of life-saving thrombolytic therapy; in the absence of such facilities, the patient should present without delay to the nearest emergency room for early therapy which should be given within the golden 1 h (Table 11-1). Fortunately, the availability of PCI has increased over the past 2 yr and is replacing thrombolytic therapy in many countries.

Pain Relief

- Pain relief must be achieved immediately and completely. **Pain** precipitates and aggravates **autonomic disturbances**, which may cause arrhythmias, hypotension, or hypertension, thus increasing the size of infarction.

Medications

1. **Morphine** is the drug of choice and should be given slowly IV.
   Dosage: Initial dose of 4–8 mg IV at a rate of 1 mg/min repeated if necessary at a dose of 2–4 mg at intervals of 5–15 min until pain is relieved. The dose is reduced or morphine

is discontinued if toxicity is observed, that is, depression of respiration, hypotension, or severe vomiting. The drug allays anxiety, relieves pain, causes venodilation, and therefore reduces preload. In addition, the drug has a favorable effect on VF threshold.

Caution: The drug is avoided or is used under close supervision if severe respiratory insufficiency is present. Severe vomiting and occasionally aspiration may increase cardiac work. Bradycardia is occasionally made worse, so care is required in patients with inferior MI in whom intense vagotonia already exists. Respiratory depression can be treated with the narcotic antagonist naloxone (Narcan) at a dose of 0.4–0.8 mg every 10–15 min as necessary to a maximum of 1.2 mg. Nausea and vomiting can be suppressed by IV metoclopramide 5–10 mg. The antiemetic should be given 5–15 min before the second injection of morphine.

The dose of the antiemetic is titrated to avoid sinus tachycardia.

a. In the United Kingdom, the pain and anxiety of AMI are managed with slow intravenous injection of **diamorphine. Dosage:** 2–5 mg IV every 4 h if needed. The drug appears to have a more euphoriant effect than morphine and is preferred physicians in the United Kingdom. An antiemetic such as metoclopramide (or, if LV function is not compromised, cyclizine) by intravenous injection should also be administered.

b. **Meperidine** (pethidine) is less effective than morphine and commonly causes sinus tachycardia. The drug is thus not generally recommended.

2. **Beta-blockers** must be given a more important place in the management of chest pain resulting from MI. Beta-blockers can be considered important second-line agents for the control of ischemic pain. This is of particular importance in patients with anterior infarction accompanied by sinus tachycardia and systolic blood pressure (BP) > 110 mmHg. Dramatic pain relief and reduction of ST segment elevation can be obtained by the administration of a beta-blocking agent. The requirement for opiates is thus reduced. In some patients, pain has been documented to be relieved by the administration of beta-blockers without concomitant use of opiates. Pain may be relieved even in the absence of sympathetic overactivity. When repeated doses of morphine are required to control pain, it is worthwhile introducing or increasing the dose of beta-blocker if there are no contraindications.
   - If there is no contraindication, metoprolol 25 mg every 12 h, increasing to 50 mg twice daily can be administered; carvedilol proved beneficial in the Carvedilol Postinfarct Survival Controlled Evaulation (CAPRICORN) study *(11)* in patients with ejection fraction (EF) < 40%.

Nonspecific Orders and Advice

1. Oxygen: 2–4 L/min.

   Considerations for the use of oxygen: 2–4 L/min of 100% oxygen by nasal prongs for 4–6 h is appropriate. Low-flow oxygen therapy is used if there is significant chronic obstructive lung disease and the arterial blood gas shows a P_{CO_2} > 45 mmHg.

   Should oxygen be used routinely? If hypoxemia is present as determined from arterial blood gas measurement, oxygen should be administered for 1–2 d or until measurements indicate the absence of hypoxemia. If measurements are not available and hypoxemia is suspected in view of clinical findings, such as the presence of LV failure (LVF), oxygen is administered. LVF causes ventilation-perfusion abnormalities and thus hypoxemia. If hypoxemia is not present, oxygen administration does not increase delivery of oxygen to tissue, and systemic vascular resistance may increase. Initiation of an IV line and administration of 5% dextrose/water keep the vein open.
2. Continuous monitoring of cardiac rhythm and heart rate. BP is measured at least every 15 min for 8 h and then every 30 min if stable.

3. Sedation: Oxazepam 15 mg (or similar agent) is given every 8 h for 2 d and then once daily, preferably at bedtime.
4. Reassurance: The patient must be reassured that the worst is over because most deaths occur before admission to hospital. This reassurance can be given by the resident staff or nurse, but it must be reinforced by the physician in charge because his or her authority is very persuasive and often relieves anxiety.
5. Diet: Nothing is given to eat or drink for the first 8 h; then if the pain is decreasing or absent, the patient can be put on a clear liquid diet for 12 h and then a light diet, potassium enriched with no added salt.
6. A stool softener: Docusate 100 mg is given three times daily.
7. Bed rest with a bedside commode. Patients should be encouraged to move the lower limbs while in bed. The patient with an uncomplicated infarct should be sitting at the side of the bed within 24 h after admission.

LIMITATION OF INFARCT SIZE AND INCREASED SURVIVAL

Timely reopening of the obstructed coronary artery is now possible with the use of PCI; where this is not readily available, thrombolytic therapy is used. In addition, the balance between myocardial perfusion and metabolic requirements must not be affected adversely by therapy. It is thus of paramount importance to avoid or correct measures that may increase infarct size, such as

- Tachycardia.
- Hypertension.
- Hypotension, in particular, hypovolemic hypotension, which may be induced by diuretics or nitrates.
- Arrhythmias.
- Hypoxemia.

Added strategies to limit infarct size and improve myocardial function and survival include

- The early administration of aspirin and clopidogrel.
- Beta-blocking agents. Current recommendations are to administer a beta-blocker as soon as possible if it is not contraindicated. Beta-blockers given within the first 3 h of onset of chest pain improve survival provided they are used orally in patients with stable BP (systolic > 105 mmHg) and there is no evidence of heart failure (HF).
- ACE inhibitors attenuate ventricular remodeling and improve adverse outcomes following AMI *(12)*. A clinical trial by Ambrosioni and colleagues *(13)* showed that zofenopril, an analog of captopril, commenced at approximately 15 h after the onset of anterior infarction and continued for 6 wk, caused a reduction in mortality and in the occurrence of severe HF at 6 wk and at 1-yr follow-up. Patients with large anterior infarcts, particularly those with previous infarction, should be commenced soon after admission on captopril 6.25 mg, increasing to 25 mg twice daily, or zofenopril 7.5 mg, increasing to 15 mg twice daily, provided the systolic BP remains >100 mmHg. ACE inhibitors are recommended in the first 24 h of an anterior MI or MI complicated by congestive HF or EF < 40% or both. The dose must be titrated to avoid hypotension. The first dose may be administered on the first hospital day if the BP is stable.
- The combination of an ACE inhibitor and a beta-blocker in patients with asymptomatic LV dysfunction provides additive benefits after MI *(11,14)*.

PERCUTANEOUS CORONARY INTERVENTION

The American College of Cardiology (ACC) guideline *(15)* **is: "If immediately available, primary PCI should be performed in patients with STEMI who can undergo PCI of the infarct artery within 12 h of symptom onset, if performed in a timely fashion (balloon inflation within 90 minutes of presentation"** (*Level of Evidence: A*) *(15).*

Policies are being mustered at all levels to ensure a door-to-balloon time of < 90 min. Various government agencies and other healthcare stakeholders expect physicians and hospitals to meet these performance standards. Unfortunately, despite active public education, triage in the United States, remains difficult, particularly because only approx 50% of patients with STEMI reach emergency rooms by ambulance.

THROMBOLYTIC THERAPY

Thrombolytic therapy is the mainstay of therapy in many countries worldwide where PCI is not immediately available.

Approximately 90% of patients with AMI are observed on coronary arteriography to have a thrombus completely occluding the infarct-related artery *(7)*. There is little doubt that coronary thrombosis is the major cause of MI and that prevention of plaque rupture and thrombosis or its immediate lysis with maintenance of a patent infarct-related artery improves short- and long-term survival.

The Italian trial of IV streptokinase (SK) (the GISSI trial) *(16)* and others have demonstrated that IV SK produces adequate reperfusion if it is **given within the first 2 h of the onset of the ischemic event** *(16,17).*

The GISSI study and ISIS-2 indicate that an IV infusion of 1.5 million U of SK over about 1 h is not particularly expensive or troublesome to give routinely, and heparin is not required.

Tissue plasminogen activator (t-PA) has several advantages over IV SK and is more effective than SK in producing higher early patency of infarct-related vessels *(18).*

The randomization of over 6000 patients in ISIS-3 and GISSI-2 indicated no real difference in early mortality between SK and t-PA, and, although there was a small trend suggestive of a slightly higher incidence of intracranial bleeding resulting from t-PA plus heparin, the total death or stroke rate with SK was approximately 11.1% and 11.1%, respectively, for tPA in ISIS-3, that is, no difference in "net clinical outcome." It is suggested, however, that in these two studies t-PA was not used optimally (very long infusion time with delay before starting heparin); heparin was used SC, when it is necessary to use heparin IV in the management of patients treated with t-PA.

This is especially important because GISSI-2 evaluated SC heparin commenced 12 h after t-PA as well as SK, and no major difference in outcome was seen. t-PA plus SC heparin is an inadequate method for use of t-PA, especially if SC heparin is delayed. IV heparin is essential to maintain patency of the infarct-related artery after the administration of tPA or tenectaplase because the raw surface of a fissured plaque is highly thrombogenic and continuous heparinization is required to prevent reocclusion.

The Global Utilization of Streptokinase and Tissue Plasminogen Activator for Occluded Coronary Arteries (GUSTO) trial studied 41,021 patients with acute infarction. The primary end point, 30-d mortality, was modestly but significantly lowered with accelerated t-PA (6.3%) versus SK (7.3%) a 14% risk reduction ($p = 0.006$) *(19).*

Not surprisingly, SK outcomes did not differ by heparin regimen.

Table 11-2
STEMI Patients at High Risk of Death

- Anterior MI
- Large infarct, extensive ST elevation
- Diabetes
- LV dysfunction, EF < 35%; HF
- Persistent systolic BP < 100 mmHg; heart rate > 100 beats/min
- New left bundle branch block
- Age > 75 yr

In the GUSTO trial, treatment times for infusion of thrombolytic therapy averaged 68 min. Currently, this delay exceeds 40 min. A delay exceeding 15 min after reaching a hospital to receive the "magic drug" is inexcusable, and hospitals will have to develop clear protocols for their emergency room physicians and staff to initiate thrombolytic therapy within 15 min of arrival. **In the United States, fewer than 50% of patients with STEMI receive thrombolytic therapy in the recommended door-to-needle or door-to-balloon time.**

The Assessment of the Safety and Efficacy of a New Thrombolytic (ASSENT)-2 trial compared single-bolus tenecteplase (TNKase) with front-loaded t-PA in 16,949 patients (20). At 30 d, mortality rates were almost identical, but in patients treated after 4 h, the mortality rate was 7% for TNKase and 9.2% for t-PA ($p = 0.018$).

In patients presenting within 4 h of symptom onset, speed of reperfusion is important, and TNKase, reteplase, or accelerated t-PA administration is preferred, particularly in patients at high risk: with anterior MI, new left bundle branch block, diabetes, and HF (Table 11-2) *(20)*. The patient of advanced age is at high risk, but there is also a higher risk of intracranial hemorrhage (ICH), and the choice of TNKase or SK should be individualized.

In patients presenting between 4 and 12 h after the onset of symptoms, the speed of reperfusion is of less importance; thus, SK and TNKase are equivalent choices. In many countries outside North America, *SK is used without heparin in the young or older patient with an inferior MI and in patients over age 75.* Individuals with acute MI in Europe, the United Kingdom, and among the >2 billion in Asia fortunately enjoy the benefits of SK. In the United States and Canada, TNKase is mostly used.

It is not logical to administer accelerated t-PA or TNKase to all patients with AMI, based on the net clinical benefit and cost effectiveness *(21)*. The choice of TNKase, t-PA, or SK is of little consequence to public health worldwide *(21)*, particularly when the **real problem is the emergency room door-to-needle time, which is still inexcusably high, in excess of 30 min**.

- The combination of SK and fondaparinux or bivaluridin without heparin deserves further RCTs. The incidence of ICH and heparin-induced thrombocytopenia can be reduced with the use of these agents.

The incidence of ICH in RCTs was reported as follows:

GUSTO II: SK 0.37, t-PA 0.72,
ASSENT-2: t-PA 0.93, TNK/t-PA, 0.94

- Analysis of the Medicare database suggests that thrombolytic therapy is harmful in patients >75 yr old *(22)*. Reportedly, the incidence of stroke is >4% for t-PA and approx 2.85% for SK in patients older than age 75.

- There appears to be a four- to fivefold greater incidence of ICH in patients >75 yr who are treated with t-PA versus SK.

Contraindications

- Existing or very recent hemorrhage; known or suspected bleeding diathesis; local tendency to bleeding (gastrointestinal disease with existing hemorrhages, translumbar aortography within the last 2 mo, recent punctures of large arteries).
- History of cerebrovascular accident with any residual disability, intracranial or intraspinal aneurysm, brain tumor, or arteriovenous malformation.
- Major surgery or serious trauma within the last 2 mo; eye surgery up to 3 mo previously; severe, poorly controlled hypertension with systolic values > 200 mmHg and/or diastolic values > 110 mmHg, but in the elderly aged > 75 yr, systolic BP > 200 mmHg or diastolic > 100 mmHg without therapy.
- Severe liver or kidney disease.
- Severe anemia.
- Disease of the urogenital tract with existing sources of bleeding.
- Diabetic proliferative retinopathy.
- Acute pancreatitis.
- Age over 75 yr with suspicion of cerebral arteriosclerotic vascular degeneration, agitation, or confusion.
- Mitral valve disease with atrial fibrillation because of a danger of embolism from the left side of the heart.
- Suspected aortic dissection.
- Allergy to SK or anistreplase or therapy with either drug from 5 d to 1 yr previously, but not contraindicated for t-PA or TNKase.
- Recent prolonged or traumatic cardiopulmonary resuscitation.
- Infective endocarditis.
- Pregnancy.

In the United Kingdom, advice on the use of thrombolytics is as follows:

- Patency of the occluded artery can be restored by PCI or by giving a **thrombolytic agent if not** contraindicated. Alteplase, reteplase, and SK need to be given within 12 h of AMI, ideally within 1 hr.
- Tenecteplase should be given within 6 h of acute MI.
- Antibodies to SK appear after 4 d, and therefore it should not be used again after this time.
- **Heparin** is used as adjunctive therapy with alteplase, reteplase, and tenecteplase to prevent rethrombosis; heparin treatment should be continued for at least 24 hr.
- Patients older than age 65 yr presenting after 12 h should not be given a thrombolytic drug; there is a high risk of cardiac rupture, particularly in women.

Drug name:	**Streptokinase**
Trade names:	Kabikinase, Streptase
Supplied:	Vials: 1.5 million IU; 750,000; 250,000; 100,000 IU
Dosage:	1.5 million IU in 100 mL 0.9% saline IV over 30–60 min

Action

SK is an enzyme derived from cultures of beta-hemolytic streptococci. SK forms an activator complex with plasminogen, converting circulating plasminogen to plasmin, which causes lysis of fibrin. Also, SK causes activation of fibrin-bound plasminogen. A patency rate of approximately 65% is expected if the usual dose of 1.5 million U is given within 3 h of onset of symptoms.

Advice and Adverse Effects

Anaphylaxis occurs in fewer than 0.5% of patients; angioneurotic edema, periorbital edema, and bronchospasm may occur. A skin test is available and can be done in the emergency room and read in 15 min.

Hydrocortisone or methylprednisolone is rarely used, because fatalities have not been reported, and reactions are easy to control with epinephrine and antihistamines. Hypotension is seen in fewer than 5% of patients and, fortunately, does not worsen with the administration of SK. The most common reaction is mild fever in 5–25% of patients, rigors, rash, flushing, and dyspnea. Hemorrhage is often confined to puncture sites and responds to pressure. Serious hemorrhage calls for discontinuation of SK and, if needed, blood products; clotting factors as well as a proteinase inhibitor such as Antagosan should be given: initially 200,000–1 million KIU, followed by 50,000 KIU/h IV until the bleeding stops.

Interactions

There is an increased risk of hemorrhage in patients who are receiving or who have been recently treated (past 5 d) with anticoagulants, indomethacin and similar antiinflammatory agents, sulfinpyrazone, allopurinol, and sulfonamides.

Drug name:	**Tissue plasminogen activator (t-PA): alteplase**
Trade names:	Activase, Actilyse (UK)
Supplied:	Vial: 10, 20, 50 mg
Dosage:	t-PA front loaded: 15-mg bolus; then 0.75 mg/kg over 30 min (not >50 mg), then 0.50 mg/kg over 60 min (not >35 mg); total dose ≤100 mg

Heparin is usually started with the t-PA infusion but can be delayed for at least 20 min after the start of t-PA and then continued to maintain the activated partial thromboplastin time (aPTT) 1.5–1.8 times control (50–75 s) for 48 h.

Action

t-PA binds specifically to fibrin. t-PA and plasminogen assemble on the fibrin surface. Fibrin increases local plasminogen concentration. Interaction occurs between t-PA and its substrate plasminogen through a cyclic fibrin bridge, resulting in activation of plasminogen to plasmin, which causes lysis of fibrin. t-PA has a very short half-life, and a 3-h infusion was used in several clinical trials up to 1990. The GUSTO trial used a 90-min infusion of t-PA.

Drug name:	**Tenecteplase**
Trade name:	TNKase
Dosage:	0.5-mg/kg bolus

TNKase is a genetically engineered triple-combination mutant of native t-PA. In ASSENT-II *(20)*, the drug caused similar mortality reduction as did t-PA in patients given the drugs at <4 h of onset, *but it was superior in patients treated at >4 h.* Rates for ICH were similar The major advantage is the ease of single-bolus injection.

Other Agents

Reteplase (Retavase, Rapilysin) is a deletion mutant of alteplase. Reteplase can be administered as a bolus injection; this is an advantage over t-PA and SK. Reteplase, however, showed only a small benefit over SK in the INJECT trial *(23)*, but it had mortality, ICH and stroke rates similar to those of t-PA in the GUSTO-III trial *(24)*. Heparin must not be given through the same IV line. **Dosage:** 10 U over 10 min; the same dose is repeated 30 min later.

ANTITHROMBINS

Low-Molecular-Weight Heparin

Enoxaparin

Enoxaparin SC is as effective as IV heparin for the prevention of adverse outcomes in patients with ACS. Major bleeding is still a concern, however. The risk for major bleeding can be reduced by decreasing the enoxaparin dose to 0.75 mg/kg once daily in patients age 75 and over and halving the dose administered once daily if the estimated glomerular filtration rate (GFR) is < 50 mL/min, as shown in the Enoxaparin and Thrombolysis Reperfusion for Acute Myocardial Infarction Treatment-Thrombolysis in Myocardial Infarction EXTRACT-TIMI 25 trial *(25)*. Importantly, the estimated GFR formula is inaccurate in patients older than 70 yr, and an adjustment must be made in patients of African origin (multiply the estimated GFR by a factor of 1.21; *see* Chapter 22 for advice on LMWH dosage).

The EXTRACT-TIMI 25 results for enoxaparin versus heparin were as follows:

- *At 30 d of follow-up:* The primary end point occurred in 12.0% of patients in the UF heparin group versus 9.0% in the enoxaparin group (17% reduction in relative risk; $p < 0.001$). There was no difference in total mortality *(25)*. Major bleeding occurred in 1.4% with UF heparin versus 2.1% with enoxaparin ($p < 0.001$). The exclusion of men with a creatinine level > 2.5 mg/dL (220 µmol/L) and women with a creatinine level > 2.0 mg/dL (177 µmol/L) was an important adjustment to prevent bleeding.
- This curtailment could have been adjusted further, however, using the suggested cutoff: for estimated GFR of 30–50 mL/min, give the 0.75-mg/kg dose once daily. If the GFR is < 30 mL/min, the latter reflects poor renal function and enoxaparin should be avoided if we are to prevent a high risk of bleeding with LMWH or fondaparinux (*see* Chapter 22).

Fondaparinux (Arixstra)

Fondaparinux is a synthetic pentasaccharide and an indirect inhibitor of activated factor X (Xa). In a comparison of fondaparinux and enoxaparin in acute coronary syndromes by the Fifth Organization to Assess Strategies in Acute Ischemic Syndromes (OASIS 5), investigators assigned 20,078 patients with ACS to either fondaparinux (2.5 mg daily) or enoxaparin (1 mg/kg twice daily) for a mean of 6 d. The primary outcome was death, MI and refractory ischemia major bleeding; and their combination at 9 d *(26)*.

- At 6 mo follow-up, the number of patients with primary-outcome events was similar in the two groups (579 with fondaparinux [5.8%] versus 573 with enoxaparin [5.7%]; hazard ratio in the fondaparinux group, 1.01 with no significant differences at 30 d).
- However, the rate of major bleeding at 9 d was 47% lower with fondaparinux than with enoxaparin (217 events [2.2%] versus 412 events [4.1%]; hazard ratio, 0.52; $p < 0.001$) *(26)*.
- Fondaparinux was associated with a significantly reduced number of deaths at 30 d (295 versus 352, $p = 0.02$) and at 180 d (574 versus 638, $p = 0.05$) *(26)*.

OASIS 6 *(10)* explored the effects of fondaparinux on mortality and reinfarction in patients with acute STEMI through an RCT of fondaparinux versus usual care in 12,092

STEMI patients. A 7–8-d course of fondaparinux was compared with either no anticoagulation or UF heparin (75% received UF heparin for less than 48 h). Sreptokinase was the main fibrinolytic used (given to 73% of those who received lytics). The primary outcome was a composite of death or reinfarction at 30 d.

- A conclusion from this trial is that fondaparinux is highly beneficial in patients in whom PCI is not available or feasible. Advantages over UF heparin include the lack of monitoring, the once-daily dose, much lower major bleeding and ICH, absence of heparin-induced thrombocytopenia (HIT), although thrombocytopenia can occur and platelet counts should be monitored. The half life is approx 15 h.
- **Dosage:** 2.5 mg SC once daily. Risk of hemorrhage is increased in patients with severe renal dysfunction, and the dose must be reduced if the estimated GFR is <50 mL/min. As advised for LMWH, the drug should be avoid if the GFR is <30 mL/min to avoid major bleeding (*see* warning for estimated GFR in patients over age 70 in the first paragraph of this section and also Chapter 22).

BETA-BLOCKERS

The salutary effects of beta-blockers are depicted in Figure 1-1. Beta-blockers cause a decrease in heart rate, BP, rate pressure product, and myocardial contractility, and they improve ventricular diastolic relaxation, thus producing a reduction in myocardial oxygen consumption. Additional benefits include the following:

- Myocardial oxygen consumption is increased by raised levels of fatty acids. Beta-blockers decrease levels of circulating free fatty acids.
- Improvement of coronary diastolic filling is achieved at a lower heart rate (*see* Chapter 1).
- Arrhythmias, including VF, which are probably induced by increased levels of catecholamine commonly present during the early phase of infarction, are prevented.

Theoretically, to achieve a favorable effect on infarct size, beta-blockers must be initiated before or within the first 3 h of infarction and certainly not later than 4 h from the onset of symptoms. Patients receiving beta-blockers before infarction appear to benefit.

Clinical trials have not adequately tested beta-blockers during the first 4 h of onset, as was done for SK and thrombolytic therapy; 4 h shows benefit with thrombolytic therapy. The Metoprolol in Acute MI (MIAMI) trial *(27)* is often quoted as showing no reduction in mortality, but the mean time to treatment was 11 h. In ISIS-1 *(28)*, 80% of patients were treated with atenolol for up to 8 h and <30% within 4 h; this approach resulted in a 15% decrease in mortality and significant prevention of myocardial rupture. Although atenolol has weak cardioprotective properties *(29)* and is expected to confer less cardioprotection than carvedilol and metoprolol, the drug showed a positive result (*see* Chapter 2, Beta-Blocker Controversies, and discussion of atenolol's poor efficacy).

Pooled trial results covering mainly 4–8 h indicated a 23% decrease in mortality occurring on d 1–2 *(1)*. Reduction of infarct size has been documented in an RCT *(30)*.

The ACC/American Heart Association (AHA) recommends beta-blocker therapy (metoprolol), given at the same time as aspirin, as soon as the diagnosis of AMI is entertained; thus, treatment should be given within 30 min after arrival at the emergency room, at which time an ECG should have been scrutinized and preparations made for PCI or administration of a thrombolytic drug.

These agents are indicated in all patients with AMI unless they are contraindicated by severe HF, heart block, bradycardia, systolic BP < 100 mmHg, or asthma. They are strongly indicated in AMI for anterior MI, with sinus tachycardia > 110 and BP > 110 mmHg. Sinus tachycardia, which is commonly present with anterior wall STEMI in the absence of HF, stimulates sensory nerves in the myocardium that initiate sympathetic overactivity and thus tachycardia and hypertension. Tachycardia lowers the VF threshold and predisposes to VF. The use of beta-blockers in this clinical situation often results in relief of chest pain and a decrease in the current of injury observed on the ECG. Beta-blockers are contraindicated, however, in patients in whom sinus tachycardia is a manifestation of HF. They are strongly indicated in AMI for

- Recurrent ischemic pain.
- LV dysfunction.
- Atrial fibrillation, rate control.
- Frequent or complex ventricular ectopy, particularly within days after MI.
- Virtually all patients from d 1 for several years, which has been proved to reduce mortality, recurrent MI, and HF. Therapy is expected to save 3–4 lives annually of 100 treated *(1)*, as indicated by the Norwegian timolol trial *(31)* and the Beta-Blocker Heart Attack Trial (BHAT) propranolol study *(32)*. Data from the Survival and Ventricular Enlargement (SAVE) trial *(13)* and CAPRICORN *(11)* indicate that beta-blockers given during acute-phase MI decrease 1-yr post-MI mortality in patients with low EF independent of the use of ACE inhibitors; the benefit from the use of both agents was additive.

Beta-blockers should be administered to all patients initially if there are no contraindications. Beta-blockade should be continued indefinitely for all patients who have residual LV dysfunction and who are at risk of ischemia.

ACE INHIBITORS

On the day of admission, after routinely recommended AMI therapies have been instituted, including aspirin, and, when appropriate, beta-blockers, and the patient has been stabilized, all patients with AMI should be considered for ACE inhibitor therapy. **There is a general agreement that high-risk patients—those with anterior MI, previous infarction, congestive HF or, in the absence of HF, an EF < 40%—should be administered an ACE inhibitor.** An RCT by Ambrosioni and colleagues *(12)*, the Survival of Myocardial Infarction Long-Term Evaluation (SMILE) study, showed that zofenopril, an analog of captopril, commenced at approximately 15 h after the onset of anterior MI and continued for 6 wk, caused a significant reduction in mortality and occurrence of severe HF at 6 wk and at 1 yr follow-up.

ACE inhibitors improve LV remodeling, prevent LV dilation, and preserve EF *(13)*. Systemic and coronary vasodilation has been suggested to limit infarct expansion and to prevent early remodeling. Patients with uncomplicated inferior MI, with EF > 40%, are unlikely to benefit significantly. Patients at high risk should receive life-long treatment.

ACE inhibitors are contraindicated in patients with systolic BP < 90 mmHg, renal failure, aortic stenosis, bilateral renal artery stenosis, a solitary kidney, and known allergy to ACE inhibitors. If ACE inhibitors are not tolerated, an angiotensin receptor blocker (ARB) is advisable (candesartan or valsartan; *see* Chapter 3).

NITRATES

IV nitrate is indicated for the relief of chest pain if more than the usual dose of an opiate is required and for the management of HF. ISIS-4 and GISSI-3 indicate that nitrates do not significantly influence survival in patients with AMI. The ISIS-4 trial *(33)* yielded an insignificant mortality reduction in patients randomized to nitrates. When data from randomized AMI trials are pooled, there is only a modest a 5.5% reduction in mortality rate with nitrate administration ($p = 0.03$). These agents are, therefore, not recommended for the routine management of acute infarction. There is an unjustifiable overuse of these agents for the management of pain during AMI.

The administration of IV nitrate requires careful monitoring to prevent harmful hypotension, reflex tachycardia, and hypoxemia. Hypotension is more common in patients who are volume-depleted by diuretics or in those with inferior and right ventricular infarction. In the latter subset, bradycardia is not uncommon. Prolonged use of IV nitrates at high infusion rates may produce significant methemoglobinemia. Avoid the use of nitrates in patients with right ventricular infarction, inferior MI with suspected posterior or right ventricular infarction, hypotension, bradycardia, and aortic stenosis.

STATINS

High-dose statins have proved to be effective in reducing morbidity and mortality rates in patients with ACS. In PROVE IT-TIMI 22 *(34)*, atorvastatin 80 mg daily decreased outcomes (*see* Chapters 17 and 22). A metaanalysis of four trials that included 27,546 patients demonstrated a 27% reduction in the odds of hospitalization for HF with intensive statin therapy in patients with ischemic cardiomyopathy *(34)*.

In PROVE IT-TIMI 22 *(35)*, atorvastatin 80 mg daily administered to patients with ACS significantly reduced the rate of hospitalization for HF (1.6% versus 3.1%; hazard ratio [HR], 0.55, 95% confidence interval [CI], 0.35–0.85, $p = 0.008$) independently of a recurrent MI or prior history of HF. Importantly, the risk of HF increased steadily with increasing quartiles of brain natriuretic peptide (BNP; $p = 0.016$ for the highest quartile compared with the lowest) *(35)*. Importantly, among patients with elevated levels of BNP (>80 pg/mL), atorvastatin administration significantly reduced the risk of HF compared with pravastatin (HR, 0.32; 95% CI, 0.13–0.8, $p = 0.014$) *(35)*.

MAGNESIUM

The Leicester Intravenous Magnesium Intervention Trial (LIMIT-2) studied 2316 patients with suspected AMI *(36,37)*. Only 60% of patients had proven infarction, and 52% of these did not receive a thrombolytic agent. Of all the trial patients, 35% were given a thrombolytic agent, and only 66% were administered aspirin. The study thus is not a comparison between magnesium (Mg^{2+}) and thrombolytic therapy. Furthermore, no indication was given of the number of patients who had probable Q-wave and non-Q-wave infarction.

ISIS-4 indicates no beneficial effects from the use of IV Mg^{2+} in acute infarction *(33)*. In ISIS-4, however, Mg^{2+} was given after thrombolytic therapy, and the 30% of patients not given a thrombolytic agent were randomized a median of 12 h from onset of symptoms. Patients given a thrombolytic agent were randomized at a median of 8 h. In LIMIT-2, Mg^{2+} was given a median of 3 h after onset of symptoms.

Experimental data indicate that a beneficial effect of Mg^{2+} is expected only if this agent is given before thrombolytic therapy, to prevent reperfusion injury *(33)*. Mg^{2+} appears to protect myocardial contractile function in models of ischemia-reperfusion injury. Because mechanical impairment of the heart, "stunning" *(38)*, develops within the first few minutes of reperfusion, Mg^{2+} if tried should be given before thrombolytic therapy.

The Magnesium in Coronaries (MAGIC) trial *(39)* in 6213 randomized patients, showed that magnesium administered IV within 6 h of onset of symptoms in high-risk patients with ST-elevation MI has no effect on 30-d mortality. The trial is conclusive, and magnesium has no role in the management of acute MI.

MANAGEMENT OF COMPLICATIONS OF INFARCTION

Arrhythmias

1. Bradycardia is common and is usually not harmful. The cautious use of atropine to correct severe bradycardia that is causing hypotension or ventricular ectopy is helpful. Atropine is given judiciously to increase the heart rate to a maximum of 60 beats/min. A slow rate is probably protective because the myocardium requires less oxygen. Overzealous use of atropine can cause sinus tachycardia and, very rarely, ventricular tachycardia (VT) or VF. Bradycardia associated with second-degree type II AV block and complete AV block unresponsive to atropine usually requires temporary pacing.
2. Tachyarrhythmias: sinus tachycardia has been adequately discussed.

VF is most common during the first 4 h of infarction and is observed in about 5.5% of patients in the first 4 h and in 0.4% of those admitted subsequently *(40)*. The incidence since the mid-1990s has been less than that quoted and appears to be related to the beneficial effects of thrombolytics, beta-blockade, and ACE inhibitors.

It is now clear that

- VF cannot be predicted accurately.
- Warning arrhythmias are misleading.
- VF can occur without warning arrhythmias and in the absence of HF or cardiogenic shock.
- VF may occur despite the adequate suppression of premature ventricular contractions (PVCs).
- Warning arrhythmias are seen frequently in those who have VF or do not go into VF.

Clearly, there is a relationship between the R-on-T phenomenon and VF, but the R-on-T phenomenon often occurs without precipitating VF. It is possible that when VF is precipitated by the R-on-T phenomenon, the VF threshold at that time has been decreased by factors such as

- Ischemia.
- Catecholamine release in the area of infarction (catecholamines increase cyclic adenosine monophosphate activity, which is believed to be important in facilitating the development of VF).
- Tachycardia (increases VF threshold).
- Hypoxemia.
- Alkalosis or acidosis.
- Hypokalemia, which lowers VF threshold (catecholamines may produce transient acute depressions in serum K^+ levels).

Lidocaine suppresses PVCs but does not sufficiently raise the VF threshold.

Management of PVCs in AMI: Most cardiologists have abandoned prophylactic lidocaine. PVCs, nonsustained VT (runs of three or more PVCs < 30 s) as warning arrhythmias, are generally ignored. Beta-blockers administered promptly to patients with MI should suffice for most of those with PVCs. This therapy has been shown to reduce the incidence of VF and death from AMI.

Prophylactic lidocaine may be important where facilities for monitoring cardiac rhythm are poor, but with heavy monitoring lidocaine is unnecessary, potentially toxic, and expensive.

Considerations against the routine use of lidocaine are as follows:

- Up to 60% of all patients admitted to the coronary care unit are found not to have AMI.
- VF occurs in about 5% of patients with acute infarcts during the early phase. It would require treating many patients not at risk and exposing many to the adverse effects of lidocaine.
- VF occurring in the coronary care unit is readily and easily managed, and no deaths usually result in this setting. Prophylactic lidocaine does not decrease mortality.
- VF may still occur despite adequate doses of lidocaine. In effect, 200 patients admitted to a coronary care unit must be treated with lidocaine to prevent VF in 5 without a significant decrease in mortality.

Dosage of lidocaine: For sustained VT, hemodynamically stable rate < 150 min: lidocaine IV initial bolus 1.0–1.5 mg/kg (75–100 mg). After 5–10 min, administer a second bolus, 1 mg/kg. Halve the dose in the presence of severe hepatic disease or reduced hepatic blood flow or a hepatically metabolized beta-blocker and in patients over age 65 yr.

The initial bolus is given simultaneously with the commencement of the IV infusion of lidocaine, so a lag between the bolus and the infusion does not occur. Commence the infusion at 2 mg/min; if arrhythmias recur, administer a bolus of 50 mg and increase the infusion rate to 3 mg/min. Carefully reevaluate the clinical situation and rationale before increasing the rate to the maximum of 4 mg/min. The maximum dose in 1 h equals 300 mg. Patients should be observed for signs of lidocaine toxicity and the dose reduced appropriately. Seizures may be controlled with diazepam.

VT: Electrical cardioversion is used if there is any hemodynamic deterioration. If the patient remains stable and VT persists, a further bolus of lidocaine is tried, followed by procainamide given as an IV 100-mg bolus: 25 mg/min; then 10–20 mg/min to 1 g in the first hour; then 1–4 mg/min.

Other arrhythmias: Atrial flutter or atrial fibrillation causing hemodynamic deterioration is converted electrically using low energy levels. If there is no hemodynamic disturbance, digoxin is administered. Esmolol may be used to control the ventricular rate.

Supraventricular tachycardia may require electrical conversion, but if there is no hemodynamic disturbance and HF is absent, esmolol or another beta-blocker is advisable.

Sinus bradycardia: Inferior and posterior MI initiates mainly vagal overactivity, which commonly causes sinus bradycardia and occasionally a nodal escape rhythm or AV block. Hypotension is often observed in this subset of patients. Bradycardia is commonly observed during the first hour of infarction *(41)*. Bradycardia may predispose to VF, especially if hypotension is present. Symptomatic bradycardia accompanied by hypotension or PVCs is managed effectively by the administration of atropine *(41,42)*. The drug should be used judiciously.

Atropine dosage: Titrated aliquots of 0.5 or 0.6 mg are given slowly IV every 3–10 min to increase the heart rate to approximately 60/min. Maximum atropine dose is 2.0 mg.

- **Caution:** Atropine in too large a dose (even 1.2 mg) or too rapid an administration may precipitate sinus tachycardia, and this is observed in about one-fifth of such patients despite careful titration. Rarely, VF may be precipitated *(43)*.

Severe bradyarrhythmias (AV block not responsive to atropine) are managed with pacing.

Heart Failure

Mild LVF is not uncommon and may resolve spontaneously. **Drug therapy** for patients unresponsive to two doses of furosemide (20, 40 mg) administered 1–2 h apart is best guided by Swan-Ganz catheterization and hemodynamic monitoring. First steps include the following:

- Furosemide is given IV 20–40 mg followed by 20–40 mg every 3–4 h if absolutely necessary. Serum K^+ must be maintained at a level > 4.5 mEq (mmol)/L.
- Morphine remains valuable.
- Sublingual, transdermal, or IV nitrate: Nitrates are useful to reduce preload when pulmonary congestion is present with a high pulmonary capillary wedge (PCW) pressure. They are contraindicated in patients with low cardiac output in the absence of a raised PCW pressure, right ventricular infarction, and cardiac tamponade and when nitroprusside is given.
- IV nitroglycerin (*see* Appendix I) or isosorbide dinitrate is given.

Any of the foregoing regimens results in clearing of symptoms of shortness of breath or pulmonary crepitations in most patients. Suggested steps for treating HF in the presence of AMI are discussed in detail in Chapter 12. IV nitrates must be used cautiously in patients with inferior or right ventricular MI, especially if associated bradycardia is present.

Oxygen: When hypoxemia is severe despite the use of 100% oxygen at 8 L/min by face mask, endotracheal intubation may be necessary. Positive pressure ventilation and/or circulatory assistance may be useful.

ACE inhibitors: These agents are recommended for the control of HF in patients with AMI.

Digitalis is generally avoided but may be tried for atrial fibrillation with uncontrolled ventricular rate in the presence of HF that has failed to clear with diuretics, nitrates, and ACE inhibitor therapy over 48 h. Digoxin levels should be maintained at 0.5–0.9 ng/mL and the serum potassium at 4–5.2 mmol/L. The drug is too weak an inotropic agent and cannot be relied on in patients with overt pulmonary edema or cardiogenic shock.

Dobutamine is usually reserved for severe HF. Nitroprusside increases cardiac output but may cause a coronary steal that is not seen with dobutamine or IV nitrates. The combination of nitroprusside and dobutamine or dopamine may be necessary. Use dobutamine for BP 80–100 mmHg; commence with a small dose, 1 μg/kg/min and slowly increase to 3–4 μg/kg/min (avoid if extreme hypotension present); use dopamine if BP is <80 mmHg. A combination of dopamine 5 μg/kg/min and dobutamine 4–5 μg/kg/min may suffice.

Because **nitroprusside** may produce a coronary steal, IV nitroglycerin is preferred. Nitroprusside is the drug of choice in patients with low cardiac output and LV filling pressure (LVFP) > 20 mmHg. If the LVFP is <15 mmHg, a reduction in stroke volume and cardiac output may occur. Infusion pump charts for dobutamine, dopamine, and nitroprusside are given in Tables 11-3 to 11-5. **Dopamine** and dobutamine do not have identical indications, and in particular situations one or the other agent may be preferred, or a combination at low doses may produce a beneficial effect.

In the management of severe HF or conditions causing hemodynamic derangements, it is vital to choose the appropriate agent or combination depending on the hemodynamic parameters. **The mean pulmonary artery pressure and the mean PCW pressure are well-recognized key parameters** (Table 11-6).

Statins: A high dose is recommended based on the conclusion from PROVE IT-TIMI 22. Atorvastatin 80 mg has been shown to decrease HF *(35)* (*see* earlier discussion).

Specialized Hemodynamic Complications

In acute severe mitral regurgitation or rupture of a papillary muscle or ventricular septum, hemodynamic deterioration is apparent. Cardiac catheterization followed by planned

Table 11-3

Dobutamine Infusion Pump Chart (Dobutamine 2 Ampules [500 mg] in 500 mL [1000 μg/mL])

Dosage	*Rate (mL/h) for different body weights (kg)*													
μg/kg/min	*40*	*45*	*50*	*55*	*60*	*65*	*70*	*75*	*80*	*85*	*90*	*95*	*100*	*105*
1.0	2	3	3	3	4	4	4	5	5	5	5	6	6	6
1.5	4	4	5	5	5	6	6	7	7	8	8	9	9	9
2.0	5	5	6	7	7	8	8	9	10	10	11	11	12	13
2.5	6	7	8	8	9	10	11	11	12	13	14	14	15	16
3.0	7	8	9	10	11	12	13	14	14	15	16	17	18	19
3.5	8	9	11	12	12	14	15	16	17	18	19	20	21	22
4.0	10	11	12	13	14	16	17	18	19	20	22	23	24	25
4.5	11	12	14	15	16	18	19	20	22	23	24	26	27	28
5.0	12	14	15	17	18	20	21	23	24	26	27	29	30	32
5.5	13	15	17	18	20	21	23	25	26	28	30	31	33	35
6.0	14	16	18	20	22	23	25	27	29	31	32	34	36	38
7.0	17	19	21	23	25	27	29	32	34	36	38	40	42	44
8.0	19	22	14	26	29	31	34	36	38	41	43	46	48	50
9.0	22	24	27	30	32	35	38	41	43	46	49	51	54	57
10.0	24	27	30	33	36	39	42	45	48	51	54	57	60	63
12.5	30	34	38	41	45	49	53	56	60	64	68	71	75	79
15.0	36	41	45	50	54	59	63	69	72	77	81	86	90	95
20.0	48	54	60	66	72	78	84	90	96	102	108	114	120	126

The above rates apply only for a 1000 mg/L concentration of dobutamine. If a different concentration must be used, appropriate adjustments in rates should be made. Usual dose range 2.5–10 μg/kg/min. Commence with 1 μg/kg/min, increase to 2 μg/kg/min, and avoid dose beyond 5 μg/kg/min.

Table 11-4
Dopamine Infusion Pump Chart
(Dopamine 400 mg in 500 mL [800 μg/mL])

Dosage (μg/kg/min)	*Rate (mL/h [pump] or drops/min [microdrip])[a] for different body weights (kg)*						
	40	*50*	*60*	*70*	*80*	*90*	*100*
1.0	3	4	5	5	6	7	8
1.5	5	6	7	8	9	10	11
2.0	6	8	9	11	12	14	15
2.5	8	9	11	12	15	17	19
3.0	9	11	14	16	18	20	23
3.5	11	13	16	18	21	24	26
4.0	12	15	18	21	24	27	30
4.5	14	17	20	24	27	30	34
5.0	15	19	23	26	30	34	38
6.0	18	23	27	32	36	41	45
7.0	21	26	32	37	42	47	53
8.0	24	30	36	42	48	54	60
9.0	27	34	41	47	54	61	68
10.0	30	38	45	53	60	68	75
12.0	36	45	54	63	72	81	90
15.0	45	56	68	79	90	101	113
20.0	60	75	90	105	120	135	150
25.0	75	94	113	131	150	169	188

The above rates apply only for an 800-mg/L concentration of dopamine. If a different concentration must be used, appropriate adjustments in rates should be made. Start at 1 μg/kg/min; ideal dose range is 5–7.5 μg/kg/min. Maximum suggested, 10 μg/kg/min. Dopamine should be given via a central line.

[a]Use chart (1) pump (mL/h) or (2) microdrip (drops/min).

Example: 60-kg patient at 2.0 μg/kg/min: pump: set pump at 9 mL/h; microdrip: run solution at 9 drops/min.

surgery provides the only chance of survival. Temporary hemodynamic stabilization may be achieved by nitroprusside and intra-aortic balloon counterpulsation.

Right Ventricular Infarction

Approximately 42% of acute inferior infarcts are accompanied by right ventricular infarction *(44)*. Patients with inferior MI and ST elevation in V4R indicating right ventricular infarction were observed to have a 31% mortality rate and 64% in-hospital complications, versus 6% and 28%, respectively, for those with inferior infarction *(45)*. The hypotension of right ventricular infarction may be confused with hypovolemic hypotension because both are associated with a low or normal PCW pressure. The markedly raised jugular venous pressure, Kussmaul's sign, absence of crepitations on examination and clear lung fields on chest radiography, a normal PCW, right atrial pressure > 10 mmHg, or a ratio of right atrial pressure to PCW pressure >0.8, in association with ECG findings of an inferoposterior MI, ST elevation in V4R, and the mean ST segment vector directed to the right and anteriorly *(46)* should suffice to establish the diagnosis. These ECG findings

Table 11-5
Nitroprusside Infusion Pump Chart
(Nitroprusside 50 mg [1 vial] in 100 mL [500 mg/L])

Dosage (μg/kg/min)	*Rate (mL/h) for different body weights (kg)* 40	50	60	70	80	90	100
0.2	1	1	1	2	2	2	2
0.5	2	3	4	4	5	5	6
0.8	4	5	6	7	8	9	10
1.0	5	6	7	8	10	11	12
1.2	6	7	9	10	12	13	14
1.5	7	9	11	13	14	16	18
1.8	9	11	13	15	17	19	22
2.0	10	12	14	17	19	22	24
2.2	11	13	16	18	21	24	26
2.5	12	15	18	21	24	27	30
2.8	13	17	20	23	27	30	34
3.0	14	18	22	25	29	32	36
3.2	15	19	23	27	31	35	38
3.5	17	21	25	29	34	38	42
3.8	18	23	27	32	36	41	46
4.0	19	24	29	34	38	43	48
4.5	22	27	32	38	43	49	54
5.0	24	30	36	42	48	54	60
6.0	29	36	43	50	58	65	72

The above rates apply only for a 500-mg/L concentration of nitroprusside. If a different concentration must be used, appropriate adjustments in rates should be made. Start at 0.2 μg/kg/min. Increase slowly. Average dose is 3 μg/kg/min. Usual dose range, 0.5–5.0 μg/kg/min.

indicate a proximal right coronary artery occlusion *(44)*. Two-dimensional echocardiography should demonstrate right ventricular akinesis or dyskinesis; intracardiac thrombi may also be detected. Radionuclide ventriculography should show a marked decrease in right ventricular EF. Differential diagnosis includes causes of a high right ventricular filling pressure—pulmonary embolism and cor pulmonale—which are identified by their clinical features and raised pulmonary artery pressure. Pericardial tamponade is distinguished by the four-chamber diastolic pressure increase typical of tamponade, as opposed to right-sided diastolic pressure increase with right ventricular infarction.

Management: Plasma volume expansion combined with inotropes such as dobutamine plus afterload-reducing agents can be life saving *(44)*. Diuretics or nitrates are positively harmful. Thrombolytic therapy is strongly indicated to ensure a patent infarct-related vessel. If hemodynamic deterioration occurs, angioplasty produces salutary effects.

Cardiogenic Shock

Cardiogenic shock usually results from extensive MI or development of mechanical defects such as rupture of a papillary muscle or ventricular septum.

Characteristic features are marked hypotension, systolic BP < 80 mmHg, marked reduction in cardiac index < 1.8 L/min/m^2, and raised PCW pressure > 18 mmHg.

Table 11-6
Choice of Pharmacologic Agents in Patients with Acute Myocardial Infarction Based on Hemodynamic Parameters

Drug effect	*Furosemide*	*IV nitrates*	*Dobutamine*	*Dopamine*	*Nitroprusside*	*ACE inhibitors*
Preload	↓	↓	—	↑	↓	↓
Afterload	—	Minimal ↓	Minimal ↓	↑	↓	↓
Sinus tachycardia	No	Yes	Minimal	Yes	Yes	No, minimal
Parameters						
Moderate heart failure PCWP ≥ 20 > 24	Yes	Yes	Yes, if BP >70	Yes, if BP < 70 and oliguria (or dobutamine)	BP > 110 and >6 h[a] postinfarction	Oral maintenance weaning nitroprusside
Severe heart failure PCWP > 4 Cardiac index > 2.5 L/min/m^2	Yes	Yes if BP > 95	Yes if BP >70	Yes if BP <70[b]	Cl < 6 h	Yes
Cardiogenic shock if BP < 95 PCWP > 18 Cardiac index < 2.5 L/min/m^2	Cl	Cl	Yes	Yes IABP	CI	RCI (*see* text)
Right ventricular infarction JVP ↑	Cl	Cl	Useful with titrated volume infusion	Relative Cl ↑ PA pressure	Cl	Cl

Yes, useful; ↓, decrease; —, no change; ↑, increase; BP, systolic blood pressure mmHg; Cl, contraindication; IABP, intraaortic balloon pump; JVP, jugular venous pressure; PCWP, pulmonary capillary wedge pressure; RCI, relative contraindication.

[a]Coronary steal during ischemic phase of infarction.

[b]Dopamine, dobutamine combination.

The insertion of a balloon flotation catheter (Swan-Ganz) is necessary for measurement of right and left filling pressures. BP should be measured by a direct intraarterial method. Systemic vascular resistance should be calculated.

Accurate determination of urinary volume output is essential. Guidelines to hemodynamic parameters include the following:

- The central venous pressure is inaccurate in the critically ill and in particular in a patient with cardiogenic shock.
- The pulmonary artery occlusive pressure (= PCW) is a reliable indicator of LVFP and is the preferred method of monitoring volume status. Normal LVFP is 8–12 mmHg. In AMI, because of reduction in LV compliance, allow a normal value of 13–18 mmHg; an LVFP of 16–20 mmHg may be necessary for optimal cardiac output.

Management

1. Hypovolemic hypotension, right ventricular infarction, cardiac tamponade, and pulmonary embolism are excluded or treated.

   Hypovolemic hypotension is a correctable condition and should be given first priority in the diagnostic checklist. Hypotension and reduced cardiac output are present with a PCW < 9 mmHg; this measurement can range from 9 to 12 mmHg and occasionally from 13 to 17 mmHg. (Right ventricular infarction is excluded by the presence of a markedly raised jugular venous pressure with a normal PCW.)

   If hypotension is present with a PCW < 17 mmHg, 50-mL IV bolus infusions of crystalloid or colloid are given with serial estimation of PCW and cardiac output.
2. Mechanical defects such as ruptured papillary muscle or ventricular septum require consultation with the cardiac surgeon. Temporary support is often attained with the combined use of nitroprusside and intraaortic balloon counterpulsation to allow catheterization.
3. Dopamine or dobutamine used alone or in combination improves hemodynamics. When the extent of myocardial damage is severe and systemic diastolic pressure remains <60 mmHg, mortality is not significantly reduced by dopamine, dobutamine, other cardiotonic agents, or vasodilators. Nitroprusside may occasionally increase cardiac output but may reduce coronary perfusion pressure.
4. Norepinephrine in doses of 2–10 mg/min may be given a trial when the systemic vascular resistance is not raised, but it does not significantly affect mortality. Norepinephrine in general is recommended only if all measures including balloon counterpulsation fail to maintain systemic arterial diastolic BP > 60 mmHg. Intraaortic balloon counterpulsation reduces afterload and increases diastolic pressure, thus improving coronary perfusion pressure.
5. Isoproterenol, methoxamine, and phenylephrine are contraindicated. The overall mortality rate is not improved by any of the suggested steps outlined.
6. Inhibition of nitric oxide synthase by L-NMMA appears promising, with rates of 50% for medical and 63% for intervention ($p = 0.027$) *(48)*.
7. Intraaortic balloon counterpulsation is needed to stabilize patients selected for angiography and revascularization.
8. PCI has a role in these critically ill patients and has resulted in an improvement in survival in this group *(49,50)*.

MANAGEMENT OF NON-ST-ELEVATION MYOCARDIAL INFARCTION

It is necessary to risk-stratify patients with NSTEMI. High-risk factors include:

1. ST segment changes in keeping with ischemia: If the ST segment burden is high the risk is increased.
2. Positive markers (troponin or CK-MB).
3. Recurrent ischemia: chest pain with further ECG changes of ischemia.
4. LV dysfunction: EF < 40% or manifest HF.

These patients should have coronary angiograms to define coronary obstructive lesions within 6–12 h of admission to an emergency room, with a maximum delay of 24 h.

The ACC/AHA diagnose NSTEMI with ECG-documented ST depression > 0.05 mm (0.05 mV) in two or more contiguous leads; the European Society of Cardiology uses ST depression of at least 0.1 mV

- Administer aspirin, beta-blocker, UF heparin, *or* LMWH (enoxaparin) and IV nitroglycerin if pain persists. High-dose statin reduces adverse outcomes, as indicated by the PROVE IT-TIMI 22 Study *(34,51)*. Atorvastatin 80 mg is usually administered to maintain LDL-C < 1.8 mmol/L (70 mg/dL). Also, the occurrence of HF is decreased *(35)*.
- Troponin testing represents a major advance in detecting small and micro-MI that may be undetected by CK-MB. Patients with positive CK-MB mass determined at admission and 6–12 h from onset have sustained an MI. Troponin T (or I) testing should be done on admission and 6–12 h after onset of symptoms (according to the European Society of Cardiology, 6–12 h after admission).

There is considerable debate concerning the best drug strategies prior to PCI.

During the years 2002–2005, platelet blockers were in vogue added to UF heparin or enoxaparin. Based on the results of several RCTs, prior to 2006 platelet receptor blockers were recommended for high-risk patients. Abciximab has proven benefit after angiography in patients selected for immediate PCI. The drug has no role outside this indication; it proved more beneficial than tirofiban in the TARGET trial *(52)*.

Eptifibatide is approved for PCI and for use during the wait before angiography, but the dose must be reduced if the GFR is <50 mL/min and avoided if it is <30 mL/min.

- The TACTICS-TIMI 18 trial indicates that tirofiban also has a role in this setting *(53)*.
- Diabetic patients benefit the most *(54,55)* from platelet receptor blocker therapy. The benefit in nondiabetic patients is minimal *(54)*, and benefit is maximal in diabetic patients when abciximab is used for PCI.
- The Clopidrogel in Unstable Angina to Prevent Recurrent Events (CURE) and PCI/CURE trials *(56,57)* established the salutary role of clopidogrel for NSTEMI and unstable angina. A 300–600-mg loading dose is advisable in combination with aspirin and should be given to virtually all patients with NSTEMI and continued at 75 mg daily for at least 9 mo regardless of PCI.
- A 600-mg loading dose of clopidogrel (Plavix), 6 h or more prior to planned PCI, is recommended. There is considerable debate regarding the dosing (300–600 mg) and the timing prior to PCI. Steinhubl et al. *(58)* point out that when a 300-mg loading dose of clopidogrel is used, little benefit is obtained compared with just 75 mg at the time of the PCI when the treatment duration is <12 h. In patients pretreated for longer durations, the optimal duration seems to approach 24 h *(58)*.

Giugliano and colleagues *(59)* emphasized the following:

- A clopidogrel loading dose of 600 mg obtains the full antiplatelet effect by 2 h *(60)*. Loading with 600 mg compared with 300 mg 4–8 h prior to PCI has been shown to be safe and has reduced the primary composite of death, MI, or target vessel revascularization significantly, from 12% to 4%, with all of the difference attributed to a reduction in post-PCI myonecrosis *(61)*.

- The Food and Drug Administration approval is for a 300-mg loading dose of clopidogrel, but the guidelines for PCI released by the European Society of Cardiology *(62)* recommend 600 mg in patients with NSTEM and unstable angina slated for immediate (<6 h) PCI.

Virtually all NSTEMI patients with positive troponin levels should undergo coronary angiograms, preferably 4–8 h after a 600-mg loading dose of clopidogrel and followed if indicated by PCI.

- In many centers in the United States, high-risk patients are taken to the cath lab within 12 h of admission; following the results of angiograms, clopidogrel is given if bypass surgery is not indicated.
- Surgery is indicated in <10% of this category of patients. Clopidogrel should be discontinued 5 d prior to surgery to prevent major bleeding because clopidogrel irreversibly inhibits ATP-induced platelet aggregation for the remaining platelets' life.

An early aggressive strategy is advisable for virtually all high-risk patients because adverse outcomes are reduced compared with conservative strategies that include PCI delayed for several days. Delays also increases patient-hospital costs. Patients graded at lower than high risk are catheterized within 48 h.

- Patients graded as low risk are discharged on a beta-blocker, aspirin, clopidogrel 75 mg, an ACE inhibitor, and high-dose statin; stress testing including nuclear studies further assess their risk and need for CT angiogram and probable PCI.

CHANGING STRATEGIES

Strategies are expected to change following the results of RCTs including the Acute Catheterization and Urgent Intervention Triage Strategy (ACUITY) trial *(63)*, which randomized 13,800 patients with NSTEMI-ACS undergoing an invasive strategy randomly to (1): UF heparin or enoxaparin with a glycoprotein (GP) IIb/IIIa blocker versus (2): bivalirudin with a GP IIb/IIIa blocker versus (3): bivalirudin with provisional use of a GP IIb/IIIa blocker (<7% received a platelet receptor blocker).

- Most important, bivalirudin administered alone without an added GP IIb/IIIa receptor blocker was as effective in reducing ischemic outcomes as was UF heparin plus a GP IIb/IIIa blocker or the study arm of enoxaparin plus a GP IIb/IIIa blocker but caused significantly (approx 50%) less major bleeding.
- Major bleeding caused by overdosing with UF heparin, LMWH, and a GP IIb/IIIa blocker is a common problem worldwide.
- Bleeding is increased in centers in which clinicians have not taken adequate precautions to lower doses in the face of age over 70 and/or renal dysfunction.
- The LMWHs, eptifibatide, and some GP IIb/IIIa blockers are eliminated by the kidneys, and caution is required.
- Bivalirudin has a short half-life of 25 min following IV infusion; the once-daily dosing without adjustment or monitoring is a remarkable feature. This agent is a major addition to our armarmentarium. Fondaparinux has proved to be effective, as indicated by OASIS-5, *(26)* and OASIS-6 *(10)*. However, adjustment must be made to fondaparinux dosing if the GFR is <40 mL/min (*see* Chapter 22).

Guidelines for PCI *(64)* and the use of heparins, antithrombins, and platelet GP IIb/IIIa receptor blockers for the management of NSTEMI patients will continue to change as a result of ongoing RCTs.

REFERENCES

1. Hamm CW, Bertrand M, Braunwald E. Acute coronary syndrome without ST elevation: Implementation of new guidelines. Lancet 2001;358:1533.
2. Thuresson M, Jarlov MB, Lindahl B, et al. Symptoms and type of symptom onset in acute coronary syndrome in relation to ST elevation, sex, age, and a history of diabetes. Am Heart J 2005;150:234–242.
3. Topol EJ. The genomic basis of myocardial infarction. J Am Coll Cardiol 2005;46:1456–1465.
4. American Heart Association: Heart Facts 2005. All Americans. Available at: http://www.americanheart.org/downloadable/heart/1106668161495AllAmAfAmHeartFacts05.pdf. Accessed July 27, 2005.
5. Willett WC. Balancing life-style and genomics research for disease prevention Science 2002;296: 695–698.
6. Wang Q, Rao S, Shen G-Q, et al. Premature myocardial infarction novel susceptibility locus on chromosome 1p34-36 identified by genome-wide linkage analysis Am J Hum Genet 2004;74:262–271.
7. Topol EJ, McCarthy J, Gabriel S, et al. GeneQuest Investigators. Single nucleotide polymorphisms in multiple novel thrombospondin genes may be associated with familial premature myocardial infarction Circulation 2001;104:2641–2644.
8. DeWood MA, Spores J, Notske R, et al. Prevalence of total coronary occlusion during the early hours of transmural myocardial infarction. N Engl J Med 1980;303:897.
9. ISIS-2 (Second International Study of Infarct Survival) Collaborative Group. Randomised trial of intravenous streptokinase, oral aspirin, both, or neither, among 17,187 cases of suspected acute myocardial infarction: ISIS-2. Lancet 1988;2:350.
10. Randomized trial. The OASIS-6 Trial Group. JAMA 2006;295:1519–1530.
11. CAPRICORN Investigators. Effect of carvedilol on outcome after MI in patients with left ventricular dysfunction; the CAPRICORN randomized trial. Lancet 2001;357:1385–1390.
12. Ambrosioni E, Borghi C, Magnani B, et al. for the Survival of Myocardial Infarction Long-Term Evaluation (SMILE) Study Investigators. The effect of the angiotensin-converting enzyme inhibitor zofenopril on mortality and morbidity after anterior myocardial infarction. N Engl J Med 1995;332:80.
13. Pfeffer MA, Braunwald E, Moye LA, et al. for the SAVE investigators. Effect of captopril on mortality and morbidity in patients with left ventricular dysfunction after myocardial infarction: Results of the Survival and Ventricular Enlargement trial. N Engl J Med 1992;327:669.
14. Vantrimpont P, Roleau JL, Chaun-Chaun W, et al. Additive beneficial effects of beta-blockers to angiotensin converting enzyme inhibitors in Survival and Ventricular Enlargement (SAVE) study. J Am Coll Cardiol 1997;29:229.
15. Antman EM, Anbe DT, Armstrong PW, et al. ACC/AHA guidelines for the management of patients with ST-elevation myocardial infarction—executive summary. J Am Coll Cardiol 2004;44:671–719.
16. GISSI: Italian Group. Effectiveness of intravenous thrombolytic treatment in acute myocardial infarction. Lancet 1986;1:397.
17. ISIS Steering Committee. Intravenous streptokinase given within 0–4 h of onset of myocardial infarction reduced mortality in ISIS-2. Lancet 1987;1:501.
18. Sheehan FH, Braunwald E, Canner P, et al. The effect of intravenous thrombolytic therapy on left ventricular function: A report on tissue-type plasminogen activator and streptokinase from the thrombolysis in myocardial infarction (TIMI phase I) trial. Circulation 1987;75:817.
19. GUSTO Investigators. An international randomized trial comparing four thrombolytic strategies for acute myocardial infarction. N Engl J Med 1993;329:673.
20. ASSENT-2 Investigators. Assessment of the Safety and Efficacy of a New Thrombolytic: Single-bolus tenecteplase compared with front-loaded alteplase in acute myocardial infarction: The ASSENT-2 double-blind randomized trial. Lancet 1999;354:716.
21. Collins R, Peto R, Baigent C, et al. Aspirin, heparin and fibrinolytic therapy in suspected acute myocardial infarction. N Engl J Med 1997;336:847.
22. Thiemann DR, Coresh J, Schulman SP, et al. Lack of benefit for IV thrombolysis in patients with MI who are older than 75 years. Circulation 2000;101:2239.
23. INJECT: International Joint Efficacy Comparison of Thrombolytics. Randomized, double blind comparison of reteplase-double bolus administration with streptokinase in acute myocardial infarction (INJECT): Trial to investigate equivalence. Lancet 1995;46:329.
24. Global Use of Strategies to Open Occluded Coronary Arteries (GUSTO-III) Investigators. A comparison of reteplase with alteplase for acute myocardial infarction. N Engl J Med. 1997;337:1118.
25. Antman EM, Morrow DA, McCabe CH, et al. Enoxaparin versus unfractionated heparin with fibrinolysis for ST-elevation myocardial infarction for the ExTRACT-TIMI 25 Investigators. N Engl J Med 2006; 354:1477–1488.

26. The Fifth Organization to Assess Strategies in Acute Ischemic Syndromes Investigators. Comparison of fondaparinux and enoxaparin in acute coronary syndromes. N Engl J Med 2006;354:1464–1476.
27. MIAMI Trial Research Group. Metoprolol in acute MI (MIAMI): A randomized placebo-controlled international trial. Eur Heart J 1985;6:199.
28. ISIS-1 Group. Randomized trial of intravenous atenolol among 16,027 cases of suspected acute myocardial infarction: ISIS-1. Lancet 1986;2:57.
29. Khan M Gabriel. Which beta blocker to choose. In: Heart Disease Diagnosis and Therapy, 2nd ed. Totowa, NJ, Humana Press, 2005, p. 55.
30. International Collaborative Study Group. Reduction of infarct size with the early use of timolol in acute myocardial infarction. N Engl J Med 1984;310:9.
31. Norwegian Multicenter Study Group. Timolol-induced reduction in mortality and reinfarction in patients surviving acute MI. N Engl J Med 1981;304:801.
32. Beta-blocker heart attack study group (BHAT). The Beta Blocker Heart Attack Trial. JAMA 1981;246: 2073.
33. Fourth International Study of Infarct Survival Collaborative Group. A randomized factorial trial assessing early oral captopril, oral mononitrate, and intravenous magnesium sulfate in 58,050 patients with suspected acute myocardial infarction. Lancet 1995;345:669.
34. Cannon CP, Braunwald E, McCabe CH, et al. Intensive versus moderate lipid lowering with statins after acute coronary syndromes. N Engl J Med 2004;350:1495–1504.
35. Scirica BM, Morrow DA, Cannon CP, for the PROVE IT-TIMI 22 Investigators. Intensive statin therapy and the risk of hospitalization for heart failure after an acute coronary syndrome in the PROVE IT-TIMI 22 Study. J Am Coll Cardiol 2006;47:2326–2331.
36. Woods KL, Fletcher S, Roffe C, et al. Intravenous magnesium sulphate in suspected acute myocardial infarction: Results of the Second Leicester Intravenous Magnesium Intervention Trial (LIMIT-2). Lancet 1992;339:1553.
37. Woods KL, Fletcher S. Long-term outcome after intravenous magnesium sulphate in suspected acute myocardial infarction: The Second Leicester Intravenous Magnesium Intervention Trial (LIMIT-2). Lancet 1994;343:816.
38. Bowli R. Mechanism of myocardial "stunning." Circulation 1990;82:723.
39. MAGIC Trial Investigators. Early administration of intravenous magnesium to high-risk patients with acute myocardial infarction in the Magnesium in Coronaries (MAGIC) Trial: A randomized controlled trial. Lancet 2002;360:1189.
40. Lawrie DM, Higgins MR, Godman MJ, et al. Ventricular fibrillation complicating acute myocardial infarction. Lancet 1968;2:523.
41. Adgey AAJ, Geddes JS, Mulholland HC, et al. Incidence, significance, and management of early bradyarrhythmia complicating acute myocardial infarction. Lancet 1968;2:1097.
42. Warren JV, Lewis RP. Beneficial effects of atropine in the pre-hospital phase of coronary care. Am J Cardiol 1976;37:68.
43. Massumi RA, Mason DT, Amsterdam EA, et al. Ventricular fibrillation and tachycardia after intravenous atropine for treatment of bradycardias. N Engl J Med 1972;287:336.
44. Wellens HJJ. Right ventricular infarction. N Engl J Med 1993;328:1036.
45. Zehender M, Casper W, Kauder E, et al. Right ventricular infarction as an independent predictor of prognosis after acute inferior myocardial infarction. N Engl J Med 1993;328:981.
46. Hurst JW. Right ventricular infarction. N Engl J Med 1994;331:681.
47. Kinch JW, Ryan TJ. Right ventricular infarction. N Engl J Med 1994;17:1211.
48. Cotter G, Kaluski E,, Blatt A, et al. L-NMMA (a nitric oxide synthase inhibitor) is effective in the treatment of cardiogenic shock. Circulation 2000;101:1358.
49. Hochman JS, Sleeper LA, Webb JG, et al. for the SHOCK investigators. Early revascularization in acute MI complicated by cardiogenic shock: Should we emergently revascularize occluded coronaries for cardiogenic shock? N Engl J Med 1999;341:625.
50. Hochman JS, Sleper LA, White HD. One year survival following early revascularization for cardiogenic shock JAMA 2001;285:190–192.
51. Ray KK, Cannon CP, Cairns R, et al. for the PROVE IT-TIMI 22 Investigators. Early and late benefits of high-dose atorvastatin in patients with acute coronary syndromes: Results from the PROVE IT-TIMI 22 trial. J Am Coll Cardiol 2005;46:1405–1410.
52. Topol EA, Moliterno DJ, Hermann HC, et al. for the TARGET investigators. Comparison of two platelet glycoprotein IIb/IIIa inhibitors, tirofiban and abciximab for the prevention of ischemic events with percutaneous coronary revascularization. N Engl J Med 2001;344:1888.

53. Cannon CP, Weintraub WS, Demopoulos LA, et al. Comparison of early invasive and conservative strategies in patients with unstable coronary syndromes treated with the glycoprotein IIb/IIIa inhibitor tirofiban. N Engl J Med 2001;344:1879.
54. Roffi M, Chew P, Mukherjee D, et al. Platelet glycoprotein IIb/IIIa inhibitors reduce mortality in diabetic patients with non ST segment elevation acute coronary syndromes. Circulation 2001;104:2767.
55. Sabatine MS, Braunwald E. Will diabetes save the platelet blockers? Circulation 2001;104:2759.
56. The Clopidogrel in Unstable Angina to Prevent Recurrent Events trial investigators. Effects of clopidogrel in addition to aspirin in patients with acute coronary syndromes without ST segment elevation. N Engl J Med 2001;345:494.
57. Mehta S, Yusuf S, Peters R, et al. Effects of pre-treatment with clopidogrel and aspirin followed by long-term therapy in patients undergoing percutaneous coronary intervention. The PCI-CURE study. Lancet 2001;358:527–533.
58. Steinhubl SR, Charnigo R, Topol EJ. Clopidogrel treatment prior to percutaneous coronary intervention: When enough isn't enough. JAMA 2006;295:1581–1582.
59. Giugliano RP, Braunwald E. The year in non-ST-segment elevation acute coronary syndromes. J Am Coll Cardiol 2005;46:906–919.
60. Hochholzer W, Trenk D, Frundi D, et al. Time dependence of platelet inhibition after a 600-mg loading dose of clopidogrel in a large, unselected cohort of candidates for percutaneous coronary intervention Circulation 2005;111:2560–2564.
61. Patti G, Colonna G, Pasceri V, et al. Randomized trial of high loading dose of clopidogrel for reduction of periprocedural myocardial infarction in patients undergoing coronary intervention. Results from the ARMYDA-2 (Antiplatelet Therapy for Reduction of MYocardial Damage during Angioplasty) study. Circulation 2005;111:2099–2106.
62. Silber S, Albertsson P, Aviles FF, et al. Guidelines for percutaneous coronary interventions: The task force for percutaneous coronary interventions of the European Society of Cardiology. Eur Heart J 2005;26: 804–847.
63. Stone GW. Acute Catheterization and Urgent Intervention Triage Strategy Trial (ACUITY). Presented at the 2006 ACC Annual Scientific Session, Mar 11–14, 2006, Atlanta, GA.
64. Smith SC Jr, Feldman TE, Hirshfeld JW Jr, et al. ACC/AHA/SCAI 2005 guideline update for percutaneous coronary intervention: A report of the American College of Cardiology/American Heart Association Task Force on Practice Guidelines (ACC/AHA/SCAI Writing Committee to Update the 2001 Guidelines for Percutaneous Coronary Intervention). J Am Coll Cardiol 2006;47:e1–121.

SUGGESTED READING

Antman EM, Morrow DA, McCabe CH, et al. Enoxaparin versus unfractionated heparin with fibrinolysis for ST-elevation myocardial infarction for the ExTRACT-TIMI 25 Investigators. N Engl J Med 2006; 354:1477–1488.

Bavry AA, Lincoff AM. Is clopidogrel cardiovascular medicine's double-edged sword? Circulation 2006; 113:1638–1640.

Beygui F, Collet J-P, Benoliel J-J, et al. High plasma aldosterone levels on admission are associated with death in patients presenting with acute ST-elevation myocardial infarction. Circulation 2006;114:2604–2610.

Calhoun DA. Aldosterone and cardiovascular disease: Smoke and fire. Circulation 2006;114:2572–2574.

Cannon CP, Braunwald E, McCabe CH, et al. Intensive versus moderate lipid lowering with statins after acute coronary syndromes N Engl J Med 2004;350:1495–1504.

Eisenstein EL, Anstrom KJ, Kong DF, et al. Clopidogrel use and long-term clinical outcomes after drug-eluting stent implantation. JAMA 2007;297:159–168.

Giugliano RP, Braunwald E. The year in non-ST-segment elevation acute coronary syndromes. J Am Coll Cardiol 2006;48:386–395.

Hirsch A, Windhausen F, Tijssen JGP for the Invasive versus Conservative Treatment in Unstable coronary Syndromes (ICTUS) investigators. Long-term outcome after an early invasive versus selective invasive treatment strategy in patients with non-ST-elevation acute coronary syndrome and elevated cardiac troponin T (the ICTUS trial): a follow-up study. Lancet 2007;369:827–835.

Hockman JS, Lamas GA, Buller CE, et al. Coronary intervention for persistent occlusion after myocardial infarction. J Engl J Med 2006;355:2395–2407.

Randomized Trial. The OASIS-6 Trial Group. JAMA 2006;295:1519–1530.

Remme WJ, Torp-Pedersen C, Cleland JGF, et al. Carvedilol protects better against vascular events than metoprolol in heart failure: results from COMET. J Am Coll Cardiol 2007; 49:963–971.

Scirica BM, Morrow DA, Cannon CP, et al. for the PROVE IT-TIMI 22 Investigators. Intensive statin therapy and the risk of hospitalization for heart failure after an acute coronary syndrome in the PROVE IT-TIMI 22 study. J Am Coll Cardiol 2006;47:2326–2331.

Scirica BM, Sabatine MS, Morrow DA, et al. The role of clopidogrel in early and sustained arterial patency after fibrinolysis for ST-segment elevation myocardial infarction. The ECG CLARITY-TIMI 28 study. J Am Coll Cardiol 2006;48:37–42.

Stevens LA, Coresh J, Greene T. Assessing kidney function—measured and estimated glomerular filtration rate. N Engl J Med 2006;354:2473– 2483.

Stone GW, McLaurin BT, Cox DA, et al. Bivalirudin for patients with acute coronary syndromes. N Engl J Med 2006;355:2203–2216.

Van Melle JP, Verbeek DEP, van den Berg MP, et al. Beta-blockers and depression after myocardial infarction: a multicenter prospective study. J Am Coll Cardiol 2006;48:2209–2214.

Von Känel, BS. Depression after myocardial infarction: Editorial. Unraveling the mystery of poor cardiovascular prognosis and role of beta-blocker therapy. J Am Coll Cardiol 2006;48:2215–2217.

12 Management of Heart Failure

THE SIZE OF THE PROBLEM

Heart failure (HF), unlike coronary heart disease (CHD), has no territorial boundaries.

- The world faces an epidemic of heart failure. The plague of HF is common in developed and in developing countries.
- Although treatment strategies have improved considerably over the past decade, improvement in outcomes remain modest and the incidence of HF is increasing. Some of this increase is owing to an aging population in all countries.
- In the United States about 5 million individuals have HF. In addition, more than half a million patients are diagnosed with a first episode of HF each year, and approximately 80% of these are over age 65.
- In the United States, HF causes more than 300,000 deaths annually *(1)* over the past 10 yr hospitalizations for HF have risen from approx 550,000 to approx 900,000 *(2)*. The cost worldwide is astronomic: in the United States more Medicare dollars are spent on the management of HF than for any other diagnosis *(3)* and this cost is estimated to be $28 billion annually.

Prevention of HF is thus crucial, and physician education concerning the most appropriate drug cocktail to prescribe is vital.

This chapter gives relevant American College of Cardiology/American Heart Association (ACC/AHA) guidelines *(4)* and class I recommendations. Class I comprises conditions for which there is evidence and/or agreement that a given therapy is useful and effective.

CAUSES OF HEART FAILURE

- The many diseases causing HF must be sought (*see* Table 12-1) and treated aggressively prior to symptomatic HF.

Basic Cause

Determine the basic cause of the heart disease. If the specific cause is present but is not recognized (e.g., surgically correctable causes: significant mitral regurgitation may be missed clinically; atrial-septal defect, arteriovenous fistula, constrictive pericarditis, and cardiac tamponade are important considerations), the possibility of achieving a complete cure, although rare, may be missed or the HF may become refractory. Cardiac tamponade and constrictive pericarditis patients may deteriorate if routine measures for treatment of HF are applied.

Note: Pulmonary edema and HF are not complete diagnoses; the basic cause and precipitating factors should be stated.

From: *Contemporary Cardiology: Cardiac Drug Therapy, Seventh Edition*
M. Gabriel Khan © Humana Press Inc., Totowa, NJ

Table 12-1
Causes of Systolic Heart Failure and Diastolic Heart Failure

Systolic Heart Failure	
Coronary heart disease	~40%[a]
Hypertensive heart disease	~40%
Valvular heart disease	~15%
Other causes	~ 5%
Diabetes	
Dilated cardiomyopathy	
Myocarditis	
Cardiotoxins	
Diastolic Heart Failure: HFPEF	
Left ventricular hypertrophy	
Hypertensive heart disease (systolic and diastolic HF)	
Chronic CHD	
Diabetes	
Myocardial fibrosis	
Cardiomyopathy	
Hypertrophic and restrictive	
Amyloid heart disease	
Sarcoidosis, hemochromatosis, metabolic storage disease	
Hypertensive hypertrophic "cardiomyopathy" of the elderly: aging heart (particularly women)	
Arrhythmogenic right ventricular dysplasia	
Constrictive pericarditis, pericardial effusion, and tamponade	
Atrial myxoma	
Systolic dysfunction is a principal cause of diastolic dysfunction.	

[a]CHD is approx 60% in the United States, but worldwide hypertension is more common, particularly in blacks and Asians.

The search for the etiology must be systematic, and the following **routine check** is suggested:

1. **Myocardial damage:**
   - Ischemic heart disease and its complications.
   - Myocarditis.
   - Cardiomyopathy.
2. **Ventricular overload:**
   - Pressure overload.
     a. Systemic hypertension.
     b. Coarctation of the aorta.
     c. Aortic stenosis.
     d. Pulmonary stenosis.
   - Volume overload.
     a. Mitral regurgitation.
     b. Aortic regurgitation.
     c. Ventricular septal defect.
     d. Atrial-septal defect.
     e. Patent ductus arteriosus.

3. **Restriction and obstruction to ventricular filling:**
   - Mitral stenosis.
   - Cardiac tamponade.
   - Constrictive pericarditis.
   - Restrictive cardiomyopathies.
   - Atrial myxoma.
4. **Corpulmonale.**
5. **Others:**
   - Arteriovenous fistula.
   - Thyrotoxicosis.
   - Myxedema.

Factors precipitating heart failure:

1. **Patient-physician problems:**
   - Reduction or discontinuation of medications.
   - Salt binge.
   - Increased physical or mental stress.
   - Obesity.
2. **Increased cardiac work precipitated by:**
   - Increasing hypertension (systemic or pulmonary).
   - Arrhythmia; digoxin toxicity.
   - Pulmonary embolism.
   - Infection, e.g., bacterial endocarditis, chest, urinary, or others.
   - Thyrotoxicosis or myxedema.
3. **Progression or complications of the basic underlying heart disease:**
   - Ischemic heart disease—acute MI, left ventricular aneurysm, papillary muscle dysfunction causing mitral regurgitation.
   - Valvular heart disease—increased stenosis or regurgitation.
4. **Blood problems:**
   - Increased volume—transfusions of saline or blood.
   - Decreased volume—overzealous use of diuretics.
   - Anemia: hemoglobin < 5 g/100 mL (50 g/L), or in cardiacs < 9 g/100 mL (90 g/L).
   - Electrolytes and acid-base problems (potassium, chloride, magnesium).
5. **Drugs that affect cardiac performance and may precipitate HF:**
   - Nonsteroidal autoinflammatory drugs (NSAIDs): indomethacin, ibuprofen (Motrin; Brufen), piroxicam (Feldene), and others.
   - Beta-blockers.
   - Corticosteroids.
   - Disopyramide, procainamide.
   - Calcium antagonists: verapamil, diltiazem, and, rarely, nifedipine.
   - Digitalis toxicity.
   - Vasodilators and antihypertensive agents that cause sodium and water retention. These agents are further likely to precipitate HF if they cause an inhibition of increase in heart rate, which is especially important in patients with severe bradycardia or sick sinus syndrome.
   - Drugs that increase afterload and increase blood pressure.
   - Adriamycin, daunorubicin, and mithramycin.
   - Alcohol, acute excess (e.g., 8 oz of gin in a period of less than 2 h causes cardiac depression and a fall in the ejection fraction [EF]).
   - Estrogens and androgens.

- Antidepressants: tricyclic compounds.
- Ephedra can cause HF.
- Chlorpropamide enhances the activity of antidiuretic hormone secretion at the renal tubular site of action.
- In addition, HF may be classified as the commonly occurring systolic HF (approx 50%) and diastolic HF (approx 25%), the managements of which have subtle and important differences. A combination of systolic HF and diastolic HF, also termed HF with preserved ejection fraction (HFPEF) exists in approx 25% of patients (*see* Table 12-1). Some would put the incidence of diastolic HF as approx 30–40%; if this is true, there is less hope for outcome improvements because there are no satisfactory or proven treatments for HFPEF. However, there are well-recognized difficulties in assessing left ventricular (LV) diastolic function, and the diagnosis should be stated as probable, or possible diastolic HF. Thus, the exact incidence awaits clarification (*see* Chapter 13, Heart Failure Controversies).

DIAGNOSIS

1. Ensure that the diagnosis is correct by critically reviewing the history, physical exam, and posteroanterior (PA) and lateral chest radiographs. Many patients are incorrectly treated for HF on the basis of the presence of crepitations at the lung bases or peripheral edema. Crepitations may be present in the absence of HF and may be absent with definite LV failure. Edema is commonly owing to causes other than cardiac. The chest radiograph may be positive before the appearance of crepitations. Edema or raised jugular venous pressure (JVP) may be absent or incorrectly assessed.
2. **Chest radiograph** confirms the clinical diagnosis. It is most important to recognize the radiologic findings of HF, listed as follows:
   - Obvious constriction of the lower lobe vessels and dilation of the upper vessels related to pulmonary venous hypertension are commonly seen in left HF, in mitral stenosis, and occasionally with severe chronic obstructive pulmonary disease (COPD).
   - Interstitial pulmonary edema: pulmonary clouding; perihilar haze; perivascular or peribronchiolar cuffing; septal Kerley A lines and more commonly B lines.
   - Effusions, subpleural or free pleural; blunting of the costophrenic angle, right greater than left.
   - Alveolar pulmonary edema (butterfly pattern).
   - Interlobar fissure thickening related to accumulation of fluid (best seen in the lateral film).
   - Dilation of the central right and left pulmonary arteries. A right descending pulmonary artery diameter > 17 mm (normal 9–16 mm) indicates an increase in pulmonary artery pressure.
   - Cardiac size: cardiomegaly is common; however, a normal heart size can be found in several conditions causing definite HF:
     a. Acute myocardial infarction (MI).
     b. Mitral stenosis.
     c. Aortic stenosis.
     d. Acute aortic regurgitation.
     e. Cor pulmonale.
   - Cardiomegaly lends support to the diagnosis, severity, and etiology of HF but has been overrated in the past. Such phrases as "no HF if the heart size on PA film is normal" are to be discarded. The heart size may be normal in the presence of severe cardiac pathology, that is, an LV aneurysm or repeated MIs that can cause hypokinetic, akinetic, or dys-

Table 12-2
Echocardiography, the Most Useful Test to Evaluate Patients with Proven Heart Failure

1. Assess left ventricular (LV) function and provide a sufficiently accurate ejection fraction (EF)[a] for guidance of therapy
2. Screen for regional or global hypokinesis
3. Gives accurate cardiac dimensions; replaces radiology for cardiac chamber dilation
4. Assess regional LV wall motion abnormalities that indicate ischemia and significant coronary heart disease
5. Assess hypertrophy, concentric or other
6. Left atrial enlargement common with valvular heart disease and an early sign of LV hypertrophy
7. Assess valvular heart disease
8. Congenital heart disease
9. Diastolic dysfunction: assess after confirmation of normal systolic function and absence of valvular disease
10. Pericardial disease, effusion, tamponade
11. Myocardial disease

[a]Gated nuclear imaging is more accurate for EF in the *absence of atrial fibrillation* but does not assess valves, hypertrophy, or items 3–11.

kinetic areas that may be observed on inspection of the chest wall but may not be detectable on PA chest radiographs. Echocardiography is often necessary as it provides the most useful information on the severity of valvular lesions, LV contractility, EF, and verification of causes of HF.

It is necessary to exclude **radiologic mimics** of cardiogenic pulmonary edema:

a. Circulatory overload.
b. Lung infection—viral and other pneumonias.
c. Allergic pulmonary edema: heroin and nitrofurantoin.
d. Lymphangitic carcinomatosis.
e. Uremia.
f. Inhalation of toxic substances.
g. Increased cerebrospinal fluid (CSF) pressure.
h. Drowning.
i. High altitude.
j. Alveolar proteinosis.

3. *BNP: Rapid testing of brain natriuretic peptide (BNP)in the emergency room* helps differentiate cardiac from pulmonary causes of acute dyspnea and has proved useful *(5)*. The popularity of BNP or amino-terminal pro-BNP as an aid to the diagnosis of HF continues to increase *(6*; *see* Chapter 13).
4. **Echocardiography** is the single most useful diagnostic test to evaluate the causes of HF and the heart function in patients confirmed to have HF clinically and radiologically (*see* Table 12-2). The echocardiographic measurement of EF carries a substantial error but should suffice for general patient management.

In patients in whom it is crucial to obtain an accurate EF, a gated radionuclide study should be requested after the results of echocardiography. Echocardiography is the key investigation because correctable causes of HF such as valvular disease, pericardial, and other problems can be rapidly documented. Adequate information on LV function is provided, e.g., a poorly contractile ventricle, and fractional shortening should suffice. An EF

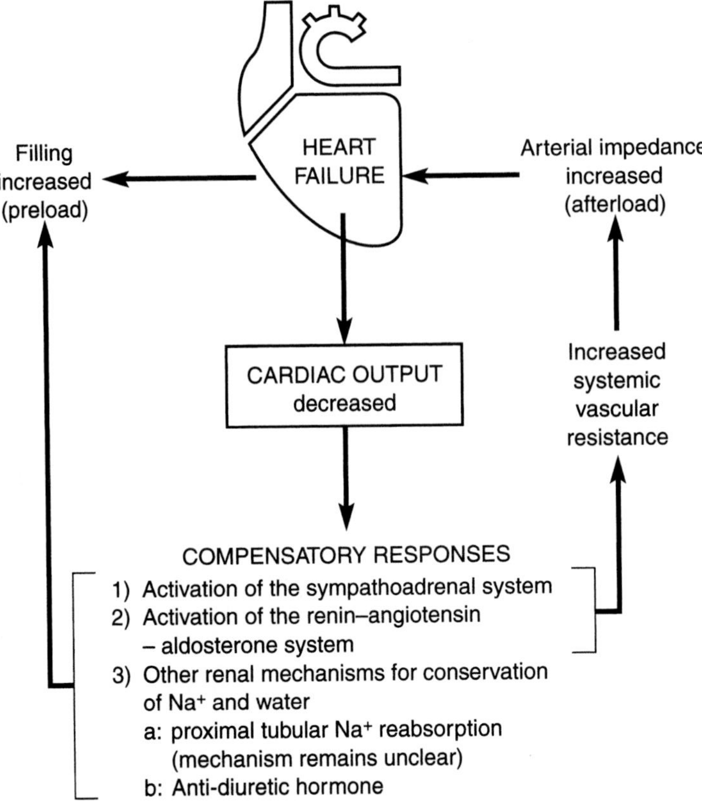

Fig. 12-1. Pathophysiology of heart failure.

< 40% is in keeping with decreased LV systolic function. Values of 20–30–35–40–45% have some meaning to those who are used to these numbers. Also, the numbers assist with reference to published articles that do not use fractional shortening. A radionuclide cardiac scan is more accurate for the determination of EF but does not evaluate hypertrophy or valvular, pericardial, and other diseases. The cost of a second test is not justifiable.

PATHOPHYSIOLOGY

- It is most important to have a clear knowledge of the pathophysiology of HF, in particular how LV work is dictated by systemic vascular resistance (SVR; *see* Fig. 12-1).
- Decrease neurohormonal activation; inhibition of the renin-angiotensin-aldosterone system.
- Inhibit LV remodeling.
- Improve myocardial hemodynamics.
- Increase cardiac output to deliver oxygenated blood to vital organs and to meet the metabolic needs of the tissues, especially during normal activities and exercise.
- The cardiac output (CO) is reduced and filling pressure is increased. The low CO results in a number of compensatory responses, as outlined in Fig. 12-1.

The following definitions are relevant:

- **Cardiac output** = stroke volume × heart rate (HR). Stroke volume is a reflection of preload (filling pressure), myocardial contractility, and afterload (arterial impedance).
- **LV work** and myocardial oxygen consumption depend on

a. HR × blood pressure (BP) (rate-pressure product).
b. BP = cardiac output × SVR.

The **resistance** or arterial impedance (afterload) against which the left ventricle must eject is an important determinant of LV workload. A reduced SVR requires less energy and less force of myocardial contraction to produce an increase in stroke volume.

SVR is automatically increased early in the development of HF and remains unchanged or increases with increasing HF. This reaction is a necessity and is a normal compensatory adjustment to maintain blood pressure and vascular homeostasis.

The compensatory adjustments are initiated by:

- Sympathetic stimulation that causes an increase in
  a. Heart rate.
  b. The force of myocardial contraction.
  c. SVR.
- Activation of the **renin-angiotensin-aldosterone system** (RAAS), which causes
  a. Intense arterial constriction and therefore an increase in SVR and blood pressure.
  b. An increase in aldosterone, which produces distal sodium and water retention.

The important proximal tubular reabsorption of sodium is believed to be caused by a combination of the preceding points and other as yet undetermined mechanisms (*see* Fig. 12-1).

- The renal response to a low CO in the normal subject is to maintain the blood pressure by causing vasoconstriction and sodium and water reabsorption (saline autotransfusion). We cannot expect the kidney to change its program when HF occurs. The kidney is behaving appropriately in the wrong circumstances. Clearly, we can prevent the kidney from carrying out its program only if we switch off the initiating cause of the renal reflex, that is, by increasing the cardiac output. Therefore, any drug that will increase CO will reduce the renal response and lower SVR and further improve CO. An alternative strategy is to reset the neurohormonal imbalance by the use of ACE inhibitors and aldosterone antagonists.

Note: Inotropic agents, digoxin or dobutamine, improve cardiac output and, therefore, cause a fall in SVR.

MANAGEMENT GUIDE

Four golden rules dictate the efficient management of HF:

1. Ensure that the **diagnosis** of HF is correct, eliminating conditions that may mimic HF.
2. Determine and treat the **basic cause** of the heart disease. The rare surgical or medical cure is worth the effort.
3. Search for the **precipitating factors**; remove or treat and prevent their recurrence to avoid further episodes of HF. Withdraw drugs known to worsen HF: NSAIDs and notably calcium antagonists *(3,6)* commonly administered to patients with hypertension and CHD.
4. The specific treatment of HF requires sound and up-to-date knowledge of the pathophysiology of HF and the actions, indications, and side effects of the pharmacologic agents used in its management.

Relieve symptoms and signs of HF by reducing raised filling pressures to near normal. Therapeutic goals:

- Shift the cardiac function curve to the left and upward, decreasing the filling pressure yet increasing stroke volume.
- Arrest or cause amelioration of the disease process.

This can be achieved by the judicious use of

- Loop diuretics.
- Angiotensin-converting enzyme (ACE) inhibitors or angiotensin II receptor blockers (ARBs).
- Beta-blockers.
- Digoxin.
- Aldosterone antagonists: spironolactone or eplerenone.
- Statins for ischemic cardiomyopathy.

VASODILATORS

ACE Inhibitors/Angiotensin II Receptor Blockers

These agents are discussed in Chapter 3. ACE inhibitors and ARBs play a major role in the management of HF.

Activation of the RAAS is an early manifestation of HF. The prime role of angiotensin II is to support systemic blood pressure by:

- Causing systemic vasoconstriction, an increase in SVR.
- Stimulation of the central and peripheral effects of the sympathetic nervous system.
- Causing retention of sodium and water in the proximal nephron and directly by stimulation of aldosterone production.
- Stimulating thirst and enhancing synthesis of vasopressin, thereby increasing total body water.

In addition, angiotensin II preserves cerebral blood flow. Renal blood flow is preserved by selective vasoconstriction of the postglomerular (efferent) arterioles. Thus, the influence of angiotensin II allows patients with severe HF to maintain blood pressure for cerebral, renal, and coronary perfusion, and relatively normal values for serum creatinine and blood urea nitrogen concentration also prevail. ACE inhibitors may cause a dramatic decrease in glomerular filtration rate and increase azotemia in patients with HF and hypotension. This deleterious effect can be minimized by reducing the patient's dependence on the renin-angiotensin system by reducing the dose of diuretic used. It is best to choose an ACE inhibitor with a short action so as to allow brief restoration of the normal homeostatic actions of the renin-angiotensin system *(7)*. Long-acting agents may produce prolonged hypotensive effects that may compromise cerebral and renal function and thus may have disadvantages in such cases compared with short-acting agents *(8)*. Initial low-dose enalapril, 2.5 mg, caused a low 3.2% incidence of hypotension in a Scandinavian study, proving the drug's safe profile *(9)*.

If ACE inhibitors or ARBs are not tolerated or are contraindicated, the combination of hydralazine/isosorbide dinitrate (ISDN) should be tried; this combination is preferred over ACE inhibitors in black patients as indicated in the Veterans Administration Heart Failure Trial (A-HeFT) *(10)*.

Data from the Veterans Administration **Vasodilator Heart Failure Trial (V-HeFT)** suggested that patients with chronic HF could be considered for treatment with hydralazine (25 mg three or four times daily) and ISDN *(11)*, but use of captopril or enalapril is preferred. In V-HeFT, the 2-yr reduction in mortality rate was 25%. Hydralazine and ISDN were poorly tolerated and were withdrawn in 19% of patients. Only 55% of patients were taking full doses of both drugs 6 mo after randomization *(12)*. Improvement in survival was observed mainly in patients with New York Heart Association (NYHA) class II HF. In this subset, 48 (24%) of 200 patients treated with enalapril and 66 (31%) of 210 patients treated with hydralazine/ISDN died *(13)*.

The Cooperative North Scandinavian Enalapril Survival Study (CONSENSUS) *(9)* showed that 6 mo of enalapril therapy produced a 40% reduction in mortality rate in patients with NYHA class IV HF. The drug, when given as a 2.5-mg initial dose, is well tolerated *(9)*.

The Studies of Left Ventricular Dysfunction (SOLVD) investigators reported a mortality rate of 35% in enalapril-treated patients with HF and an EF < 35% *(14)* and a mortality rate of 40% in the placebo group. Enalapril reduced the number of hospitalizations. The prevention arm of SOLVD did not show a significant improvement in the survival rate of patients with EF < 3 5% but without overt HF *(14)*. Unfortunately, 65% of patients in SOLVD were more than 4 wk post-MI. Thus, the study cannot be generalized to all patients with HF.

Plasma renin levels are usually normal in patients with HF in NYHA class I and II, and ACE inhibitors may not be logical therapy at this stage. When these patients are treated with diuretics, however, plasma renin levels increase and ACE inhibitors may produce salutary effects. In these situations not all patients benefit from ACE inhibitor therapy; it is estimated that approx 50% of patients may improve in LV function, but survival data are not available except in postinfarction patients. ACE inhibitors decrease LV hypertrophy, an important cause of diastolic dysfunction that predisposes to the late phase of the failing ventricle. In the last phase of HF, both systolic and diastolic dysfunctions prevail. Although ACE inhibitors have not proved useful in patients with mainly diastolic dysfunction, they can be used to prevent this condition. ACE inhibitors are not indicated as monotherapy for patients with HF with CHD or hypertension.

Dosage

Patients with very severe HF who are taking diuretics often have hyponatremia and high plasma renin activity. These patients are likely to respond dramatically to ACE inhibitors but with an associated profound fall in blood pressure. Thus, in this subset of patients, it is necessary to discontinue diuretics and nitrates for 2–3 d and to initiate very-low-dose captopril or enalapril therapy. The patient should be kept in bed for up to 3 h following captopril administration. Captopril 6.25 mg is given twice daily for 1–2 d, increasing the dose slowly to 6.25 mg three times daily and then 12.5 mg twice or three times daily if systolic BP is >100 mmHg; at this stage, a low dose of diuretic is commenced. A captopril dose of 25 mg three times daily is often sufficient to provide benefit. It may require 1–3 wk to achieve the dosage proved effective in clinical trials. Maximum dose is 50 mg three times daily.

The physician must not be put off by mild hypotension (BP 90–100 mmHg) and must be prepared to give ACE inhibitors a fair trial. Many weeks of treatment may be required before clinical improvement becomes manifest. Pooled studies of a number of randomized placebo-controlled trials with other vasodilators compared with ACE inhibitor therapy in patients with severe HF showed a significant improvement in survival in groups treated with ACE inhibitors *(15,16)*. Only captopril reduced wall stress and improved functional class in 18 patients with dilated cardiomyopathy *(17)*.

Post-MI Heart Failure with Left Ventricular Dysfunction

The following studies have tested the effect of ACE inhibitors:

- In the Survival and Ventricular Enlargement (SAVE) trial, 36,630 post-MI patients were screened, but only 2231 of the 8938 patients with EF ≤ 40% were randomly assigned. Follow-up at 3.5 yr showed a 37% reduction in the risk of developing HF and a 22% decrease in the risk of requiring hospitalization for HF *(18)*. There was no significant reduction in mortality rates.

- In the Acute Infarction Ramipril Efficacy (AIRE) study, ramipril was shown to improve prognosis in post-MI patients with clinical evidence of HF *(19)*.

Drug name:	**Captopril**
Trade name:	Capoten
Supplied:	12.5, 25, 50, 100 mg
Dosage:	*See* text

Dosage

Withdraw diuretics and other antihypertensives for 24–48 h; then give a test dose of 3–6.5 mg and then the same dose twice daily, increasing to 12.5 mg two or three times daily, preferably 1 h before meals (on an empty stomach).

The maximum suggested daily dose is 75–150 mg.

In renal failure, the dose interval is increased according to the creatinine clearance (*see* Chapter 3 for a detailed account of adverse effects, cautions, interactions, and pharmacokinetics).

Drug name:	**Enalapril**
Trade names:	Vasotec, Innovace (UK)
Supplied:	2.5, 5, 10, 20 mg
Dosage:	2.5-mg test dose; 8–12 h later start 2.5 mg twice daily, increasing over days to weeks to 10–20 mg once or twice daily

Contraindications, side effects, and other considerations are discussed in Chapter 3 (*see* Table 3-1). Notably, the drug's onset of action is delayed 2–4 h as opposed to captopril (½–1 h). Thus, an initial effect on hypotension is observed within 1 h after captopril dosing and at about 2½ h with enalapril *(17)*. Withdrawal of diuretics does not always prevent marked hypotension or syncope *(20)*, so caution is required with captopril and enalapril. In the Scandinavian study, a 2.5-mg initial dose caused a 3.2% withdrawal of patients and a 31% reduction in the 1-yr mortality rate *(9)*.

A RCT indicates that 20 mg of enalapril is as beneficial as 60 mg daily for HF treatment *(21)*.

Drug name:	**Lisinopril**
Trade names:	Prinivil, Zestril, Carace (UK)
Supplied:	5, 10, 20, 40 mg
Dosage:	2.5-mg test dose, then titrate dosage; 5–10 mg once daily, average 10–20 mg daily. If no hypotension or adverse effects, the dose may be increased to 30–35 mg daily

The high dose was used in the Assessment of Treatment with Lisinopril and Survival (ATLAS) study *(22)*. Unfortunately, the ATLAS study compared 2.5–5 mg with 32.5–35 mg lisinopril daily. It would make more clinical sense to have compared the dose commonly used by cardiologists in clinical practice (i.e., 10–20 mg) as the low dose. The results of the study showed a marginal difference; the high dose decreased modestly the risk of hospitalization but not total mortality.

For other ACE inhibitors and ARBs, *see* Chapter 3. ARBs are advisable if ACE inhibitors are not tolerated *(23,24)*.

Drug name:	**Hydralazine**
Trade name:	Apresoline
Supplied:	25, 50 mg
Dosage:	25 mg (average 50 mg) three times daily, max. 200 mg daily

Hydralazine is an effective vasodilator useful mainly when combined with oral nitrates, as shown in V-HeFT I *(12)*.

V-HeFT II indicated that hydralazine with ISDN is inferior to ACE inhibitor therapy in achieving improved survival in patients with NYHA class II HF. Thirty-three percent of patients cannot tolerate the drug because of headaches, dizziness, and other side effects, and of the remaining 66% only half derive some benefit *(25)*. Adverse effects were similar in V-HeFT I and II. Hydralizine/ISDN may be used if an ACE inhibitor or ARB is contraindicated. In A-HeFT, the combination significantly reduced mortality and hospitalizations in patients of African origin (*see* Chapter 22).

Amlodipine

The Prospective Randomized Amlodipine Survival Evaluation (PRAISE)-2 study showed that amlodipine caused neither benefit nor harm in patients with CHF. The result of PRAISE-1 was the result of chance. In PRAISE-2, amlodipine increased the occurrence of pulmonary edema in patients with low EF *(26)*. Calcium antagonists should not be used in the treatment of HF or in patients with EF < 40%.

DIURETICS

Indications and Guidelines

Heart failure precipitated by acute MI: In this situation, the cautious use of titrated doses of furosemide usually suffices.

Furosemide 20–40 mg intravenously (IV) followed by 40 mg, 30 min to 1 h later, is given. If symptoms persist, diuresis is not established, and the BP is stable, 80 mg is given.

Ensure that the serum K^+ level remains normal; do not wait to see it fall to <3.5 mEq (mmol)/L before adding potassium chloride (KC1).

In patients with moderate and severe HF who are predicted to have recurrent bouts of HF and who are receiving digitalis, give furosemide 80–160 mg daily. Occasionally, bumetanide produces a greater diuresis than furosemide.

The combination of furosemide and hydrochlorothiazide or **metolazone** *(27)* increases diuresis and should be given a trial in patients refractory to furosemide or other loop diuretics. In patients with **refractory HF with severe renal failure**, furosemide 160–320 mg along with metolazone may be required to promote adequate diuresis.

Note that the diuretic and antihypertensive actions of furosemide and thiazides are reduced by drugs that are prostaglandin inhibitors, in particular indomethacin and other NSAIDs.

Torsemide (Demadex): 10–20 mg IV. Maximum single dose 100–200 mg

Bumetamide: 1.0 mg, maximum 4–8 mg.

ALDOSTERONE ANTAGONISTS

Figure 12-1 indicates the role of increased aldosterone production in the pathophysiology of HF. (*See* also Chapter 7, New Concepts.)

It is necessary to block aldosterone completely because it causes

- Na and water retention. This effect continues when the effects of short-acting, poorly absorbed loop diuretics, such as furosemide, have dissipated.
- K^+ and Mg loss.
- Myocardial and vascular fibrosis.
- Norepinephrine release and increased myocardial uptake of norepinephrine that can contribute to sudden death; myocardial fibrosis that contributes to progressive HF.
- Although aldosterone antagonists have proved successful in reducing adverse outcomes in patients with HF, their use in patients with impaired renal function is a risk factor for hyperkalemia.
- Most important, elderly patients with a serum creatinine in the normal range often have renal impairment, and the various formulas for assessing glomerular filtration rate (GFR) have drawbacks, particularly in patients older than age 70.

Drug name:	**Spironolactone**
Trade name:	Aldactone
Supplied:	25 mg
Dosage:	Initial 12.5 mg if serum assess K^+ 5.0 or less and reassess in 3 d and at 1 wk; if $K^+ < 5.0$ mEq/L, give 25 mg once daily Reassess at 1 mo then every 3 mo: maintain K^+ 4 to maximum 5.0 mEq/L (mmol/L) Use cautiously with close monitoring of serum potassium in patients with serum creatinine 1.2–1.5 mg/dL (106–133 μmol/L) or estimated GFR 50–60 mL/min. Avoid in patients with more severe renal dysfunction: estimated GFR or creatinine clearance < 40 mL/min. The ACC/AHA advises < 30 mL/min

- A major breakthrough is the strong recommendation to add 25 mg spironolactone (Aldactone) in patients with class III and IV HF because the drug caused a 30% reduction in the risk of death among this class of patients with EF < 35% treated with loop diuretics, an ACE inhibitor, and digoxin. Hospitalization for recurrent HF was significantly reduced *(28)*. Unfortunately, the dosage of ACE inhibitor used was smaller than that used in modern clinical practice: mean dose captopril 63 mg, enalapril 15 mg, lisinopril 14.3 mg.
- Spironolactone causes gynecomastia and other androgenic effects, and eplerenone, which does not have these effects, has proved effective in a RCT.
- The dose of spironolactone used in the Randomized Aldactone Evaluation (RALES) trial was 25 mg *(28)*.
- **Caution** is required in patients with abnormal renal function and in type II diabetes with hyporeninemic hypoaldosteronism because severe hyperkalemia may ensue.
- If the serum K^+ reaches 5.0– 5.1 mEq/L, the dose of ACE inhibitor should be decreased and loop diuretic increased before reducing the 25-mg dose of spironolactone.
- Serum K^+ should be evaluated at 3 d and 1–2 wk after starting treatment and then about 3 monthly. If the K^+ reaches 5.1 mEq/L, spironolactone should be discontinued. **Caution:** Spironolactone or eplerenone should be used with close monitoring of serum potassium in patients with serum creatinine 1.2–1.5 mg/dL (106–133 μmol/L) or estimated GFR 49–59 mL/min *(28a)*.

- Avoid in patients with more severe renal dysfunction: estimated GFR or creatinine clearance < 40 mL/min. The ACC/AHA advises <30 mL/min.
- Elderly patients with a creatinine 1.2–1.4 mg/dL (102–123 μmol/L) within the normal range may have a markedly reduced creatinine clearance (estimated GFR) of 49–59 mL/min.

In patients age > 75 yr, a normal serum creatinine does not indicate normal renal function. It is necessary to assess the GFR.

- However, caution is needed because the formula to determine estimated GFR gives inaccurate results in patients older than age 70; in blacks a correction is required: multiply by 1.2.
- Avoid concomitant use of NSAIDS or cyclooxygenase-2 inhibitors.

Drug name:	**Eplerenone**
Trade name:	Inspra
Dosage:	If baseline K^+ < 5.1 mEq/L, 12.5 mg once daily Assess K^+ in 3 d and at 1 wk; if <5.0 mEq/L, increase to 25 mg once daily. Reassess K^+ at 1 mo then every 3 mo: maintain K^+ 4 to maximum 5.1 mEq/L (mmol/L) Max. 50 mg once daily Use cautiously with close monitoring of serum potassium in patients with serum creatinine 1.2–1.5 mg/dL (106–133 μmol/L) or estimated GFR 49–59 mL/min Avoid in patients with more severe renal dysfunction: GFR or creatinine clearance < 40 mL/min. The ACC/AHA advises < 30 mL/min; see above cautions for spironolactone in the elderly

- Avoid concomitant use of NSAIDS or cyclooxygenase-2 inhibitors.

BETA-BLOCKERS

- Three beta-blocking drugs have been approved for the management of HF: carvedilol, metoprolol extended release (Toprol XL), and bisoprolol.
- Beta-blockers play a major role in the management of patients with HF and are strongly recommended for the management of class I–III HF and also for compensated class IV patients.
- Beta-blocker therapy is initiated as soon as possible after the diagnosis of HF provided the patient is free from fluid overload.

Some specialists have advocated the commencement of a beta-blocker prior to ACE inhibition in the hypotensive patient because this may cause an improvement in LV function, thus allowing initiation (or an increase in dosage) of the ACE inhibitor *(29)*.

- They are most effective in patients with ischemic heart disease and dilated cardiomyopathy *(30)*.
- Transmyocardial measurements have documented that the failing human heart is exposed to increased adrenergic activity. Chronic adrenergic activation has adverse effects on the natural course of heart muscle disease *(31,32)*.
- These agents partially block RAAS and augment atrial and brain natriuretic peptide.
- It is often forgotten that beta-blockers significantly reduce renin secretion from the juxtaglomerular cells of the kidney, which causes a decrease in angiotensin levels and reduced aldosterone production; this action adds to their life-saving potential.
- Beta-blockers decrease renin and aldosterone production, which contributes to their life-saving potential in patients with HF, but a mild increase in K^+ may occur and potentiate that caused by spironolactone or eplerenone.

Drug name:	**Carvedilol**
Trade names:	Coreg, Eucardic (UK)
Supplied:	12.5, 25 mg
Dosage:	3.125-mg test dose and then twice daily after food for 1–2 wk; increase to 6.25 mg twice daily wk 3–4; then 9.375 mg twice daily during weeks 5–8; then if tolerated 12.5 mg twice daily. Increase slowly to the highest level tolerated; max. 25 mg twice daily. *See* text for further advice

Dosage (Further Advice)

- Carvedilol should be taken with food to slow the rate of absorption and reduce the incidence of orthostatic effects. If dizziness, lightheadedness, or hypotension occur, the dose of diuretic or ACE inhibitor should be reduced to allow up-titration of carvedilol or other beta-blocker. If symptoms persist, the dose of carvedilol should be reduced.
- In an RCT *(33)*, this drug resulted in a 67% reduction in mortality rate in patients with HF treated with diuretics and an ACE inhibitor; almost all patients were taking digoxin**.** The Carvedilol Postinfarct Survival Controlled Evaluation (CAPRICORN) study *(34)* in patients after MI with a mean EF of 33% found a 23% relative reduction in mortality, identical to the result of a metaanalysis of 22 long-term RCTs in post-MI patients. Notably, a similar benefit—a 2.3% absolute reduction in risk—was observed in SAVE, AIRE, and TRACE with ACE inhibitors, i.e., 43 patients treated to save one life.
- The Carvedilol Prospective Randomized Cumulative Survival Study (COPERNICUS) trial *(35)* studied 2289 patients with severe HF, EF 16–24%, *but free from overt fluid retention* or recent treatment with IV diuretics or positive inotropic drugs. The results showed a highly significant 35% reduction in all-cause mortality with carvedilol (*see* Chapter 22).

Beta-blocking drugs such as carvedilol have proved useful in improving survival and decreasing the number of hospitalizations for worsening HF. The drug is as effective as an ACE inhibitor in this setting. Carvedilol is indicated for the management of NYHA class II–III HF; the drug has not been adequately tested in patients with class IV HF. Compensated class IV HF patients free of fluid overload have shown benefit and should be treated, judiciously, with carvedilol with up-titration of doses over 4–6 wk.

Drug name:	**Metoprolol succinate** **Extended release** **Metoprolol CR/XL**
Trade names:	Betaloc, Lopressor, Toprol XL
Supplied:	50, 100 mg
Dosage:	12.5 mg test dose and then once daily for 2 wk; then 25 mg; titrate over 4–8 wk to 100 mg usual maintenance dose; max. 200 mg once daily

In a randomized trial in 338 patients with HF from dilated cardiomyopathy, metoprolol prevented clinical deterioration and improved symptoms and cardiac function *(36)*. The Metoprolol Extended-Release Randomized Intervention Trial in Heart Failure (MERIT-HF) trial involving patients with class II and III HF, mean EF 28%, resulted in risk reduction of 33% for total mortality or worsening HF *(37)*.

This agent was used in combination with diuretics, **digoxin**, and ACE inhibitors.

In a randomized trial in 50 patients with HF caused by ischemic heart disease, metoprolol 25–100 mg daily when added to standard HF therapy resulted in

- A decrease in the number of hospital admissions.
- Improved functional class.
- Increased EF.
- A greater increase in exercise duration compared with placebo *(37)*. It is known that beta-blocking agents cause a decrease in sudden cardiac deaths and increased survival in post-MI patients, and this beneficial result may be obtained in patients with varying grades of HF.

Bisoprolol (Zebeta, Monocor)

In the Cardiac Insufficiency Bisoprolol Study II (CIBIS II) *(38)*, bisoprolol resulted in a significant decrease in mortality in patients with NYHA class III HF and EF < 35%. CIBIS II involved 2647 patients aged 18–80 yr with class III or IV HF. Study patients received ACE inhibitor and diuretic (digitalis was allowed) for at least 2 mo prior to bisoprolol or placebo. Bisoprolol, initial dose 1.25 mg daily, was titrated at weekly intervals in 1.25-mg increments for 4 wk and then up to a maximum of 10 mg daily. Bisoprolol therapy reduced all-cause mortality by 32% ($p = 0.00005$) and sudden death by 45% ($p = 0.001$). A 30% reduction in hospitalization occurred in the bisoprolol-treated group. Treatment withdrawals in the bisoprolol-and placebo-treated patients were similar (approx 15%).

Drug name:	**Bisoprolol**
Trade names:	Zebeta, Monocor
Dosage:	1.25 mg test dose; then once daily; increase in 2–3 wk to 3.75 mg; at 5–6 wk if tolerated 5-mg maintenance dose At >12 wk, if needed max. dose 10 mg provided that the BP is >120 mmHg systolic and heart rate > 55 beats/min

INOTROPIC AGENTS

Drug name:	**Digoxin**
Trade name:	Lanoxin
Supplied:	0.625, 0.125, 0.25 mg
Dosage:	*See* text

Digoxin (Lanoxin) is the most reliable digitalis preparation and is used by the majority of physicians. Remarks are confined to this drug.

Indications

- Atrial fibrillation with uncontrolled ventricular response is the most clear-cut indication.
- HF related to poor LV contractility. These patients usually have a third heart sound gallop (S3), crepitations over the lung fields, and EF < 35%.
- A failure of diuretics and vasodilator therapy. Hypotension often limits the use of vasodilators in patients with severe HF and a low EF. Digoxin has a role in this category of patients.

Digoxin is indicated for all patients with impaired systolic function and NYHA class III, and IV HF *(39)*. Patients with NYHA class II HF are often managed with diuretics and ACE inhibitors, and recurrence of HF is an indication for the addition of digoxin.

- Ahmed and colleagues did a comprehensive *post hoc* analysis of the Digitalis Investigation Group (DIG) trial *(40)*. Digoxin showed a reduction in mortality and hospitalization for HF *(40)*.

Digoxin is not usually recommended, or is of limited value, for the management of HF resulting from or accompanied by:

- Acute MI, except from d 2 if HF is not easily controlled by furosemide, nitrates, ACE inhibitor, dobutamine, or nitroprusside.
- Advanced first-degree, second-degree, and complete atrioventricular (AV) block. (It is preferable with second- and third-degree AV block to pace the patient and then use digitalis.)
- Patients with low EF, sinus rhythm, and no history of HF symptoms.
- The use of digoxin to minimize symptoms in patients with HF with preserved EF is not well established.
- Mitral stenosis, normal sinus rhythm.
- Hypertrophic cardiomyopathy (HCM), except if HF is moderate or severe. (The drug is potentially dangerous in HCM.)
- Sick sinus syndrome; it is advisable to put in a permanent pacemaker and then commence beta-blocker therapy.
- Cor pulmonale, except for the management of atrial fibrillation with a fast ventricular response or in patients with added severe LV failure exhibiting a low cardiac output and both central and peripheral cyanosis.

A study by Arnold and colleagues *(41)* demonstrated that patients with proven HF show improvement in hemodynamics during acute and long-term administration as well as during exercise. Withdrawal of digoxin in that study produced a significant increase in pulmonary capillary wedge pressure, heart rate, and SVR and a fall in stroke work index and EF. After acute retreatment, all parameters improved, including exercise hemodynamics.

Gheorghiade and colleagues *(42)* have confirmed these hemodynamic effects of digoxin. In a double-blind placebo-controlled study of patients with documented HF and no reversible etiology, 16 of the 46 patients deteriorated between 4 d and 3 wk after stopping digoxin *(43)*.

Analysis of the Digoxin Study

The effect of digoxin on mortality and morbidity in patients with HF was reported in 1997 *(39,40)*. The results of this study provided some answers to 200 yr of controversy regarding the use of digitalis.

Digoxin was assigned to 3397 patients, and 3403 received diuretics and an ACE inhibitor. The mean EF was 28% ± 9%. The average follow-up was 37 mo. Fewer patients in the digoxin group were hospitalized for worsening HF: 26.8% versus 34.7% in the placebo group ($p < 0.001$; *see* Table 12-3).

- The study did not show a significant decrease in total mortality. **Digoxin, however, did not cause an increase in mortality.** In fact, there was a trend toward a decrease in the risk of death attributed to worsening HF ($p = 0.06$).
- **Most important, the risk associated with the combined outcome of death related to HF or hospitalization related to HF was significantly lower in the digoxin group (1041 versus 1291 patients, $p < 0.01$; *see* Table 12-3) and was similar to that observed in SAVE and SOLVD attributed to the benefits of ACE inhibitor.**
- Unfortunately, *the study included only 2% class IV and 30% class III patients. Digoxin is expected to benefit class III–IV patients; this subset was not well represented in the study.* Digoxin is strongly indicated in class III–IV HF and in patients with EF < 30%.
- Fortunately, the study showed that in patients with EF < 0.30, death or hospitalization related to worsening HF occurred in 428 of 1127 in the digoxin group and in 556 of 1130 in the placebo group, a 23.0% reduction. In patients with NYHA class III HF, death or hospitaliza-

Table 12-3
Effect of Digoxin on Mortality and Morbidity in Patients with Heart Failure

	Digoxin (n = 3397)	*Placebo (n = 3403)*	*% reduction*	*p*	*Risk ratio*[a]
Worsening CHF	910	1180	22.9	<0.001	
Death plus CHF	1041	1291	19.3	<0.001	
Death owing to worsening CHF	394	449		0.06	
Death or hospitalization owing to CHF EF < 0.25	428/1127	556/1130	23.0		0.68 (0.60–0.70)
Class III or IV Class IV only 2% of study group	438/1118	552/1105	20.6		0.70 (0.61–0.79)
Cardiothoracic ratio > 0.55	441/1176	567/1170	22.2		0.69 (0.61–0.79)

[a]Values in parentheses are 95% confidence intervals. CHF, congestive heart faillure; EF, ejection fraction.
Modified from the Digitalis Investigation Group. The effect of digoxin on mortality and morbidity in patients with heart failure. N Engl J Med 1997;336:525.

tion occurred in 438 of 1118 in the digoxin group and in 552 of 1105 in the placebo group, a 20.6% reduction (risk ratio 0.70 [95% confidence [CI] interval 0.61–0.79]). A 19% reduction was observed for the risk of death, CHF, or hospitalization ($p = 0.001$).

- A 22% decrease in death or hospitalization was observed in patients with cardiothoracic ratio > 0.55. The study indicated that digoxin significantly decreases death or hospitalization caused by worsening HF in patients with class II–III and IV HF with EF < 0.25 or with cardiothoracic ratio > 0.55. The enalapril CONSENSUS study showed an increased survival rate in class IV patients treated over 6 mo with enalapril added to diuretics and digoxin.
- *Currently we strongly recommend this drug in patients with class III and IV HF, with EF < 30%, and with increased LV volume and cardiothoracic ratio > 0.55. This is advisable particularly if the systolic blood pressure is <100 mmHg caused by ACE inhibitors and beta-blockers. Digoxin does not cause a decrease in BP. However, digoxin levels must remain in the range 0.5–1 ng/mL.*

Is the Combination of Digoxin and ACE Inhibitors Necessary?

The Randomized Assessment of Digoxin on Inhibitors of ACE (RADIANCE) study included 178 patients with chronic HF and sinus rhythm who were clinically stable with diuretics, an ACE inhibitor, and digoxin *(44)*. Most patients (70%) were in NYHA class II. In patients withdrawn from digoxin for 3 months, there was a sixfold worsening of HF. Patients taking a placebo had a higher incidence of deterioration and worsening HF (23 versus 4 patients) and more deterioration in quality of life. The dose of digoxin in the RADIANCE study was 0.38 mg daily, and serum digoxin levels ranged from 0.9 to 2.0 ng/mL.

- Digoxin favorably alters the neurohormonal imbalance that contributes to HF. It is, therefore, rational to use the triple combination of diuretics, ACE inhibitors, and digoxin to manage LV failure and improve symptoms, survival, and quality of life in virtually all patients with class III–IV HF.
- A salutary interaction of digoxin and spironolactone: These two now have an important role in the management of class III and IV HF. Na entry into Na channels in myofibroblasts is enhanced by aldosterone and is the trigger for myocardial fibrosis.

Table 12-4
Conditions in Which There is an Increased Sensitivity to Digoxin and Conservative Dosing is Recommended

Elderly patients (age > 70 yr)
Renal dysfunction; creatinine > 1.2 mg/dL (106 μmol/L)
Estimated GFR < 50 mL/h
Thin patients, low skeletal mass
Hypokalemia
Hyperkalemia
Hypoxemia
Acidosis
Acute myocardial infarction
Hypomagnesemia
Hypercalcemia
Hypocalcemia
Myocarditis
Hypothyroidism
Amyloidosis

- When digoxin is added, there is a reduction in fibrosis because digoxin blocks sodium-potassium adenosine triphosphatase (Na^+,K^+-ATPase) and thus decreases Na entry into fibroblasts and decreases fibrosis. *In the spironolactone study, 72% of patients received digoxin.*

Mechanism of Action

1. Digoxin increases the force and velocity of myocardial contraction in both the failing and the nonfailing heart. It inhibits the function of the sodium pump, resulting in an increase in intracellular sodium accompanied by an increase in cellular calcium. Digoxin causes the Frank-Starling function curve to move upward and to the left, i.e., an improved ventricular function curve. Improvement in cardiac output produces a favorable alteration of the compensatory responses of HF including the neurohormonal response (*see* Fig. 12-1).
2. **Electrophysiologic effects:**
   a. Decreases conduction velocity in the AV node, i.e., the drug sets up a "traffic jam" in the AV node, producing an important reduction in ventricular response in atrial fibrillation.
   b. Increases the slope of phase 4 diastolic depolarization and therefore increases automaticity of ectopic pace makers.
3. **Vasoconstrictor:** The drug has a mild vasoconstrictor effect that increases total systemic resistance. In the failing heart, however, the drug increases cardiac output, which counteracts the reflex stimulation of the sympathetic and angiotensin systems, resulting in vasodilation and a fall in total systemic resistance, i.e., afterload reduction.

Dosage Considerations

Before writing an order for digoxin, review the indications and reassess renal function and conditions that increase sensitivity (Table 12-4).

1. **Loading Dose (Initial Dose)**
   For adults and children over 10 yr and in the absence of conditions that may increase sensitivity—**initial 0.5–1 mg orally**, given as follows:

- *Slow method:* 0.5 mg immediately and 0.25 mg every 12 h for two doses (1 mg/24 h).

OR

- 0.25 mg twice daily for 2 d and then maintenance depending on age and renal function.

Note: A low skeletal mass means less binding to skeletal muscle receptors, and therefore a smaller loading dose is required in the thin or elderly patient and in women. For a more **rapid effect** (e.g., atrial fibrillation, heart rate 130–150/beats/min) give 0.5 mg immediately and then 0.25 mg every 6 h for two or three doses.

Intravenous: Mainly for atrial fibrillation, heart rate >150/beats/min in the absence of digoxin therapy within the last 2 wk. Give either:

- 0.75 mg IV slowly over 5 min and then 0.25 mg every 2 h for two doses, under electrocardiography (ECG) cover, reassessing the patient before each dose is given. A total dose of 1.25–1.5 mg is often necessary.

OR

- 0.75–1.25 mg as an infusion over 2 h or more, which is advised in the United Kingdom when rapid control is needed.

2. **Maintenance Dose**

Digoxin is mainly excreted unchanged by the kidney, with an average half-life of 36 h. In normal renal function, as a general rule give the following:

- Age < 70 yr: 0.25 mg daily, preferably at bedtime.
- Age > 70 yr: 0.125 mg daily, and reduced dose if renal impairment is present, to maintain a level of 0.5 to maximum 1 ng/mL.

Note: Atrial fibrillation with a fast ventricular response may require 0.125 mg daily or twice weekly in addition to the preceding dose.

Caution:

- Serum digoxin levels > 1.0 ng/mL appear to increase mortality in women. The dose should be 0.152 mg daily or less to achieve a level of 0.6–1 ng/mL.
- In renal failure, the dose interval is increased depending on the creatinine clearance. The serum creatinine level is not an accurate measure of the creatinine clearance. It is advisable to estimate the GFR. Despite such calculations, digoxin toxicity may develop if renal dysfunction is present. Digoxin is best avoided in patients with moderate degree of renal failure: estimated GFR < 30 mL/h.
- The use of digitalis in the presence of moderate or severe renal failure represents a controversial area because the risk of toxicity is common.

The bioavailability of digitalis is reduced in malabsorption syndrome and by the following drugs:

- Cholestyramine, colestipol.
- Neomycin.
- Antacids.
- Metoclopramide.
- Diphenylhydantoin.
- Phenobarbital.
- Phenylbutazone.

Serum Digoxin Levels and Interactions

Low therapeutic or even subtherapeutic digoxin levels < 1.0 ng/mL do not exclude toxicity. Beneficial effects are observed in the low range 0.5–1.1 ng/mL; toxicity is rare if levels are thus maintained. Determinations should be made no earlier than 6 h after the last dose of digoxin. If digoxin is given at night, a serum level can be obtained at steady state on the following morning, and the drug dosage can be modified when the patient is seen during the day.

Values of 2 ng/mL (2.6 nmol/L) may be associated with toxicity, and in some patients levels of 2–3 ng/mL may not indicate toxicity. Patients must never be allowed to have levels greater than 2 ng/mL μg/L. There are several limitations to these statements:

- The sensitivity of the myocardium and conducting system is important.
- Sensitivity of the radioimmunoassay is between 0.2 and 0.4 ng/mL digoxin. Values can differ (up to 30%).
- **Spironolactone causes falsely raised values.**
- Atorvastatin, quinidine, calcium antagonists, and amiodarone increase serum digoxin levels. Decreased renal elimination of digoxin results from a quinidine-induced decrease in tubular secretion of digoxin *(46)*. Verapamil causes a significant increase in digoxin levels that may result in severe bradycardia or asystole *(47)*. Interaction with diltiazem is minimal and with nifedipine insignificant. Amiodarone reduces clearance of digoxin and causes a 25–75% increase in digoxin levels. A reduction of the dose of digoxin by 50% is recommended when quinidine, quinine, verapamil, or amiodarone is given concurrently *(48)*.

Clinical studies indicate that there is no clear-cut serum level that establishes the presence of toxicity. The serum digoxin level is useful when interpreted relative to the serum potassium level and the clinical situation. The serum K^+ concentration increases with digitalis toxicity.

If digoxin toxicity is suspected, it is advisable to discontinue digoxin if:

- Serum digoxin level is >1.1 ng/mL with a serum K^+ level of 2.5–3.5 mEq (mmol)/L.
- Serum potassium level is <2.5 mEq (mmol)/L. In this case, digoxin should be withheld regardless of the serum digoxin concentration.

Potassium depletion must be corrected before recommencing digoxin.

This seems a reasonable course of action because there are other treatments for the management of HF.

Digitalis Toxicity

- The incidence of digoxin toxicity decreased during the 1990s, and toxicity occurs in about one episode for every 20 yr of treatment. In large digoxin trials, adverse effects have been no different than with placebo.
- *The incidence of toxicity is rare with the lowered dose currently advised.*
- The ECG may be nonspecific, but symptoms may provide enough clues, especially when combined with knowledge of the results of the serum creatinine or creatinine clearance and the maintenance dose of digoxin. This information should enable the physician to reach a decision about whether or not the patient has digoxin toxicity. There is no need to await notification of digoxin levels. If you suspect toxicity, withhold the drug for at least 48 h—there are other effective treatments for HF, and withholding a few doses of digoxin will not be detrimental.

Symptoms of Toxicity

- **Gastrointestinal:** anorexia, nausea, vomiting, diarrhea, and weight loss.
- **Central nervous system:** visual hallucinations, mental confusion, psychosis, restlessness, insomnia, drowsiness, and extreme weakness; blue-green-yellow vision, blurring of vision, and scotomas.

Cardiac Dysrhythmias

1. **Ventricular premature beats:** bigeminal or multifocal.

2. **AV block:**
   a. Second degree (Wenckebach).
   b. Atrial tachycardia with AV block, ventricular rate commonly 90–120/min, so often missed clinically, and the ECG may be misread because the P-waves can be buried in the T-waves. Be on the alert when there is steady moderate tachycardia without obvious cause.
   c. Rarely, complete heart block.
   d. A very slow ventricular response < 50/min; an intermittently regular rhythm at a slow rate in a patient with atrial fibrillation.
3. **Tachycardias:**
   a. Nonparoxysmal junctional tachycardia with AV dissociation or accelerated AV junctional rhythm.
   b. Ventricular tachycardia and ventricular fibrillation.
4. **Bradyarrhythmias:**
   a. Sinus bradycardia alone is a poor predictor of toxicity.
   b. Sinus arrest and sinoatrial block.

Management of Toxicity

General measures:

- Stop the drug.
- Discontinue diuretics or, if they are necessary, use a potassium-sparing diuretic or ample K supplements.
- Measure serum digoxin levels and serum K.
- Recheck the dose used and correlate with weight, age, and creatinine clearance.
- Record baseline ECG. If arrhythmia is present, monitor the cardiac rhythm.
- Search for and correct factors that can precipitate digitalis toxicity, e.g., physician error, giving too big a dose in the presence of renal insufficiency or hypokalemia.

Hyperkalemia may be owing to digitalis toxicity, and it is believed to result from inhibition by digitalis of the Na^+,K^+-ATPase enzyme causing a release of intracellular potassium into the extracellular space. Other predisposing factors are as listed in Table 12-2. Advise the patient in the future to bring all medications, to be rechecked at each hospital or office visit.

Tachyarrhythmias: Ventricular tachycardia, multifocal premature ventricular contractions (PVCs), and atrial tachycardia with block are managed as follows:

1. **Potassium intravenously:** 40–60 mEq (mmol) in 1 L of normal or half-normal saline is given over 4 h, except:
   a. In patients with a raised serum K^+ concentration (>5 mEq (mmol)/L).
   b. In renal insufficiency.
   c. In patients with AV block because increasing K^+ concentration may increase the degree of the AV block.

   If more than 10 mEq (mmol)/h of KC1 is infused, cardiac monitoring is necessary. KC1 in 5% dextrose/water is used if HF is present.
2. **Lidocaine; lignocaine** is reasonably effective for the management of ventricular tachycardia and multifocal PVCs. The short duration of action and relatively low toxicity are major advantages. A bolus of 1–1.5 mg/kg is given simultaneously with a continuous infusion of 2–3 mg/min.
3. **Phenytoin** may be effective in the management of digitalis-induced ventricular arrhythmias but should be reserved for nonresponders to lidocaine or K^+ because more careful supervision is required during its administration and severe toxic side effects do occur.

Dosage: IV 250 mg at a rate of 25–50 mg/min given in 0.9% saline through a caval catheter or utilizing a central vein Phenytoin is useful as it depresses ventricular automaticity without slowing intraventricular conduction. The decrease in AV conduction produced by digitalis may be reversed. The drug has a relatively mild negative inotropic effect in comparison with procainamide or disopyramide.

Caution:

- Hypotension, heart block, asystole, and ventricular fibrillation have occurred, especially with increase in the infusion rate of phenytoin.
- 250-mg vials contain 40% propylene glycol as a diluent with a pH of 11. Do not mix with dextrose. Pain, inflammation, or venous thrombosis may occur.

4. Magnesium deficiency may coexist with hypokalemia. Magnesium sulfate parenterally may be indicated.
5. Beta-blockers are reserved for nonresponders to measures 1–4. The drug may be useful for PVCs or supraventricular tachycardia (SVT) in the absence of AV block. The use of beta-blockers has appropriately dwindled with the advent of digoxin-specific Fab antibody.

Bradyarrhythmias: Sinoatrial dysfunction causing syncope or hemodynamic deterioration can be managed with atropine IV 0.4, 0.5, or 0.6 mg every 5 min to a maximum of 2.4 mg. Failure to respond to atropine is an indication for temporary pacing.

Cardioversion: Ventricular fibrillation requires the usual energy levels (200 joules, if necessary up to 320 joules). IV amiodarone is of value in the management of recurrent ventricular fibrillation. If other arrhythmias are life threatening, phenytoin or lidocaine followed if necessary by cardioversion using a low energy of 5–20 joules initially is tried.

Drug name:	**Digoxin Immune Fab (Digoxin-specific antibody)**
Trade name:	Digibind
Supplied:	Vial 40 mg (38 mg UK)
Dosage:	2–6 vials; infusion of six vials (228–240 mg) is adequate to reverse most cases of toxicity; *see* text for further advice

Dosage (Further Advice)

Up to 20 vials have been used to treat patients with overdose. *See* product monograph on calculated dosage based on body weight, serum digoxin level, or, with overdose, the amount ingested.

Treatment of digitalis intoxication with digoxin-specific Fab antibody fragments: There is little doubt that this method of treatment is effective for the management of life-threatening arrhythmias not responding to conventional therapy. The treatment is especially useful in the presence of hyperkalemia. Skin testing to avoid allergic reactions to the digoxin-specific Fab from sheep is recommended. The drug is available as Digibind in the United Kingdom and as Digitalis Antidote BM in Europe.

In a multicenter study, digoxin-specific Fab antibody fragments administered to 150 patients with potentially life-threatening digitalis toxicity resulted in an 80% amelioration of symptoms *(49)*. Response to treatment was observed within 20 min, and up to 75% of patients obtained a beneficial result in 1 h. Approximately 3% of patients are expected to have a recurrence, especially if the dose of Fab is inadequate. Adverse effects are rare. Allergic reactions occur in less than 1%; hypokalemia is found in less than 5% and must be anticipated and treated vigorously.

Beta-Stimulants

Drug name:	**Dobutamine**
Dosage:	250 mg/20 mL vial—diluted in 5% dextrose/water and infused at a rate of 2.5–10 μg/kg/min. For dobutamine infusion pump chart, *see* Chapter 11 and Appendix I

Dobutamine is a direct myocardial beta$_1$- and a mild beta$_2$-stimulant. The positive inotropic effect is equal to that of isoproterenol.

In patients with HF, the drug causes a large increase in cardiac output, which is equal to that seen after nitroprusside administration *(50)*. The reduction in SVR with dobutamine may rarely cause **hypotension**, and the drug is contraindicated in patients who are hypotensive.

Increase in cardiac output occurs with only minimal increase in heart rate at infusion rates < 5 μg/kg/min.

Dobutamine increases cardiac output while reducing left ventricular filling pressure (LVFP) with little or no increase in heart rate or blood pressure. Except at low doses, dopamine produces an increase in LVFP, heart rate, SVR, and blood pressure and therefore increases myocardial oxygen demand. Dobutamine is thus superior to dopamine in patients with a very high LVFP. Advantages of dobutamine include a short half-life < 3 min, which allows rapid dissipation of adverse effects.

Importantly low doses are currently advised: 1 μg/kg/min with increase to 2 μg; a dose of 5 μg/kg/min is often excessive. This lower recommended dose avoids adverse effects.

- Dopamine increases SVR, and cardiac output may not increase despite its inotropic effect. In patients with peripheral vascular disease, gangrene of the digits may be precipitated.

ACC/AHA GUIDELINES

The following recommendations were extracted from the 2005 ACC/AHA practice guidelines (*see* Table 12-5); Fig. 12-2 gives an algorithm for the management of HF.

Recommendations for Patients at High Risk of Developing HF (Stage A)

Class I = the therapy is effective.

- Control of systolic and diastolic hypertension in accordance with recommended guidelines (*Level of Evidence: A [4])*.
- Treatment of lipid disorders in accordance with recommended guidelines (*Level of Evidence: A*).
- ACE inhibition in patients with a history of atherosclerotic CVD, diabetes mellitus, or hypertension and associated cardiovascular risk factors *(Level of Evidence: A)*.
- Avoidance of patient behaviors that may increase the risk of HF (e.g., smoking, alcohol consumption, and illicit drug use) (*Level of Evidence: C* = no RCT; experts' opinion only).

Recommendations for Patients with Cardiac Structural Abnormalities but Without Signs and Symptoms of HF (Stage B)

Class I recommendation

In addition to all recommendations given for Stage A, administer the following:

Table 12-5
Stages of Heart Failure[a]

Stage	*Description*	*Examples*
A	Patients at high risk of developing HF because of the presence of conditions that are strongly associated with the development of HF. Such patients have no identified structural or functional abnormalities of the pericardium, myocardium, or cardiac valves and have never shown signs or symptoms of HF.	Systemic hypertension; coronary artery disease; diabetes mellitus; history of cardiotoxic drug therapy.
B	Patients who have developed structural heart disease that is strongly associated with the development of HF but who have never shown signs or symptoms of HF.	Left ventricular hypertrophy or fibrosis; left ventricular dilatation or hypocontractility; asymptomatic valvular heart disease; previous myocardial infarction.
C	Patients who have current or prior symptoms of HF associated with underlying structural heart disease.	Dyspnea or fatigue: patients who are undergoing treatment for prior symptoms of HF.
D	Patients with advanced structural heart disease and marked symptoms of HF at rest despite maximal medical therapy and who require specialized interventions.	Patients who are frequently hospitalized for HF or cannot be safely discharged from the hospital; patients in the hospital awaiting heart transplantation; patients at home receiving continuous intravenous support for symptom relief or being supported with a mechanical circulatory assist device; patients in a hospice setting for the management of HF.

[a]Modified from ACC/AHA practice guidelines, 2005.
HF, heart failure.

- Beta-blockers and ACE inhibition for patients with a recent or remote history of MI regardless of presence of HF or EF. An ARB can be used for all patients intolerant to an ACE inhibitor for all categories.
- ACE inhibition in patients with a reduced EF and absence of HF whether or not they have experienced an MI.
- Valve replacement or repair for patients with hemodynamically significant valvular stenosis or regurgitation and no symptoms of HF.

Recommendations for Treatment of Symptomatic HF Patients with Left Ventricular Systolic Dysfunction (Reduced EF) (Stage C)

Class I

- Diuretics in patients who have evidence of fluid retention.
- ACE inhibition in all patients; or ARB if intolerant.
- Commence early therapy with beta-adrenergic blockade: carvedilol, bisoprolol, or metoprolol succinate (extended release Toprol XL) in all stable patients. Patients should have no evidence of fluid retention and should not have required treatment recently with an intravenous positive inotropic agent.

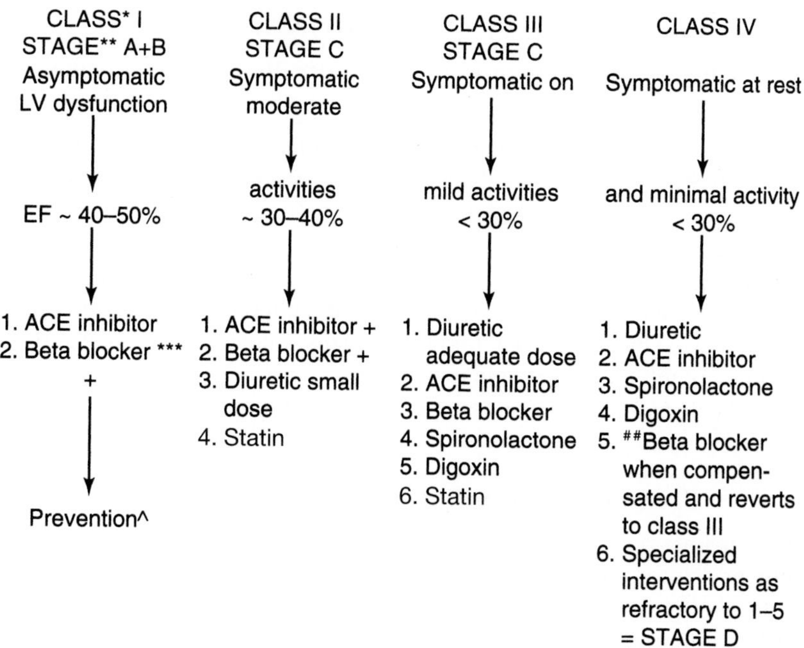

*New York Heart Association functional classification.

**ACC/AHA stages of HF "is intended to complement but not replace" NYHA functional classification.

#Beta blocker not FDA approved for CLASS IV but as soon as the patient reaches a compensated state free of overt fluid retention, a trial of beta blocker slow dose titration is advisable (see text for COPERNICUS).

^**Optimize control of: BP, lipid and thyroid disorders, diabetes, smoking, alcohol abuse, weight and stress levels, atrial fibrillation and tachycardias, and timely correction of valvular lesions.

***Class I stage B: CHD, hypertension, atrial fibrillation **needs beta blockade**.

##eplerenone.

Fig. 12-2. Algorithm for the treatment of heart failure.

Digoxin for patients with current or prior HF is a class IIa recommendation. *See* earlier discussion under digoxin and use in patients with HF with low EF and cardiothoracic ratio > 0.55; also *see* Chapter 13, Heart Failure Controversies. This is a clinical situation in which digoxin causes salutary effects and is particularly useful in patients with low systolic pressures < 100 mmHg and in whom ACE inhibitors and beta-blockers cause further lowering of blood pressure.

- Withdrawal of drugs known to affect the clinical status of patients adversely (e.g., NSAIDS, most antiarrhythmic drugs, and all calcium channel blocking drugs).
- Aldosterone antagonists: spironolactone in patients with recent or current class IV HF, preserved renal function, and a normal potassium concentration (*see* earlier discussion under spironolactone).

1. Exercise training as an adjunctive approach to improve clinical status in ambulatory patients.
2. Angiotensin receptor blockade in patients who cannot be given an ACE inhibitor because of cough or angioedema.
3. A combination of hydralazine and a nitrate in patients who are being treated with digitalis, diuretics, and a beta-blocker and in whom an ACE inhibitor or ARB is contraindicated. This combination is particularly useful in patients of African origin, as shown in A-HeFT (*see* Chapters 13 and 22).

MANAGEMENT OF PULMONARY EDEMA

Pulmonary edema is not a diagnosis. Its cause is usually cardiogenic or noncardiogenic.

Cardiogenic

- Usually owing to LV failure, often caused by to complications of ischemic heart disease, tachyarrhythmias, hypertension, valvular heart disease, or congestive dilated cardiomyopathy.
- Mitral stenosis and, rarely, left atrial myxoma.

OR

Noncardiogenic

- Adult respiratory distress syndrome in which there is altered alveolar-capillary membrane permeability caused by pneumonia, toxins, allergens, smoke inhalation, gastric aspiration, radiation pneumonitis, hemorrhagic pancreatitis.
- Other causes include drugs, narcotic overdose, severe hypoalbuminemia, uremia, neurogenic and lymphangitic carcinomatosis.

Treatment of Cardiogenic Pulmonary Edema

1. **Oxygen**, to maintain an adequate PO_2.
2. **Morphine** or diamorphine, provided severe respiratory insufficiency is absent, because either drug may cause respiratory depression or even arrest.

   Dosage: A dilute solution of morphine sulfate 1 mg/mL is administered IV at a rate of **1 mg/min** in a dose of 3–5 mg. Repeat as needed at 15- to 30-min intervals to a total dose of 10–15 mg. The average patient may require 30 mg in 24 h. **Diamorphine** 2–5 mg, repeated once if necessary, is often used in the United Kingdom. The beneficial effects of the opiates result from:

   a. venous pooling and therefore preload reduction.
   b. the allaying of anxiety and reduction in tachypnea.
   c. an increase in ventricular fibrillation threshold.

   Vomiting and aspiration should be avoided. An antiemetic such as cyclizine or metoclopramide 5 mg is useful when given 15 min before the dose of morphine is repeated. **Naloxone** (Narcan) 0.4 mg IV repeated at 4-min intervals is given if respiratory depression occurs (maximum 1.2 mg).
3. **Furosemide 40–80 mg IV** slowly repeated in 30 min if symptoms persist and the blood pressure is stable.

   Warning: In patients with normal or low blood volume, an initial dose of 40 mg or more may cause severe hypotension, especially when morphine and nitrates are used concomitantly. Improvement in dyspnea usually occurs within 10 min of furosemide administration as a result of its venodilator action. Failure to respond to the second dose is an indication for preload- or afterload-reducing agents.
4. **Nitroglycerin** (glyceryl trinitrate) can be of immediate benefit. Nitroglycerin is given sublingually along with a transdermal preparation. In severe pulmonary edema IV nitrate or nitroprusside is indicated.

Important Considerations and Added Therapy

1. **The cardiac rhythm** must be determined immediately because atrial fibrillation or ventricular tachycardia may be the cause of the pulmonary edema. Ventricular tachycardia may be reversed by a bolus of lidocaine. Arrhythmias may quickly respond to electrical cardioversion.
2. If severe hypertension is present, nitroprusside or an ACE inhibitor is useful.
3. Dobutamine should be tried if mild hypotension is present. Nesiritide may cause hypotension and renal dysfunction; also, increased mortality appears to be a concern (*see* Chapter 13).

4. Rotating venous tourniquets are rarely necessary but should be considered if the preceding steps fail. Only three of the four tourniquets should be inflated 10 mmHg above the diastolic pressure, and one must be released every 15 min.
5. If **hypotension** is present, dopamine 2.5–10 μg/kg/min and nitrate are indicated.
6. If **atrial fibrillation or supraventricular tachycardia** is present and electrical cardioversion cannot be utilized, digoxin has a definite role in the early management. For patients in normal sinus rhythm, digitalis may be withheld until more is known about the underlying cause of heart disease and the rationale for its use.
7. **Aminophylline** is a nonspecific treatment and is often overprescribed. The drug may cause cardiac arrhythmias. Nausea and vomiting related to the combination of morphine and aminophylline may occur. If bronchospasm and diaphragmatic fatigue are prominent features, aminophylline should be tried. **Loading dose:** 2–5 mg/kg, slowly over 20 min. **Maintenance**: Continuous infusion 0.3–0.6 mg/kg/h. A slightly smaller dose must be used in elderly people, in those with HF, and with the concomitant use of drugs that raise theophylline blood levels.
8. **Endotracheal intubation** and mechanical ventilation are recommended for patients with respiratory failure ($PO_2 < 50$ mmHg or $PCO_2 > 50$ mmHg).
9. **Positive end-expiratory pressure** (PEEP) may improve oxygenation and decrease intra-alveolar fluid. However, PEEP reduces cardiac output and may cause hypotension.

REFERENCES

1. O'Connell JB, Bristow M. Economic impact of heart failure in the United States: Time for a different approach. J Heart Lung Transplant 1999;13:S107.
2. Haldeman GA, Croft JB, Giles WH, Rashidee A. Hospitalization of patients with heart failure: National Hospital Discharge Survey. Am Heart J 1999;137:352.
3. Hunt SH, Baker DW, Chin MH, et al. ACC/AHA guidelines for the evaluation and management of chronic heart failure in the adult: Executive summary: A report of the American College of Cardiology/ American Heart Association Task Force on practice guidelines. J Am Coll Cardiol 2001;38:2101.
4. Hunt SA, Abraham WT, Chin MH, et al. ACC/AHA 2005 guideline update for the diagnosis and management of chronic heart failure in the adult—summary article: A report of the American College of Cardiology/American Heart Association Task Force on Practice Guidelines (Writing Committee to Update the 2001 Guidelines for the Evaluation and Management of Heart Failure). J Am Coll Cardiol 2005;46: 1116–1143.
5. Maisel AS, Krishnaswamy P, Nowak RM, et al. Rapid measurement of B-type natriuretic peptide in the emergency diagnosis of heart failure. N Engl J Med 2002;347:161.
6. Wilson Tang WH, Francis GS. The year in heart failure. J Am Coll Cardiol 2005;46:2125–2133.
7. Packer M. Is the renin-angiotensin system really unnecessary in patients with severe chronic heart failure?: The price we pay for interfering with evolution. J Am Coll Cardiol 1985;6:171.
8. Packer M, Lee WH, Yushak M, et al. Comparison of captopril and enalapril in patients with severe chronic heart failure. N Engl J Med 1986;315:847.
9. CONSENSUS: Consensus Trial Study Group. Effects of enalapril on mortality in severe congestive heart failure: Results of the Cooperative North Scandinavian Enalapril Survival Study (Consensus). N Engl J Med 1987;316:1429.
10. A-HeFT: Taylor AL, Ziesche S, Yancy C, et al. Combination of isosorbide dinitrate and hydralazine in blacks with heart failure. N Engl J Med 2004;351:2049–2057.
11. Cohn JN, Archibald DG, Francis GS, et al. Veterans Administration Cooperative Study on Vasodilator Therapy of Heart Failure: Influence of prerandomization variables on the reduction of mortality by treatment with hydralazine and isosorbide dinitrate. Circulation 1987;75(IV):IV–49.
12. Cohn JN, Archibald DG, Ziesche S, et al. Effect of vasodilator therapy on mortality in chronic congestive heart failure. Results of a Veterans Administration Cooperative Study. N Engl J Med 1986;314: 1547.
13. V-HeFTII: Cohn JN, Johnson G, Ziesche S, et al. A comparison of enalapril with hydralazine-isosorbide dinitrate in the treatment of chronic congestive heart failure. N Engl J Med 1991;325:303.

14. SOLVD Investigators. Effect of enalapril on survival in patients with reduced ventricular ejection fractions and congestive heart failure. N Engl J Med 1991;325:293.
15. Furberg CD, Yusuf S. Effect of vasodilators on survival in chronic congestive heart failure. Am J Cardiol 1985;55:1110.
16. Furberg CD, Yusuf S. Effect of drug therapy on survival in chronic congestive heart failure. Am J Cardiol 1988;62:41A.
17. Agostoni PG, De Gasare N, Doria E, et al. Afterload reduction: A comparison of captopril and nifedipine in dilated cardiomyopathy. Br Heart J 1986;55:391.
18. SAVE: Pfeffer MA, Braunwald E, Moye LA, et al. for the SAVE Investigators. Effect of captopril on mortality and morbidity in patients with left ventricular dysfunction after myocardial infarction. Results of the Survival and Ventricular Enlargement trial. N Engl J Med 1992;327:669.
19. AIRE: Acute Infarction Ramipril Efficacy (AIRE) Study Investigators. Effect of ramipril on mortality and morbidity of survivors of acute myocardial infarction with clinical evidence of heart failure. Lancet 1993;342:821.
20. Cleland JGF, Dargie HJ, McAlpine H, et al. Severe hypotension after first dose of enalapril in heart failure. BMJ 1985;291:1309.
21. Nanas JN, Alexopoulos G, Anastasiou-Nana MI, et al. Outcome of patients with congestive heart failure treated with standard versus high doses of enalapril: A multicenter study. J Am Coll Cardiol 2000;36:2090.
22. ATLAS Study Group. Packer M, Poole-Wilson PA, Armstrong P, et al. Comparative effects of low and high doses of angiotensin-converting inhibitor, lisinopril, on morbidity and mortality in chronic heart failure. Circulation 1999;100:2312.
23. CHARM: Granger CB, McMurray JJV, Yusuf S, et al. for the CHARM Investigators and Committees. Effects of candesartan in patients with chronic heart failure and reduced left ventricular systolic function intolerant to angiotensin converting enzyme inhibitors; the CHARM-alternative trial. Lancet 2003;362: 772–776.
24. Cohn JN, Tognoni G. A randomized trial of the angiotensin-receptor blocker valsartan in chronic heart failure. N Engl J Med 2001;345:1667–1675.
25. Walsh WF, Greenberg BH. Results of long-term vasodilator therapy in patients with refractory congestive heart failure. Circulation 1981;64:499.
26. PRAISE: Packer M, O'Connor CM, Ghali JK, et al. Effect of amlodipine on morbidity and mortality in severe chronic heart failure. For the Prospective Randomized Amlodipine Survival Evaluation Study Group. N Engl J Med 1996;335:1107.
27. Kiyingi A, Field MJ, Pawsey CC, et al. Metolazone in treatment of severe refractory congestive cardiac failure. Lancet 1990;336:29.
28. RALES: Pitt B, Zannad F, Remme WJ, et al. for the Randomized Evaluation Study Investigators: The effect of spironolactone on morbidity and mortality in patients with severe heart failure. N Engl J Med 1999;341:709.
28a. Stevens LA, Coresh J, Green T. Assessing kidney function—measured and estimated glomerular filtration rate. N Engl J Med 2006;354:2473–2483.
29. Hass GJ, Abraham WT. The challenge of heart failure. J Am Coll Cardiol 2005;46:2052–2053.
30. Khan M Gabriel, Goodwin JF. Cardiomyopathy. In: Heart Disease, Diagnosis and Therapy. Baltimore, Williams & Wilkins, 1996.
31. Bristow MR, Kantrowitz NE, Ginsburg R, et al. Beta-adrenergic function in heart muscle disease and heart failure. J Mol Cell Cardiol 1985;17:41.
32. Waagstein F, Hjalmarson A, Swedberg K, et al. Beta-blockers in dilated cardiomyopathies: They work. Eur Heart J 1993;173(Suppl A).
33. Packer M, Bristow MR, Cohn JN, et al. The effect of carvedilol on morbidity and mortality in patients with chronic heart failure. N Engl J Med 1996;334:1349.
34. CAPRICORN Investigators. Effect of carvedilol on outcome after myocardial infarction in patients with left-ventricular dysfunction. Lancet 2001;357:1385.
35. Packer M, Coats JS, Fowler MB, et al. for the Carvedilol Prospective Randomized Cumulative Survival Study Group: Effect of carvedilol on survival in severe chronic heart failure. N Engl J Med 2001;344:1651.
36. Waagstein F, Bristow MR, Swedberg K, et al. for the Metoprolol in Dilated Cardiomyopathy (MDC) Trial Study Group. Beneficial effects of metoprolol in idiopathic dilated cardiomyopathy. Lancet 1993; 342:1441.
37. MERIT/HF: The Metoprolol CR/XL Randomized Intervention Trial in Congestive Heart Failure: Effects of controlled-release metoprolol on total mortality, hospitalizations, and well-being in patients with heart failure. JAMA 2000;283:1295.

38. CIBIS-II: The Cardiac Insufficiency Bisoprolol Study II (CIBIS-II). A randomized trial. Lancet 1999;353: 9–13.
39. The Digitalis Investigation Group. The effect of digoxin on mortality and morbidity in patients with heart failure. N Engl J Med 1997;336:525.
40. Ahmed A, Rich MW, Love TE, et al. Digoxin and reduction in mortality and hospitalization in heart failure: A comprehensive post hoc analysis of the DIG trial. Eur Heart J 2006;27:178–186.
41. Arnold SB, Byrd RC, Meister W, et al. Long-term digitalis therapy improves left ventricular function in heart failure. N Engl J Med 1980;303:1443.
42. Gheorghiade M, St Clair J, St Clair C, et al. Hemodynamic effects of intravenous digoxin in patients with severe heart failure initially treated with diuretics and vasodilators. J Am Coll Cardiol 1987;9:849.
43. Dobbs SM, Kenyon WI, Dobbs RJ. Maintenance digoxin after an episode of heart failure: Placebo-controlled trial in outpatients. BMJ 1977;1:749.
44. Packer M, Gheorghiade M, Young JB, et al. for the RADIANCE study. Withdrawal of digoxin from patients with chronic heart failure treated with angiotensin-converting-enzyme inhibitors. N Engl J Med 1993;329:1.
45. Packer M, Cohn JN. Consensus recommendations for the management of chronic heart failure. Am J Cardiol 1999;83:1A.
46. Schenck-Gustafsson K, Jublin-Dannfelt A, Dahlquist R. Renal function and digoxin clearance during quinidine therapy. Clin Physiol 1982;2:401.
47. Zatuchni J. Verapamil-digoxin interaction. Am Heart J 1984;108:412.
48. Marcus FI. Pharmacokinetic interactions between digoxin and other drugs. J Am Coll Cardiol 1985;5: 82A.
49. Antman EM, Wenger TL, Butler VP, et al. Treatment of 150 cases of life-threatening digitalis intoxication with digoxin-specific Fab antibody fragments. Circulation 1990;82:1744.
50. Mikulic E, Cohn JN, Franciosa JA. Comparative hemodynamic effects of inotropic and vasodilator drugs in severe heart failure. Circulation 1977;56:528.
51. Little WC. Enhanced load dependence of relaxation in heart failure: Clinical implications. Circulation 1992;85:2326.
52. Little WC, Cheng CP. Diastolic dysfunction. Cardiol Rev 1998;6:231.
53. Meier-Ewert HK, Gaasch WH. What is diastolic heart failure and how do we treat it? ACC Curr J Rev Nov/Dec:52, 2001.

SUGGESTED READING

Ahmed A, Rich MW, Love TE, et al. Digoxin and reduction in mortality and hospitalization in heart failure: a comprehensive post hoc analysis of the DIG trial. Eur Heart J 2006;27:178–186.

Bhatia RS, Tu JV, Lee DS. Outcome of heart failure with preserved ejection fraction in a population-based study. N Engl J Med 2006;355:260–269.

Davis BR, Piller LB, Cutler JA, et al. for the Antihypertensive and Lipid-Lowering Treatment to Prevent Heart Attack Trial (ALLHAT) Collaborative Research Group. Role of diuretics in the prevention of heart failure: The Antihypertensive and Lipid-Lowering Treatment to Prevent Heart Attack Trial. Circulation 2006;113:2201–2210.

deGoma EM, Vagelos RH, Fowler MB. Emerging therapies for the management of decompensated heart failure. J Am Coll Cardiol 2006;48:2397–2409.

Gheorghiade M, Dirk J. van Veldhuisen, Colucci WS. Contemporary use of digoxin in the management of cardiovascular disorders. Circulation 2006;113:2556–2564.

Greenberg B, Mehra MR. All patients with heart failure and intraventricular conduction defect or dyssynchrony should not receive cardiac resynchronization therapy. Circulation 2006;114:2685–2691.

Hass GJ, Abraham WT. The challenge of heart failure. J Am Coll Cardiol 2005;46:2052–2053.

Jhund P, McMurray JV. Does aspirin reduce the benefit of an angiotensin-converting enzyme inhibitor?: Choosing between the Scylla of observational studies and the Charybdis of subgroup analysis. Circulation 2006;113:2566–2568.

Nanas JN, Matsouka C, Karageorgopoulos D, et al. Etiology of anemia in patients with advanced heart failure. J Am Coll Cardiol 2006;48:2485–2489.

Owan TE, Hodge DO, Herges RM. Trends in prevalence and outcome of heart failure with preserved ejection fraction. N Engl J Med 2006;355:251–259.

Pfeffer MA. Editorial Comment. Blood pressure in heart failure: A love-hate relationship. J Am Coll Cardiol 2007;49:40–42.

Ramasubbu K, Mann DL. The emerging role of statins in the treatment of heart failure. J Am Coll Cardiol 2006; 47:342–344.

Remme WJ, Torp-Pedersen C, Cleland JGF, et al. Carvedilol protects better against vascular events than metoprolol in heart failure: research from COMET. J Am Coll Cardiol 2007;49:963–971.

Scirica BM, Morrow DA, Cannon CP, et al. for the PROVE IT-TIMI 22 Investigators. Intensive statin therapy and the risk of hospitalization for heart failure after an acute coronary syndrome in the PROVE IT-TIMI 22 STUDY. J Am Coll Cardiol 2006;47:2326–2331.

Stevens LA, Coresh J, Greene T. Assessing kidney function—measured and estimated glomerular filtration rate. N Engl J Med 2006;354:2473–2483.

Takemoto Y, Hozumi T, Sugioka K, et al. Beta-blocker therapy induces ventricular resynchronization in dilated cardiomyopathy with Narrow QRS complex. J Am Coll Cardiol 2007;49:778–783.

Tang WH, Francis GS. The year in heart failure. J Am Coll Cardiol 2006;48:2575–2583.

Taylor AL, Ziesche S, Yancy C, et al. Combination of isosorbide dinitrate and hydralazine in blacks with heart failure. N Engl J Med 2004;351:2049–2057.

13 Heart Failure Controversies

MANAGEMENT OF HEART FAILURE PRESERVED EJECTION FRACTIONS (HFPEF)

The prevalence of heart failure (HF) rises from 2% to 3% at age 65 to more than 50% in persons older than age 80. Many of these patients have HFPEF. The condition is not uncommon in elderly women, most of whom have hypertension, diabetes mellitus, or both and often coronary heart disease (CHD). However, CHD more commonly causes systolic heart failure (SHF). Atrial fibrillation is common in the elderly, and ventricular rates even when not very rapid (120–140) may precipitate HF with a preserved ejection fraction (EF).

Is it preferable to adopt the term HFPEF rather than diastolic HF? Not all patients with HFPEF show definite diagnostic diastolic abnormalities. Controversies abound, however, among the experts.

Mauer et al. *(1)* stated that HF with normal ejection fraction (HFNEF) is preferred over the term diastolic heart failure (DHF) mainly because

- Doppler-derived diastolic parameters do not provide specific information on intrinsic passive diastolic properties; thus, diastolic dysfunction cannot be diagnosed *reliably* by Doppler echocardiography.
- Delayed relaxation and/or stiffened passive properties may not be the unifying pathophysiologic mechanisms in all patients who present with HF and normal EF.

Nonetheless, abnormal diastolic function is a common cause of HFPEF.

Oh et al. *(2)* criticized Mauer and colleagues and emphasized that diastolic HF is easily diagnosed by echocardiography in a patient with a preserved left ventricular (LV)EF with evidence of abnormal relaxation, decreased compliance, increased filling pressure, and normal LV dimensions. However, Oh et al. describe the situation that exists in most sophisticated diagnostic laboratories with highly trained echocardiographers and clinicians and that does not represent the real world of medicine.

The American College of Cardiology/American Heart Association (ACC/AHA) guidelines of 2001 stated that it is difficult to be precise about the diagnosis of diastolic HF *(3)*. This difficulty still exists in 2007 and is unlikely to change substantially in the near future. The incidence of this condition is stated to be approx 33% or more of all HF patients. Allowing for diagnostic errors, the incidence is probably <25% for all patients with HFPEF. More than 66% of HFPEF instances are represented by DHF.

The diagnosis of definite diastolic HF can be made if typical signs, symptoms, and radiologic features of HF, as well as elevated brain naturietic peptide (BNP), are documented in the presence of normal LV systolic function within 1–2 d of the episode, in the absence of valvular disease or atrial fibrillation and there is objective evidence of diastolic dysfunction at *echocardiographic assessment:* EF > 50%; abnormal LV relaxation, filling, diastolic distensibility, or stiffness and normal LV volumes.

From: *Contemporary Cardiology: Cardiac Drug Therapy, Seventh Edition*
M. Gabriel Khan © Humana Press Inc., Totowa, NJ

The diagnosis of probable diastolic HF can be made by using the criteria of Vasan and Levy criteria *(4)*. A study by Zile and colleagues *(5)* indicated that it is possible to make the diagnosis of definite diastolic HF provided that there is evidence of mild LV hypertrophy.

- The ACC/AHA guidelines of 2005 note the controversy by stating that there have been several proposed criteria by which clinicians and investigators may define HFPEF *(6)*:
- The diagnosis is based on the finding of typical symptoms and signs of HF in a patient with a normal LVEF and no valvular abnormalities on echocardiography.
- A definitive diagnosis requires the finding of: an elevated LV filling pressure in a patient with normal LV volumes and contractility; usually the rate of ventricular relaxation is slowed *(6)*.
- **It is surprising that the magic number for normal EF is not stated in the guidelines; it would be wise to use >50% as a cutoff rather than 45%, allowing for errors in echocardiographic assessment.**
- **In addition, it is crucial to** exclude other possible explanations or disorders that may present in a similar manner.

Differential diagnosis and mimics include:

- Incorrect diagnosis or incorrect measurement of EF. *The echocardiographic assessment of EF is fraught with errors but remains a useful guide to diagnosis and management of systolic HF.*
- *Valvular disease.*
- Pericardial constriction and left atrial myxoma *are rare and do not genuinely represent HFPEF; in this setting there is simply restriction to ventricular filling.*
- Episodic or reversible systolic HF, *which is not uncommon.*
- Severe hypertension *can cause both systolic HF and HFPEF.*
- Myocardial ischemia *more commonly causes systolic HF but can cause a combination of both types of HF and rarely pure HFPEF.*
- Cor pulmonale.
- Diastolic dysfunction of uncertain origin.

Age and the diseases listed appear to cause changes in crosslinking of intercellular connective tissue. The heart fills less and empties less, and the percentage ejected may be relatively normal but the stroke output and cardiac index are decreased; thus, the renin-angiotensin-aldosterone system (RAAS) is stimulated. Systolic dysfunction impairs the ability of the left ventricle to relax and fill at low pressure *(7)*. Thus, systolic dysfunction is a principal cause of diastolic dysfunction *(8)*.

Treatment

There are no tested proven therapies for HFPEF or for most patients who have DHF. Importantly, the treatment of HFPEF is treatment of the cause. With systolic HF, medications help considerably to improve outcomes versus DHF, in which medications are unproved except for symptomatic improvement enhanced by judicious diuretic therapy.

The following are the ACC treatment guidelines *(6)*, *with my additions in italics.*

In the absence of randomized controlled trials (RCTs), the management of patients with HFPEF is based on the following:

- *The judicious* use of diuretics (class I) recommended *to relieve symptoms.*
- Beta-blockers *decrease heart rate and the longer diastolic interval might improve ventricular filling* (class II).
- Angiotensin-converting enzyme (ACE) inhibitors (class II) may be used to minimize symptoms of HF but with a level of evidence (C) *that does not mean they are well-established therapy.*

- Digoxin receives a similar class IIb recommendation (level of evidence C).
- The main reliance is on improved control of blood pressure (BP), reduction in heart rate in patients with atrial fibrillation and aggressive management of CHD.
- There is no mention of the use of aldosterone antagonists. Spironolactone and eplerenone provide salutary effects on ventricular function and I strongly recommend their use as we await the results of RCTs. (*See* Chapters 7 and 12.)
- **Caution:** Because a decrease in preload exists, the overzealous use of preload-reducing agents, including loop diuretics, ACE inhibitors, and nitrates, may cause hemodynamic and clinical deterioration. Usually dosages are 50–75% lower than those used for systolic HF, and diuretics except eplerenone 25 mg may not be required except during the symptomatic congestive phase that may last a few weeks. Loop diuretics are contraindicated in pericardial diseases and restrictive cardiomyopathy and relatively contraindicated in hypertrophic cardiomyopathy (HCM) and in hypertensive HCM of the elderly with impaired ventricular relaxation *(9)*.

Prevention is Crucial

- Aggressive drug therapy is important to control BP, as is prevention of left ventricular hypertrophy (LVH): low-dose ACE inhibitors, beta-blockers, and diuretics including 25 mg eplerenone or spironolactone prevent and cause regression. Calcium antagonists and alpha-blockers do not.

Drug Treatment of Diastolic HF is Governed by the Underlying Disease: Hypertensive LVH and Chronic CHD

1. A diuretic at low dosage: approx 50% lower than for systolic HF, e.g., furosemide 40 mg daily for a few days, then 20 mg daily during the congestive phase, and then on alternate days.
2. An ACE inhibitor, also at low dosage, approx 50% less than for systolic HF, can speed the rate of LV relaxation and improve diastolic function.
3. A beta-blocker low dose to decrease heart rate, which allows a longer diastolic filling phase. Beta-blockers are necessary to influence the underlying disease favorably, e.g., ongoing ischemia in CHD. Ischemia contributes to diastolic dysfunction. However, beta-blockers slow the rate of LV relaxation and may impair diastolic function. Also they can be dangerous in patients with chronotropic incompetence. Consideration should be given to insertion of a permanent pacemaker in those with chronotropic insufficiency who are otherwise not able to tolerate beta-blockade
4. Spironolactone and eplerenone can favorably modify myocardial collagen and the development of fibrosis and have a role in therapy. RCTs are under way. A 25-mg dose of spironolactone or eplerenone 25–50 mg is advisable (*see* cautions for use in Chapter 7 and later in this chapter).
5. Digoxin is not generally recommended except for patients with atrial fibrillation to control rate and in patients with mixed SHF and HFPEF (*see* digoxin discussion in Chapter 12).
   - HCM, restrictive infiltrative disease, constrictive pericarditis, amyloid, and other diseases in the absence of hypertension and LVH are difficult to treat with drugs: hypotension and deterioration may be precipitated by diuretics, nitrates, and ACE inhibitors; calcium antagonists have no role *(10)*.

DIGOXIN IS NOT USEFUL FOR HFPEF: TRUE OR FALSE?

The guidelines have demoted digoxin to a class IIa recommendation *(6)*. Ahmed et al. *(11)* did a comprehensive *post hoc* analysis of the randomized controlled Digitalis Investigation Group trial ($n = 7788$) *(12)* and focused on 5548 patients: 1687 with digoxin levels drawn randomly at 1 mo, and 3861 placebo patients, alive at 1 mo.

Findings: Digoxin at 0.5–0.9 ng/mL reduced mortality and hospitalizations in all HF patients, including those with HFPEF. At higher serum concentration, digoxin reduced HF hospitalization but had no effect on mortality or all-cause hospitalizations.

Importantly, digoxin is the only HF agent that does not decrease BP. Systolic BP < 100 mmHg is a common problem in clinical practice when proven agents (ACE inhibitor, diuretic, and beta-blocker) are combined. Digoxin provides salutary effects including reduction in mortality and hospitalizations for recurrent HF in patients with SHF class III–IV with enlarged LV provided levels are maintained at 0.5–0.9 ng/mL.

IS CHARM-PRESERVED A CLEAR STUDY OF HFPEF?

It must be emphasized that the EF should be >50% determined within 3 d of the episode of HF to be diagnostic of HFPEF. Thus, Candesartan in Heart Failure Assessment in Reduction of Mortality (CHARM)-Preserved *(13)*, which studied patients with EF > 40%, was not a true study of patients with HFPEF. An EF of 40–45% cannot be assumed to be normal LV systolic function.

- CHARM-Preserved randomized 3025 patients with EF > 40%. There was an 18% reduction in the number of patients with investigator-reported hospitalizations for HF with candesartan (230 versus 279, $p = 0.017$), but there was no decrease in deaths *(13)*.
- The primary end points of cardiovascular disease (CVD) death and hospitalization were not met (11%, $p = 0.051$; total hospitalization, 912 patients versus 922, $p = 0.99$). Thus, CHARM-Preserved is flawed.

DOES AN ACE INHIBITOR COMBINED WITH AN ARB IMPROVE OUTCOMES?

The Valsartan Heart Failure Trial (Val-HeFT) compared valsartan (160 mg/d) + ACE inhibitor with placebo in approx 5000 patients with class II–III HF. There was a 28% reduction in hospitalization for HF, but no reduction in mortality *(14)*.

- Importantly, in 794 patients given an ACE inhibitor, a beta-blocker, and valsartan, there was a significant increase in mortality (129 versus 97 deaths; hazard ratio [HR], 1.42; 95% confidence interval [CI], 1.09–1.85, $p = 0.009$), compared with 806 patients treated with an ACE inhibitor, a beta-blocker and placebo. Beta-blocker therapy is an integral component of HF therapy. An angiotensin receptor blocker (ARB) added to ACE inhibitor/beta-blocker therapy is not advisable. Extensive RAAS blockade appears to be harmful *(14)*.

CHARM-Added *(15)* used the same entry criteria as Val-HeFT: mainly patients with class III HF and virtually no class IV patients.

- Enalapril, lisinopril, captopril, and ramipril were given. The mean daily doses of these drugs in the candesartan group were 16.8, 17.7, 82.2, and 6.8 mg, respectively; in the placebo group they were 17.2, 17.7, 82.7, and 7.3 mg, respectively.
- The trialists stated that they thought 96% of patients in each group were receiving optimum doses of ACE inhibitor at randomization.
- In addition, a subclinical low dose of ACE inhibitor was used. The trial results, therefore are not clinically acceptable.
- 483 (38%) patients in the candesartan group and 538 (42%) in the placebo group experienced the primary outcome of cardiovascular death or admission to hospital for CHF (unadjusted HR 0.85; 95% CI, 0.75–0.96; $p = 0.011$).
- Cardiovascular death in the treated group was 302 (23.7%) versus 347 (27.3%) in the placebo group, a nonclinically significant reduction of 12.5%.

- In patients treated with beta-blockers in addition to an ACE inhibitor, 175 (25%) of 702 died in the candesartan group, and 195 (27%) of 711 died in the placebo group (HR, 0.88; 95% CI, 0.72–1.08; $p = 0.22$) *(15)*. Perhaps the combination is not as dangerous as was observed with valsartan, but harmfulness cannot be excluded.
- Hyperkalemia was observed in 3% of treated patients and 1% in the placebo arm; caution is required.
- The combination of an ACE inhibitor and an ARB is not advisable. Also, patients should not receive aldosterone antagonists when this combination is used because the incidence of hyperkalemia is significantly increased. It is more beneficial to add an aldosterone antagonist to an ACE inhibitor than to add an ARB.

ALDOSTERONE ANTAGONISTS: USEFUL BUT HARMFUL?

In the Randomized Aldactone Evaluation Study (RALES), spironolactone 12.5–37.5 mg daily added to ACE inhibitor therapy for patients with class IV HF symptoms or class III symptoms and recent hospitalization decreased the risk of death from 46% to 35% (30% relative risk reduction) over 2 yr, with 35% reduction in HF hospitalization *(16)*. Serum creatinine was below 2.5 mg/dL (220 μmol/L) in the main trial.

- Eplerenone in patients with LVEF < 40% and clinical evidence of HF or diabetes mellitus within 14 d of myocardial infarction (MI) decreased mortality from 13.6% to 11.8% at 1 yr *(17)*. Hyperkalemia occurred in 5.5% of those treated with eplerenone compared with 3.9% in the placebo arm. Hyperkalemia occurred in 10.1% versus 4.6% of patients with estimated creatinine clearance < 50 mL/min.

My advice is as follows:

- *In HF patients treated with an ACE inhibitor or ARB, aldosterone antagonists should be used with caution and with close monitoring of estimated glomerular filtration rate (GFR) in patients with a serum creatinine of 1.2–1.4 mg/dL (104–124 μmol/L), especially in diabetics and the elderly; it is advisable to obtain an estimated GFR. A 24-h urine collection for creatinine clearance is rarely required, but some caution is needed because the estimated GFR can be somewhat erroneous in patients over age 70 and in blacks.*
- *Aldosterone antagonists should not be combined with ACE inhibitors in patients with estimated GFR < 50 mL/min. Monthly monitoring of K^+ is advisable if used when the estimated GFR range is 50–60 mL/min, a finding that is common after age 70.*
- It is now recognized that an aldosterone antagonist should not be combined with an ACE inhibitor in patients with more severe renal dysfunction: a serum creatinine > 1.5 mg/dL (132 μmol/L) or estimated GFR < 50 mL/min. Hyperkalemia is more frequent in type 2 diabetics with hyporeninemic hypoaldosteronism, and the combination of an aldosterone antagonist and an ACE inhibitor or an ARB is particularly harmful in the setting of significant renal impairment.

HEART FAILURE IN BLACKS: DO DIFFERENCES EXIST?

- Heart failure has a 50% higher incidence in the black population than is observed in the general population.
- ACE inhibitors have not shown as great a benefit in black patients with HF as found in the white population. Also, angioedema is more common in black versus white patients treated with ACE inhibitors.
- In the Veterans Administration Heart Failure Trial (VHeFT), hydralazine combined with isosorbide dinitrate was not shown to be significantly effective in reducing cardiac mortality in mainly white patients (*see* Chapter 12).

An RCT of 1050 black patients with class III/IV HF was conducted using isosorbide dinitrate and hydralazine along with a standard HF regimen. Treatment resulted in a 43% decrease in total mortality, which led to premature termination of the trial. Time to first hospitalization was improved *(18)*.

The combination of isosorbide dinitrate and hydralazine has a role in white patients with HF if ACE inhibitors and ARBs are contraindicated.

SHOULD THE ROLE OF NATRIURETIC PEPTIDES BE EXPANDED?

The peptide is produced by both ventricles in response to increased wall stretch, volume overload, and hypertrophy. B-type natriuretic peptide (BNP) or amino-terminal pro-BNP has found a niche as an aid to the diagnosis of HF *(19)*.

- However, is this test overused? Are costs justified? Is this test needed if there is a clear clinical diagnosis with radiologic confirmation of HF, and a cause for HF is identified? The test is most useful in patients who present with acute dyspnea of unknown etiology, and particularly in those with probable HFPEF.

  Consider the following:

- Age and female gender increase BNP levels.
- Levels decrease with obesity because BNP is metabolized by adipose tissue.
- A decrease in body mass index is accompanied by an increase not only in BNP but also in NT-pro-BNP.
- Decreased excretion from the kidney contributes to the elevated BNP in HF patients with renal dysfunction, especially in patients with an estimated GFR < 60 mL/min. Importantly, >75% of individuals older than age 70 have an estimated GFR < 55 mL/min, and HF is a disease of the elderly.
- In studies of BNP, an estimated one in four study participants had a BNP level of 100–500 pg/mL, and approx 33% of these patients were subsequently determined to not have HF *(19)*.

There are probably no false-positive BNP levels. If the BNP is elevated, consider the following:

- HF.
- A pulmonary-related problem: pulmonary embolism or other conditions causing right ventricular stretch increase levels.
- The kidneys are not eliminating it, particularly in the elderly patient.
- Severe myocardial ischemia may cause higher levels.
- Anemia: higher levels are found in anemia.
- Reduction in body mass.
- Assay types and demographics.

The Systolic Heart Failure Treatment Supported by BNP (STARS-BNP) trial indicated that a BNP-guided strategy of HF management resulted in improved clinical end points *(20,21)*, but costs must be justified.

IS NESIRITIDE A USEFUL ADDITION?

Patients who cannot be weaned from intravenous to oral therapy may require continuous infusion of dobutamine or nesiritide. The use of the peptide nesiritide is limited to patients who are hospitalized with acute decompensated HF. Nesiritide may cause renal dysfunction *(22)*, however, and appears to increase mortality *(23)*. Also, the drug causes hypotension, which limits its use.

ARE STATINS RECOMMENDED FOR PATIENTS WITH HEART FAILURE?

The PROVE IT-TIMI 22 study randomized 4162 patients, stabilized after acute coronary syndrome (ACS), to either intensive statin therapy (atorvastatin 80 mg) or moderate statin therapy (pravastatin 40 mg). Hospitalization for HF occurring more than 30 d after randomization was determined during a mean follow-up of 24 mo. Levels of BNP were measured at baseline *(24)*.

- Atorvastatin 80 mg significantly reduced the rate of hospitalization for HF (1.6% versus 3.1%; HR, 0.55; 95% CI, 0.35–0.85; $p = 0.008$) independently of a recurrent MI or prior history of HF *(24)*.
- The risk of HF increased steadily with increasing quartiles of BNP (HR, 2.6; 95% CI, 1.2–5.5; $p = 0.016$ for the highest quartile compared with the lowest). Among patients with elevated levels of BNP (>80 pg/mL), treatment with atorvastatin significantly reduced the risk of HF compared with pravastatin (HR, 0.32; 95% CI, 0.13–0.8; $p = 0.014$) *(24)*.
- Scirica and colleagues concluded that intensive statin therapy reduces the risk of hospitalization for HF after ACS with the most gain in patients with elevated levels of BNP *(24)*.

The evidence for high-dose statin therapy inpatients with nonischemic HF, however, awaits the results of further studies. In a study by Sola et al. *(25)*, the use of atorvastatin in patients with nonischemic HF improved LVEF and attenuated adverse LV remodeling. The effects on soluble levels of several inflammatory markers with atorvastatin suggest, in part, mechanisms by which statins might exert their beneficial effects in nonischemic HF *(25)*.

Ramasubbu and colleague point out that there are several ongoing large-scale clinical outcome trials in HF patients (Controlled Rosuvastatin Multinational Trial in Heart Failure [CORONA], Gruppo Italiano per lo Studio della Sopravvivenza nell'Insufficienza Cardiaca [Italian Group for the Study of Survival in Cardiac Insufficiency; GISSI-HF], and RosUvastatiN Impact on Ventricular Remodelling Lipids and Cytokines [UNIVERSE]). These should provide a more definitive answer to the expanded use of statins in HF patients *(26)*.

REFERENCES

1. Mauer MS, Spevack D, Burkhoff D, Kronzon I. Diastolic dysfunction: Can it be diagnosed by Doppler echocardiography? J Am Coll Cardiol 2004;44:1543–1549.
2. Oh, JK, Hatle L, Tajik AJ, et al. Diastolic heart failure can be diagnosed by comprehensive two-dimensional and Doppler echocardiography. J Am Coll Cardiol 2006;47:500–506.
3. ACC/AHA guidelines for the evaluation and management of chronic heart failure in the adult: Executive summary. J Am Coll Cardiol 2001;8:2101.
4. Vasan RS, Levy D. Defining diastolic heart failure. A call for standardized diagnostic criteria. Circulation 2000;101:2118.
5. Zile M, Brutsaert D. New concepts in diastolic dysfunction and diastolic heart failure: Part I. Diagnosis, prognosis, and measurements of diastolic function. Circulation 2002;105:1387–1393.
6. Hunt SA, Abraham WT, Chin MH, et al. ACC/AHA 2005 guideline update for the diagnosis and management of chronic heart failure in the adult—summary article. A report of the American College of Cardiology/American Heart Association Task Force on Practice Guidelines (Writing Committee to Update the 2001 Guidelines for the Evaluation and Management of Heart Failure). J Am Coll Cardiol 2005;46:1116–1143.
7. Little WC, Cheng CP. Diastolic dysfunction. Cardiol Rev 1998;6:231.
8. Meier-Ewert HK, Gaasch WH. What is diastolic heart failure and how do we treat it? ACC Curr J Rev Nov/Dec:52, 2001.
9. Topol EJ, Traill TA, Fortuin NJ. Hypertensive hypertrophic cardiomyopathy of the elderly. N Engl J Med 1985;312:277.

10. Khan M Gabriel. Cardiomyopathy. In: Heart Disease, Diagnosis and Therapy. Totowa, NJ, Humana Press, 2005, pp. 443–470.
11. Ahmed A, Rich MW, Love TE, et al. Digoxin and reduction in mortality and hospitalization in heart failure: A comprehensive post hoc analysis of the DIG trial. Eur Heart J 2006;27:178–186.
12. Eichhorn EJ, Gheorghiade M. Digoxin—new perspective on an old drug. N Engl J Med 2002;47:1394.
13. Yusuf S, Pfeffer MA, Swedberg K, et al. Effects of candesartan in patients with chronic heart failure and preserved left-ventricular ejection fraction: The CHARM-Preserved Trial. Lancet 2003;362:777–781.
14. Cohn JN, Tognoni G. A randomized trial of the angiotensin-receptor blocker valsartan in chronic heart failure. N Engl J Med 2001;345:1667–1675.
15. McMurray JJV, Östergren J, Swedberg K, Granger CB. Effects of candesartan in patients with chronic heart failure and reduced left-ventricular systolic function taking angiotensin-converting-enzyme inhibitors: The CHARM-Added trial. Lancet 2003;362:767–771.
16. Pitt B, Zannad F, Remme WJ, et al. for the Randomized Evaluation Study Investigators. The effect of spironolactone on morbidity and mortality in patients with severe heart failure. N Engl J Med 1999;341: 709.
17. Pitt B, Remme W, Zannad F, et al. for the Eplerenone Post-Acute Myocardial Infarction Heart Failure Efficacy and Survival Study Investigators. Eplerenone, a selective aldosterone blocker, in patients with left ventricular dysfunction after myocardial infarction. N Engl J Med 2003;348:1309–1321.
18. Taylor AL, Ziesche S, Yancy C, et al. Combination of isosorbide dinitrate and hydralazine in blacks with heart failure. N Engl J Med 2004;351:2049–2057.
19. Maisel AS, Krishnaswamy P, Nowak RM, et al. Rapid measurement of B-type natriuretic peptide in the emergency diagnosis of heart failure. N Engl J Med 2002;347:161.
20. Jourdain P, Funck F, Gueffet P, et al. Benefits of BNP plasma levels for optimizing therapy: The Systolic Heart Failure Treatment supported by BNP multicenter randomised trial (STARS-BNP). (abstr) J Am Coll Cardiol 2005;45(Suppl A):3A.
21. Wright SP, Doughty RN, Pearl A, et al. Plasma amino-terminal pro-brain natriuretic peptide and accuracy of heart-failure diagnosis in primary care: A randomized, controlled trial. J Am Coll Cardiol 2003; 42:1793–1800.
22. Sackner-Bernstein JD, Skopicki HA, Aaronson KD. Risk of worsening renal function with nesiritide in patients with acutely decompensated heart failure Circulation 2005;111:1487–1491.
23. Sackner-Bernstein JD, Kowalski M, Fox M, Aaronson K. Short-term risk of death after treatment with nesiritide for decompensated heart failure: A pooled analysis of randomized controlled trials. JAMA 2005;293:1900–1905.
24. Scirica BM, Morrow DA, Cannon CP, et al, for the PROVE IT-TIMI 22 Investigators. Intensive statin therapy and the risk of hospitalization for heart failure after an acute coronary syndrome in the PROVE IT-TIMI 22 Study. J Am Coll Cardiol 2006;47:2326–2331.
25. Sola S, Mir MQS, Lerakis S, et al. Atorvastatin improves left ventricular systolic function and serum markers of inflammation in nonischemic heart failure. J Am Coll Cardiol 2006;47:332–337.
26. Ramasubbu K, Mann DL. The emerging role of statins in the treatment of heart failure. J Am Coll Cardiol 2006;47:342–344.

SUGGESTED READING

Calhoun DA. Aldosterone and cardiovascular disease: smoke and fire. Circulation 2006;114:2572–2574.

Gheorghiade M, van Veldhuisen DJ, Colucci WS. Contemporary use of digoxin in the management of cardiovascular disorders. Circulation 2006;113:2556–2564.

Ramasubbu K, Mann DL. The emerging role of statins in the treatment of heart failure. J Am Coll Cardiol 2006;47:342–344.

Scirica BM, Morrow DA, Cannon CP, et al, for the PROVE IT-TIMI 22 Investigators. Intensive statin therapy and the risk of hospitalization for heart failure after an acute coronary syndrome in the PROVE IT-TIMI 22 Study. J Am Coll Cardiol 2006;47:2326–2331.

Stevens LA, Coresh J, Greene T. Assessing kidney function—measured and estimated glomerular filtration rate. N Engl J Med 2006;354:2473–2483.

Taylor AL, Ziesche S, Yancy C, et al. Combination of isosorbide dinitrate and hydralazine in blacks with heart failure. N Engl J Med 2004;351:2049–2057.

14 Management of Cardiac Arrhythmias

The rational basis of antiarrhythmic therapy ideally requires a knowledge of

1. **The mechanism of the arrhythmia:**
   - Disturbances in impulse generation (enhanced automaticity or ectopic tachyarrhythmia).
   - Disturbances of impulse conduction (reentrant arrhythmias). Most of the evidence suggests that reentry is the mechanism for sustained ventricular tachycardia (VT).
   - The site or sites where such disturbances are present.
2. **The mode of action of the drug** with which control of the arrhythmia is to be attempted.
3. **The clinical situation:**
   - Acute, persistent or paroxysmal.
   - Associated with a low blood pressure < 90 mmHg, congestive heart failure (CHF), or distressing symptoms.
   - Associated with cardiac pathology, accessory pathway or secondary to hypoxemia, acute blood loss, electrolyte or acid-base imbalance, extracardiac conditions as diverse as thyrotoxicosis, chronic obstructive pulmonary disease, or acute conditions such as pyrexial illness, pneumothorax, or even rupture of the esophagus.

Prevention of episodes of arrhythmia and treatment of the acute attack are considered separately.

Except in emergency, the first step in therapy is to remove or correct a precipitating cause when this is feasible, thus reducing the need for antiarrhythmic medication. Precipitating factors include heart failure (HF), ischemia, digoxin toxicity or administration of beta-stimulants or theophylline, sick sinus syndrome, atrioventricular (AV) block, thyrotoxicosis, hypokalemia, hypomagnesemia, hypoxemia, acute blood loss, acid-base disturbances, and infection.

Not all arrhythmias require drug treatment, and the need for therapy is considered carefully for each individual bearing in mind the limited effectiveness of drugs and the occurrence of adverse effects, which is particularly important during long-term management—and the occasional unexpected proarrhythmic effect of some drugs.

In addition, especially in the management of ventricular arrhythmias that are difficult to control, it is important to achieve target plasma concentrations known to be associated with suppression of the arrhythmia. This requires careful titration of dosage dictated by salutary effects and sometimes by concentration monitoring.

Note: Plasma concentration for some drugs does not reflect the full activity of the drug or metabolites.

This chapter concentrates mainly on clinical advice rather than on details of electrophysiology.

From: *Contemporary Cardiology: Cardiac Drug Therapy, Seventh Edition*
M. Gabriel Khan © Humana Press Inc., Totowa, NJ

Table 14-1
Electrophysiologic Classification of Antiarrhythmic Drugs

Class	*Drugs*	*Duration of action potential*
I Membrane-stabilizing, inhibit fast sodium channel Restriction of sodium current	A. Quinidine	Slightly prolonged (slows phase 0 of the action potential)
	Disopyramide	
	Procainamide	
	B. Lidocaine	Shortened[a] (minimal slowing of phase 0)
	Mexiletine	
	Aprindine	
	Phenytoin	
	Tocainide	
	C. Flecainide	Unaffected or slight effect (slow phase 0)
	Lorcainide	
	Encainide	
	Propafenone	
II Inhibit sympathetic stimulation	Beta-blockers	
III Delayed repolarization	Amiodarone	Prolonged as major action
	Bretylium	
	Bethanidine	
	Clofilium	Prolongation of the effective refractory period
	Sotalol	
IV Calcium antagonists		
Inhibit slow calcium channel	Verapamil	
Restriction of calcium current	Diltiazem	

[a]Controversial.

Modified from Vaughan Williams EM. Classification of antiarrhythmic drugs. In Sandhoe E, Flensted-Jensen E, Olesen KH, eds. Symposium on Cardiac Arrhythmias. Sodertalje, Sweden: AB Astra, 1970, p 449.

CLASSIFICATION

Antiarrhythmic drugs may be considered from three distinct points of view:

1. According to their **site of action**.
2. According to their **electrophysiologic action** on isolated cardiac fibers (classes I–IV, as proposed by Vaughan Williams *[1]*; Table 14-1). Vaughan Williams indicated that class IB drugs are rapidly attached to sodium channels during the action potential. Thus, few channels are available for activation at the commencement of diastole and the effective refractory period (ERP) is prolonged. During diastole, however, the drugs are rapidly detached. At the end of diastole, most channels are drug free. Thus, there is no slowing of conduction velocity in the ventricle or His-Purkinje system. Class IC drugs detach very slowly from their binding to the channels during diastole. This action eliminates some sodium channels, producing slower conduction; ERP is not prolonged. Class IA drugs are intermediate between classes IB and IC. Note that this classification is based on drug action rather than the drugs themselves. Amiodarone has class I, II, and III actions. Experience during the past 20 yr indicates that drug actions are much more complex than those given in this classification, but the classification is retained because it has been used worldwide for over 30 yr and it simplifies our understanding of drug action.
3. The Sicilian Gambit classification is based on identification of the mechanism, determination of the vulnerable parameter of the arrhythmia most susceptible to modification, definition of the target likely to affect the vulnerable parameter, and selection of an anti-

arrhythmic that will modify the target *(2)*. Any classification scheme tends to be arbitrary and should not be accepted by all.

DIAGNOSIS OF ARRHYTHMIAS

The following advice on diagnosis is confined to relevant clinical clues and is of necessity brief. The diagnosis is usually established by careful examination of multiple leads of the electrocardiogram and information derived from carotid massage as appropriate in doubtful cases.

Arrhythmias with NARROW QRS Complex (3)

1. **REGULAR**
   - *Ventricular rate 100–140/min:* Consider **sinoatrial tachycardia**. P-wave morphology is identical to that during normal sinus rhythm. The arrhythmia accounts for about 5% of cases of supraventricular tachycardia (SVT).

     or

     Paroxysmal atrial tachycardia (PAT) with block: The P wave is often buried in the preceding T wave.
   - *Ventricular rate 140–240/min:* Consider AV **nodal reentrant tachycardia** (>70% of regular SVTs). Retrograde P waves are usually buried within the QRS or at the end of the QRS complex, with a short R-P interval causing pseudo-S waves in II, III, AVF and pseudo r^1 that mimics Rsr^1 in V_1

     or

     Wolff-Parkinson-White (WPW) syndrome with AV reentry (about 15% of SVTs)

     or

     atrial flutter

     or

     ectopic atrial tachycardia.
2. **IRREGULAR**
   a. Atrial fibrillation (AF).
   b. Atrial flutter (when AV conduction is variable).
   c. Multifocal atrial tachycardia (chaotic atrial tachycardia). Varying P-wave morphology, P-P intervals vary, atrial rate 200–130/min.

Arrhythmias with WIDE QRS Complex (3)

1. **REGULAR rhythm**

   VT or SVT with functional aberrant conduction. SVT with preexisting bundle branch block, and preexcited tachycardia (SVT with anterograde conduction over an accessory pathway).

   Regular wide QRS tachycardia is considered VT if the following clues apply *(4)*:

- Predominantly negative QRS complexes in the precordial leads V_4 to V_6: diagnostic for VT *(4)* (Fig. 14 –1).
- Presence of a QR complex in one or more of the precordial leads V_2 to V_6: certainly VT *(4)*.
- Absence of an RS complex in all precordial leads: negative QRS complexes in all precordial leads V_1 to V_6: negative concordance V_1 to V_6 = VT (Fig. 14-1).
- AV relationship different from 1:1: more QRS complexes than P waves; consider VT.

Consider SVT with aberrant conduction only in the absence of any of (a) or (b) and with the following present:

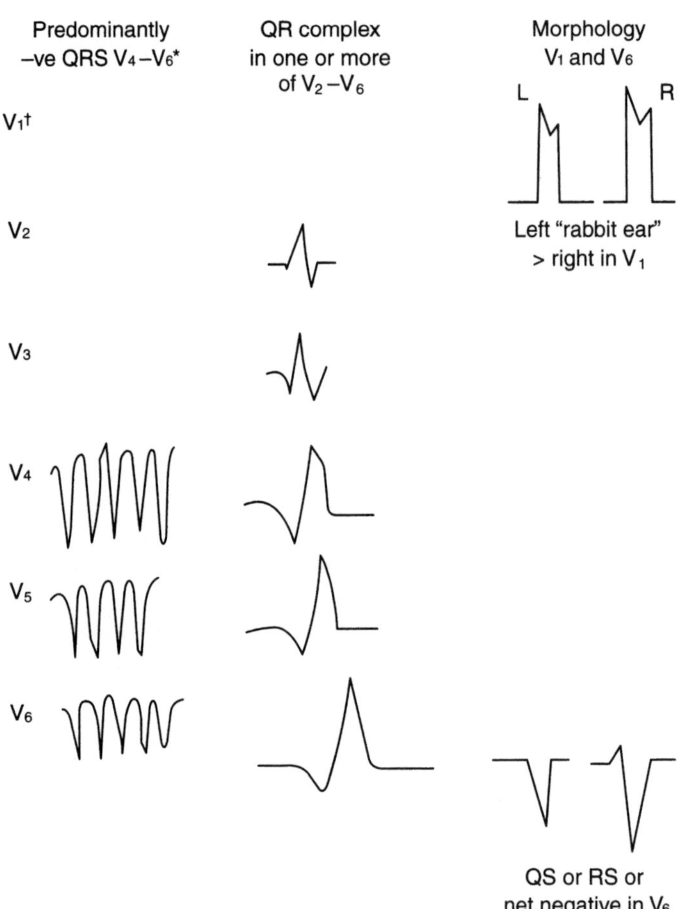

Fig. 14-1. Electrocardiographic hallmarks of ventricular tachycardia. *, Or concordant negativity in leads V_1 to V_6; positive concordance in leads V_1 to V_6 can be caused by ventricular tachycardia or Wolff-Parkinson-White antidromic (preexcited) tachycardia. †It is necessary to study the entire 12-lead tracing with particular emphasis on leads V_1 to V_6; lead 2 may be useful for assessment of P waves and AV dissociation. From Khan M Gabriel. On Call Cardiology, 3rd ed. Philadelphia, WB Saunders/ Elsevier, 2006.

QRS morphology similar to intraventricular conduction defect (IVCD) apparent on electrocardiography (ECG) while not in tachycardia:

- In basic sinus rhythm

or

- Visible on atrial ectopic beats = **SVT with aberrant conduction**. Fixed relationship with P waves, or the presence of a q in V_6, suggests but does not prove a supraventricular origin.
- Other clues in favor of VT include lead V_6: QS or rS; r:S ratio less than 1. Lead V_1, V_2: if the tachycardia has an LBBB shape and an r wave that is smaller than the r when in sinus rhythm, or notched or slurred downslope of the S wave; left "rabbit-ear" taller than the right.

Alternative diagnoses to VT or SVT with aberrance:

a. Atrial flutter and WPW conduction.
b. WPW tachycardia (rare type with anterograde conduction, through accessory pathway, preexcited tachycardia).

2. **IRREGULAR rhythm**

Atrial fibrillation (AF) and WPW syndrome with a rapid conduction, rate 200–300/min. *Note:* The rapidity of the ventricular response (**regular** or **irregular, narrow** or **wide**) should alert the physician to the diagnosis of WPW. AV block or dissociation excludes the presence of a bypass tract.

- AF and IVCD; a previous ECG is needed for comparison.

MANAGEMENT OF SUPRAVENTRICULAR ARRHYTHMIAS

AV Nodal Reentrant Tachycardia (AVNRT)

SVT usually arises from reentry mechanisms involving the AV node (AVNRT) and occasionally an accessory pathway, AV reciprocating tachycardia (AVRT), the sinus node, or the atrium. Consequently, drug therapy is directed toward slowing or blocking conduction at some point within the reentry circuit. Whenever the AV node or sinus node is involved directly in the reentry circuit, as is usually the case, SVT is frequently terminated by maneuvers or drugs that increase vagal activity or drugs that slow the velocity of propagation of impulses in the region of the sinoatrial (SA) or AV nodes.

AVNRT in patients aged < 35 yr usually occurs in an otherwise normal heart, with a good prognosis. It may occur in patients with organic heart disease, e.g., ischemic or rheumatic heart disease, and can be life threatening. The episode is characterized by an abrupt onset and termination. The heart rate varies from 140 to 240/beats/min and the rhythm is regular.

Termination of the Acute Attack of AVNRT

Vagal Maneuvers. Many patients learn to terminate the arrhythmia by gagging or by the Valsalva maneuver (expiration against a closed glottis) or Müller maneuver (sudden inspiration against the closed glottis) or facial immersion in cold water. The Valsalva maneuver is effective in approx 50% of patients with AVNRT.

Warning. Eyeball pressure has also been used to cause reflex vagal stimulation but is not recommended as retinal detachment may occur.

Carotid sinus massage either causes a reversion to sinus rhythm or has no effect at all. This all-or-none effect is in contrast to the slowing that results when atrial flutter or fibrillation is present. Carotid sinus massage is not recommended in the elderly or in patients with known carotid artery disease. In patients over age 35 yr, if a history of carotid disease is suggested by transient ischemic attacks or carotid bruits on auscultation, do not massage the carotid.

The patient must be supine with the head slightly hyperextended and turned a little toward the opposite side. Locate the right carotid sinus at the angle of the jaw. Using the first and second fingers, apply firm pressure in a circular or massage fashion for 2–6 s. Carotid massage is discontinued immediately upon termination of the arrhythmia because prolonged asystole may otherwise supervene in rare patients.

If unsuccessful, massage the left carotid sinus.

Warning. Never massage for more than 10 s and do not massage the right and left carotid simultaneously.

In some patients, restoration of sinus rhythm is clearly a matter of great urgency because of hemodynamic deterioration or angina, and direct current (DC) cardioversion is performed either before any drug is given or when the need becomes apparent following unsuccessful drug therapy.

Drug Management in the Acute Situation

1. **Adenosine** (Adenocard) 0.05–0.25 mg/kg given IV is an effective and relatively safe agent for the termination of acute reentrant SVT. Adenosine terminates AVNRT and AVRT in up to 90% of cases *(5,6)*. The 6-mg and 12-mg doses cause a 60–80% and 90–95% termination, respectively. The drug has both therapeutic and diagnostic value *(5)*.

   The drug has replaced verapamil when very rapid conversion of the arrhythmia is required, as in cases with HF or hemodynamic compromise, thus avoiding DC countershock in many individuals *(3,5)*. It can be given to patients with known SVT and aberration; little harm ensues if the diagnosis is in fact VT, whereas verapamil use is detrimental *(3)*.

   Nonetheless the drug is contraindicated in patients with a wide QRS complex tachycardia unless the diagnosis of SVT with aberrancy is certain *(7)*.

   The drug has no appreciable hypotensive or negative inotropic effect and slows AV nodal conduction.

   Dosage: Usually IV bolus 6 mg (0.05–0.25 mg/kg) over 2 s, rapidly flushed into a **peripheral vein**, should cause reversion to sinus rhythm in 1 min; the action of the drug is only about ½ min and, if needed, a 12-mg second bolus injection is given approximately 2 min after the first injection. A further 12-mg dose may be repeated in 3–5 min, as the arrhythmia occurs in 10–33% of cases. The very short half-life, less than 2 s, allows rapid dose titration to be achieved. Adenosine has been safely given centrally by means of a catheter positioned in, or near, the right atrium. The initial dose should be 3 mg followed every minute by 6, 9, and 12 mg until termination of the tachycardia *(8)*. Chest pain occurs more frequently with central injections than with peripheral administration (17% versus 10%).

   Interactions: Dipyridamole potentiates the effects of adenosine. Thus, the dose of adenosine must be reduced in patients taking dipyridamole including Aggrenox; significant hypotension may be caused by the combination. Theophylline is an antagonist.

   Adverse effects: Transient headache, facial flushing, and dyspnea, but bronchospasm may last more than a half-hour in **asthmatics**. The drug has minor proarrhythmic effects and may cause atrial and ventricular premature beats; rarely SVT or atrial flutter may degenerate to AF *(8)*. Atrial flutter is not an indication for adenosine; 1:1 conduction and extreme tachycardia may ensue.

   Contraindications: Asthma, severe chronic obstructive lung disease (COPD), wide QRS complex if the diagnosis of SVT with aberrancy is uncertain and in heart transplant recipients.

2. **Verapamil** IV is effective in more than 90% of episodes of AVNRT (narrow complex); here there is no question of VT, so the drug is safe provided the contraindications listed below are excluded. The drug has proved useful in patients with normal hearts and without the following complications:
   - Hypotension.
   - Known WPW syndrome or suspicion of WPW in view of very fast ventricular response > 220/min.
   - Acute myocardial infarction (MI), CHF, or cardiomegaly (*see* Table 14-2).
   - Left ventricular dysfunction, ejection fraction (EF) < 40%.
   - Sinus or AV node disease.
   - Wide QRS tachycardia (>0.10 s) (*see* Fig. 14-1).
   - Suspected digitalis toxicity.
   - Beta-blockade present.

   In these situations, adenosine is the drug of choice *(3,5,6)*.

   Contraindications: Verapamil is contraindicated in patients with wide QRS tachycardia, WPW syndrome, severe hypotension, HF, known sick sinus syndrome, digitalis toxicity, and concurrent use of beta-blockers or disopyramide.

Table 14-2
Classification of Drug Actions on Arrhythmias Based on Modification of Vulnerable Parameter

Mechanism	*Arrhythmia*	*Vulnerable parameter effect*	*Drugs (effect)*
Automaticity			
Enhanced normal	Inappropriate sinus tachycardia	Phase 4 depolarization (decrease)	Beta-adrenergic blocking agents
	Some idiopathic ventricular tachycardias		Na^+ channel blocking agents
Abnormal	Atrial tachycardia	Maximum diastolic potential (hyperpolarization)	M_2 agonist
		Phase 4 depolarization (decrease)	Ca^{2+} or Na^+ channel blocking agents
			M_2 agonist
	Accelerated idioventricular rhythms	Phase 4 depolarization (decrease)	Ca^{2+} or Na^+ channel blocking agents
Triggered activity			
EAD	Torsades de pointes	Action potential duration (shorten)	Beta-adrenergic agonists; vagolytic agents (increase rate)
		EAD (suppress)	Ca^{2+} channel blocking agents; Mg^{2+}; beta-adrenergic blocking agents
DAD	Digitalis-induced arrhythmias	Calcium overload (unload)	Ca^{2+} channel blocking agents
		DAD (suppress)	Na^+ channel blocking agents
	Right ventricular outflow tract ventricular tachycardia	Calcium overload (unload)	Beta-adrenergic blocking agents;
		DAD (suppress)	Ca^{2+} channel blocking agents adenosine

(continued)

Table 14-2 (Continued)

Mechanism	*Arrhythmia*	*Vulnerable parameter effect*	*Drugs (effect)*
Automaticity			
Reentry—Na^+ channel-dependent			
Long excitable gap	Typical atrial flutter	Conduction and excitability (depress)	Type 1A, 1C Na^+ channel blocking agents
	Circus movement tachycardia in WPW	Conduction and excitability (depress)	Type 1A, 1C Na^+ channel blocking agents
	Sustained uniform ventricular tachycardia	Conduction and excitability (depress)	Na^+ channel blocking agents
Short excitable gap	Atypical atrial flutter	Refractory period (prolong)	K^+ channel blocking agents
	Atypical atrial fibrillation	Refractory period (prolong)	K^+ channel blocking agents
	Circus movement tachycardia in WPW	Refractory period (prolong)	Amiodarone, sotalol
	Polymorphic and uniform ventricular tachycardia	Refractory period (prolong)	Type IA Na^+ channel blocking agents
	Bundle branch reentry	Refractory period (prolong)	Type IA Na^+ channel blocking agents, bretylium
	Ventricular fibrillation	Refractory period (prolong)	
Reentry—Ca^{2+} channel-dependent			
	AV nodal reentrant tachycardia	Conduction and excitability (depress)	Ca^{2+} channel blocking agents
	Circus movement tachycardia in WPW	Conduction and excitability (depress)	Ca^{2+} channel blocking agents
	Verapamil-sensitive ventricular tachycardia	Conduction and excitability (depress)	Ca^{2+} channel blocking agents

WPW, Wolff-Parkinson-White syndrome; DAD, delayed after depolarization; EAD, early after depolarization.

From Task Force of the Working Group on Arrhythmias of the European Society of Cardiology: The Sicilian Gambit: A new approach to the classification of antiarrhythmic drugs based on their actions on arrhythmogenic mechanisms. Circulation 1991;84:1831. Copyright 1991, American Heart Association.

Dosage: IV 0.075–0.15 mg/kg, i.e., 5–10 mg, is given slowly over 1–2 min. The depressant effect on the AV node may persist for up to 6 h, and a second dose may produce complications. If the arrhythmia persists following Valsalva maneuver or right carotid massage or recurs without hemodynamic deterioration in patients with a normal heart, a second dose not exceeding 5 mg may be considered after 30 min. If restoration of sinus rhythm is clearly urgent, adenosine is tried, and then, if needed, DC conversion. **IV infusion** 1 mg/min to a total of 10 mg or 5–10 mg over 1 h; 100 mg in 24 h.

Prolongation of AV conduction induced by verapamil can be reversed by atropine. Calcium gluconate or chloride is useful in the management of hypotension, circulatory collapse, or asystole owing to sinus arrest or AV block. Atropine may be of value in this situation.

3. **Propranolol** 1 mg IV given slowly and repeated every 5 min to a maximum of 5 mg; the usual dose required is 2–4 mg. **Metoprolol** is given in a dose of 5 mg at a rate of 1–2 mg/min repeated after 5 min if necessary to a total dose of 10–15 mg.
4. **Digoxin:** Because the effect of digoxin takes more than 2 h to appear, it is not often advised when rapid restoration of sinus rhythm is required.
5. **Diltiazem IV** is as effective as verapamil and causes fewer adverse effects; both agents cost approximately $15 per treatment compared with $100 for two 6-mg doses of adenosine. Diltiazem has a role in patients who have well-defined SVT.

   Dosage: Initial bolus 0.25 mg/kg over 2 min; if needed, rebolus 0.35 mg/kg.
6. **Phenylephrine** (Neo-Synephrine) is an alpha-sympathetic agonist. The drug is now rarely used because of better alternatives, especially adenosine. The drug has a role only in young patients with a normal heart, when adenosine has failed, when the blood pressure is <90 mmHg, and when cardioversion is considered undesirable. The resulting increase in blood pressure stimulates the baroreceptor reflexes and increases vagal activity, often resulting in termination of the arrhythmia.

   Contraindications: Patients with MI, severe cardiac pathology, and narrow-angle glaucoma.

   Dosage: Phenylephrine is administered as repeated IV bolus injections; 0.1 mg is diluted with 5 mL 5% dextrose and water (D/W) and given over 2 min. Blood pressure is measured at 30-s intervals. Arterial blood pressure must not be allowed to exceed 140 mmHg. Sufficient time (1–2 min) should elapse after each bolus to allow the blood pressure to return to its baseline value before subsequent doses are administered.

   Dose range: 0.1–0.5 mg. Higher doses have been used but are not recommended. Administration by IV drip infusion may result in variation in drug rates that may cause an unacceptable increase in blood pressure.

Chronic Maintenance of AVNRT

Recurrent prolonged or frequent episodes may require chronic drug therapy. The following may be tried:

1. **Digoxin.** This drug is especially useful in patients with left ventricular dysfunction (LV) and in those with resting systolic blood pressure < 110 mmHg in whom beta-blockers, verapamil, or diltiazem may cause symptomatic hypotension or bradycardia. Also, the drug is inexpensive and available as a one-a-day tablet. It is not used in patients with WPW syndrome.
2. **A beta-blocker.** Choose a once-daily preparation: 50 mg, metoprolol succinate sustained release (Toprol XL) 50 mg. If AVNRT recurs on this regimen, verapamil 80–120 mg orally usually aborts the attack within 1 h and avoids bothersome emergency room visits.
3. **Digoxin plus a one-a-day beta-blocker** may be necessary in patients resistant to (1) and (2).
4. **Verapamil** 80–120 mg three times daily, **Isoptin** SR 120–180 mg daily, and **diltiazem** (Cardizem CD) 180–240 mg are effective in <50% of patients. This is an expensive regimen, and compliance may be a problem.

5. **Flecainide** (200–400 mg daily) has been shown to decrease freedom from recurrent tachycardia in up to 80% of patients, compared with 15% in individuals administered placebo. Pooled studies indicate that flecainide is effective in approximately 77% of patients with AVNRT and in 66% of those with AVRT.
6. **Amiodarone**, low dose, may be used in refractory cases before contemplating ablative therapy of an accessory pathway.
7. **Pill in the pocket: No prophylactic treatment** is given.
   At the onset of an episode, the patient takes:
   - Verapamil 80–120 mg or a beta-blocker e.g., metoprolol tartrate (rapid acting) or bisoprolol 5 mg orally.
   - Flecanide

   or

   - The combination of diltiazem and propranolol terminated 80% of SVT episodes within 2 h of administration *(9)*.

These regimens are safe and efficacious in patients with normal hearts. Recurrent AVNRT resistant to pharmacologic therapy should prompt consideration of catheter ablation.

Multifocal Atrial Tachycardia (Chaotic Atrial Tachycardia)

This arrhythmia is caused by frequent atrial ectopic depolarizations. The arrhythmia is characterized by variable P-wave morphology and P-P and PR interval. The atrial rate is usually 100–130/min, and the ventricular rhythm is irregular. The diagnosis is made by demonstrating three or more different P-wave morphologies in one lead. The arrhythmia is usually precipitated by acute infections, exacerbation of COPD, electrolyte and acid-base imbalance, theophylline, beta$_1$-stimulants, and, rarely, digitalis toxicity. Digitalis is usually not effective, and treatment of the underlying cause is most important. If the ventricular response is excessively rapid, slowing may be achieved with verapamil given orally. Magnesium sulfate is an effective alternative if verapamil is contraindicated. Adenosine is ineffective.

Paroxysmal Atrial Tachycardia (PAT) with Block

Episodes are usually associated with severe cardiac or pulmonary disease. PAT is a common manifestation of digitalis toxicity. The atrial rate is commonly 180–220/min. AV conduction is usually 2:1. The rhythm is usually regular. The ventricular rate of 90–120/min may not cause concern, and the P waves are often buried in the preceding T wave, so the diagnosis is easily missed.

If the ventricular rate is 90–120/min and the serum potassium (K^+) level is normal, digoxin and diuretics should be discontinued, and often no specific treatment is required. If the serum K^+ concentration is <3.5 mEq (mmol)/L and a high degree of AV block is absent, IV potassium chloride 40 mEq (mmol) in 500 mL 5% D/W is given over 4 h through a central line. If the serum K^+ level is <2.5 mEq (mmol)/L, KC1 is best given in normal saline to improve the serum potassium level quickly.

Other therapies are outlined under treatment of digitalis toxicity.

Atrial Premature Contractions

Atrial premature contractions (APCs) often occur without apparent cause. Recognized causes include stimulants, drugs, anxiety, hypoxmia, HF, ischemic heart disease, and other cardiac pathology. APCs in themselves require no drug therapy. Treatment of the underlying cause is usually sufficient. In patients with no serious underlying cardiac disease, reassurance is of utmost importance. Stimulants such as caffeine, theophylline, nicotine, nicotinic acid, and other cardiac stimulants as well as alcohol should be avoided.

When heart or pulmonary disease is present, APCs may predict runs of SVT, AF, or atrial flutter, and the resulting increase in heart rate may be distressing to the patient. Digoxin may be useful and, rarely, disopyramide may be necessary. If mitral valve prolapse is associated, sedation or a beta-blocker may be useful.

Atrial Flutter

Underlying heart disease is usually present; however, hypoxemia owing to a pneumothorax, atelectasis, and other noncardiac causes may precipitate the arrhythmia. Atrial flutter tends to be unstable, either degenerating into AF or reverting to sinus rhythm.

The atrial rate is usually 240–340/min. The ventricular rate is often 150/min with an atrial rate of 300, i.e., 2:1 conduction. Therefore a ventricular rate of 150/min with a regular rhythm should alert the clinician to a diagnosis of atrial flutter. The sawtooth pattern in lead II should confirm the diagnosis. Carotid sinus massage may increase the degree of AV block, slow the ventricular response, and reveal the sawtooth P waves as opposed to P waves separated by isoelectric segments in PAT with block. Rarely a 1:1 conduction with a rapid ventricular response is seen, especially in patients with preexcitation syndromes or in patients receiving a class 1 antiarrhythmic agent.

Treatment

Atrial flutter is easily converted to sinus rhythm by synchronized DC shock at low energies of 25–50 joules. Electrical cardioversion is often indicated and should be performed if the patient is hemodynamically compromised or if the ventricular response is >200/min or the patient is known or suspected to have WPW syndrome.

If the patient is hemodynamically stable with a ventricular response < 200/min, propranolol may be used to slow the ventricular response. The benefit of propranolol or metoprolol is that patients who can undergo electrical cardioversion may do so easily, whereas following digoxin DC shocks have been reported to be hazardous. If underlying heart disease is present, digoxin has a role in the acute and chronic management. Digoxin converts atrial flutter to AF, and the ventricular response is nearly always slowed to an acceptable level provided sufficient digoxin is used. Removal of underlying causes may be followed by spontaneous reversion to sinus rhythm. Verapamil or diltiazem is effective in slowing the ventricular response and may occasionally cause conversion to sinus rhythm. Digoxin, verapamil, and beta-blockers are contraindicated in patients with WPW syndrome presenting with atrial flutter. Quinidine, procainamide, or disopyramide must not be used alone for the conversion of atrial flutter to sinus rhythm because these drugs, especially quinidine, increase conduction in the AV node and may result in a 1:1 conduction with a ventricular response exceeding 220/min. If quinidine is administered, it must be preceded by adequate digitalization to produce a sufficient degree of AV block.

Propafenone and flecainide have been shown to convert atrial flutter to sinus rhythm in 20% and 33% of patients, respectively *(3)*.

Atrial Fibrillation

AF is the most common sustained arrhythmia observed in clinical practice. In most patients, drug action to control the ventricular response provides adequate therapy. In some patients it may be necessary to achieve reversion to sinus rhythm with drugs or DC conversion.

A ventricular response < 80/min in an untreated patient should raise the suspicion of disease of the AV node or concomitant sick sinus syndrome, particularly in the elderly. AF with a slow ventricular rate that becomes regular, indicative of the presence of a junctional pacemaker, should raise the suspicion of digitalis toxicity.

Atrial Fibrillation of Recent Onset

In acute AF, with a fast ventricular rate, especially if there is hemodynamic compromise or with rates exceeding 220/min, WPW syndrome may be the cause, and drugs that block the AV node are contraindicated. Drug therapy to slow the ventricular response in patients with AF, in whom conduction using the accessory pathway can be excluded, includes the following:

1. **Diltiazem** IV is the drug of choice for urgent rate control in patients with AF; a constant IV infusion brings the ventricular response under control reliably. Sinus rhythm is achieved in only about 15%, and hypotension occurs in up to 33% of patients. Diltiazem IV followed by **procainamide** IV bolus may cause reversion to sinus rhythm.
2. **Esmolol** slows the rate adequately over 20 min, and sinus rhythm may ensue. The drug causes hypotension in up to 40% of patients. Esmolol and digoxin are effective, and hypotension is much less common than when esmolol alone is used. Digoxin appears to protect from hypotension.
3. **Ibutilide** (Corvert). Ibutilide fumarate injection is indicated for the conversion of AF or flutter to sinus rhythm.

   Dose: A 1-mg dose is given over 10 min with cardiac monitoring for patients > 60 kg (0.01 mg/kg < 60 kg); a 1-mg dose is repeated in 20 min.

   Caution: The drug should not be used in patients with a low serum potassium level or prolonged QT interval because torsades de pointes (TDP) may be precipitated. There is a 5% incidence of torsades in patients with ischemic heart disease. If AF is of less than 2 days' duration, anticoagulants are not indicated; in patients with AF persistent for more than 2 d, anticoagulants are recommended for 4 wk, and then conversion is attempted.

   Caution: Stop the infusion as soon as AF converts to sinus rhythm or if new or worsening ventricular arrhythmias develop. The patient with continuous cardiac rhythm monitoring should be observed for at least 4 h following infusion or until the QT interval has returned to baseline. If the arrhythmias do not terminate within 10 min of the end of the initial infusion, a second 10-min infusion of 1 mg may be administered 10 min after completion of the first infusion. QT interval should not be >440 ms, and the serum potassium level should be above 4 mEq (mmol)/L. Ibutilide is a methane sulfonamide derivative with structural similarities to sotalol *(10)*; its primary mechanism of action is a class III effect.

   Interactions: Do not administer to patients taking sotalol or amiodarone.
4. **Dofetillde** (Tikosyn) is a methane sulfonamide drug similar to ibutilide but is administered orally and inhibits only the rapid component of the delayed rectifier potassium current, whereas ibutilide also has an effect on the early fast inward Na^+ current.

   Indications: Oral therapy for conversion of and maintenance of sinus rhythm after conversion in patients with persistent highly symptomatic AF or atrial flutter. The drug is not useful in paroxysmal AF.

   Dosage: *See* product monograph.

   Adverse effects and precautions are similar to those for ibutilide, with a 3.3% incidence of torsades.

Contraindications include:

- QT interval > 440 ms.
- Thyrotoxicosis.
- CHF, renal failure.
- The presence of drugs that increase the QT interval.
- Calcium antagonists, cimetidine.

5. **Azimilide** is a newer agent undergoing clinical trials because it appears to be more effective and has fewer side effects than ibutilide and dofetilide; also, it can be used IV for conversion or orally for long-term prevention, with a distinctly lesser incidence of torsades (1% versus 3%). The difficult to manage paroxysmal AF may benefit. It is tolerated in renal dysfunction.

Paroxysmal Atrial Fibrillation

The patient should be anticoagulated to prevent embolization. IV disopyramide (not approved in the United States) or procainamide given with digoxin may restore sinus rhythm in <33%. If the rate <150 is well tolerated, it is advisable to observe the rhythm for 8–12 h because spontaneous rhythm is common, particularly if the patient has taken an extra dose of sotalol (40–80 mg) prior to coming to the emergency room. DC cardioversion should be immediately available if drug therapy fails, when the ventricular rate is rapid, or when hypotension and HF ensue. **For the prevention of recurrent episodes**: sotalol low dose 40–60 mg is beneficial in 40–50% of patients. Although low-dose amiodarone is more effective than sotalol (approx 75%) and pulmonary side effects run approx 3%, other side effects may emerge. Clinical trial results are awaited for azimilide.

Chronic Atrial Fibrillation

In most patients with chronic AF of more than 1 year's duration, slowing of the ventricular response will suffice.

- **A beta-blocker is a good choice** even in patients with class I–III HF or asymptomatic LV dysfunction.
- Verapamil or a beta-blocker slows the ventricular rate during exercise, whereas digoxin often fails to do so. Verapamil SR has a role in selected cases but may cause constipation or other adverse effects and is considerably more expensive than digoxin. **Beta-blockers are preferred.**
- The combination of digoxin and bisoprolol 5 mg or metoprolol long acting (Toprol XL) 50 mg is often beneficial.
- **Sotalol is not advisable for chronic AF** because the drug may cause conversion to sinus rhythm in a few patients, which may lead to an increase in thromboembolism; also, sotalol carries a risk of TDP and is no more effective than other beta-blockers in controlling the ventricular rate. The three drugs are contraindicated in patients with WPW syndrome and AF or atrial flutter.
- **Digoxin** is inexpensive and is suitable in many elderly people who do not engage in much physical activity. If the patient is asymptomatic, the rate at rest is <80, and on a 4-min walk the rate is <110, digoxin should suffice, particularly if a beta-blocker has caused tiredness; verapamil should be avoided in the elderly because it causes bothersome constipation and may cause HF in some. The ventricular rate may be slow in the elderly because of concomitant AV node disease. **Sick sinus syndromes should be anticipated, and pacing may be considered.**

Synchronized DC Cardioversion

The advisability of attempting DC conversion of AF is always considered carefully.

In selected acute cases, reversion to sinus rhythm may be warranted. One should first consider whether it would be worthwhile to restore sinus rhythm with DC conversion. The question is necessary because reversion to sinus rhythm may cause embolization or AF may recur because the underlying heart disease is unchanged. The incidence of embolization following cardioversion is about 2%.

Except in special circumstances, cardioversion is usually contraindicated in patients with:

- AF of duration >1 yr.
- Valvular heart disease in patients due to undergo surgery within the next few weeks.
- Digitalis-induced arrhythmias.
- Sick sinus syndrome.
- Advanced AV block.
- Left atrium > 5 cm, as sinus rhythm is usually not maintained.

If AF is of <48 hours' duration, anticoagulants are believed not to be necessary. If AF is of >3 days' duration, administer warfarin for 3 wk before and for 8–12 wk after elective cardioversion. Digoxin is maintained for the period before conversion and is interrupted 24–48 h before conversion. Sotalol or quinidine is commenced immediately after conversion when there is believed to be a high probability of recurrence of AF. Sotalol is more effective than quinidine in the prevention of recurrent AF and for the maintenance of sinus rhythm (see below) *(3)*. Amiodarone may be commenced before conversion if this drug is selected.

Cardioversion is considered only when conditions contraindicating its use are absent or the patient's life is threatened by the rapidity of the ventricular response or loss of atrial transport function, such as

- Heart rate >150/min believed to be causing HF, chest pain, or cardiogenic shock.
- Patients with hypertrophic cardiomyopathy or severe aortic stenosis (in whom atrial transport function is of great importance).
- AF in patients with WPW syndrome.

Rate Control versus Rhythm Control

No clear advantage exists between rhythm control and rate control.In five RCTs no significant differences were recorded in primary end points. Adverse outcomes with a rhythm-control approach were seen in the two largest studies *(11,12)*. None of the benefits expected from rhythm control were documented, unfortunately. The strongest risk factor for stroke was a lack of anticoagulation, because of the tendency to stop anticoagulants in patients who reverted to sinus rhythm, resulting in increased stroke rate.

The Role of Anticoagulants

Approximately 70% of AF occurs at age 65–85. The risk of stroke in patients with AF who have one or more risk factors for stroke is approx 5%, and anticoagulants are recommended to keep the International Normalized Ratio (INR) at 2 to 3 (*see* Fig. 14-2). Bleeding occurrence is associated in virtually all cases with an INR > 3.

Risk factors include:

- Significant valvular heart disease, particularly mitral stenosis and moderate mitral regurgitation, LV dysfunction, HF, hypertension, prior stroke or transient ischemic attack, and age > 75 yr.

In patients < 65 yr with lone AF (no cardiac abnormality risk factors), the risk of stroke is low (<1%), and coated acetylsalicylic acid (ASA) 325 mg is recommended. In patients

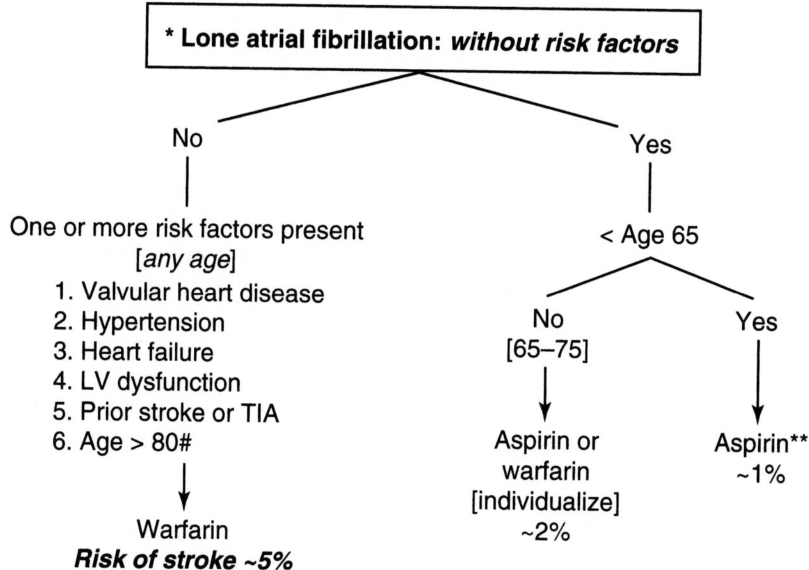

*Normal heart clinically and on echocardiography.
**No proof that it is protective but risk is low.
#Very high risk/stroke but high risk of intracranial bleed: INR must be kept <3, range 1.8 to 2.8.

Fig. 14-2. Guidelines for the prevention of embolic stroke in patients with chronic or paroxysmal atrial fibrillation.

age 65–75 with lone AF, the risk is approx 2%, and ASA versus warfarin should be determined on an individual basis because trials have not yielded clear answers. All patients with risk factors should receive anticoagulants, but patients older than 75 have an increased risk of intracranial hemorrhage and the INR should be closely monitored to keep it between 1.8 and 2.8.

Arrhythmias in Wolff-Parkinson-White Syndrome

Patients with WPW syndrome may present with atrial flutter or AF as well as with AVRT. During sinus rhythm the short PR interval and delta wave are characteristic.

A circus movement through the AV node with retrograde conduction along the accessory bundle, reaching the AV node again via the atria, produces the typical AVRT pattern. This variety usually responds to verapamil. However, verapamil should not be given to prevent paroxysmal tachycardia until proven safe by electrophysiologic (EP) testing because the drug has been reported to accelerate the ventricular response following the development of AF or atrial flutter *(2)*.

In some patients with AF or flutter with WPW conduction, the impulses are conducted at high frequency through the accessory pathway. A rapid ventricular response of 240–300/min can occur with a risk of precipitating ventricular fibrillation. The rapidity of the ventricular response should alert the clinician to the diagnosis of WPW syndrome. In this subset of patients with WPW syndrome, drugs that block impulses through the AV node (digoxin, verapamil, diltiazem, and beta-blockers) do not slow the response and are contraindicated. Furthermore, digoxin and verapamil may dangerously accelerate the ventricular rate. Verapamil or digoxin may precipitate VF.

DC conversion is indicated, and drugs that block conduction in the bypass tract—flecainide, disopyramide, procainamide, aprindine, propafenone, and especially amiodarone *(2)*—slow the response. IV amiodarone can rarely increase the ventricular rate or cause hypotension and caution is required. Lidocaine could occasionally increase the ventricular response in patients with WPW syndrome presenting with AF or flutter. EP testing is advisable in symptomatic patients and in those with AF, flutter, or rates exceeding 220/min. Patients shown to be at risk of sudden death should have the bypass tract obliterated cryothermally or by other ablation techniques that produce a cure. Fortunately, serious life-threatening arrhythmias are rare. Asymptomatic patients in whom the delta wave disappears rarely have problems.

VENTRICULAR ARRHYTHMIAS

Ventricular arrhythmias are best considered under benign, potentially fatal, and fatal arrhythmias.

Premature Ventricular Contractions: Benign Arrhythmias

The Cardiac Arrhythmia Suppression Trial (CAST) *(13)* indicated that treatment of post-MI PVCs and potentially fatal arrhythmias with flecainide or encainide caused an increase in mortality. Beta-blockers are the only safe antiarrhythmic agents that have been shown to improve survival in patients with postinfarction ventricular arrhythmias regardless of their ability to suppress PVCs. Amiodarone has been shown to have a modest beneficial effect.

Consideration 1. The significance of PVCs as risk markers for sudden death varies enormously according to the clinical context.

- There is no evidence as yet that suppression of PVCs reduces the incidence of sudden death.
- The numerous antiarrhythmic agents all possess the capacity to produce serious side effects or arrhythmias, sometimes worse than the arrhythmias that they are supposed to suppress.
- The added cost and inconvenience to the patient can be a burden and may not be justifiable.

Consideration 2. The correlation between the suppression of PVCs or lack of it with suppression of recurrent VT is limited. This holds for PVCs in pairs (salvos of two) or triplets (salvos of three—nonsustained VT).

PVCs in the presence of the otherwise normal heart require no therapy.

Treatment of PVCs Associated with Cardiac Pathology

1. The management of PVCs occurring in the acute phase of MI is discussed in Chapter 11.
2. There is suggested evidence that patients 10–16 d post-MI with frequent PVCs > 10/h have an increased 1-yr mortality rate *(14)*. Treatment of this subset, which represents about 25% of post-MI patients, may reduce mortality, but antiarrhythmic agents other than beta-blockers have not been proved to be effective or safe *(2,14)*.

VENTRICULAR TACHYCARDIA

VT is a regular wide QRS complex tachycardia. In general, consider regular wide QRS complex tachycardia as ventricular unless there is strong evidence to the contrary; if there is doubt about the diagnosis (VT versus SVT with aberrant conduction), treat as VT; the accurate diagnosis of VT is sometimes difficult. The salient diagnostic points for VT were discussed earlier in this chapter (*see* Fig. 14-1).

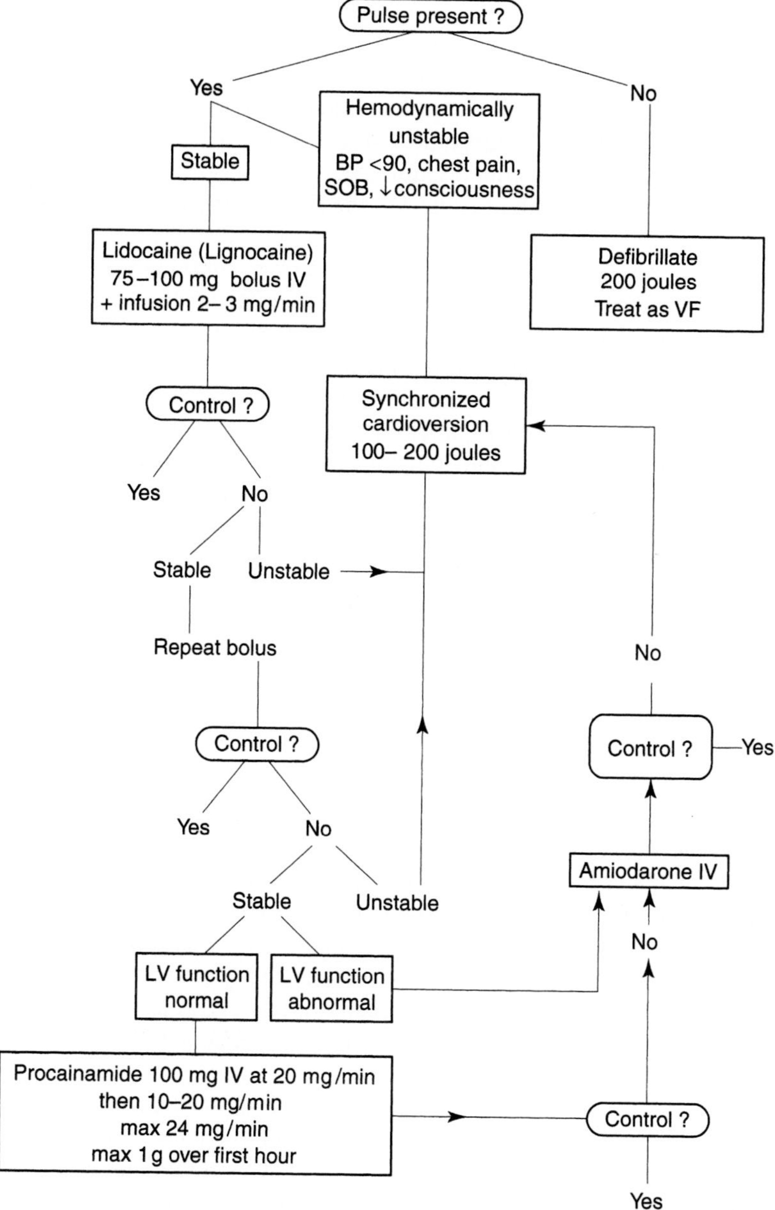

Fig. 14-3. Management of sustained ventricular tachycardia. BP, blood pressure; SOB, shortness of breath; VF, ventricular fibrillation. (From Khan M Gabriel. Arrhythmias. In: Heart Disease, Diagnosis and Therapy. Totowa, NJ, Humana Press, 2005.

In the treatment of VT, cardioversion is frequently employed, especially in patients with acute MI or when the rate is over 200/min or there is hemodynamic disturbance or coronary insufficiency.

The management of sustained VT is given in Fig. 14-3. Drugs are used cautiously to terminate the attack because of the combined effect of the arrhythmia and the drug on blood pressure. Cardioversion is immediately available during drug treatment. It is quite legitimate to use DC conversion as first-line elective therapy:

- Lidocaine (lignocaine). If there is a failure to respond, try:
  - Procainamide.
  - Disopyramide.
  - Flecainide (perhaps second choice in the United Kingdom).
- If hemodynamic deterioration occurs at any stage during the use of the antiarrhythmics, synchronized DC shock is immediately utilized.
- If VT occurs during the first 48 h of acute MI, the IV antiarrhythmic is continued for 24 h after conversion.
- If VT occurs after 48 h post-MI in the absence of recurrence of infarction or ischemic pain, it is likely that a permanent irritable focus possibly associated with an aneurysm is present. The arrhythmia is abolished with IV lidocaine or other agents, and an oral antiarrhythmic is commenced within a few hours and maintained for a minimum of 3–6 mo.
- It is advisable to initiate therapy with beta-blockers if there is evidence of painful or silent ischemia or recent infarction. A beta-blocking agent is worthy of trial in sustained or non-sustained VT. **Beta-blockers** are antiischemic and can reduce symptoms and prevent VT regardless of their effect on ventricular ectopy. In addition, they have been demonstrated to reduce post-MI mortality and mortality in patients with CHF, a harbinger of fatal arrhythmias.
- Bigger's division of ventricular arrhythmias into benign and malignant forms has merit *(14)*.

Fatal Ventricular Arrhythmias

- VF outside hospital.
- Recurrent sustained VT.
- Torsades de pointes.

Treatment is obviously necessary in these three categories.

1. **VF outside hospital:** The survivors of outside-hospital VF represent a therapeutic dilemma. There are no clear answers to therapy; they are best managed by finding an agent or combination of agents that are effective on EP testing or a trial of amiodarone. Patients who survived an episode of out-of-hospital VF in the absence of acute infarction were enrolled in the Conventional versus Amiodarone Drug Evaluation (CASCADE) study *(15)*. The trial comprised 113 patients treated with amiodarone and 115 given conventional antiarrhythmics. At 4-yr follow-up, the amiodarone-treated group showed improved survival and received fewer shocks from an implanted defibrillator; syncope followed by a shock from a defibrillator was less common.
2. **Recurrent sustained VT:** The choice of an oral antiarythmic depends on the physician's clinical experience and formulated policy with respect to the use of particular drugs and EP testing. EP testing may result in selection of a drug or combination that is more efficacious than empirical therapy *(17,18)* and that does not include amiodarone or sotalol. Clinical studies support the empirical use of amiodarone and sotalol to prevent recurrent VT and sudden death, especially in patients with CHD and previous infarction *(16)*. Amiodarone does not appear to be as effective in patients with HF or hypertrophic cardiomyopathy, and sotalol has not been sufficiently studied (*see* discussion under amiodarone and sotalol). In a nonrandomized study *(17)*, 3 of 44 patients in the group receiving therapy guided by EP studies died suddenly, compared with 8 of 18 patients receiving therapy not guided by EP studies. Also, patients who were asymptomatic without inducible sustained VT, and who were untreated, had a low probability of sudden death *(17)*.

   A beta-blocker, disopyramide or mexiletine, may be tried first, followed by drug combinations, and then amiodarone. It is necessary to monitor the serum potassium (K^+) level, magnesium, and Q-T interval during antiarrhythmic therapy. A beta-blocker is often valuable in combination with other agents such as mexiletine but is not recommended for use in association with disopyramide and is often unnecessary when amiodarone is selected. Metoprolol or sotalol is commonly used. Amiodarone combined with mexiletine may also prove successful in refractory recurrent life-threatening VT.

3. **Torsades de pointes** is a life-threatening arrhythmia and is associated with prolongation of the QT interval. The rate is usually 200–250/min. The amplitude and shape of the QRS complexes progressively vary, and they are dramatically spindle-shaped. The peaks of the R-wave direction change from one side to the other of the isoelectric line. This twisting appearance resulted in the name torsades de pointes. The normally conducted complexes show a prolonged QT interval or a prominent U wave. The QT interval is usually >500 ms. QTc is not an important measurement. The episode of TDP commonly lasts 5–30 s and may end with a return to normal rhythm, extreme bradycardia, or ventricular standstill or may degenerate to VF. The patient usually complains of syncope. Palpitations may be present.

   The many precipitating causes of TDP include *(19,20)*:

   - Antiarrhythmics: quinidine, disopyramide, procainamide, sotalol, rarely amiodarone *(21)*, and especially combinations of amiodarone with quinidine or disopyramide *(22)*, but in the absence of hypokalemia, amiodarone does not appear to cause torsades. The drug has been used successfully to treat torsades and can be used as treatment of arrhythmias in patients who have had recurrent TDP *(21,23)*.
   - Coronary vasodilators: prenylamine and lidoflazine.
   - Astemizole, terfenadine, and pentamidine.
   - Psychotropic: tricyclic antidepressants and phenothiazines.
   - Electrolyte disturbances: hypokalemia and hypomagnesemia.
   - Bradycardia owing to complete heart block, sinoatrial block, or sinus bradycardia.
   - Congenital QT prolongation syndromes (with or without deafness).

   Rare causes include subarachnoid hemorrhage, ischemic heart disease, mitral valve prolapse, and liquid protein diet.

   Treatment. Because TDP is a brady-dependent arrhythmia, accelerating the heart rate is the simplest and quickest method to shorten the QT interval and usually results in control of the attacks.

   Temporary atrial or ventricular pacing (AV sequential pacing is preferable to ventricular pacing) should be instituted as soon as possible. Pacing rates within the range of 70–90/min are usually effective. Occasionally, higher rates up to 120/min are required. While preparing for pacing or when pacing is not available, a trial of isoproterenol IV infusion 2–8 μg/min may be given, and control is sometimes achieved within a few minutes. Isoproterenol is contraindicated in acute MI, angina, or severe hypertension. If pacing is not readily available, other possible therapies include atropine, IV propranolol, or bretylium. **Magnesium sulfate bolus injection**, 2 g (10 mL of a 20% solution) over 1 min, causes reversion to sinus rhythm in some patients, particularly in patients with an acquired form of TDP *(24–26)*.

   In the congenital prolonged QT syndrome, beta-blockers are of proven value, and a dose of propranolol 40–60 mg three times daily is often effective. Phenytoin has a role if beta-blockers are contraindicated. For resistant cases, permanent pacing plus beta-blockers or left stellate ganglionectomy is of value.

   Treatment of the acquired prolonged QT syndrome is correction of the underlying cause and avoidance of the class I antiarrhythmics, especially quinidine, disopyramide, procainamide, and sotalol.

   A short-coupled variant of TDP has been described by Leenhardt and colleagues *(27)*. This variant responds to verapamil IV and not to beta-blockers or amiodarone. Because of the high incidence of sudden death in this variant of torsades, an ICD is strongly recommended *(27)*.

ANTIARRHYTHMIC AGENTS

Class IA

Drug name:	**Quinidine**
Supplied:	Quinidine sulfate: 200, 300 mg Quinidine bisulfate: 250 mg
Dosage:	*See* text

The use of quinidine has decreased greatly since 1975, especially since the advent of other antiarrhythmic agents. The drug has been shown to increase cardiac mortality, and its use will decline further *(2,28,29)*.

Dosage

Quinidine sulfate: 200 mg test dose to detect hypersensitivity reactions. If there are no adverse effects, give 200–400 mg every 3 h for three or four doses, then 6-hourly. Introduce controlled-release preparations only after suppression of the arrhythmia. Quinidine bisulfate (Biquin, Kinidin Durules): 250 mg; usual maintenance 500 mg twice daily. Sustained-release tablets: Quinaglute Dura-Tabs 324 mg; 1–2 tablets, two or three times daily.

Action

Quinidine inhibits the fast sodium channel, slows phase 0 of the action potential, and depresses spontaneous phase 4 diastolic depolarization. Quinidine also inhibits the outward K^+ current and thus prolongs the duration of the action potential. Type I agents in general are potent local anesthetics on nerves and produce a depressant effect on myocardial membrane. The added antivagal action can cause acceleration of AV nodal conduction.

Pharmacokinetics

- Absorption from the gut is about 70%.
- Peak plasma concentrations are achieved in 1–3 h.
- The half-life is 7–9 h, but slow-release preparations are available. In liver or renal disease the half-life is increased; in HF the half-life is relatively unchanged.
- Protein binding is 80–90%.
- Metabolized mainly in the liver by hydroxylation; a small amount is excreted by the kidneys.
- Plasma levels for antiarrhythmic effects are 2–5 μg/mL (3–5.5 μmol/L).

Advice, Adverse Effects, and Interactions

Sinus arrest, SA block, AV dissociation, excessive QRS and QT prolongation with the precipitation of TDP or other reentry arrhythmias can occur. The risk of torsades may be decreased by giving quinidine only to patients with a normal serum K^+ level and a QT interval < 400 ms *(8,30)*. Other adverse effects include nausea, vomiting and diarrhea, and thrombocytopenia. The idiosyncratic reaction and rate precipitation of ventricular fibrillation, especially in those undergoing medical cardioversion for AF, are well known.

The drug decreases **ventricular fibrillation threshold**, and it does not seem reasonable to give priority to a drug that may increase the risk of VF. Quinidine may precipitate VT and cardiac arrest *(31)*. The drug is contraindicated in WPW syndrome associated with atrial flutter or AF. Quinidine increases the serum digoxin level, and the digoxin dose should be decreased by 50%. The effect of coumarin anticoagulants is enhanced.

Drug name:	**Disopyramide**
Trade names:	Norpace, Rythmodan, Dirythmin SA (UK)
Supplied:	Ampules: 100 mg in 5 mL 100, 150 mg and controlled release (CR-SR) *See* text for further details
Dosage:	Oral: 300 mg initially, and then 100–150 mg every 6 h; max. 200 mg every 6 h Sustained action: 150–300 mg twice daily IV: 2 mg/kg over 15 min and then 1–2 mg/kg by infusion over 45 min (max. 300 mg in first hour; 800 mg daily); maintenance 0.4 mg/kg/h

Sustained release: Norpace CR 150 mg. Rythmodan Retard 250 mg; Dirythmin 100–150 mg; Dirythmin SA 150 mg.

Action

Actions are similar to those of quinidine, but the drug has considerably more anticholinergic activity. Thus, urinary retention, constipation, and worsening of glaucoma are bothersome adverse effects.

Hemodynamic

The drug has a very significant negative inotropic effect, which is much greater than that of any other available antiarrhythmics. CHF may be precipitated, and this is a major drawback to the use of the drug in patients with poor ventricular function.

Pharmacokinetics

- Absorption from the gut is adequate; bioavailability is about 80%.
- Peak plasma concentration is achieved in 1–2 h. The therapeutic range is 2–5 mg/L (2–5 μg/mL, 6–12 (μmol/L).
- Half-life 6–8 h.
- 50% of the drug is excreted unchanged by the kidney; about half is metabolized, and the metabolites may have some activity. One metabolite is powerfully anticholinergic.

Indications

The drug is indicated for the management of VT in the acute setting. It is used after trials of other agents such as lidocaine and procainamide have resulted in failure. The drug along with other class I agents does not decrease the incidence of VF in the acute phase of MI and does not reduce the incidence of cardiac death in the post-MI patient. Disopyramide acts selectively on the accessory bundle and may result in a clinically useful decrease in ventricular response or may terminate the episode of atrial flutter or fibrillation in WPW syndrome. The drug may be combined with digoxin in the management of supraventricular arrhythmias. The drug has a limited role in the management of recurrent ventricular arrhythmias and in general is not administered in combination with other antiarrhythmic agents, apart from digoxin. Disopyramide appears to have a role in the management of hypertrophic cardiomyopathy because of its negative inotropic effect.

Advice, Adverse Effects, and Interactions

- Do not use in the presence of severe renal failure or HF or in patients with poor LV contractility.
- Glaucoma, myasthenia gravis, hypotension, and significant hypertrophy of the prostate causing urinary retention are contraindications.

HF, sinus node depression, dry mouth, and blurred vision are not uncommon sequelae. TDP or VF may also occur. Do not use in combination with diltiazem or verapamil.

Drug name:	**Procainamide**
Trade names:	Pronestyl, Procanbid
Supplied:	Oral capsules: 250, 375, 500 mg Sustained release (Procanbid): 500, 1000 mg tablets IV ampules: 100 mg/mL, 10 mL vial
Dosage:	*See* text

The drug is indicated for the acute management of VT when lidocaine fails.

Dosage

IV 100-mg bolus at a rate of 20 mg/min, and then 10–20 mg/min, maximum 24 mg/min *(32)*, to a maximum of 1 g over the first hour. Maintenance 1–4 mg/min. IV doses exceeding 24 mg/min commonly cause hypotension *(32)*. Oral 500-mg loading dose then 375–500 mg every 3 h for 24–48 h, and then sustained-release tablets: 500–1000 mg every 12 h. Oral use should be limited to a maximum of 6 mo.

Pharmacokinetics

- Absorption is about 85%.
- Half-life is about 3–5 h.
- Rapid renal elimination occurs, and plasma metabolism is by hydroxylation.
- The therapeutic plasma level is 4–8 mg/L (4–8 μg/mL or 17–34 μmol/L). Toxic levels range from 8 to 10 mg/L with severe toxicity about 16 mg/L (16 μg/mL or 67 μmol/L).

Indications

- The drug may cardiovert acute-onset AF. Digoxin treatment is recommended as a pretreatment because procainamide can accelerate AV conduction. An increase in ventricular rate to >226/min can be life-threatening. The maximum rate of administration is 24 mg/min.
- The acute management of VT unresponsive to the second bolus of lidocaine and AF with anterogradely conducting accessory pathway.

Advice, Adverse Effects, and Interactions

- The drug has a mild to moderate negative inotropic effect and can precipitate HF.
- VT or VF may occur, or recur, at least in part as a result of the drug's proarrhythmic effects.
- Lupus syndrome occurs in about one-third of patients after 6 mo of therapy; agranulocytosis may occur after prolonged treatment and appears to be more common with the slow-release formulation *(33)*.
- Avoid combination with angiotensin-converting enzyme (ACE) inhibitors because of enhanced immune effects. Cimetidine increases procainamide levels by inhibiting renal clearance.

Contraindications include AV block, hypotension, HF, and severe renal failure.

Cautions include asthma and myasthenia gravis. Reduce the dose or increase the dose interval in renal impairment.

Class IB

Drug name:	**Lidocaine; Lignocaine**
Trade names:	Xylocaine, Xylocard
Supplied:	Prefilled syringes: 5 mL, 50 mg/5 mL (1%); 10 mL, 100 mg/10 mL (1%). For dilution: 1 g/25 mL In the UK: lignocaine 0.2% in dextrose, 2 mg/mL, 500 mL or 1 L container; Xylocard 20 mg/mL, 5-mL syringe = 100 mg
Dosage:	*See* text

Lidocaine is the standard agent for suppression of ventricular arrhythmias associated with acute MI or cardiac surgery.

Dosage

IV: initial bolus 1.0–1.5 mg/kg (75–100 mg). After 5–10 min, administer a second bolus of 0.75–1.0 mg/kg. Halve dose in the presence of severe hepatic disease or reduced hepatic blood flow as in cardiogenic shock, severe HF, during concurrent cimetidine administration, and in patients over age 65 yr. Blood levels are increased by concomitant administration of hepatic metabolized beta-blockers and halothane.

The initial bolus is given simultaneously with the commencement of the IV infusion of lidocaine so that a lag between the bolus and the infusion does not occur. Commence the infusion at 2 mg/min. If arrhythmias recur, administer a third bolus of 50 mg and increase the infusion rate to 3 mg/min. Carefully reevaluate the clinical situation and rationale before increasing the rate to the maximum of 4 mg/min. **Maximum** dose in 1 h = 300 mg, IM 400 mg.

Preparation of IV infusion: 1 g lidocaine for IV use is added to 500 mL or 1 L of 5% D/W.

Action

The major action is depression of spontaneous phase 4 diastolic depolarization. There is little effect on action potential duration or conduction in normal circumstances, but conduction in diseased myocardium or following premature stimulation may be depressed. The drug is more effective in the presence of a relatively high serum K^+ level, so hypokalemia should be corrected to obtain the maximum effect of lidocaine or other class I antiarrhythmics.

Pharmacokinetics

A single bolus is effective for only 5–10 min. Clearance is related to the hepatic blood flow and to hepatic function. Clearance is prolonged in the elderly in cardiac failure and hepatic disease. Therapeutic blood levels are 1.4–6 mg/L (1.4–6 μg/mL or 6–26 μmol/L). Central nervous system side effects, including seizures, may occur at concentrations >5 mg/L.

Indications

The main indication for lidocaine is in the acute management of VT. In the early **post-MI patient**, proven prophylactic therapy requires the use of high doses of lidocaine. Prophylactic lidocaine remains controversial *(2,34)*, and is not cost-effective; most centers in the United States and Europe do not routinely use the drug (*see* Chapter 11.) IM lidocaine is efficacious but must be given to about 250 patients with suspected MI to save one from VF *(35)*.

Ventricular arrhythmias owing to **digitalis intoxication**, phenolthiazines, or tricyclic antidepressants are managed effectively by lidocaine. Lidocaine crosses the placenta after IV or epidural administration. The drug appears to be safe during pregnancy if used in the smallest effective dose for the suppression of VT *(36)*.

Advice, Adverse Effects, and Interactions

Lidocaine has little hemodynamic effect. High concentrations may cause bradycardia and hypotension. Rare sinus arrest occurs in patients with sinus node dysfunction. Lidocaine has precipitated complete heart block in patients with impaired atrioventricular conduction. Nausea, vomiting, dizziness, twitching, and grand mal seizures may occur with repeated bolus injections in patients with impaired hepatic function.

Contraindications. The presence of grade 2 or 3 AV block or nodal or idioventricular rhythm. Lidocaine may suppress necessary escape foci in these rhythms and produce cardiac arrest.

Drug name:	**Mexiletine**
Trade name:	Mexitil
Supplied:	Ampoules: 10 mL, 25 mg/mL Capsules: 150, 200, 250 mg
Dosage:	IV (not in the USA): 100–250 mg at 25 mg/min followed by infusion of 250 mg as a 0.1% solution over 1 h, 125 mg/h for 2 h, then 500 mg/min Oral: initial dose 200–400 mg, followed after 2 h by 200–250 mg every 8 h (every 12 h in hepatic or severe renal failure, HF, or acute Ml). Maximum dose 900 mg daily

Mexiletine is a primary amine that is fairly effective after IV and oral administration in the management of ventricular arrhythmias. Some studies indicate a lack of effectiveness and a high incidence of minor adverse effects *(37,38)*, but low proarrhythmic effects.

Actions

Mexiletine has class IB activity. EP effects are similar to those of lidocaine. There is no significant effect on LV contractility.

The drug has a relatively mild negative inotropic effect, and this is an advantage in patients with HF.

Pharmacokinetics

- Oral absorption is adequate.
- Peak plasma concentrations are achieved in 2–4 h.
- Half-life is 9–12 h and may be **prolonged to 19–26 h** in patients with HF, acute MI, and liver dysfunction.
- About 15% of the drug is excreted unchanged in the urine, so the dose interval is increased in severe renal impairment to avoid toxicity.
- Effective plasma concentrations: 0.75–2.0 mg/L (0.75–2 μg/mL or 3.5–9.3 μmol/L).

Advice, Adverse Effects, and Interactions

Hypotension, bradycardia and transient AV block, and precipitation of arrhythmias owing to proarrhythmic effect may occur. Mexiletine is lipophilic and enters the brain, so neurologic side effects are common, especially confusional state, tremor, diplopia, paresthesia, ataxia, and nystagmus. Side effects occur in up to 70% of patients *(39)*. Indigestion is common, but liver damage rarely occurs. Phenytoin and rifampin reduce plasma levels.

Contraindications. Severe LV failure, cardiogenic shock, hypotension, bradycardia, sinus node disease, AV block conduction defects, hepatic or severe renal failure, and epilepsy.

Drug name:	**Phenytoin; Diphenylhydantoin**
Trade name:	Epanutin
Supplied:	5-mL ampule, 50 mg/mL
Dosage:	*See* text

Dosage

IV: 3.5–5 mg/kg at a rate not exceeding 50 mg/min via caval catheter. Repeat after 10 min if required. Do not exceed a rate of 50 mg/min. **Maximum** of 500 mg in 1 h. **Maximum** dose 1 g in 24 h. Dilute in 0.9% NaCl. Flush the vein immediately with normal saline to avoid thrombosis. **Oral** 500 mg daily for 2 d, and then 300–400 mg daily. However, chronic administration is not recommended because of the drug's poor antiarrhythmic effect. The drug is not approved by the Food and Drug Administration for use as an antiarrhythmic.

Action and Pharmacokinetics

Phenytoin accelerates conduction by increasing the initial rapid phase of the action potential in Purkinje fibers. The drug also depresses phase 4 diastolic depolarization. The half-life of the drug is 24 h, and therapeutic plasma levels are 10–20 μg/mL (40–80 μmol/L). Reduce dosage in the presence of hepatic or renal disease.

Indications

The drug is no longer indicated in digitalis-induced arrhythmias. The drug is occasionally useful in the prolonged QT syndromes when beta-blockers are contraindicated, or it is occasionally combined with a beta-blocker. Indications are restricted because of the potential hazards of IV administration.

Advice, Adverse Effects, and Interactions

Well-known central nervous system effects, hypotension, HF, and, rarely, respiratory depression may occur. Note that the drug is supplied in 250-mg vials with diluent containing 40% propylene glycol with a pH of 11. The drug precipitates if mixed with an alkaline solution such as dextrose.

Contraindications. Complete heart block and HF. Do not administer concomitantly with dopamine or lidocaine.

Class IC

Drug name:	**Flecainide**
Trade name:	Tambocor
Supplied:	400, 600 mg (UK 100, 200 mg)
Dosage:	100 mg twice daily, increasing if needed to 200 mg twice daily, reducing the dose after 3–5 d if possible Elderly: 50 mg twice daily, max. 100 mg twice daily; reduce dose in renal or hepatic dysfunction

Action

The drug has class IC activity.

Pharmacokinetics

- Flecainide is well absorbed and is metabolized.
- The half-life is about 20 h; half-life is prolonged with renal failure. Therapeutic levels are 400–800 mg/mL.

Advice, Adverse Effects, and Interactions

The drug is effective in suppressing ventricular premature beats and nonsustained VT and blocks the accessory pathways in WPW syndrome. The drug is poorly effective against sustained VT, especially in patients with ventricular dysfunction. In this subset, the drug increases the frequency of sustained VT that is poorly tolerated and difficult or impossible to terminate even with prolonged resuscitation *(40)*. Flecainide is effective in the prevention of recurrent AVNRT and AVRT (*see* above) *(41,42)*. An overall efficacy for long-term control of PSVT (81% for AVNRT and 74% for AVRT) has been observed *(41)*. Another study indicated that flecainide was effective in 74% of cases of AVNRT and in 66% of AVRT *(42)*. The incidence of such serious drug-induced arrhythmia is about 20%. Among 588 patients, 33 developed new or worsened VT or VF, and there was difficulty resuscitating some patients. Other side effects include precipitation of or worsening HF, dizziness, and visual problems.

Contraindications. Patients with CHF or LV dysfunction, benign or potentially fatal ventricular arrhythmias.

Drug name:	**Propafenone**
Trade names:	Rythmol, Arythmol (UK)
Supplied:	150, 225, 300 mg
Dosage:	Oral: For patients > 70 kg, 150 mg three times daily after meals; lower dose in elderly or patients < 70 kg; increase if needed in 3–7 d to 300 mg two or three times daily IV (not in the USA): 2 mg/kg followed by an infusion of 2 mg/min Administer under hospital supervision with ECG monitoring and blood pressure assessment

The increase in mortality rate owing to flecainide observed in the CAST study has caused the drug to be removed from use for benign or potentially fatal ventricular arrhythmias. Flecainide is occasionally used for the prevention of atrial flutter or fibrillation or acute conversion, but **caution** is necessary because 1:1 conduction may occur as with quinidine if treatment with digoxin is not enforced *(2)*.

Action

This class IC drug blocks the fast sodium channel; membrane-stabilizing activity; prolongation of the PR interval owing to blocking at the AV node; prolongation of the PR and QRS intervals owing to prolonged ventricular conduction but with no effect on QT. The drug has additional mild beta-blocking effects *(43)*.

Pharmacokinetics

- The oral preparation is nearly completely absorbed but is subjected to extensive first-pass metabolism.

- Bioavailability ranges from 5% to 12% for the 150- and 300-mg tablets used in the United States.
- Peak plasma concentration is observed within 2–3 h of administration.
- The plasma half-life is 2–12 h, and about 95% of the drug is protein bound. Therapeutic plasma concentrations are highly variable: 0.2–3.0 μg/mL. Genetic variations in propafenone metabolism may explain the variable plasma half-life and poor circulation between plasma levels and therapeutic response *(43,44)*.

Advice, Adverse Effects, and Interactions

The drug is useful in the management of ventricular arrhythmias *(43.45–51)*. Suppression of ventricular arrhythmias has been documented in several studies *(43,45–51)*, but late proarrhythmic effects are unknown, as with other class IC agents. Propafenone is effective for some supraventricular arrhythmias, including WPW syndrome *(52,53)*. The drug has a low proarrhythmic effect. The incidence of proarrhythmias appears lower than observed with encainide or flecainide, but fatal VT has been reported *(54)*. Prolongation of the PR and QRS interval and conduction defects occur, as with other class IC agents *(55)*. Other side effects include dizziness, lightheadedness, disturbance of taste, nausea, constipation, and abdominal discomfort; rare hepatitis and lupus-like reactions have been reported *(56)*. Side effects occurred in about 33% of patients *(57)*. Single reports of granulocytopenia and agranulocytosis have occurred. The precipitation of TDP is rare, and the drug was capable of controlling two cases of torsades *(47)*.

Interactions. Propafenone may potentiate the effect of warfarin. Digoxin levels are increased from 35% at 450 mg propafenone daily to 85% at 900 mg daily. The negative inotropic effect of beta-blockers or calcium antagonists is additive. The drug must be used under strict supervision in combination with these agents. The drug has been combined with quinidine, procainamide, and amiodarone at reduced doses.

Contraindications

- The drug has a negative inotropic effect, precipitates HF *(57)*, and is contraindicated in patients with HF or severe impairment of ventricular function.
- Disease of the sinus node, AV or bundle branch block, severe bradycardia, marked hypotension, cardiogenic shock, severe chronic obstructive lung disease.
- Benign and potentially fatal ventricular arrhythmias similar for encainide and flecainide as influenced by the CAST study *(12)*.

Class II: Beta-Blockers

Action

From the EP standpoint, beta-blockers produce depression of phase 4 diastolic depolarization. Sympathetically mediated acceleration of impulses through the AV node are blocked, and beta-blockers are therefore effective in abolishing arrhythmias induced or exacerbated by increased catecholamine levels. There is a variable but often fairly potent effect on ventricular arrhythmias that may be abolished if they result from increased sympathetic activity such as may occur in myocardial ischemia and other situations. Beta-blockers cause a significant increase in VF threshold. Intravenous propranolol *(58)*, metoprolol, and timolol have been shown to reduce the incidence of VF during acute infarction. Beta-blockers and amiodarone are the only antiarrhythmics proved to reduce cardiac mortality. They suppress VT without complete suppression of VPCs. The frequency of VT was reduced by at least 75% in 8 of 17 patients receiving 50 mg atenolol daily *(59)*. The drug was more effective in suppressing VT than in suppressing ventricular ectopy *(59)*.

Drug name:	**Sotalol**
Trade names:	Betapace, Sotacor, Beta-Cardone (UK)
Supplied:	40, 80, 160 mg
Dosage:	40–80 mg once or twice daily; max. 240 mg, rarely 320 mg daily

Sotalol is a unique beta-blocker with additional class III activity. The drug is a more effective antiarrhythmic agent than other beta-blockers.

After DC cardioversion of AF, sotalol is as effective as quinidine in maintaining sinus rhythm and is better tolerated. In 98 patients with post-DC cardioversion of AF, sotalol 160–320 mg daily provided maintenance of sinus rhythm in 52%, and in 85 quinidine-treated patients sinus rhythm was maintained in 48% *(10)*. Twenty-six percent of the quinidine group and 11% of the sotalol group withdrew because of adverse effects.

Sotalol is useful for the management of paroxysmal AF (*see* earlier discussion of AF). The drug is not recommended for slowing the ventricular rate in patients with chronic AF because other beta-blockers have similar beneficial effects, but they do not carry the risk of TDP.

Sotalol is effective in suppressing ventricular couplets and frequent ventricular ectopy *(60)*. In a randomized study, a 99% reduction in ventricular couplets was achieved with sotalol and 49% with propranolol *(60)*.

In small nonrandomized studies with up to 18 mo of follow-up, sotalol therapy has caused reduction in the recurrence of sustained VT and VF *(16)*. In a study of 16 patients with recurrent sustained VT refractory to an average of 4.8 antiarrhythmic agents *(61)*, sotalol was effective at high dosage, 320–960 mg daily, in suppressing inducible sustained VT. Arrhythmias refractory to other antiarrhythmic agents including amiodarone have shown a beneficial response to sotalol administration *(16)*. Patients evaluated with noninvasive or invasive means exhibit efficacy with sotalol similar to that of those treated empirically. Thus, both sotalol and amiodarone can be used as empirical therapy in patients with life-threatening ventricular arrhythmias.

A head-to-head comparison of sotalol and amiodarone was carried out by the Amiodarone versus Sotalol Study Group *(62)*. This multicenter trial studied 59 patients with documented VT who had failed a class I agent. Patients were randomly assigned to amiodarone and sotalol. At 1-yr follow-up, there was no significant difference between the groups. Treatment failures (death, recurrent ventricular arrhythmias, and side effects) were similar (13 of 29 with sotalol and 14 of 30 with amiodarone). The author and the majority of cardiologists recommend sotalol rather than amiodarone as the first-choice class III agent for the management of life-threatening ventricular arrhythmias including after cardiac arrest.

In the Electro-Physiologic Study versus Electrocardiographic Monitoring (ESVEM) study *(63)*, sotalol was superior to six sodium channel-blocking antiarrhythmic agents. The actuarial probability of a recurrence of ventricular arrhythmia and the risk of death from any cause, from a cardiac cause, and from arrhythmia were significantly lower in patients treated with sotalol *(63)*. Sotalol should not be used with potassium-wasting diuretics or other agents that cause hypokalemia or prolong the QT interval because TDP may be precipitated. Torsades caused by sotalol do occur, albeit rarely, in the absence of hypokalemia. A case of torsades occurring in a patient with a serum potassium level of 4.0 mmol/L and therapeutic sotalol concentration, failing to respond to conventional therapy including electrical cardioversion 15 times during a 12-h period, responded within an hour of dialysis *(64)*.

The incidence of TDP is approx 2% and is similar to that observed with quinidine *(11)*. Of a total of 1288 patients treated with sotalol in controlled trials, 27 experienced TDP (2%) *(65)*.

Class III

Drug name:	**Amiodarone**
Trade names:	Cordarone, Cordarone X (UK)
Supplied:	Tablets: 200 mg; ampules: 150 mg
Dosage:	*See* text

Amiodarone is a benzofuran derivative that has two atoms of iodine and structural similarities to thyroxine (T_4) and triiodothyronine (T_3). The drug was originally developed in Belgium as a coronary vasodilator for the treatment of angina.

Dosage

IV (indicated only for recurring VF, unstable VT): 5 mg/kg over 2 h via a central line, maximum 1.2 g/24 h. Repeat if needed for 2 d, for life-threatening arrhythmias. Severe hypotension may occur with the IV preparation; this may be owing to its solvent. Oral: a low-dose regimen is used: 200 mg three times daily for 1 wk reduced to 200 mg twice daily for a further week or two, and then maintenance of 200 mg daily or the minimum dose required to control the arrhythmia after 4 wk. A 5 d/wk regimen may suffice in some. The total daily dose of drug should be lower in patients with HF. After 4 wk, aim for a serum level of 2 μg/mL amiodarone and 2 μg/mL of the active metabolite desethyl amiodarone *(66)*. Initial loading with IV amiodarone 5 mg/kg followed by oral dosing can shorten the time to optimal arrhythmic control *(67)*.

Action

Electrophysiologic and antiarrhythmic effects: oral administration of amiodarone lengthens the action potential duration and thus the ERP in all cardiac tissues including accessory pathways. The drug has been labeled a class III antiarrhythmic agent because of the aforementioned major action. Its effects, however, overlap those of other classes of antiarrhythmics, e.g., class IA. Amiodarone produces potent sodium channel blockade during phases 2 and 3 of the cardiac action potential. Thus, the drug depresses myocardial and His-Purkinje conduction.

The salutary antiarrhythmic effects are accompanied by a consistent lengthening of the QT interval *(66,68)*. The latter effect, if conspicuous, may arouse suspicion of imminent side effects such as precipitation of VF or TDP. EP studies do not consistently predict the drug's clinical effect on ventricular arrhythmias. Horowitz and colleagues *(69)* and others *(70,71)* noted a predictable effect.

Hemodynamic consequences are usually negligible. Vasodilation produces a mild decrease in systemic vascular resistance. There is a very mild negative inotropic effect, and in clinical practice the drug does not usually precipitate HF *(68–73)*, except in rare circumstances associated with cardiac slowing.

Pharmacokinetics

- Absorption from the gut is about 50%; bioavailability ranges from 22% to 86%. The drug undergoes extensive hepatic metabolism. Peak plasma levels are reached 6–8 h after an oral dose. The therapeutic effect is not well defined by plasma levels. However, after 4 wk of therapy, levels between 1.0 and 2.5 μg/mL appear to be associated with therapeutic effect and lowered toxicity.

- The volume of distribution is high (approx 5000 L). The drug is almost completely bound to protein and binds extensively with virtually all body tissues. The concentration in the myocardium is 10–15 times that in plasma, and the concentration in the liver, lung, and adipose tissue is much higher. Because of the large volume of distribution, the drug is preferably given as a loading dose when used orally, if prompt control of arrhythmia is required *(73)*.
- Rosenbaum and colleagues *(74)* have shown that, when the drug is administered orally, action depends on tissue stores and not on plasma levels. Others have demonstrated some relation between plasma levels and effect, and this measurement may be useful in guiding dosage.
- Half-life is 30–110 d. Therapeutic effect generally occurs within 10–15 d of oral therapy but may take 3–6 wk with the use of low loading doses. At high loading doses a response may be seen within 48 h. Activity persists for more than 50 d after stopping the drug.

Indications

The drug is used for the management of refractory life-threatening arrhythmias. In patients with fatal arrhythmias, recurrent cardiac arrest, and HF, amiodarone therapy is justifiable *(2,58)*. In the United Kingdom, but not in the United States, the drug is indicated for the management of patients with WPW syndrome who have life-threatening arrhythmias and is given IV in these situations.

The drug given IV via a central line is useful in the management of AF and VT *(76)* and is also beneficial with refractory VT caused by digitalis toxicity. IV administration has been shown to be useful in critically ill patients with VT-VF *(77)*, and the drug appears to be effective in over 66% of refractory cases of recurrent VT-VF *(78)*. A metaanalysis indicates that prophylactic amiodarone reduces the rate of sudden death in high-risk patients with recent MI or CHF with an overall reduction of 13% *(79)*.

Clinical studies of interest include the following:

1. In the Basel Antiarrhythmic Study of Infarct Survival (BASIS) during the 1-yr follow-up, there were only five deaths in the amiodarone-treated patients, 12 deaths in patients treated with class LA drugs, and 15 deaths in the control group ($p < 0.05$) *(80)*.
2. The Canadian and European Myocardial Amiodarone Trials (CAMIAT and EMIAT *[81]*) did not show significant mortality reduction with the administration of amiodarone. In the Canadian Implantable Defibrillation Study (CIDS), the ICD surprisingly failed to demonstrate a significant survival benefit over amiodarone; at 3 yr, 60% of ICD patients were receiving a beta-blocker compared with 25% for amiodarone (*see* Suggested Reading).
3. In the CASCADE study, amiodarone-treated patients who had survived an episode of VF in the absence of acute MI showed improved survival *(15)*.
4. The Cardiac Arrest Study Hamburg (CASH) in patients following cardiac arrest has shown the ICD to be superior to amiodarone. After 2 yr of follow-up, there was a 37% reduction in overall mortality rate among patients assigned to ICD compared with drug therapy; metoprolol, however, was as good as amiodarone in decreasing the mortality rate for up to 2 yr following cardiac arrest.

Advice, Adverse Effects, and Interactions

1. Corneal microdeposits of yellow-brown granules occur in 50–100% during long-term therapy. They do not affect vision, are reversible on discontinuing the drug, and constitute clinical evidence of the drug's impregnation. Periodic eye examinations are recommended

during long-term use. There is some evidence that the deposits can be diminished by withdrawal of therapy for 1–2 wk or by ophthalmic drops containing sodium-iodine heparinate; optic neuritis and blindness have been reported.

2. Rashes, especially photosensitivity; permanent grayish blue discoloration of the skin occurs in over 10% of patients after approx 18 mo of high-dose therapy but is rare with current low-dose regimens. On discontinuing amiodarone, the discoloration regresses. Patients should be advised to use a sunscreen and to shield their skin from light.
3. Mild bradycardia, but rare precipitation of severe brady-arrhythmia in patients with sick sinus syndrome, may occur. Asystole and sinus arrest have occurred in patients with therapeutic serum concentrations of amiodarone.
4. Precipitation of TDP is rare and occurs mainly in patients with hypokalemia and with drugs that prolong the QT interval. Amiodarone has been used successfully to treat TDP *(82)* but cannot be recommended as first-line *(83)* or second-line treatment.
5. Pulmonary infiltrates and pulmonary fibrosis occur in 5–20% of patients receiving chronic doses, 400–800 mg/d *(84,85)*. Pulmonary toxicity occurred in 6% of 145 patients given an average dose of 845 mg for 2 wk, and then an average of 410 mg daily for 18 mo *(86)*, but the incidence is <1% with the low dosage advised earlier in this chapter *(2)*. Periodic pulmonary function tests, in particular diffusion capacity (DCO), reveal early cases. Discontinuation of amiodarone and steroid therapy causes regression of pulmonary complications in some patients.
6. Hypothyroidism or hyperthyroidism occurs in about 3–7% of patients. The T_4 concentration is mildly raised, the T_3 level is very mildly decreased, and there is a marked rise in reverse T_3 levels in patients without clinical thyroid disturbance.
7. Proximal muscle weakness and neurologic problems, especially ataxia, are not uncommon.
8. Gastrointestinal symptoms and increase in transaminase levels are seen (10–20%). Hepatitis is rare. After 5 yr of amiodarone therapy, approx 50% of adult patients *(87)* and treated children *(88)* are observed to be continuing successfully on the drug.
9. **Drug interaction** with anticoagulants has been well documented. Amiodarone potentiates the actions of oral anticoagulants, and the combination may lead to serious bleeding *(89)*. The maintenance dose of warfarin should be halved when amiodarone and warfarin are used together. There is evidence that amiodarone increases plasma **quinidine** levels. The combination of these two agents, both of which tend to prolong the QT interval, is not recommended. A significant interaction between amiodarone and digoxin occurs. Serum digoxin concentration usually doubles, but ventricular dysrhythmias are suppressed by amiodarone. Halve the dose of digoxin when the two drugs are given together. The combination of amiodarone and verapamil or diltiazem should be avoided because severe depression of SA and AV nodes may occur. Interactions have been noted with flecainide, phenytoin, and theophylline.

   Drugs that prolong the QT interval should not be combined with amiodarone: sotalol, class IA antiarrhythmics, tricyclic antidepressants, and phenothiazines.

   Caution: Potassium-losing diuretics must not be given concomitantly, as torsades may be precipitated.

A 5-yr follow-up of 242 amiodarone-treated patients *(90)* revealed the following: 59% adverse effects and withdrawal in 26%; 25% discontinued the drug. Few patients tolerated the drug on a long-term basis. In addition, blindness appears to be a rare but alarming adverse effect. Before commencing amiodarone, the physician must be aware of the amiodarone withdrawal problem *(73)* If the drug is discontinued because of a serious side effect, the effect may persist for months. Also, other antiarrhythmics then used may interact with amiodarone.

Bradyarrhythmias

Bradyarrhythmias that cause hemodynamic disturbances and are symptomatic or life-threatening and unresponsive to optimal doses of atropine require pacing.

Update: a recent study indicates that statin therapy may decrease the risk of atrial fibrillation; this would be a remarkable advance, if proved to prevent some cases of the most common and serious arrhythmias observed in clinical practice.

REFERENCES

1. Vaughan Williams EM. Classification of antiarrhythmic drugs. In: Sandhoe E, Flensted-Jensen E, Olesen KH (eds). Symposium on Cardiac Arrhythmias. Sodertalje, Sweden, AB Astra, 1970, p 449.
2. Task Force of the Working Group on Arrhythmias of the European Society of Cardiology. The Sicilian Gambit. A new approach to the classification of antiarrhythmic drugs based on their actions on arrhythmogenic mechanisms. Circulation 1991;4:1831.
3. Khan M Gabriel. Arrhythmias. In: Heart Disease, Diagnosis and Therapy. Totowa, NJ, Humana Press, 2005.
4. Steurer G, Gursoi S, Frey B, et al. Differential diagnosis on the electrocardiogram between ventricular tachycardia and preexcited tachycardia. Clin Cardiol 1994;17:306.
5. DiMarco JP, Miles W, Akhtar M. Adenosine for paroxysmal supraventricular tachycardia: Dose ranging and comparison with verapamil. Assessment in placebo-controlled, multicenter trials. Ann Intern Med 1990;113:104.
6. Rankin AC, McGovern BA. Adenosine or verapamil for the acute treatment of supraventricular tachycardia? Ann Intern Med 1991;114:513.
7. Delacrétaz E. Supraventricular tachycardia. N Engl J Med 2006;354:1039–1051.
8. Jaeggi E, Chiu C, Hamilton R, et al. Adenosine induced atrial pro arrhythmia in children. Can J Cardiol 1999;15:169.
9. Alboni P, Tomasi C, Menozzi C, et al. Efficacy and safety of out-of-hospital self-administered single-dose oral drug treatment in the management of infrequent, well-tolerated paroxysmal supraventricular tachycardia. J Am Coll Cardiol 2001;37:548–553.
10. Murray KT. Ibutilide. Circulation 1998;97:493.
11. Opolski G, Torbicki A, Kosior DA, et al. Rate control vs rhythm control in patients with nonvalvular persistent atrial fibrillation: the results of the Polish How to Treat Chronic Atrial Fibrillation (HOT CAFE) Study. Chest 2004;126:476–486.
12. Wyse DG, Waldo AL, DiMarco JP, et al. Atrial Fibrillation Follow-up Investigation of Rhythm Management (AFFIRM) Investigators. A comparison of rate control and rhythm control in patients with atrial fibrillation. N Engl J Med 2002;347:1825–1833.
13. Ruskin JN. The cardiac arrhythmia suppression trial (CAST). N Engl J Med 1989;321:385.
14. Bigger JT. Definition of benign versus malignant ventricular arrhythmias: Targets for treatment. Am J Cardiol 1983;52:47C.
15. Green HL, for the CASCADE Investigators. The CASCADE study: Randomized antiarrhythmic drug therapy in survivors of cardiac arrest in Seattle. Am J Cardiol 1993;72:70F.
16. Nora M, Zipes DP. Empiric use of amiodarone and sotalol. Am J Cardiol 1993;72:62F.
17. Buxton AE, Marchlinski FE, Flores BT, et al. Non-sustained ventricular tachycardia in patients with coronary artery disease: Role of electro-physiological study. Circulation 1986;75:1178.
18. Josephson ME. Treatment of ventricular arrhythmias after myocardial infarction. Circulation 1986;74:653.
19. Smith WM, Gallagher JJ. “Les torsades de pointes”: An unusual ventricular arrhythmia. Ann Intern Med 1980;93:578.
20. Stratmann HG, Kennedy HL. Torsades de pointes associated with drugs and toxins: Recognition and management. Am Heart J 1987;113:1470.
21. Lazzara R. Amiodarone and torsades de pointes. Ann Intern Med 1989;111:549.
22. Mattioni TA, Zheutlin TA, Sarmiento JJ, et al. Amiodarone in patients with previous drug-mediated torsade de pointes. Ann Intern Med 1989;111:574.
23. Rankin AC, Pringle SD, Cobe SM. Acute treatment of torsades de pointes with amiodarone: Proarrhythmic and antiarrhythmic association of QT prolongation. Am Heart J 1990;19:185.
24. Tzivoni D, Banai S, Schuger C, et al. Magnesium sulfate therapy for sustained monomorphic ventricular tachycardia. Circulation 1988;77:392.

25. Allen BJ, Brodsky MA, Capparelli EV, et al. Magnesium sulfate therapy for sustained monomorphic ventricular tachycardia. Am J Cardiol 1989;64:1202.
26. Ben-David J, Zipes DP. Torsades de pointes and proarrhythmia. Lancet 1993;341:1578.
27. Leenhardt A, Glasser E, Burguera M, et al. Short-coupled variant of torsade depointes: A new electrocardiographic entity in the spectrum of idiopathic ventricular tachyarrhythmias. Circulation 1994;89:206.
28. Cohn IS, Jick H, Cohen SI. Adverse reactions to quinidine in hospitalized patients: Findings based on data from the Boston Collaborative Drug Surveillance Program. Prog Cardiovasc Dis 1977;20:151.
29. Grace AA, Camm AJ. Drug therapy. Quinidine. N Engl J Med 1998;338:35.
30. Bauman JL, Beuerfeind RA, Hoff JV, et al. Torsades de pointes due to quinidine: Observations in 31 patients. Am Heart J 1984;107:425.
31. Ruskin JN, McGovern B, Garan H, et al. Antiarrhythmic drugs: A possible cause of out-of-hospital cardiac arrest. N Engl J Med 1983;309:1302.
32. Huang SK, Marcus FI. Antiarrhythmic drug therapy of ventricular arrhythmias. Curr Prob Cardiol 1986; 11:179.
33. Ellrodt AG, Murata GH, Riedinger MS, et al. Severe neutropenia associated with sustained release procainamide. Ann Intern Med 1984;100:197.
34. MacMahon S, Collins, R, Peto R, et al. Effects of prophylactic lidocaine in suspected acute myocardial infarction. JAMA 1988;260:1910.
35. Koster RW, Dunning AJ. Intramuscular lidocaine for prevention of lethal arrhythmias in the prehospitalization phase of acute myocardial infarction. N Engl J Med 1985;313:1105.
36. Rotmensch HH, Elkayam U, Frishman W. Antiarrhythmic drug therapy during pregnancy. Ann Intern Med 1983;98:487.
37. Palileo EV, Welsch W, Hoff J, et al. Lack of effectiveness of oral mexiletine in patients with drug-refractory paroxysmal sustained ventricular tachycardia. Am J Cardiol 1982;50:1075.
38. Poole JE, Werner JA, Brady GH, et al. Intolerance and ineffectiveness of mexiletine in patients with serious ventricular arrhythmias. Am Heart J 1986;112:322.
39. Campbell RWF. Medical intelligence: drug therapy, mexiletine. N Engl J Med 1987;316:29.
40. Roden DM, Woosley RL. Drug therapy: Flecainide. N Engl J Med 1986;315:36.
41. Anderson JL, Jolivette DM, Fredell PA. Summary of efficacy and safety of flecainide for supraventricular arrhythmias. Am J Cardiol 1988;62:62D.
42. Benditt DG, Dunnigan A, Buetikofer J, et al. Flecainide acetate for long-term prevention of PSVT. Circulation 1991;83:345.
43. Siddoway LA, Roden DM, Woosley RL. Clinical pharmacology of propafenone. Pharmacokinetics, metabolism and concentration-response relations. Am J Cardiol 1984;54:9D.
44. Siddoway LA, Thompson KA, McAllister BC, et al. Polymorphism of propafenone metabolism and disposition in man: Clinical and pharmacokinetic consequences. Circulation 1987;75:785.
45. Prystowsky EN, Heger JJ, Chilson DA, et al. Antiarrhythmic and electrophysiologic effects of oral propafenone. Am J Cardiol 1984;54:26D.
46. Naccarella F, Bracchetti D, Palmieri M, et al. Propafenone for refractory ventricular arrhythmias: Correlation with drug plasma levels during long-term treatment. Am J Cardiol 1984;54:1008.
47. Conmel P, Leclercq J, Assayag P. European experience with the antiarrhythmic efficacy of propafenone for supraventricular and ventricular arrhythmias. Am J Cardiol 1984;54:60D.
48. Heger JJ, Hubbard J, Zipes D, et al. Propafenone treatment of recurrent ventricular tachycardia: Comparison of continuous electrocardiographic recording and electrophysiologic study in predicting drug efficacy. Am J Cardiol 1984;54:40D.
49. Chilson DA, Heger JJ, Zipes DP, et al. Electrophysiologic effects and clinical efficacy of oral propafenone therapy in patients with ventricular tachycardia. J Am Coll Cardiol 1985;5:1407.
50. Podrid JP, Lown B. Propafenone: A new agent for ventricular arrhythmia. J Am Coll Cardiol 1984;4:117.
51. Naccarella F, Bracchetti D, Palmieri M, et al. Comparison of propafenone and disopyramide for treatment of chronic ventricular arrhythmias: Placebo-controlled, double-blind randomized crossover study. Am Heart J 1985;109:833.
52. Breithardt G, Borggrefe M, Wiebringhaus E, et al. Effects of propafenone in the Wolff-Parkinson-White syndrome: Electrophysiologic findings and long-term follow-up. Am J Cardiol 1984;54:29D.
53. Ludmer PL, McGowan NE, Antman EM, et al. Efficacy of propafenone in Wolff- Parkinson-White syndrome: Electrophysiologic findings and long term follow-up. J Am Coll Cardiol 1987;9:1357.
54. Nathan AW, Bexton RS, Hellestrand KG, Camm AJ. Fatal ventricular tachycardia in association with propafenone, a new class IC antiarrhythmic agent. Postgrad Med J 1984;60:155.

55. Hodges M, Salerno D, Granrud G. Double-blind placebo-controlled evaluation of propafenone in suppressing ventricular ectopic activity. Am J Cardiol 1984;54:45D.
56. Guindo J, De La Serna AR, Borja J, et al. Propafenone and a syndrome of lupus erythematosus type. Ann Intern Med 1986;104:589.
57. Podrid PH, Cytryn R, Lown B. Propafenone noninvasive evaluation of efficacy. Am J Cardiol 1984; 54:53.
58. Norris RM, Barnaby PF, Brown MA, et al. Prevention of ventricular fibrillation during acute myocardial infarction by intravenous propranolol. Lancet 1984;2:883.
59. Fenster PE, Reynolds D, Horowitz LD, et al. Atenolol for ventricular ectopy: A dose response study. Clin Pharmacol Ther 1987;41:118.
60. Kubac G, Klinke WP, Grace M. Randomized double blind trial comparing sotalol and propranolol in chronic ventricular arrhythmia. Can J Cardiol 1988;4:355.
61. Singh SN, Cohen A, Chen Y, et al. Sotalol for refractory sustained ventricular tachycardia and nonfatal cardiac arrest. Am J Cardiol 1988;62:399.
62. Amiodarone vs. Sotalol Study Group. Multi-centre randomized trial of sotalol vs. amiodarone for chronic malignant ventricular tachyarrhythmias. Eur Heart J 1989;10:685.
63. Mason JW, on behalf of the ESVEM investigators. A comparison of 7 anti-arrhythmic drugs in patients with ventricular tachyarrhythmia. N Engl J Med 1993;329:452.
64. Singh SN, Lazin A, Cohen A, et al. Sotalol-induced torsades de pointes successfully treated with hemodialysis after failure of conventional therapy. Am Heart J 1991;121:601.
65. Soyka LF, Wirtz C, Spangenberg RB. Clinical safety profile of sotalol in patients with arrhythmias. Am J Cardiol 1990;65(Suppl):74A.
66. Somberg JC. Antiarrhythmic drags: Making sense of the deluge. Am Heart J 1987;113:408.
67. Kerin NZ, Blevins RD, Frumin H, et al. Intravenous and oral loading versus oral loading alone with amiodarone for chronic refractory ventricular arrhythmias. Am J Cardiol 1985;55:89.
68. Nademanee K, Singh BN, Hendrickson J, et al. Amiodarone in refractory life-threatening ventricular arrhythmias. Ann Intern Med 1983;98:577.
69. Horowitz LN, Greenspan AM, Spielman SR, et al. Usefulness of electrophysiologic testing in evaluation of amiodarone therapy for sustained ventricular tachyarrhythmias associated with coronary heart disease. Am J Cardiol 1985;55:367.
70. Naccarelli GV, Fineberg NS, Zipes DP, et al. Amiodarone: Risk factors for recurrence of symptomatic ventricular tachycardia identified at electrophysiologic study. J Am Coll Cardiol 1985;6:814.
71. McGovern B, Hasan G, Malacoff RF, et al. Long-term clinical outcome of ventricular tachycardia or fibrillation treated with amiodarone. Am J Cardiol 1984;53:1558.
72. Kaski JC, Girotti LA, Messuti H, et al. Long-term management of sustained, recurrent, symptomatic ventricular tachycardia with amiodarone. Circulation 1981;64:273.
73. Mason JW. Drug therapy: Amiodarone. N Engl J Med 1987;316:455.
74. Rosenbaum MB, Chiale PA, Halpern MS, et al. Clinical efficacy of amiodarone as an antiarrhythmic agent. Am J Cardiol 1976;38:934.
75. Nademandee K, Hendrickson JA, Cannon DS, et al. Control of refractory life threatening ventricular tachyarrhythmias by amiodarone. Am Heart J 1981;101:759.
76. Hohnloser SH, Meinertiz T, Dammbacher T, et al. Electrocardiographic and antiarrhythmic effects of intravenous amiodarone: Results of a prospective, placebo-controlled study. Am Heart J 1991;91:89.
77. Ochi RP, Goldenberg IF, Airnquist A, et al. Intravenous amiodarone for the rapid treatment of life-threatening ventricular arrhythmias in critically ill patients with coronary artery disease. Am J Cardiol 1989;64: 599.
78. Weiss JJ, Nademanee K, Stevenson WG, et al. Ventricular arrhythmias in ischemic heart disease. Ann Intern Med 1991;114:784.
79. Amiodarone Trials Meta-Analysis Investigators. Effect of prophylactic amiodarone on mortality after acute myocardial infarction and in congestive heart failure: Meta-analysis of individual data from 6500 patients in randomised trials. Lancet 1997;350:1417.
80. Burkhart F, Pfisterer M, Kiowski W, et al. Effect of antiarrhythmic therapy on mortality in survivors of myocardial infarction with asymptomatic complex ventricular arrhythmias: Basel Antiarrhythmic Study of Infarct Survival (BASIS). J Am Coll Cardiol 1990;16:1711.
81. Julian DG, Camm AJ, Frangin G, et al. Randomised trial of effect of amiodarone on mortality in patients with left ventricular dysfunction after recent myocardial infarction: EMIAT. Lancet 1997;349:667.
82. Rankin AC, Pringle SD, Cobbe SM. Acute treatment of torsades de pointes with amiodarone proarrhythmic and antiarrhythmic association of QT prolongation. Am Heart J 1990;119:185.

83. Rankin AC, Pringle SD, Cobbe SM, et al. Amiodarone and torsades de pointes. Am Heart J 1990;120: 1482.
84. Morady F, Sauve MJ, Malone P, et al. Long-term efficacy and toxicity of high-dose amiodarone therapy for ventricular tachycardia or ventricular fibrillation. Am J Cardiol 1983;52:975.
85. Marchlinski FE, Gansher TS, Waxman HL, et al. Amiodarone pulmonary toxicity. Ann Intern Med 1982; 98:839.
86. Myers M, Peter T, Weiss D, et al. Benefit and risks of long-term amiodarone therapy for sustained ventricular tachycardia/fibrillation: Minimum of three-year follow-up in 145 patients. Am Heart J 1990;119:8.
87. Herre JM, Sauve MJ, Malone P, et al. Long-term results of amiodarone therapy in patients with recurrent sustained ventricular tachycardia or ventricular fibrillation. J Am Coll Cardiol 1989;13:442.
88. Guccione P, Paul T, Garson A. Long-term follow-up of amiodarone therapy in the young: Continued efficacy, unimpaired growth, moderate side effects. J Am Coll Cardiol 1990;15:1118.
89. Hamer A, Peter T, Mandel WJ, et al. The potentiation of warfarin anti-coagulation by amiodarone. Circulation 1982;65:1025.
90. Smith WM, Lubbe WF, Whitlock RM, et al. Long-term tolerance of amiodarone treatment for cardiac arrhythmias. Am J Cardiol 1986;57:1288.

SUGGESTED READING

Alboni P, Tomasi C, Menozzi C, et al. Efficacy and safety of out-of-hospital self-administered single-dose oral drug treatment in the management of infrequent, well-tolerated paroxysmal supraventricular tachycardia. J Am Coll Cardiol 2001;37:548–553.

15 Cardiac Arrest

Approximately a quarter million individuals die suddenly from cardiac arrest (CA) in the United States each year before they reach a hospital *(1)*. It is relevant that approx 50% of patients with ventricular fibrillation (VF) survive cardiopulmonary resuscitation (CPR) versus <10% for other rhythms, represented by asystole and pulseless electrical activity (PEA). The incidence of VF in most surveys of CA is approx 50%. Thus immediate defibrillation remains the mainstay of therapy for CA, and this concept is endorsed by the American Heart Association (AHA) 2005 guidelines *(2–4)*.

There are only two cardiac arrest rhythms *(2–5)*:

1. Ventricular fibrillation/pulseless ventricular tachycardia (VF/VT). VF is defined as a pulseless chaotic disorganized rhythm with an undulating irregular pattern that varies in size and shape and a ventricular waveform > 150/min.
2. Non-VF/VT: asystole and PEA.

Always assume VF or pulseless VT *(6)*, as indicated above.

Individuals who can be saved from cardiac arrest are usually in VF or pulseless VT; thus, the earliest possible delivery of defibrillation is the single most effective intervention necessary to save victims of sudden cardiac death *(7,8)*.

The widespread distribution of automatic external defibrillators (AEDs) will help to accomplish early defibrillation programs. The endorsement of this policy by the Emergency Cardiac Care Committee of the AHA as part of the "Chain of Survival Concept" will do much for the development of more efficient resuscitative teams in the United States and, it is hoped, all countries where the incidence of sudden cardiac death is high. The AHA endorses the position that all first-responding emergency personnel, both hospital and nonhospital (e.g., physicians, nurses, emergency medical technicians, paramedics, firefighters, volunteer emergency personnel) be trained and permitted to operate a defibrillator, which should be readily available in all emergency ambulances or emergency vehicles that engage in the care of and transit of cardiac patients *(8)*. Modern biphasic defibrillators have a high first-shock efficacy in more than 90% *(9,10)*; thus, VF is usually eliminated with one shock of 360 joules with biphasic or monophasic defibrillators; the latter are being phased out.

In a study of 168 consecutive cases of sudden coronary death (within 6 h of onset of symptoms), Davies *(11)* showed that 74% had a recent coronary thrombotic lesion. These patients had warning chest pain prior to arrest. In 52 patients without chest pain or infarction, 48% had coronary thrombi. In patients with previous infarction, the absence of warning chest pain before arrest selects for a primary arrhythmia caused by preexisting hypertrophy or scarring, or both. In a study of successfully resuscitated cardiac arrest victims, 40 of 84 (48%) had coronary artery occlusion on angiography; successful angioplasty was achieved in 28 of 37 of these patients *(12)*. Cardiac deaths in young athletes

From: *Contemporary Cardiology: Cardiac Drug Therapy, Seventh Edition*
M. Gabriel Khan © Humana Press Inc., Totowa, NJ

are usually caused by hypertrophic cardiomyopathy *(13)* (35%) and anomalous origin of the left main coronary artery from the right sinus of Valsalva (20%). Other conditions causing sudden cardiac death include prolonged QT syndrome; right bundle branch block and ST segment elevation in leads V_1 to V_3 have been shown to be a marker for sudden death in patients without structural heart disease.

The 2005 AHA Guidelines for CPR emphasize the following ***(2–4)*****:**

- There were insufficient data to recommend CPR before defibrillation for all victims of VF CA.
- Lay rescuers should use the AED as soon as it is available.
- In the first minutes of VF CA, ventilation is not as important as chest compressions. Rescuers should push hard, push fast, allow full chest recoil, minimize interruptions in compressions, and defibrillate promptly when appropriate *(2)*.
- A 30:2 ratio is recommended to simplify training in one-rescuer or two-rescuer CPR for adults and all lay rescuer resuscitation. The combination of inadequate and interrupted chest compressions and excessive ventilation rates reduces cardiac output and coronary and cerebral blood flow and diminishes the likelihood of a successful resuscitation attempt *(2–4)*.
- *For infants and children asphyxial arrest* is usually the cause of CA. Thus a compression-ventilation ratio of 15:2 is recommended for two-rescuer CPR. This will result in the delivery of more rescue breaths for combating asphyxia.
- When multiple rescuers are present, one rescuer can perform CPR while the other readies the defibrillator, thereby providing both immediate CPR and early defibrillation.
- A change from a three-shock sequence to one shock followed immediately by CPR.
- The consensus recommendation for initial and subsequent monophasic waveform doses is 360 joules.
- Modern biphasic defibrillators have a high first-shock efficacy (defined as termination of VF for at least 5 s after the shock), averaging more than 90% *(9,10)*, so that VF is likely to be eliminated with one shock.
- Following defibrillation, rescuers should not interrupt chest compressions to check circulation (e.g., evaluate rhythm or pulse) until after approximately 2 min of CPR.
- In the **Emergency Cardiovascular Care (ECC) Guidelines 2000**, pulse and rhythm checks were recommended after each shock. These recommendations contributed to prolonged interruptions in chest compressions. To minimize these interruptions in chest compressions:
- The **2005 AHA Guidelines for CPR and ECC** recommend that rescuers resume CPR beginning with chest compressions *immediately* after a shock, without an intervening rhythm (or pulse) check *(2–4)*. Perhaps it is more logical after a 30:2 cycle to verify the rhythm, because if it is VF, defibrillation should proceed following the 30:2 cycle. If a rhythm other than sinus rhythm is restored, do not assess the pulse; instead, start compressions immediately.

LIFE-SAVING PROCEDURES

Responsiveness

Check responsiveness. If the patient is unresponsive, commence a strategy of CAB (instead of the old ABC method), as follows:

- C = circulation.
- A = airway.
- B = breathing.
- The CAB concept was used in some parts of Europe over the past two decades and was described in the first edition of *Cardiac Drug Therapy* (1984).

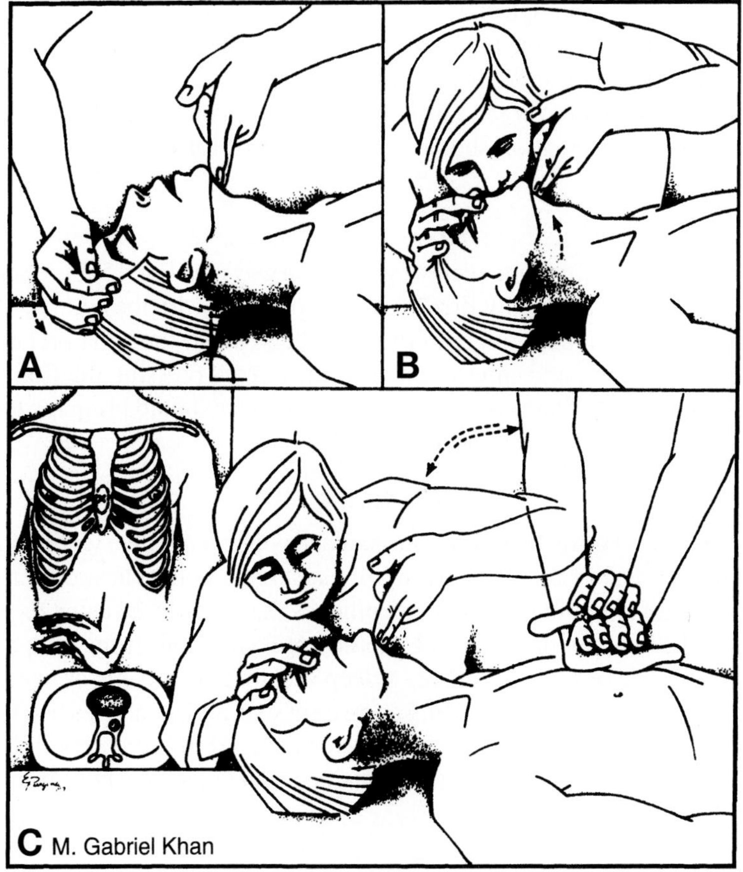

Fig. 15-1. Basic life support.

Circulation

External chest compression is instituted to provide a circulation as soon as possible. The new AHA guidelines *(2–4)* emphasize:

- In the first minutes of VF CA, ventilation does not appear to be as important as chest compressions.
- A 30:2 ratio is recommended to simplify training in one-rescuer or two-rescuer CPR for adults and all lay rescuer resuscitation.
- The combination of inadequate and interrupted chest compressions and excessive ventilation rates reduces cardiac output and coronary and cerebral blood flow and diminishes the likelihood of a successful resuscitation attempt.

Place the heel of one hand over the lower half of the sternum but at least 1½ inches (two finger-breadths) away from the base of the xiphoid process. The heel of the second hand is positioned on the dorsum of the first, both heels being parallel. The fingers are kept off the rib cage (*see* Fig. 15-1). If the hands are applied too high, ineffective chest compression may result, and fractured ribs are more common with this hand position.

The arms are kept straight at the elbow (locked elbows), and pressure is applied as vertically as possible. The resuscitator's shoulders should be directly above the victim's sternum. The rescuer should compress in the center of the chest at the nipple line.

Chest compressions are straight down and thus easily carried out by forceful movements of the shoulders and back, so the maneuver is less tiring. The sternum is depressed 1½–2 inches toward the spine using the heel of both hands.

CPR should never be interrupted for more than 5 s. This interval should be sufficient to allow defibrillation. Cessation should not exceed 30 s for endotracheal intubation.

Airway

Open the airway.

Use the head-tilt/chin-lift maneuver to open the airway (*see* Fig. 15-1). Place one hand on the victim's forehead and apply firm backward pressure with the palm to tilt the head back. Put the index and middle finger of the other hand under the bony part of the lower jaw. Lift the chin forward and support the jaw, thus avoid pressing the fingers into the soft tissue under the chin. The head-tilt/chin-lift maneuver should bring the teeth almost together and maintain dentures in position *(14)*.

Breathing

Assessment—determine breathlessness: place your ear over the victim's mouth and nose. If you do not hear or feel the flow of air escaping and the chest does not rise and fall, the victim is not breathing. The rescuer pinches the nose closed using the thumb and index finger of the hand on the forehead, thereby preventing air from escaping through the victim's nose. The rescuer then takes a deep breath and seals his or her lips around the outside of the victim's mouth, creating an airtight seal, and then gives two full breaths, allowing the chest to deflate totally between each breath. From 1 to 1½ seconds per breath should be allowed to provide good chest expansion and decrease the possibility of gastric distension *(14)*.

The Precordial Thump

The beneficial effects of the precordial thump have been supported by a clinical study *(14)*. The thump is utilized in specific monitored situations *(15)*:

The thump is likely to restore normal rhythm only if delivered within 30 s of the onset of the arrhythmia. Thus use only for witnessed sudden cardiac arrest (SCA).

- Patients with monitored VF.
- The thump if properly applied immediately in patients with pulseless VT may cause cardioversion and may be tried in a monitored arrest if a defibrillator is not immediately available.
- Ventricular asystole due to heart block. (A thump may, rarely, produce a QRS complex.) Thus, a thump may be tried during preparation for pacing.
- In witnessed cardiac arrests within 30 s, if a monitor and/or defibrillator is unavailable. Nothing is lost, and gain may ensue *(15)*.
- In patients with VT who have a pulse (i.e., not a cardiac arrest): if the trial of a cough is ineffective, a thump may be utilized but only if a defibrillator is available; a thump can induce VF or standstill.

During cardiac arrest, the first thump may stop an episode of VT or VF, *but the next thump may produce ventricular standstill.* Assume VF or pulseless VT; **therefore use only one thump**.

Thump Technique

Commence with the fist held about 10 inches above the sternum and deliver a sharp firm blow directed at a point two-thirds of the way down the sternum *(15)*. Use the lower fleshy portion of the fist. A precordial thump was considered a class I recommendation by the International Liason Committee on Resuscitation (ILCOR), but the AHA considers the thump an optional technique in a monitored arrest.

Oxygen

Supplemental oxygen at 100% concentration is given as soon as possible through a bag-valve mask or endotracheal tube. Note that oxygen by nasal prongs attains an oxygen concentration of only 24–40% with a flow rate of 6 L/min. Plastic face masks can provide 50–60% oxygen with an oxygen flow rate of 10 L/min.

Defibrillation

The following points need to be borne in mind for successful defibrillation:

1. Defibrillation should be accomplished as quickly as possible.
2. Paddle placement should be as follows: One paddle electrode is positioned to the right of the upper sternum below the clavicle (right second intercostal space). The other paddle is placed to the left of the left nipple with the center of the electrode in the midaxillary line. In the United Kingdom, the latter paddle is placed over the points designated as V_4 and V_5 for the electrocardiogram—a little outside the position of the normal apex beat. The paddle should be placed at least 5 inches away from a pacemaker generator.
3. An appropriate gel (i.e., one known to have a low impedance) should be used. Jelly tends to spread during chest compression, and subsequent shocks may arc across the chest surface. Conducting gel pads are preferred to jelly but should be removed between shocks.
4. Heavy arm pressure must be applied on each paddle.
5. Defibrillation should take place when the victim's phase of ventilation is in full expiration.
6. **Energy setting:**
   AHA panel and ILCOR recommendations:
   - First shock 360 joules.
   - Subsequent shocks: 360 joules.
7. Both paddle buttons should be discharged simultaneously.

A review article by Eisenberg and Mengert *(16)* emphasized some common errors in CPR:

- Defibrillation errors: Synchronized mode is accidentally selected before defibrillation is attempted; thus no shock is delivered.
- The operator believes that lead I, II, or III is being displayed when in fact the selection is set to paddles and asystole is falsely displayed.
- Considerable chest hair should be shaved off where the paddles are to be placed, and smeared gel across the chest should be toweled off.

Procedure for Defibrillation*

Defibrillation should be accomplished at the earliest opportunity when VF is present. Nonsynchronized countershock is also indicated for the treatment of VT in an unconscious patient with no effective circulation when preparation for synchronized cardioversion may cause an unnecessary delay.

The following is a protocol for appropriate use of defibrillation in an arrest situation.

---

1. **Initiate basic life support (BLS) and summon defibrillation equipment and assistance.** If a properly prepared defibrillator is immediately available in a monitored situation, defibrillation should be performed at once prior to initiation of BLS, unless a precordial thump has been successful in restoring an effective rhythm and cardiac output.
2. **Delegate BLS responsibilities to qualified assistants, but monitor the effectiveness.** Continuity of effective BLS cannot be overemphasized. If adequate help is available, an intravenous (IV) lifeline should be started at this time and supplemental oxygen administered.
3. **Evaluate cardiac rhythm.** Turn on monitor power, apply conductive medium to paddles, and evaluate rhythm with the quick-look paddles. Continuous monitoring using patient leads should be initiated when possible without interruption of the resuscitation effort.
4. **If VF is present:** The following steps should be accomplished, interrupting BLS as briefly as possible:
   a. Apply additional conductive medium to paddles if needed.
   b. Turn on defibrillator power (be certain defibrillator is not in synchronous mode).
   c. Select energy and charge the capacitor.
   d. Properly place paddles on the chest with a slight twist to distribute the conductive medium.
   e. Recheck rhythm on monitor.
   f. Clear area and check that no personnel are directly or indirectly in contact with the patient. The operator must ensure that he or she is not touching the patient when the shock is delivered.
   g. Apply firm arm pressure (approximately 10 kg or 25 lb) on each paddle with a squeezing action. (Do not lean on paddles—they may slip.)
   h. Deliver countershock by depressing both paddle discharge buttons simultaneously. (If no skeletal muscle contraction is observed, check equipment.)
5. Chest compressions 30: 2 then **assess** for an organized rhythm.
   a. If VF persists, repeat the countershock as soon as possible. Continue CPR during any delays.
   b. If an organized rhythm has been restored, immediately check for an effective pulse. *If no pulse is present, resume BLS.*
6. **Additional ACLS procedures:** If a second countershock is unsuccessful in terminating VF, CPR should be continued.

Ventricular asystole causing cardiac arrest indicates a poor prognosis. BLS is initiated, atropine and epinephrine are given, and defibrillation may be tried because VF may masquerade as asystole. The monitoring electrodes should be rotated from their original position to ensure that VF is not present. Asystole or electromechanical dissociation is usually owing to irreversible myocardial damage and inadequate myocardial perfusion; pacing is ineffective in this setting.

Resume defibrillation attempts: use 360-joule (or equivalent biphasic) shocks after each medication or after each minute of CPR. Acceptable patterns: CPR-drug-shock (repeat) or CPR-drug-shock-shock-shock (repeat).

DRUG THERAPY

The AHA guidelines emphasize the following *(2–4)*:

- **Vasopressors, antiarrhythmics, and sequence of actions during treatment of cardiac arrest:**
- Despite the widespread use of epinephrine and several studies of vasopressin, no placebo-controlled study has shown that any medication or vasopressor given routinely at any stage during human cardiac arrest increases rate of survival to hospital discharge.

- A metaanalysis of five randomized out-of-hospital trials showed no significant differences between vasopressin and epinephrine for return of spontaneous circulation, death within 24 h, or death before hospital discharge *(17)*. A proposal to remove all recommendations for vasopressors was considered but not approved in the absence of a placebo versus vasopressor trial and the presence of laboratory evidence documenting the beneficial physiologic effects of vasopressors on hemodynamics and short-term survival *(2–4)*.

There was no evidence that routine administration of any antiarrhythmic drug during human cardiac arrest increased rate of survival to hospital discharge. One antiarrhythmic, amiodarone, improved short-term outcome (i.e., survival to hospital admission) but did not improve survival to hospital discharge compared with placebo *(18)* and lidocaine *(19)*.

- Given this lack of documented effect of drug therapy in improving long-term outcome from cardiac arrest, the sequence for CPR deemphasizes drug administration and reemphasizes basic life support.

Current AHA advice on drug therapy *(2–4)* is as follows:

- **Amiodarone** (class IIb) 300 mg IV push (cardiac arrest dose). If VF/pulseless VT recurs, consider administration of a second dose of 150 mg IV. Maximum cumulative dose: 2.2 g over 24 h.
- **Lidocaine** (class indeterminate) 1.0–1.5 mg/kg IV push. Consider repeat in 3–5 min to a maximum cumulative dose of 3 mg/kg. A single dose of 1.5 mg/kg in cardiac arrest is acceptable.
- **Magnesium sulfate** 1–2 g IV in polymorphic VT (torsades de pointes) and suspected hypomagnesemic state.
- **Procainamide** 30 mg/min in refractory VF (maximum total dose: 17 mg/kg) is acceptable but not recommended because prolonged administration time is unsuitable for cardiac arrest.

Drug name:	**Epinephrine; adrenaline**
Trade name:	Adrenalin
Supplied:	Prefilled syringes: 10 mL (1 mg in 1:10,000 dilution) Ampules: 1 mL (1 mg in 1:10,000 dilution)
Dosage:	IV: 1 mg, 0.01 mg/kg (10 mL of a 1:10,000 solution) repeated at 3–5-min intervals as needed; ILCOR recommendation is every 3 min. Give a 20-mL flush of IV fluid to ensure delivery of the drug centrally Tracheobronchial: 1 mg, 10 mL of a 1:10,000 solution. *See* text for further advice

Epinephrine is of paramount importance in the management of cardiac arrest and is one of the most frequently used drugs; other agents are being tested.

Dosage (Further Advice)

The epinephrine solution can be instilled directly into the tracheobronchial tree through an endotracheal tube. Chest compression should be interrupted for no more than 30 s while epinephrine is introduced through the endotracheal tube. Positive-pressure ventilation is then applied and chest compression resumed.

Intracardiac injections of any type should be avoided. Give epinephrine by the intracardiac route only if neither IV nor intratracheal route is possible. Hazards of intracardiac injections include

- Interruption of chest compression.
- Cardiac tamponade.

- Coronary artery laceration.
- Intramyocardial injection, which with epinephrine can cause intractable VF.
- Pneumothorax.

Infusion. Epinephrine 1 mg in 250 mL 5% dextrose/water: rate 1 μg/min, increase to 3–4 μg/min.

Indications

- Fine VF that is rendered more amenable to removal by countershock.
- VF that does not respond to electrical countershock.
- Asystole and pulseless idioventricular rhythms.
- Electromechanical dissociation.

1. Epinephrine should continue to be used as the primary vasopressor for the management of cardiac arrest. Epinephrine is an alpha- and beta-adrenergic agonist. Therefore:
   a. It stimulates spontaneous cardiac contractions.
   b. Peripheral vascular effects cause a marked increase in systemic vascular resistance (SVR), resulting in an increased aortic diastolic perfusion pressure and thus improving coronary blood flow. It is relevant that epinephrine constricts peripheral vessels but preserves flow to vital organs, and, importantly, coronary artery dilation occurs.
2. Isoproterenol is contraindicated in the treatment of cardiac arrest.

Drug name:	**Vasopressin**
Dosage:	40 U IV single dose, one time only.
Indication:	Only for VF/ pulseless VT; if no response in 5 min, resume epinephrine IV 1 mg

Drug name:	**Amiodarone**
Dosage:	300 mg IV push. If VF/pulseless VT recurs; 150 mg IV; max. 2.2 g over 24 h

Drug name:	**Sodium bicarbonate**
Supplied:	Prefilled syringes: 50 mL of an 8.4% solution = 50 mEq (mmol); or 50 mL of a 7.5% solution = 44.6 mEq (mmol)
Dosage:	IV bolus 50 mEq (mmol); (50 mL of an 8.4% solution; 1 mL = 1 mEq (mmol)/mL) Usual initial dose 1 mEq (mmol)/kg; then administer half this dose every 10 min if necessary

Advice, Adverse Effects, and Interactions

Sodium bicarbonate is no longer recommended for routine use except for preexisting hyperkalemia. Prompt ventilation of the lungs is essential for excretion of CO_2 and is the most effective method of combating acidosis. Priority should be given to early defibrillation and adequate ventilation through endotracheal intubation and the use of epinephrine.

The adverse effects outweigh the minor benefits of bicarbonate administration.

1. Bicarbonate increases intracellular CO_2 in ischemic myocardium. Furthermore, the resulting intracellular acidosis causes depression of myocardial contractility.
2. Bicarbonate can inactivate the required salutary effects of epinephrine when the two are given concomitantly.

3. Increases in pH shift the oxyhemoglobin saturation curve, thus inhibiting the release of oxygen.
4. Bicarbonate-induced alkalosis may precipitate malignant arrhythmias.
5. Marked increase in serum sodium levels and an osmotic load are undesirable.
6. Central venous pH and PCO_2 are better predictive parameters than arterial blood gases. Because arterial blood gases are potentially misleading and their use is unsubstantiated, reliance on them should be reduced. **Bicarbonate may be used** as a class IIa, IIb recommendation:
   a. Known bicarbonate-responsive acidosis.
   b. Tricyclic overdose.
   c. Long arrest: After about 10 min of ventilation including intubation, defibrillation, and the use of epinephrine.
   d. On return of circulation after long arrest.

Drug name:	**Atropine**
Dosage:	Cardiac arrest (asystole): 1 mg IV, especially for asystole, repeated in 2–5 min if necessary to max. 3 mg (0.04 mg/kg) Severe bradycardia: 0.5 mg every 5 min, max. 2 mg

Atropine enhances the rate of discharge of the sinoatrial node and improves atrioventricular conduction.

INDICATIONS

The drug is of value in the management of bradyarrhythmias associated with cardiac arrest. In this setting the dose is much larger than in the acute myocardial infarction patient with bradycardia.

An increase in oxygen consumption caused by atropine is not relevant in victims of cardiac arrest, and the potential for adverse reactions to a dose of 1 mg of atropine is so slight that its use is to be encouraged.

- Severe sinus bradycardia with hypotension.
- High-degree atrioventricular block.
- Slow idioventricular rates.
- Asystole may respond to atropine while preparations are being made for pacing.

Drug name:	**Lidocaine; Lignocaine**
Trade names:	Xylocaine, Xylocard
Dosage:	IV bolus of 75–100 mg (1–1.5 mg/kg) with a simultaneous infusion at 2 mg/min. Repeat bolus of 50 mg in 5–10 min and if needed increase the infusion rate to 3 mg/min; *see* text for further advice

INDICATIONS

- Following defibrillation, lidocaine is used to prevent further recurrence of VF and is partially effective therapy. Lidocaine is as effective as bretylium and is the drug of choice for the treatment of VT and the prevention of VF *(13)*.
- Management of ventricular tachycardia.

DOSAGE (FURTHER ADVICE)

The maximum infusion rate should not be continued for more than 3 h; a maximum of 4 mg/min is used only after careful consideration of side effects. In the presence of HF, decreased hepatic blood flow, or in the elderly, halve the dose.

Beta-Blockers

Beta-blockers have a role in patients with recurrent VF *(19,20)*. If lidocaine or bretylium fails and several countershocks are required, an intravenous **beta-blocker may occasionally be useful, especially with electrocution**. In general, beta-blockers as well as all other agents that have a negative inotropic effect should be avoided in cardiac arrest.

Drug name:	**Propanolol**
Trade name:	Inderal
Dosage:	USA: 1 mg IV over 5 min every 5 min; max. 5 mg UK: 1 mg over 2 min every 2 min; max. 5 mg

Drug name:	**Calcium chloride**
Supplied:	10-mL prefilled syringe or ampule of 10% calcium chloride containing 15.6 mEq (mmol) calcium; 1 mL = 100 mg
Dosage:	IV: 2.5–5 mL of a 10% solution (5–7 mg/kg)

Calcium chloride is no longer recommended. No benefit is derived from the use of calcium in cardiac arrest except in the management of severe hyperkalemia, hypocalcemia, calcium antagonist toxicity, and weaning from cardiopulmonary bypass. Calcium chloride administration may cause dangerous increases in serum calcium levels (range, 12–18 mg/dL [3–4.5 mmol/L]). In addition, digitalis is often used by cardiac patients, and a raised serum calcium concentration is potentially dangerous in patients taking digitalis.

Calcium gluconate, 10 mL of a 10% solution, is mainly used in the United Kingdom.

Magnesium sulfate is reported to expedite ventricular defibrillation; for polymorphic VT (torsades de pointes), dosage, 1–2 g IV.

REFERENCES

1. Cobb LA, Fahrenbruch CE, Olsufka M, Copass MK. Changing incidence of out-of-hospital ventricular fibrillation, 1980–2000. JAMA 2002;288:3008–3013.
2. The AHA guidelines (Circulation 2005;112:IV-206–IV-211). International Liaison Committee on Resuscitation. 2005 International Consensus on Cardiopulmonary Resuscitation and Emergency Cardiovascular Care Science with Treatment Recommendations. Circulation 2005;112:III-1–III-136.
3. Zaritsky A, Morley P. 2005 American Heart Association Guidelines for Cardiopulmonary Resuscitation and Emergency Cardiovascular Care. Editorial: The evidence evaluation process for the 2005 International Consensus on Cardiopulmonary Resuscitation and Emergency Cardiovascular Care Science With Treatment Recommendations. Circulation 2005;112:III-128–III-130.
4. Hazinski MF, Nadkarni VM, Hickey RW, O'Connor R, Becker LB, Zaritsky A. Major changes in the 2005 AHA Guidelines for CPR and ECC: Reaching the tipping point for change. Circulation 2005;112: IV-206–IV-211.
5. Klock W, Cummins RO, Chamberlain D, et al. An advisory statement from the Advanced Life Support Working Group of the Internal Liaison Committee on Resuscitation: The universal advanced life support algorithm. Circulation 1997;95:2180.
6. Guidelines 2000 for Cardiopulmonary Resuscitation and Emergency Cardiovascular Care. The AHA in collaboration with the International Liaison Committee on Resuscitation. Circulation 2000;102(Suppl): 1–142.
7. Kerber RE. Statement on early defibrillation from the Emergency Cardiac Care Committee, American Heart Association. Circulation 1991;83:2233.
8. Nichol G, Hallstrom AP, Kerber R, et al. American Heart Association Report on the Second Public Access Defibrillation Conference, April 17–19, 1997. Circulation 1998;97:1309.

9. White RD, Blackwell TH, Russell JK, Snyder DE, Jorgenson DB. Transthoracic impedance does not affect defibrillation, resuscitation or survival in patients with out-of-hospital cardiac arrest treated with a non-escalating biphasic waveform defibrillator. Resuscitation 2005;64:63.
10. Morrison LJ, Dorian P, Long J, et al. Out-of-hospital cardiac arrest rectilinear biphasic to monophasic damped sine defibrillation waveforms with advanced life support intervention trial (ORBIT). Resuscitation 2005;66:149–157.
11. Davies MJ. Anatomic features in victims of sudden coronary death; coronary artery pathology. Circulation 1992;85(Suppl 1):1.
12. Spaulading CM, Joly LM, Rosenberg A, et al. Immediate coronary angiography in survivors of out-of-hospital cardiac arrest. N Engl J Med 1997;336:1629.
13. Moron BJ. The young competitive athlete with heart disease. Cardiol Rev 1997;5:220.
14. Emergency Cardiac Care Committee and Subcommittees, American Heart Association. Guidelines for cardiopulmonary resuscitation and emergency cardiac care. JAMA 1992;268:2171.
15. Caldwell G, Millar G, Quinn E, et al. Simple mechanical methods for cardioversion: Defence of the precordial thump and cough version. BMJ 1985;291:627.
16. Eisenberg MS, Mengert T. Cardiac resuscitation. N Engl J Med 2001;44:1304.
17. Aung K, Htay T. Vasopressin for cardiac arrest: A systematic review and meta-analysis. Arch Intern Med 2005;165:17–24.
18. Kudenchuk PJ, Cobb LA, Copass MK, et al.. Amiodarone for resuscitation after out-of-hospital cardiac arrest due to ventricular fibrillation. N Engl J Med. 1999;341:871–878.
19. Dorian P, Cass D, Schwartz B, Cooper R, Gelaznikas R, Barr A. Amiodarone as compared with lidocaine for shock-resistant ventricular fibrillation. N Engl J Med. 2002;346:884–890.
20. Sloman G, Robinson JS, McLean K. Propranolol (Inderal) in persistent ventricular fibrillation. BMJ 1965; 1:895.
21. Rothfeld EL, Lipowitz M, Zucker IR, et al. Management of persistently recurring ventricular fibrillation with propranolol hydrochloride. JAMA 1968;204:546.

SUGGESTED READING

Angelos MG, Menegazzi JJ, Callaway CW. Bench to bedside: Resuscitation from prolonged ventricular fibrillation. Acad Emerg Med 2001;8:909–924.

Cooper JA, Cooper JD, Cooper JM. Cardiopulmonary resuscitation: history, current practice, and future direction. Circulation 2006;114:2839–2849.

Ewy G. Cardiocerebral resuscitation: the new cardiopulmonary resuscitation. Circulation 2005;111:2134–2142.

Hallstrom A, Cobb L, Johnson E, Copass M. Cardiopulmonary resuscitation by chest compression alone or with mouth-to-mouth ventilation. N Engl J Med 2000;342:1546-1553.

Hazinski MF, Nadkarni VM, Hickey RW, O'Connor R, Becker LB, Zaritsky A. Major changes in the 2005 AHA Guidelines for CPR and ECC: Reaching the tipping point for change. Circulation 2005;112:IV-206–IV-211.

International Liaison Committee on Resuscitation. 2005 International Consensus on Cardiopulmonary Resuscitation and Emergency Cardiovascular Care Science with Treatment Recommendations. Circulation 2005; 112:III-1–III-136.

Ornato JP, Peberdy MA. Measuring progress in resuscitation: it's time for a better tool. Circulation 2006;114: 2754–2756.

SOS-KANTO study group. Cardiopulmonary resuscitation by bystanders with chest compression only (SOS-KANTO): an observational study. Lancet 2007;369:920–926.

Tang W, Snyder D, Wang J, et al. One shock versus three-shock defibrillation protocol significantly improves outcome in a porcine model of prolonged ventricular fibrillation cardiac arrest. Circulation 2006;113: 2683–2689.

Weiss JN, Garfinkel A, Karagueuzian HS, Qu Z, Chen PS. Chaos and the transition to ventricular fibrillation: A new approach to antiarrhythmic evaluation. Circulation 1999;99:2819-2826.

Zaritsky A, Morley P. 2005 American Heart Association Guidelines for Cardiopulmonary Resuscitation and Emergency Cardiovascular Care. Editorial: The evidence evaluation process for the 2005 International Consensus on Cardiopulmonary Resuscitation and Emergency Cardiovascular Care Science with Treatment Recommendations. Circulation 2005;112:III-128–III-130.

16 Management of Infective Endocarditis

Infective endocarditis (IE) most often results from bacterial infection, but infections caused by fungi, *Coxiella,* or *Chlamydia* are not rare. Infection usually involves heart valves not always previously known to be abnormal, in particular a bicuspid aortic valve, mitral valve prolapse, or (rarely) a septal defect or ventricular aneurysm. Coarctation of the aorta, patent ductus arteriosus, aneurysms, or arteriovenous shunts may be the site of infective endarteritis. Prosthetic valves may be involved, and infection at the site of implantation of foreign material including devices poses a particularly difficult problem.

- The old fashioned terms acute and subacute bacterial endocarditis (SBE) are still clinically useful, although they no longer hold prominence because pathogens such as *Staphylococcus aureus* and streptococci can cause either fulminant or indolent disease in different patients.
- The term SBE or subacute IE used in a patient who is not critically ill refers to a subacute syndrome, with minimal signs of toxicity, which is usually caused by viridans streptococci, enterococci, coagulase-negative staphylococci, or gram-negative coccobacilli *(1)*. These organisms cause a slow, low-grade infection that evolves clinically over weeks to months, thus allowing the clinician to delay therapy for a few days while awaiting the results of blood cultures and other diagnostic tests.
- Acute IE is accompanied by marked toxicity with progression over days to a few weeks resulting in valvular destruction, hemodynamic deterioration, heart failure (HF), and metastatic infection *(1)* and is caused mainly by *S. aureus, which carries about a 40% rate of HF.*

Rheumatic valvular heart disease is now uncommon in developing countries, and IE is encountered mainly in patients with prosthetic heart valves, biscupid aortic valves, particularly in men over age 60, and degenerative valvular disease (aortic sclerosis). Mitral valve prolapse (MVP) accounts for approx 18% of native valve IE, with an increased risk in men older than 45. The risk of IE in patients with MVP is significant mainly if a regurgitant murmur is heard or if there is documented thickening of valve leaflets > 5 mm. Intravenous (IV) drug abusers represent a special group with right-sided IE.

CLASSIFICATION AND DIAGNOSIS

A logical classification of IE is as follows:

- Native valve IE; acute or subacute presentation.
- Prosthetic valve IE.
- Right-sided endocarditis, observed particularly in IV drug users.
- Culture-negative IE.

Diagnostic Guidelines

Diagnostic criteria are as follows *(2)*:

- Conformation of persistent bacteremia resulting from organisms.
- Evidence of cardiac valvular involvement: documentation of vegetation, new murmur of valvular regurgitation, or paravalvular abscess.

From: *Contemporary Cardiology: Cardiac Drug Therapy, Seventh Edition*
M. Gabriel Khan © Humana Press Inc., Totowa, NJ

- Supporting findings include: fever, risk factors for IE, vascular or immune complex phenomena, or intermittent bacteremia or fungemia.

The diagnosis of IE requires a high index of suspicion. The condition should be considered and carefully excluded in all patients with a heart murmur and pyrexia of undetermined origin. The Duke criteria utilize echocardiographic findings as a major criterion for diagnosis and have merit for diagnosis of native valve endocarditis; the utility of the Duke criteria has not yet been adequately assessed, however, for suspected prosthetic valve endocarditis. Diagnosis is made in the majority by blood cultures and echocardiography. Two-dimensional transthoracic endocardiography (TTE) can miss 25% of vegetations <10 mm and 75% of those <5 mm. Transesophageal echocardiography (TEE) is superior; it is crucial for the diagnosis and management of endocarditis and is more sensitive than TTE for detecting vegetations and cardiac abscess.

High-risk echocardiographic features include *(2)*:

- Large and/or mobile vegetations.
- Valvular insufficiency.
- Suggestion of perivalvular extension.
- Secondary ventricular dysfunction.

Need for Surgery

- Heart failure is an immediate indication. Features that suggest potential need for surgical intervention *(2)* are as follows:
- Abcess formation.
- Staph infection.
- Persistent vegetation after systemic embolization.
- Anterior mitral leaflet vegetation, particularly with size > 10 mm.
- One or more embolic events during first 2 wk of antimicrobial therapy.
- Increase in vegetation size > 1.5 cm despite appropriate antimicrobial therapy.
- Acute aortic or mitral insufficiency with signs of ventricular failure.
- Valve perforation or rupture, valvular dehiscence, or fistula.
- Large abscess or extension of abscess despite appropriate antimicrobial therapy.
- New heart block.
- Combination of large vegetation size and positive antiphospholipid antibody.

Precipitating and Predisposing Factors

- If prior to **dental work,** the usual organism producing IE is *S. viridans* or, rarely, *S. faecalis.* If an acute presentation emerges after dental work, one must suspect *Staphylococcus* or the extremely rare *Fusobacterium,* which is not uncommon in gingival crevices and the oropharynx.
- With **genitourinary instrumentation** or in other surgical procedures, gram-negative bacteria are the rule.
- Prosthetic heart valve.
- Narcotic addicts: mainly right heart endocarditis, owing to *S. aureus, Pseudomonas aeruginosa, P. cepacia,* and *Serratia marcescens.*

Blood Cultures

Adequate cultures and as wide as possible a range of sensitivities must be obtained. Approximately 90% of the causative organisms can be isolated if there has been no previous antibiotic therapy. The past two decades have seen an increasing incidence of staphylococci and enterococci, often resistant to penicillin. The incidence of gram-negative organisms has also increased. If the organism is to be isolated at all, four to six blood cultures carry a 98% chance of success.

Three separate sets of blood cultures should be taken, each from a separate venipuncture site, over 24 h *(3)*. Ten milliliters of blood drawn should be put in each of two blood culture bottles, one containing aerobic and the other anaerobic medium *(4)*.

If the presentation is acute and the patient's status is critical with a high suspicion of *S. aureus* infection, another view is to take four blood cultures over a period of 1–2 h, after which antibiotic treatment should begin and should on no account be withheld pending a bacteriologic diagnosis. The presence of echocardiographically visible vegetations greatly increases the urgency of commencing treatment, as does the presence of infection on prosthetic valves.

Aids in identifying the organism:

- Cultures must be incubated both aerobically and anaerobically; the latter is necessary especially for *Bacteroides* and anaerobic streptococci.
- Serological tests (complement fixation tests (CFTs)) are of value in patients with *Brucella, Candida, Cryptococcus, Coxiella,* or *Chlamydia.*
- Examination of a Gram stain of the "buffy" coat of the peripheral blood.
- In cases other than group A *Streptococcus,* it is advisable to monitor the serum bactericidal titer (SBT) 1:8 or higher, the minimum inhibitory concentration (MIC), and the minimum bactericidal concentration (MBC).

A discussion of the case with the microbiologist is often helpful. Some organisms such as *Haemophilus influenzae* and variants of streptococci require enriched media. *Neisseria gonorrhoeae* and *N. meningitidis* require 5–10% of CO_2, and *Pseudomonas* grows poorly in unvented bottles. Fungi require a medium containing broth and soft agar and are seldom identified by culture. The culture of an arterial embolus may reveal a fungal etiology.

THERAPY

Initial choice of appropriate antibiotic prior to laboratory determination of the infecting organism is guided by the following parameters:

1. **Native valve:** A subacute presentation, SBE, is caused by *S. viridans* in approximately 80%, *S. faecalis* in 10%, and other organisms in 10%.
2. **Native valve, elderly endocarditis:** *S. faecalis* is commonly seen, but *S. viridans* is implicated in about 50% of cases.
3. **Prosthetic valve endocarditis.**
   - Early infection after operation is usually caused by *Staphylococcus epidermidis or S. aureus.*
   - Late after operation the organisms are similar to those seen in SBE or acute endocarditis with the additional probability of fungal infection, but *S. epidermidis* is not uncommon. Following abdominal surgery, gram-negative and anaerobic infections are not uncommon.
4. **Acute bacterial endocarditis** (ABE) is usually caused by *S. aureus.*
5. **Endocarditis in narcotic addicts:** right-sided endocarditis.
6. **Culture-negative endocarditis** is often caused by:
   - The usual bacterial organisms, which are masked by previous antibiotic therapy.
   - Slow-growing penicillin-sensitive streptococci with fastidious nutritional tastes.
   - *Coxiella* and *Chlamydia.*

Table 16–1
Treatment of *Staphylococcus aureus* Endocarditis

Type	*Antibiotic*	*Dosage*
Native valve	Nafcillin +	2 g IV every 4 h for 6 wk
	optional Gentamicin	1–1.4 mg/kg IV every 8 h for 1 wk
Methicillin-resistant staphylococci	Vancomycin	15 mg/kg IV every 12 h for 6 wk
Prosthetic valve	Nafcillin +	2 g every 4 h for >6 wk
	Rifampin	300 mg orally every 8 h for 6 wk
	Gentamicin	1–1.4 mg/kg IV every 8 h for 2 wk
Methicillin-resistant staphylococci	Vancomycin +	15 mg/kg IV every 12 h for 6 wk
	Rifampin	300 mg orally every 8 h for >6 wk
	Gentamicin	1–1.4 mg/kg IV every 8 h for 2 wk

Consider patients with culture-negative endocarditis under two categories:

- Those with negative blood cultures associated with recent antibiotic therapy.
- Those infected with microorganisms that are difficult to grow in routinely used blood culture media.

S. aureus *Endocarditis*

***This most harmful organism* accounts for nearly all cases of native valve acute bacterial endocarditis and approx 50% of prosthetic valve IE.**

For **penicillinase**-producing staphylococci, nafcillin, oxacillin, or flucloxacillin with the optional addition of gentamicin is given for 6 wk, the latter for only 1 wk (*see* Table 16-1). An aminoglycoside is not added in the United Kingdom. Other regimens advised for penicillinase-producing staphylococci include

- Vancomycin.
- Cephalosporins: cephalothin, cephradine, cefuroxime.
- Rifampin plus aminoglycoside.
- Rifampin plus cloxacillin.
- Rifampin plus vancomycin.
- Clindamycin and cephalosporin.

Vancomycin and cephalothin are effective alternatives when penicillin is contraindicated. Cephalothin is more active than other cephalosporins against *S. aureus*. Clindamycin is relatively effective but is not advisable because it is bacteriostatic or less bactericidal than penicillin or cephalosporins; also, pseudomembranous colitis may supervene. If metastatic infection is present, rifampin is usually added at a dose of 600–1200 mg daily and continued until abscesses are drained and excised. For methicillin-resistant staphylococci, vancomycin 1 g every 12 h is the treatment of choice. Care should be taken in patients over age 65 yr and/or those with renal impairment or eighth nerve dysfunction. Vancomycin serum levels should be maintained at <50 μg/mL. There appears to be no advantage in adding an aminoglycoside or rifampin. If vancomycin is contraindicated, no suitable alternatives have been tested: trimethoprim-sulfamethoxazole (Bactrim, Septra) has been used with some success. Rifampin must not be used alone because resistant strains quickly emerge. Fusidic acid 500 mg four times daily with rifampin has been used and provides a reasonable alternative.

Generally, 4–6 wk of antibiotic therapy is considered adequate for methicillin-resistant staphylococci, but some patients require extended treatment.

Prosthetic Valve Endocarditis

Methicillin-resistant strains are common, and vancomycin is the agent of choice. Combination with an aminoglycoside and rifampin improves the cure rate but increases the incidence of drug toxicity and resistant strains. The infection is usually invasive, destructive, and often difficult to eradicate, with a mortality rate exceeding 50%. TEE is crucial for the diagnosis. Prognosis is poor, especially if HF supervenes; thus, surgery is frequently necessary.

Native Valve Endocarditis Caused by **Staphylococci**

Oxacillin-Susceptible Strains

Nafcillin or oxacillin 12 g/24 h IV in 4–6 equally divided doses for 6 wk.

Oxacillin-Resistant Strains

Vancomycin 30 mg/kg per 24 h IV in 2 equally divided doses for 6 wk. Adjust vancomycin dosage to achieve 1-h serum concentration of 30–45 μg/mL and trough concentration of 10–15 μg/mL *(2)*.

Native Valve Endocarditis Caused by **S. viridans** *and* **Streptococcus bovis** *Sensitive to Penicillin*

- **Native valve endocarditis and other forms of subacute IE are commonly treated as outpatient situations, but it is advisable to commence antibiotic treatment in hospital for 1 wk and then proceed to outpatient therapy.**

In patients < 65 yr old with normal renal function:
18–30 million U/24 h IV either continuously or in 6 equally divided doses plus gentamicin 1 mg/kg every 8 h for 4–6 wk *(2)*

or

Ampicillin 12 g/24 h IV in 6 equally divided doses for 4–6 wk *(2)*.

The use of ceftriazone constitutes the biggest advance in antibiotic therapy during the past two decades.

Ceftriaxone 2 g IV or IM once daily can be given to selected patients as **outpatient therapy for 4 wk.**

- Native valve: 4-wk therapy recommended for patients with symptoms of illness ≤3 mo; 6-wk therapy recommended for patients with symptoms >3 mo *(2)*.
- In patients older than 65 yr and/or in those with renal impairment or impairment of eighth cranial nerve function: Crystalline penicillin G sodium; 12–18 million U/24 h IV either continuously or in 4 or 6 equally divided doses for 4 wk

or

- Ceftriaxone sodium: 2 g/24 h IV/IM in 1 dose, for 4 wk *(2)*.

Prosthetic Valve Endocarditis Caused by Susceptible **S. viridans** *or* **S. bovis** *Infections*

Penicillin and gentamicin should be given for 4–6 wk at doses given above with close monitoring for gentamicin toxicity.

S. viridans or *S. bovis* relatively resistant to penicillin should be treated with ampicillin and gentamicin for **4 wk** and then amoxicillin orally 500 mg every 6 h for 2 wk. In patients **allergic to penicillin**, give vancomycin 12.5 mg/kg every 12 h.

Vancomycin may cause ototoxicity, thrombophlebitis, or nephrotoxicity. Thus, an approximate cephalosporin may be used cautiously except in patients who have had angioedema, anaphylaxis, or definite urticarial reactions to penicillin. *S. bovis* accounts for about 20% of cases of penicillin-sensitive streptococcal endocarditis. *S. bovis* bacteremia usually arises in patients with gastrointestinal lesions, in particular inflammatory bowel disease, bleeding diverticula, polyposis, villous adenoma, and (rarely) carcinoma of the colon. Thus, gastrointestinal investigations should be undertaken to exclude these lesions.

Native Valve Enterococcal Endocarditis

Therapy of native valve enterococcal endocarditis *(2)* remains difficult.

IV ampicillin 1.5–2 g every 4 h or penicillin 3–6 million units every 4 h plus gentamicin 1–1.4 mg/kg every 8 h for 4–6 wk

or

Ceftriaxone sodium 2 g/24 h IV/IM in 1 dose for 4 wk plus gentamicin 3 mg/kg per 24 h IV in 3 equally divided doses for 2 wk.

Enterococcal endocarditis is usually caused by *S. faecalis* and rarely by *S. faecium* or *S. durans.* These organisms are relatively resistant to most antibiotics. Penicillin and vancomycin are only bacteriostatic, and in this situation many strains are resistant to penicillin as well as streptomycin.

Vancomycin dose: 30 mg/kg per 24 h IV in 2 equally divided doses not to exceed 2 g/ 24 h. Vancomycin therapy is recommended only in the presence of normal renal function and for patients unable to tolerate penicillin or ceftriaxone therapy *(2)*.

No single antibiotic consistently produces bactericidal activity against enterococci in vivo or in vitro. However, bactericidal synergy between the penicillins and streptomycin or gentamicin has been well documented. Thus, antibiotic combinations are necessary to eradicate the infection. A combination of penicillin or ampicillin and/or gentamicin is standard therapy. There is some evidence that amoxicillin is more rapidly bactericidal than ampicillin and may be more active against *S. faecalis.* Gentamicin is more effective than streptomycin and is more conveniently given IV. Thus, it is the aminoglycoside of choice.

Enterococcal endocarditis in the penicillin-allergic patient: A combination of vancomycin and gentamicin for 6 wk is recommended, notwithstanding the potential toxicity of the combination. Unfortunately, “third-generation” cephalosporins are relatively inactive against enterococci.

Other Bacteria Causing IE

Other bacteria and suggested antibiotics include:

- Nutritionally variant viridans streptococci (NVVS), for example, *Streptococcus mitis, S. anginosis,* and other strains may be missed if blood cultures are not quickly subcultured on special media that support the growth of NVVS. These organisms were believed to be the cause of some cases of “culture-negative” endocarditis. Treatment is similar to that for enterococcal endocarditis with ampicillin or penicillin and gentamicin for 4–6 wk.
- *H. influenzae* and *H. parainfluenzae* are best treated with ampicillin and gentamicin IV for 6 wk or more.
- *P. aeruginosa:* Tobramycin with carbenicillin is one combination of value.

- *P. cepacia* is often sensitive to trimethoprim-sulfamethoxazole.
- *Chlamydia psittaci* endocarditis is very rare. Treatment includes the use of tetracycline. Doxycycline 200 mg orally daily was used successfully in a reported case *(5)*, although valve replacement is suggested as necessary in most cases.
- The Q fever organism is difficult to eradicate with tetracycline. A combination of cotrimoxazole and rifampin is advisable, but surgery may be finally required.

Right-Sided Endocarditis

IE in IV drug users is right sided in approx 63% and is caused by *Staphylococcus* in approx 77%, streptococci in approx 5%, and enterococci in only approx 2%; it is polymicrobial in approx 8% with absence of fungi. By contrast, left-sided IE occurs in approx 37% with approx 23% caused by *Staphylococcus*, approx 15% by streptococci, >24% by enterococci, gram-negatives by approx 13%, and fungi by approx 12%. Right-sided endocarditis has increased in incidence because of IV drug abuse. *S. aureus* is the commonest infecting organism, followed by *P. aeruginosa* in some cities and, less commonly, streptococci, *Serratia marcescens*, gram-negatives, and *Candida*. The tricuspid valve is commonly affected and occasionally the pulmonary valve. The murmur of tricuspid regurgitation is commonly missed; the murmur can be augmented by deep inspiration and hepatojugular reflux. Also, pleuropneumonic symptoms may mask and delay diagnosis.

Therapy: Empirical therapy is commenced as outlined earlier and adjusted when culture and sensitivities are available. TEE differentiation of vegetations into less or greater than 1.0 cm diameter is helpful in directing surgical intervention *(6)*. Vegetations < 1.0 cm are usually cured by antibiotic therapy for 4–6 wk, as well as about two-thirds of cases seen with vegetations > 1.0 cm. If in the latter category fever persists beyond 3 wk without a cause such as abscess, phlebitis, drug fever, or inadequate antibiotic levels *(6)*, valve replacement should be contemplated.

Gentamicin and Tobramycin

Dosage. 1.5–2 mg/kg loading dose and then 3–5 mg/kg daily in divided doses every 8 h.

predose level (trough)	<2 μg/mL (2 mg/L)
postdose level (peak)	<10 μg/mL (10 mg/L)

The normal dose interval every 8 h can vary (e.g., every 24 h), depending on creatinine clearance, age, sex, and lean body weight. Despite the use of nomograms, errors are not unusual and it is advisable to have repeated aminoglycoside serum concentrations (ASCs) to achieve adequate peak levels and therefore therapeutic success without causing nephrotoxicity or ototoxicity. Gentamicin trough concentrations >2 mg/L appear to be more important than high peak concentrations in the causation of ototoxocity *(7)*.

The usual recommended dose of gentamicin of 3 mg/kg/d may not achieve optimal peak and trough ASCs in more than 50% of patients with normal renal function. In young adults the dose may need to be given every 6 h. **Do not rely** on the serum creatinine level as an estimate of glomerular filtration rate (GFR). If the estimated GFR is 40–70 mL/min, give the dose every 12 h; 20–39 mL/min every 24 h; and 5–19 mL/min every 48 h. Beyond age 70 the estimated GFR formula is inaccurate. **Caution is needed to avoid toxicity effects of these antibiotics. In such difficult cases, it is advisable to obtain the assistance of an ID specialist and to warn the patient of the dangers of the therapy.**

Troughs and Peaks. The trough ASC is best taken immediately before the dose and the peak 30 min after the end of an IV infusion. If the ASC **trough** is **too high** (>2 μg/mL), extend the dosing interval. If the **peak** is **too high** (>10 μg/mL), decrease the dose. Peak levels must not exceed 14 μg/mL (14 μg/L).

Fungal Endocarditis

Major predisposing factors for the development of fungal endocarditis are previous valve surgery and IV drug abuse. Most commonly infection is caused by *Candida* (66%) or occasionally *Aspergillus* or *Histoplasma,* and rarely *Coccidioides* and *Cryptococcus.* Except for *Candida,* fungi are difficult to grow from blood cultures. Thus, diagnosis may be difficult. Sometimes the diagnosis is made from examination of an arterial embolus. Serological tests (CFT) for *Candida, Histoplasma,* and *Cryptococcus* are useful in monitoring therapy and may be the clue to deep fungal infection.

The diagnosis of fungal endocarditis is often impossible to establish. The clinical circumstances (e.g., previous prolonged course of antibiotics) sometimes lead to suspicion, as does failure to detect other organisms or failure to respond to other antimicrobial agents.

Amphotericin exerts antifungal activity by binding to ergosterol in fungal cell walls.

DOSAGE (FURTHER ADVICE)

Side effects can be minimized by IV administration of hydrocortisone 100 mg and diphenhydramine 50 mg before each dose. Monitor renal function, blood count, and platelets. Hypokalemia and hypomagnesemia may occur.

Drug name:	**Amphotericin B**
Trade names:	Amphocil, Fungizone
Dosage:	IV: 1-mg test dose over 4 h; if tolerated, give 10-mg dose in 500 mL 5% dextrose over 12 h and then 0.25 mg/kg/d. Increase by 0.25 mg/kg/d to reach 0.5–1 mg/kg/d. Usually 25–50 mg is given in 500 mL 5% dextrose over 6 h once daily. Maximum dose range: 35–50 mg/d. **Do not** exceed 90 mg/d. *See* text for further advice

If the organism is sensitive to flucytosine (5-fluorocytosine), this drug can be added in a dose of 37.5 mg/kg every 6 h (dose and interval to be altered, depending on creatinine clearance). When used in combination with flucytosine, the dose of amphotericin B should be reduced to 0.3 mg/kg/d *(8).*

The toxicity of the drugs and the resistance of the organisms often necessitate valve replacement, especially in patients with a prosthetic valve. Valve replacement is strongly recommended. The prognosis is generally poor.

Histoplasma is the only infection that is often successfully managed medically.

Anticoagulant Therapy in Endocarditis

- Avoid heparin except when absolutely necessary.
- If warfarin is used, keep the prothrombin time to 1.25–1.5 times the normal control value or the International Normalized Ratio (INR) to 2–3. This may be necessary in patients with prosthetic heart valves who were previously taking anticoagulants.

Indications for Surgery

The decision to operate and the timing of operation are of critical importance, especially in patients with prosthetic heart valves and most patients with gram-negative endocarditis.

Heart Failure

HF is associated with a grave prognosis with medical or surgical therapy. In the presence of HF, the decision to delay surgery to prolong the duration of preoperative antibiotic therapy carries with it the risk of permanent ventricular failure. and is not recommended *(2)*. Evaluation with TEE helps to delineate the causes and severity of HF.

Suggested indications for **early surgical intervention** are:

- The development of or deterioration in left or right heart failure. Native valve endocarditis complicated by HF has a high mortality rate that can be improved significantly by early surgical intervention.
- Sudden onset or worsening of aortic or mitral incompetence with precipitation of HF.
- Patients with prosthetic valve endocarditis: Advise surgical intervention after infection has been brought under control because of the poor chance of achieving a long-term cure with antibiotics alone. Immediate surgery without delay for
  - Precipitation of HF.
  - Dehiscence.
  - Abscess formation.
  - Fungal infection, especially of a prosthetic valve, is virtually never cured medically and requires early intervention.
  - Gram-negative infection (most cannot be cured with antibiotics).
  - Resistant organism or recurrent infection.
- Accessible mycotic aneurysms.
- Most patients with left-sided gram-negative endocarditis are **rarely completely cured** with antibiotics and may present a difficult decision.
- Rare organisms, e.g., *Brucella* or Q fever (*Coxiella*), known to be difficult to eradicate and showing no response after 3 wk of treatment.
- Relapse after 6 wk of adequate medical therapy.
- Aneurysm of the sinus of Valsalva.
- Septal abscess (suggested by increasing degree of atrioventricular block).
- Valve ring abscesses.
- Patients with repeated arterial embolization. (Embolization, Osler nodes, change in murmur, or congestive heart failure may develop, however, during adequate medical therapy or when treatment/cure has been established.) Right-sided endocarditis is associated with a 70–100% incidence of pulmonary emboli; such recurrent emboli are not an indication for surgery *(6)*.

PROPHYLAXIS OF BACTERIAL ENDOCARDITIS

Bacterial endocarditis is hard to prevent. Endocarditis occurred in 6% of 304 patients with prosthetic valves undergoing 390 procedures without prophylaxis. No cases of endocarditis occurred in 229 patients undergoing 287 procedures with prior prophylaxis *(9)*. Only about 20% of cases of IE are believed to be of dental origin *(10)*, and in approx 60% of cases the portal of entry cannot be identified *(10)*.

In over 40% of cases, infection occurs on valves not known to be abnormal, especially on bicuspid aortic valves and in patients with MVP. Except for prosthetic valves, prophylaxis is aimed at streptococci, which account for only about 65% of all cases of endocarditis.

Prophylaxis is not indicated for dental work in cardiac patients with pacemakers, implantable cardioverter-defribillators (ICDs), and stents.

The American Heart Association (AHA) guidelines include the following:

- General prophylaxis: amoxicillin (adults): 2.0 g; children 50 mg/kg administered orally 1 h before the procedure.
- For patients unable to take oral meds, give ampicillin 2 g Im or IV; children 50 mg/kg IM or IV within 30 min before the procedure.
- For patients allergic to penicillin: clindamycin is recommended 600 mg for adults; children 20 mg/kg IV **within 30 min** before procedure; or azithromycin 500 mg for adults; children 15 mg/kg orally 1 h before procedure.

Prophylactic regimens for genitourinary, or gastrointestinal procedures are as follows:

- High-risk patients should be given ampicillin 2 g IM or IV plus gentamicin 1.5 mg/kg not to exceed 120 mg within 30 min of starting the procedure; 6 h later ampicillin 1 g IM or IV or amoxicillin 1 g orally.
- For high-risk patients and for patients allergic to penicillin or amoxicillin give vancomycin 1 g IV over 1–2 h; complete the infusion within 30 min of starting the procedure.

REFERENCES

1. Karchmer AW. Infective endocarditis. In: Braunwald E. Heart Disease. Philadelphia, WB Saunders, 2005, pp. 1633–1643.
2. Baddour LM, Wilson WR, Bayer AS, et al. Infective Endocarditis Diagnosis, Antimicrobial Therapy, and Management of Complications: A Statement for Healthcare Professionals from the Committee on Rheumatic Fever, Endocarditis, and Kawasaki Disease, Council on Cardiovascular Disease in the Young, and the Councils on Clinical Cardiology, Stroke, and Cardiovascular Surgery and Anesthesia, American Heart Association—Executive Summary: *Endorsed by the Infectious Diseases Society of America.* Circulation 2005;111:3167–3184.
3. Bayer AS, Bolger AF, Taubert KA, et al. Diagnosis and management of IE and its complications. Circulation 1998;8:2936.
4. Towns ML, Reller LB. Diagnostic methods as current best practices and guidelines for isolation of bacteria and fungi in infective endocarditis. Infect Dis Clin North Am 2002;16:363.
5. Walker LJE, Adgey AAJ. Successful treatment by doxycycline of endocarditis caused by ornithosis. Br Heart J 1987;57:58.
6. Robbins MT, Soeiro R, Frishman WH, et al. Right–sided valvular endocarditis: Etiology, diagnosis, and an approach to therapy. Am Heart J 1986;111:128.
7. Reeves D. The frequency of ototoxicity—a review of the literature. In: Richardson RG (ed). Round Table Discussion on Gentamicin and Tobramycin (R Soc Med Int Congr Symp Ser 4, p 45). London, Academic Press, 1978.
8. Cohen J. Antifungal chemotherapy. Lancet 1982;2:1323.
9. Horstkotte D, Sick P, Bircks W, et al. Effectiveness of antibiotic prophylaxis to prevent prosthetic valve endocarditis: evidence in humans. J Am Coll Cardiol 1991;71:2125.
10. MacMahon SW, Hickey AJ, Wilcken DEL, et al. Risk of infective endocarditis in mitral valve prolapse with and without precordial systolic murmurs. Am J Cardiol 1986;58:105.

SUGGESTED READING

Baddour LM, Wilson WR, Bayer AS, et al. Infective Endocarditis Diagnosis, Antimicrobial Therapy, and Management of Complications: A Statement for Healthcare Professionals from the Committee on Rheumatic Fever, Endocarditis, and Kawasaki Disease, Council on Cardiovascular Disease in the Young, and the Councils on Clinical Cardiology, Stroke, and Cardiovascular Surgery and Anesthesia, American Heart Association—Executive Summary: *Endorsed by the Infectious Diseases Society of America.* Circulation 2005;111:3167–3184.

Lewin MB, Otto CM. The bicuspid aortic valve: adverse outcomes from infancy to old age. Circulation 2005;111:832–834.

Moreillon P, Que YA. Infective endocarditis. Lancet 2004;363:139–149.

17 Management of Dyslipidemias

This chapter covers the following areas:

- The salient points related to diagnosis of dyslipidemias and advance beyond the National Cholesterol Education Program (NCEP) guidelines *(1)*.
- The revolutionary **statins**: the changes in management of dyslipidemia based on the proven effectiveness of statins in achieving goal low-density lipoprotein (LDL-C) levels and improvement in survival. In patients with coronary heart disease (CHD), statins result in an approximately 29% decrease in risk of cardiac death and about 20% decrease in total mortality. The decrease in the risk of mortality provided by statins is equal to that observed with angiotensin-converting enzyme (ACE) inhibitors, whereas the combined effects of estrogens, antioxidants, folic acid, vitamin E, and herbal remedies are insignificant, and their effects are unfairly exploited, to the detriment of patients who are thus deprived of proven mortality- and morbidity-reducing agents. It is not surprising, therefore, that >40% of individuals who require aggressive control of dyslipidemia are not receiving adequate treatment. *Goal LDL-C must be achieved if we are to stem the plague of CHD.*
- **LDL-C–HDL-C goal:** *Agents that decrease LDL-C to goal and also increase high-density lipoprotein (HDL-C) levels by >20% are ideal agents.* Although fibrates significantly increase HDL-C, they only modestly decrease LDL-C *and rarely achieve goal LDL-C levels.* Fortunately, newer statins such as atorvastatin and rosuvastatin have been shown to decrease LDL-C by 40–50% and virtually always achieve goal levels except in patients with genetic familial hyperlipidemia.
- For the first time, a randomized controlled trial (RCT) has shown that rosuvastatin 40 mg daily, by maintaining an LDL-C cholesterol < 60 mg/dL (1.6 mmol/L), resulted in regression of coronary atheroma. This was A Study to Evaluate the effect of Rosuvastatin On Intravascular ultrasound-Derived coronary atheroma burden (ASTEROID) *(2)*.
- New acute coronary syndrome (ACS) indication: A powerful LDL-C-reducing agent should be prescribed within hours of admission. There is now supporting evidence from Pravastatin or Atrovastatin Evaluation and Infection Therapy-Thrombolysis in Myocardial Infarction (PROVE IT-TIMI) 22 trial *(3)* and other RCTs *(4)* that statins used early in the treatment of ACS at a high dose (atorvastatin 60–80 mg daily) significantly reduce coronary artery disease (CAD) outcomes.
- On admission to hospital, <20% of patients are expected to have LDL-C < 100 mg/dL (2.6 mmol/L with ACS goal < 1.9 mmol/L, optimally <60 mg/dL (1.6 mmol/L).
- The plieotropic effects of statins are salutary. Early statin therapy ameliorates vasoconstriction and other detrimental effects of endothelial dysfunction that prevail during this common syndrome. C-reactive protein (CRP) levels are reduced *(5)*.
- The rationale for prescribing other hypolipidemic agents (resins, fibrates, nicotinic acid, and combination therapy) is put in perspective for practitioners.

From: *Contemporary Cardiology: Cardiac Drug Therapy, Seventh Edition*
M. Gabriel Khan © Humana Press Inc., Totowa, NJ

Table 17-1
Guidelines for the Management of Elevated LDL-C Cholesterol: When to Use Drug Therapy

	Coronary artery disease or diabetes?		
	*NO**		
*Yes***	*Several risk factors*	*Average risk (one or two risk factors)*	*Low risk*
LDL-C	LDL-C	LDL-C	LDL-C
>100mg/dL	>130 mg /dL	>160 mg /dL	190 mg/dL
(2.5 mmol/L)	(3.5 mmol/L)	(4 mmol/L)	(5 mmol/L)
Drug therapy	Drug therapy	Consider drug therapy	Consider drug therapy
Goal	Goal	Goal	Goal
<70 mg/dL	<100 mg/dL	<120 mg/dL	<130 mg/dL
(<1.8 mmol/L)	(<2.6 mmol/L)	(<3.1 mmol/L)	(<3.5 mmol/L)
very high risk***			
<1.6 mmol/L			
<60 mg/dL			

LDL-C, low-density lipoprotein cholesterol.
*No CAD or diabetes.
**CAD or diabetes.
***Acute coronary syndrome.

DIAGNOSIS

Persons with a marked increase in serum levels of cholesterol to >350 mg/dL (9 mmol/L) represent a very small group of individuals in the population at very high risk for developing atherosclerotic coronary disease. Less than 20% of these individuals (0.1% of the population) have a genetic abnormality, characterized by cellular LDL-C receptor deficiency *(6)*. Thus, emphasis is now correctly placed on the vast population of individuals with a total serum cholesterol concentration in the range of 200–270 mg/dL (5.5–7 mmol/L), in whom the majority of heart attacks occur (*see* Table 17-1). A serum cholesterol level that carries minimal risk for CHD and is regarded as the ideal value is in the range of 130–160 mg/dL; an ideal LDL-C level is <100 mg/dL (2.6 mmol/L) for all adults ages 20–80 with CHD or at least one risk factor. In the majority this ideal is difficult to achieve without drug therapy.

Conversion Formula for mg to mmol

- **LDL-C** is calculated by the laboratory utilizing the total cholesterol (TC) and >12-h fasting triglyceride (TG) as follows: LDL-C mg/dL = TC – HDL-C – (TG ÷ 5). For LDL-C using mmol/L, divide by 2.2 instead of 5. If the TG level is >400 mg/dL (4 mmol/L), the calculation is not valid.
- To convert total-C, LDL-C, or HDL-C from mg/dL to mmol/L, divide by 38.5 or multiply by 0.02586.

Secondary Causes of Dyslipidemias

A *secondary cause* commonly accounts for dyslipidemia, and the following conditions must be sought and treated or regulated:

- Dietary
- Diabetes mellitus

- Hypothyroidism
- Nephrotic syndrome
- Chronic liver disease
- Obesity
- Dysgammaglobulinemia (monoclonal gammopathy)
- Obstructive jaundice
- Biliary cirrhosis
- Pancreatitis
- Excess alcohol consumption
- Estrogens/progesterone
- Glycogen storage disorders
- Lipodystrophy
- Medications

1. **Dietary:** Excessive carbohydrate intake; weight gain; increased saturated fat or alcohol intake.
2. **Diseases:** Diabetes mellitus, hypothyroidism, pancreatitis, nephrotic syndrome, liver disease (obstructive jaundice, biliary cirrhosis), and monoclonal gammopathy.
3. **Medications:** Oral contraceptives and diuretics may unfavorably alter cholesterol and HDL-C cholesterol. The serum lipid alterations produced by beta-blockers have been exaggerated and perhaps exploited. Acebutolol with weak intrinsic sympathomimetic activity (ISA) caused no significant changes in total or HDL-C cholesterol at 24 mo.

In the Norwegian timolol multicenter study, timolol decreased total cardiac and sudden deaths regardless of the drug effects on serum lipid levels *(7)*. Some studies indicate that non-ISA beta-blockers cause no significant alteration of HDL-C *(8)*, whereas others indicate a small decrease of 5%. There is no evidence to support the notion that a 5% decrease in HDL-C increases risks. The variable and mild decrease in the HDL-C (1–7%) caused by a beta-blocking drug should not persuade against their use because these agents have important salutary effects *(9)* and a proven role in prolongation of life. Thus, when needed, it is advisable to combine a beta-blocker with statin in patients at high risk for CHD events. Beta-blockers may increase triglyceride levels in some individuals. The evidence linking triglycerides with an increased risk of CHD remains elusive. Raised levels of triglycerides appear to be a significant risk factor in women. In patients under age 60 yr, if triglyceride levels measured 6 mo after commencement of a beta-blocker show >30% increase or a decrease in HDL-C >10%, then a weak ISA beta-blocker (e.g., acebutolol) or other therapy should be substituted.

DIETARY THERAPY

Dietary therapy is necessary in all patients with hyperlipidemia. In individuals without evidence of CHD or cardiovascular disease, drugs are utilized only after a concerted effort by the physician and patient to lower serum cholesterol adequately. In patients with CHD and LDL-C cholesterol levels > 3.4 mmol/L (130 mg/dL), dietary therapy is necessary along with drug therapy. Fortunately, raised levels of triglycerides are virtually always controlled by carbohydrate and alcohol restriction, weight reduction, and exercise.

1. **Phase I diet:** Fat intake reduced to 30% of food energy with approximately 15% from saturated fats and 10% from polyunsaturated. Cholesterol intake should be <300 mg, carbohydrate 55%, and protein 15% of calories daily. This modification is recommended for the general population.

2. **Phase III:** Intake of fat 20%, approx 7% total daily calories from saturated fats, cholesterol 100–150 mg, carbohydrate 65%, and protein 15% of calories. The ratio of polyunsaturated fat to saturated fat (P/S) should be near 1.0. The recommendations in the United Kingdom are not as restrictive. For the general population or those at risk: intake of fat 35%, with saturated fat 11% of food energy. Polyunsaturated acids should reach 7% with P/S ratio about 0.45% *(10)*. The UK panel claims that the effects on the population of a P/S ratio of 1.0 or beyond are unknown *(10)*.

In constructing diets, the following points should be considered. A marked increase in carbohydrate intake may decrease HDL-C levels. Most studies show that saturated and monounsaturated fats raise the HDL-C cholesterol concentration; *high consumption of polyunsaturated fats lowers the level of HDL-C (11). A reduction in saturated fat intake from 35–40% to 20–25% of energy intake lowers HDL-C cholesterol concentration irrespective of the type of fat (11).* Depending on the dose, marine (n-3 polyunsaturated) oils may increase HDL-C cholesterol levels and decrease serum cholesterol and TG levels and platelet aggregation *(12)*. The favorable effects are not consistent, and occasionally a fall in HDL-C concentration occurs *(13,14)*. Diets containing 200 g of mackerel raised HDL-C levels in two studies *(15,16)*. However, 1 or 2 g of fish consumed twice weekly for 3 mo produced no changes in HDL-C in a large group of subjects *(17)*.

Olive oil containing oleic acid appears to have protective effects, but scientific proof is needed.

Favorable effects on serum lipids, in particular the HDL-C/LDL-C cholesterol ratio, should be achieved by restriction of total fat intake to about 30% of food energy and by substitution of saturated fats by monounsaturated fats, marine oils, and a moderate intake of vegetable polyunsaturated fats *(11)*. An increased intake of "nonpolluted" fish and marine oils provides omega-3 fatty acids, which appear to be cardioprotective: sock-eye salmon, Atlantic herring, rainbow trout, albacore tuna. Care is needed to avoid overindulgence because marine oils also contain a significant amount of cholesterol. One hundred grams of codliver oil contain approximately 19 g of omega-3 fatty acids but 570 mg of cholesterol *(18)*. One hundred grams of salmon or herring or commercial fish body oils contain approximately 485, 766, and 600 mg cholesterol, respectively. *Noncholesterol foods with abundant omega-3 fatty acids include purslane* (Portulaca oleracea) *(19), common beans, soybeans, walnuts, walnut oil, wheat germ oil, butternuts, and seaweed.*

- A Mediterranean-type diet is strongly recommended: no day without fruit; abundant fresh vegetables, olive oil, avocado, more fiber, fish, nuts, and less meat; butter and cream replaced by polyunsaturated/monounsaturated margarine, *non-trans* fatty acids. A trial comparing a **Mediterranean-based alpha-linolenic acid-rich diet** with a postinfarct low-fat diet in the secondary prevention of CHD reported a risk ratio of 0.24 for cardiovascular death and 0.30 for total mortality in the linolenic acid group at 27 mo of follow-up *(20)*. The Lyon Heart Study confirms post-myocardial infarction (MI) protection *(21)*.
- **Nuts** such as almonds, walnuts, hazelnuts, and pecans are high in beneficial poly- and monounsaturated fat as well as arginine, the precursor of nitric oxide (NO), which causes vasodilation. Arginine/NO appears to improve endothelial dysfunction and may improve performance in some patients with claudication and also angina *(22)*. Daily consumption of nuts is cardioprotective.
- ***Trans fatty acids*** increase LDL-C and must be curtailed. Major sources of food containing *trans* isomers include margarine, cookies (biscuits), cake and white bread, shortening, some margarine, fried foods, and cookies prepared with these fats *(24)*. The effect of intake of *trans* fatty acids was evaluated in the Nurses Health Study of 85,095 women without diag-

nosed CHD, stroke, or dyslipidemia in 1980. At 8-yr follow-up, intake of *trans* isomers was directly related to the risk of CHD *(24)*.

- *Plant stanols/sterols* can augment cholesterol management, and a margarine is available that may cause a small but significant lowering of LDL-C.

GUIDELINES FOR DRUG THERAPY

- The assignment to three categories of risk by the Adult Treatment Panel (ATP) III includes an important 10-yr risk score of >20% or <20%, which is clinically helpful. Because approx 66% of diabetics die of cardiovascular disease, they are considered CHD risk equivalent and to have a 10-yr risk for a CHD event >20%; so do patients with abdominal aortic aneurysm (AAA), peripheral vascular disease (PVD), and significant carotid disease.
- *Guidelines for drug therapy are given in Table 17-1.*

STATINS

The management of dyslipidemia has been revolutionized with the expanded use of statins (3-hydroxy-3-methylglutaryl coenzyme A (HMG CoA) reductase inhibitors). The more powerful LDL-C-lowering agents, atorvastatin and the new rosuvastatin, are effective in reducing

- LDL-C cholesterol to goal levels.
- Mortality in patients with CHD.
- The incidence of MI in patients with CHD.
- The degree of obstructive atheroma in coronary arteries as indicated by follow-up coronary angiography.
- The risk of stroke.
- Regression in atheroma volume; *see* ASTEROID trial *(3)*.

Pleiotropic effects of statins include

- Antithrombotic.
- Antiinflammatory: decreased C-RP.
- Antioxidants reduced ischemia and endothelial dysfunction.
- Reduction of calcific aortic stenosis.
- Improvement in congestive heart failure.
- A decrease in occurrence of atrial fibrillation?

Available statins include atorvastatin, fluvastatin, lovastatin, simvastatin, pravastatin, and (in 2003) rosuvastatin. The Cholesterol and Recurrent Events (CARE) study involved post-MI patients with cholesterol concentration in the low range (209 ± 17 mg/dL); there was no decrease in total mortality rate *(23)*. The number of fatal MIs was 38 versus 24 (p = 0.07), yet there was a relative risk reduction of 37%. Thus, clinicians should not accept percentage relative risk reduction as significant if the p value is not expressed or is 0.05 or greater. Note that breast cancer occurred in 12 pravastatin-treated patients versus 1 in the control group (p = 0.002). It is important in women to evaluate the use of statins, particularly in patients who have a positive family history of breast cancer.

In the Long-Term Intervention with Pravastatin in Ischemic Disease (LIPID) study, pravastatin reduced the risk for CHD mortality by 24% ($p < 0.001$), reduced the risk for any death by 22%, and significantly reduced nonfatal MIs and coronary revascularization *(48)*.

In the West of Scotland Study, in so-called healthy Scottish men with a mean cholesterol level of 272 mg/dL, total mortality was not significantly decreased; only nonfatal MIs were decreased significantly *(26)*. Thus, it is not justifiable to apply the results of the West of

Scotland trial to healthy men with cholesterol concentration in the range of 200–250 mg/dL. Approximately 38 million adults in the United States have high total cholesterol concentrations of 6.2 mmol/L (240 mg/dL) *(25)*, according to National Cholesterol Education Program (NCEP) action limits for the general population *(6,25,26)*.

The available statins possess **subtle differences**:

- The only hydrophilic agent excreted by the kidney is pravastatin. Thus, fewer adverse effects occur from drug interactions compared with lipophilic statins, which are hepatically metabolized.
- Lipophilic agents (atorvastatin, lovastatin, and simvastatin) are hepatically metabolized. Interactions may occur with cimetidine, cyclosporine, and other agents that use the cytochrome P-450 pathway (3A4).
- Rosuvastatin and fluvastatin engage hepatic 2C9; thus, caution is required particularly with cyclosporine, warfarin, and phenytoin.
- Fibrinogen: Atorvastatin has been shown to raise fibrinogen levels by 22% *(27)*.

The statins are competitive inhibitors of HMG-CoA reductase, the key enzyme catabolizing the early rate-limiting step in the biosynthesis of cholesterol within the hepatocyte. The lowering of intracellular cholesterol levels, resulting in a small increase in the number of receptors on the hepatocyte through the process of upregulation, results in increased clearance of circulating LDL-C cholesterol and a decrease in total serum cholesterol levels. In susceptible individuals, HMG-CoA reductase inhibitors are currently the most potent, best tolerated cholesterol-lowering agents.

Effect of simvastatin on coronary atheroma: The Multi-Centre Anti-Atheroma Study (MAAS) *(28)* indicated that 20 mg simvastatin daily over 4 yr reduced dyslipidemia and slowed progression of diffuse and focal coronary atherosclerosis. In a study evaluating the efficacy of intensive dietary therapy, alone or combined with lovastatin in outpatients with hypercholesterolemia, the level of HDL-C cholesterol fell by 6% during the low-fat diet and rose by 4% during treatment with lovastatin ($p > 0.001$) *(29)*.

Contraindications include hepatic dysfunction and concomitant use of nicotinic acid or fibrates, cyclosporin, other cytotoxic drugs, and erythromycin and similar antibiotics. They are also contraindicated in pregnancy, in women of childbearing age, and during lactation.

Advice and Adverse Effects

Increase in hepatic transaminases greater than three times the upper limit of normal occurs in 1–2% of patients receiving average maintenance and maximum dosages of these agents, respectively.

Monitoring of transaminase levels should be done every 4 mo, and the drug should be discontinued if levels of these enzymes are raised. If drug treatment is considered essential, patients with an increase less than three times normal can be observed at least twice monthly. Increases of up to fivefold with or without myalgia occur in up to 3% of patients, and levels >10 times normal with myalgia are observed in <1%. Myalgia without an increase in creatine kinase (CK) concentration is not uncommon.

- Severe **myositis** with rhabdomyolysis with the risk of renal failure has occurred with the combination of HMG-CoA reductase inhibitors with **gemfibrozil and also with cyclosporin**.
- **It is advisable to give the individual administered a statin a requisition for an emergency blood test for CK and creatinine and a urinalysis if muscle pains occur without associated upper respiratory tract infection (URTI) symptoms. The statin is discontinued immediately pending results of these tests.**

- Myopathy has been noted with **erythromycin combination**, and other antibiotic interactions in seriously ill patients may ensue. Angioedema has been reported. **Caution:** it is necessary to discontinue these lipid-lowering agents during serious intercurrent illness and sepsis when other drugs are being used.
- The anticoagulant effect of warfarin may be slightly enhanced by simvastatin administration, and digoxin levels may show a small increase: approx 10% for simvastatin and approx 20% for atorvastatin.
- Headaches are bothersome in up to 10% of patients. A switch from one HMG-CoA reductase inhibitor to another may resolve headaches, chest or abdominal pain, or rash. Thrombocytopenia has been reported.
- Lens opacities have been noted only in dogs given very high doses of these agents but have not been observed in patients. Current clinical data indicate that these agents do not cause cataracts *(30)*, but long-term effects beyond 15 yr are unknown.
- HMG-CoA reductase inhibitors are less effective in patients with familial hypercholesterolemia because these individuals have very low or absent LDL-C receptor activity. In these patients, combination therapy is necessary.

Drug name:	**Lovastatin**
Trade name:	Mevacor
Supplied:	10, 20, 40 mg
Dosage:	10–20 mg once daily with the evening meal; *see* text for further advice

Check serum cholesterol level after 8 wk and then three or four times monthly, with estimation of transaminase and CK levels at each visit. Increase the dose, if needed, to 40 mg once daily. The drug is more effective when given with the evening meal, as cholesterol biosynthesis occurs mainly at night *(31)*; thereafter, if needed, increase to 60 mg to a maximum of 80 mg daily in two divided doses.

Low-dose lovastatin (10 mg daily) appears to be highly effective for the management of hypercholesterolemia in most postmenopausal women.

Drug name:	**Simvastatin**
Trade name:	Zocor
Supplied:	5, 10, 20, 40, 80 mg
Dosage:	5 or 10 mg with evening meal. Monitor hepatic transaminases and CK in 3–4 mo with repeat serum cholesterol; if needed, increase to 20 mg once daily; max. 60 mg daily

This widely used statin has been proved in an RCT to decrease total mortality significantly. The Scandinavian Simvastatin Survival Study (4S), carried out in patients with CHD and cholesterol concentrations of 5.5–8 mmol/L (210–310 mg/dL) showed a 29% reduction in the total mortality rate *(32)*.

Drug name:	**Pravastatin**
Trade names:	Pravachol, Lipostat
Supplied:	10-, 20-, 40-mg tablets
Dosage:	10–20 mg with evening meal, increasing in 3–4 mo as required; max. 40 mg daily, with the same precautions as for lovastatin. Do not use if renal failure is present; maximum dose 10 mg in the elderly or if the GFR is 50–70 mL/min.

Results of the Pravastatin Limitations of Atherosclerosis in the Coronary Arteries (PLAC) I trial *(33)* indicate that pravastatin therapy reduced progression of CHD by 40% compared with placebo and caused a 54% reduction in fatal and nonfatal infarctions. The study included 408 patients with a <50% angiographically determined coronary stenosis. Patients were randomly assigned to pravastatin or placebo and followed up for 3 yr with repeated angiography performed in 323 patients and determination of clinical events. Baseline characteristics: cholesterol level of about 230 mg/dL (5.9 mmol/L), LDL-C cholesterol of 162–165 mg/dL (4.2–4.3 mmol/L), HDL-C cholesterol of 41 mg/dL (1.1 mL/L). After 3 yr of treatment, LDL-C cholesterol was reduced 28%, and an 8% increase in HDL-C cholesterol was observed. There were 15 new lesions in the pravastatin group, compared with 33 in the placebo patients. It appears that pravastatin inhibits platelet mural thrombosis at the site of arterial injury. A histologic study of patients' arteries showed that pravastatin decreased platelet formation in the arterial wall in hypercholesterolemic patients.

Drug name:	**Atorvastatin**
Trade name:	Lipitor
Supplied:	Tablets: 10, 20, 40, 60, 80 mg
Dosage:	10–40 mg daily after the evening meal; max. 80 mg

- Atorvastatin 10, 40, and 80 mg has been shown to cause a 38%, 46%, and 54% decrease in LDL-C cholesterol, respectively.
- The drug causes a 13–32% decrease in TG levels and is the only statin recommended for the management of mixed dyslipidemia.
- In the Atorvastatin Versus Revascularization Treatments (AVERT) study, treatment with 80 mg atorvastatin caused a 36% reduction in nonfatal MI, revascularization, and worsening angina compared with patients receiving angioplasty followed by usual care. In the Myocardial Ischemia Reduction with Aggressive Cholesterol Lowering (MIRACL) study, atorvastatin reduced early recurrent ischemic events in non-ST-elevation MI (NSTEMI) ACS patients treated within 14 d of an event *(4)*. In PROVE-IT TIMI 22, ACS patients showed a significant reduction in CAD outcomes when treated with atorvastatin 80 mg daily *(3)*.

Advice and Interactions

Flatulence and headaches occurred in 2% of patients in trials; otherwise the drug has a low side effect profile.

- As with other statins metabolized by the cytochrome P-450 system (3A4), interactions occur with grapefruit juice and agents such as cimetidine and erythromycin series of antibiotics, and digoxin levels may increase 20%.
- Warfarin is not affected,
- It is advisable to stop the drug (or other statins) for a few days during acute infections, major surgery, acute renal failure, and seizure activity.

Drug name:	**Rosuvastatin**
Trade name:	Crestor
Supplied:	10, 20, 40 mg
Dosage:	10–40 mg once daily. Do not use if severe renal failure is present. Use maximum 10 mg/d in patients age > 70 of if GFR is 50–70 mL/min.

Rosuvastatin is a powerful statin that has been shown to cause a 40–65% reduction in LDL-C and a significant increase in HDL-C *(3)* beyond that of atorvastatin The drug avoids the cytochrome P-450, 3A4 pathway, resulting in no interactions with drugs that use this pathway,

- However, cytochrome P-450, 2C9 is involved; thus caution is required, particularly with cyclosporine, warfarin, and phenytoin. Lovastatin, simvastatin, and atorvastatin use the 3A4 pathway. Rosuvastatin and fluvastatin engage 2C9.
- Warning: The active metabolite is approx 90% fecal and 10% renal eliminated. In individuals with renal failure, GFR < 30 mL/min there is a threefold increase in plasma concentrations and the drug is contraindicated. Caution is also needed in those with GFR 31–50 mL/min and in individuals older than age 70 who may have a normal serum creatinine but a GFR 50–60 mL/min.

Rosuvastatin at 20–40 mg daily should allow more patients to attain LDL-C goals and perhaps significant HDL-C improvements. A 12.4% increase in HDL-C levels has been noted after 18 mo of therapy with rosuvastatin.

COMBINATION THERAPY

The combination of an HMG-CoA reductase inhibitor with a bile acid-binding resin results in a further lowering of serum cholesterol levels. Both groups of lipid-lowering agents increase LDL-C receptor activity by different mechanisms. Concomitant use of simvastatin 40 mg daily and cholestyramine 8 g twice daily was more effective than simvastatin alone in lowering serum cholesterol concentration (37% versus 29%) and LDL-C cholesterol levels (45% versus 37%) in a 1-yr study. Similar effects have been reported for fluvastatin, lovastatin, and pravastatin. When one is combining the two groups of lipid-lowering agents, the HMG-CoA reductase inhibitor must be given 1 h before or 4 h after the bile acid-binding resin. Hoeg and colleagues *(34)* compared the safety and efficacy of six different treatment regimens for severe hypercholesterolemia. Neomycin-niacin, cholestyramine, and lovastatin had the most favorable therapeutic response. Only these three regimens increased HDL_2 cholesterol levels. However, only lovastatin treatment was free of adverse effects. The neomycin-niacin combination therapy caused unpleasant adverse effects *(34)*. The combination of lovastatin and colestipol resulted in a 36% reduction in serum cholesterol, a 48% decrease in LDL-C, and a 17% increase in HDL-C cholesterol levels *(35)*. The combination of probucol and cholestyramine caused about a 30% lowering of the LDL-C cholesterol concentration *(36)*.

The combination of fluvastatin with niacin was studied in 38 patients randomly assigned to fluvastatin and niacin and 36 patients allocated to placebo plus niacin and followed up for 15 wk *(37). The combination offluvastatin and niacin* caused a 40% decrease in LDL-C cholesterol and about a 30% increase in HDL-C cholesterol levels. Myositis, rhabdomyolysis, and myopathy did not occur during the study. Although the combination proved safe in this study, it is not recommended for general use and, if necessary, should be used with extreme caution and close monitoring.

Fluvastatin 20–40 mg with bezafibrate 400 mg was studied in 18 patients for 56 wk *(38)*. LDL-C cholesterol level decreased by 19% and 27% with 20 mg and 40 mg fluvastatin daily, respectively, and by 31% and 35%, respectively, with combination therapy: fluvastatin 20, 40 mg plus bezafibrate.

Pravastatin, combined with gemfibrozil, was studied in 32 patients for about 53 wk *(39)*. Myopathy or myositis was not observed during the study. Nonetheless, these combinations have not been studied in large clinical trials with long-term follow-up, and caution is advised when such combinations are administered to patients. Several deaths occurred when cerivastatin (now withdrawn) was combined with fibrates; some deaths were caused by the use of too high a dose of the drug, >0.4 mg. Colesevelam (Welchol), may be combined with a statin.

Cholesterol Absorption Inhibitors

Drug name:	**Ezetimibe**
Trade names:	Zetia, Ezetrol (C)
Supplied:	Tablets, 10 mg
Dosage:	10 mg once daily, with or without food

Ezetimibe is a new class of cholesterol absorption inhibitors.

The drug localizes and appears to act at the brush border of the small intestine and inhibits cholesterol absorption. The administration of Zetia will render resins obsolete. Ezetimibe 10 mg combined with simvastatin 40 mg resulted in a mean LDL-C lowering of 20%. Combination with a statin further decreases LDL-C. The drug is a welcome addition to our armamentarium.

Cholestyramine and colestipol are bile acid-binding resins. They are not absorbed in the gastrointestinal tract and act by binding bile salts in the intestine. This action is believed to cause increasing cholesterol catabolism to bile acids as well as increased cholesterol biosynthesis. The statins and ezetimibe have rendered these agents obsolete.

Advice, Adverse Effects, and Interactions

Cholestyramine can cause a 10–15% reduction in serum cholesterol levels. Very few patients tolerate the drug, and most refuse and/or take half the prescribed dose after 1 yr of therapy. Palatability can be improved by mixing the product with orange juice or the newer Questran Light; orange flavor appears to have better acceptance by patients. In practice, only about a 10% reduction in cholesterol is achieved. In the Lipid Research Clinic Primary Prevention Trial (LRCPPT) *(40)*, mean falls of 14% and 8% were observed at 1 and 7 yr, respectively. This modest reduction in serum cholesterol concentration was associated with a 19% reduction in risk ($p < 0.05$) of the primary end point—definite CHD death and/or definite nonfatal MI. However, there was a nonsignificant (7%) reduction of all-cause mortality.

Constipation can be severe; gritty taste, nausea, bloating, abdominal cramps, mild steatorrhea, and malabsorption can cause nutritional deficiency, especially of fat-soluble vitamins. Hypoprothrombinemia has been reported, and a mild increase in triglycerides may occur.

Contraindications and Cautions. Complete biliary obstruction. Supplements of fat-soluble vitamins and folate required with high doses.

Drug Interaction. Interference with absorption of digoxin, anticoagulants and an increase in the excretion of digitoxin. Other medications including HMG-CoA reductase inhibitors, thiazides, and thyroxine should be given 1 h before or 4 h after administration of cholestyramine or colestipol.

Divistyramine, a lipid-lowering drug that is available in some European countries, appears to cause fewer abdominal cramps and has a less gritty taste than cholestyramine.

NICOTINIC ACID

Drug name:	**Nicotinic acid; Niacin**
Supplied:	50, 100, 250 mg (500 mg US)
Dosage:	100 mg three times daily with meals for 1 wk and then 200 mg three times daily for 1–4 wk; average 500 mg three times daily; *see* text for further advice

Nicotinic acid inhibits lipolysis of adipose tissue. Also, the drug inhibits secretion of lipoproteins from the liver, causing a reduction in LDL-C and TGs.

Advice, Adverse Effects, and Interactions

Adverse effects include flushing, pruritus, nausea, abdominal pain, diarrhea, significant hepatic dysfunction and cholestatic jaundice, exacerbation of diabetes mellitus, hyperuricemia and exacerbation of gouty arthritis, palpitations, arrhythmias, dizziness, and rashes.

Cautions. Hypotension may occur in combination with other medications. Do not combine with HMG-CoA reductase inhibitors (statins). **Avoid in patients with AMI, heart failure (HF), gallbladder disease, past history of jaundice, liver disease, peptic ulcer, and diabetes mellitus. Hepatic necrosis has been reported and because of the adverse effects with little gain for patients, the drug is not recommended by the author and it should not be combined with statins.**

Nicotinic acid mainly reduces triglyceride levels, and doses of 3–4 g daily cause about a 25% increase in HDL-C cholesterol concentration.

Dosage (Further Advice)

The dose recommended in most standard texts is 2–4 g daily—an amazing number of tablets, 12–20 per day, unless sustained-release tablets are available, although these have an even higher adverse effect profile. **A case of fulminant liver failure has been reported in a patient soon after switching from nicotinic acid tablets taken for 1 yr to a sustained-release preparation *(41)*.**

FIBRATES

Drug name:	**Gemfibrozil**
Trade name:	Lopid
Supplied:	Tablets: 600 mg (capsules: 300 mg UK, Canada)
Dosage:	300–600 mg ½ h before morning and evening meals

Gemfibrozil is a chemical homolog of clofibrate but differs somewhat in mechanism of action and therapeutic effect. The drug decreases production of very low-density lipoprotein (VLDL) triglyceride and enhances its clearance.

The lipid-lowering effect is as follows:

- 11% reduction in serum cholesterol concentration.
- 30–50% reduction in the level of triglycerides *(42)*.
- 10% increase in HDL-C cholesterol concentration *(42)*.

Occasionally, the total cholesterol level is only mildly reduced. However, an increase in plasma prekallikrein and kininogen levels is constant and may confer a fibrinolytic effect.

The Helsinki Heart Study *(42)* randomly assigned 4080 asymptomatic men aged 40–55 yr to a group treated with gemfibrozil 600 mg twice daily and another group receiving placebo. At the end of 5 yr, 45 deaths had occurred in the gemfibrozil group and 42 in the placebo group, a nonsignificant decrease in cardiac mortality. However, 40 nonfatal myocardial infarcts occurred in the gemfibrozil group and 61 in the placebo group, a 34% reduction in nonfatal MIs.

Advice, Adverse Effects, and Interactions

Side effects include epigastric pain and bloating in 5–10%; rarely, rash and eczema. A mild increase in hepatic enzymes of 3–10% and rarely a mild increase in blood sugar levels occurs.

Cautions. Contraindications and interactions are the same as for clofibrate. The lithogenic activity appears to be slightly lower than that of clofibrate. Thus, the drug resembles clofibrate with, however, fewer side effects and causes a significant increase in HDL_2 cholesterol levels. Do not combine with HMG-CoA reductase inhibitors (statins).

Drug name:	**Bezafibrate**
Trade names:	Bezalip, Bezalip Mono
Supplied:	200 mg (Mono 400 mg)
Dosage:	200 mg three times daily with or after food Mono formulation: 1 tablet daily in the evening

Drug name:	**Fenofibrate**
Trade names:	Lipidil Supra
Supplied:	100, 145 mg
Dosage:	100–145 mg once daily with the main meal; max. 100 mg in renal dysfunction, with monitoring. **Avoid if creatinine** > 1.5 mg/dL 132 μmol/L or estimated GFR < 60 mL/min

This drug has been shown to decrease LDL-C cholesterol levels by up to 15% and to increase HDL-C concentration by about 20%. Advice, adverse effects, and cautions are similar to those listed under gemfibrozil. In the FIELD trial *(43)* (*see* Chapter 22), fenofibrate did not significantly reduce the risk of the primary outcome of coronary events. It did reduce total cardiovascular events, mainly owing to fewer nonfatal MIs.

CONCLUSIONS

- There is ample evidence to support the strong recommendation to commence statin therapy immediately on admission in patients with acute STEMI, NSTEMI, and unstable angina.
- Aggressive therapy with statins regardless of lipid levels has salutary effects on endothelial dysfunction that worsens vasoconstriction and induces platelet aggregation. Statins have an important role as antiatherogenic agents. They stabilize the atherosclerotic fibrous cap by increasing its collagen content. A thin, fragile cap is prone to rupture. The survival of vascular smooth muscle cells (VSMCs) and their unique ability to form tough collagen are essential to heal the plaque or maintain its stability. Plaque rupture or fissuring is dictated by the presence of a poorly formed thin fibrous cap, a lipid-rich core, and an abundance of inflammatory cells (macrophages) that are associated with a host of problems related to plaque stabilization. Indeed, atherosclerosis has an important unique nonspecific inflammatory component that contributes to growth and rupture of atheroma.
- It is not surprising to observe the increasing importance attached to high CRP levels found in patients with ACS *(5,44)*. Unfortunately, the inflammatory reaction does not appear to

be driven by organisms that can be eradicated with antibiotics. Trials using antibiotics have not resulted in salutary effects; *see* Chapter 22.

- It must be reemphasized that the inflammatory response observed is nonspecific, is probably a response to endothelial injury, and does not have an infective basis.
- Pravastatin does not inhibit VSMC proliferation and has been shown to have a salutary effect on the inflammatory process.
- In the CARE study *(45)*, pravastatin reduced CRP levels by 38% compared with placebo, but 12 cases of breast cancer occurred in 2079 treated patients compared with one case in the placebo arm ($p = 0.002$; *see* Table 17-2).
- In the LIPID study, pravastatin decreased total mortality from 14.1% to 11% (relative risk reduction was 33% [$p < 0.001$]) and death from CHD from 8.3% to 6.4% (relative risk reduction 24% [$p < 0.00$]). There was no increase in the number of newly diagnosed breast cancers in the pravastatin group.
- In the TNT trial *(46)*, intensive lipid-lowering therapy with 80 mg of atorvastatin daily in patients with stable CAD provided significant clinical benefit beyond that afforded by treatment with 10 mg of atorvastatin· The mean level of LDL-C was reduced to 77 mg/dL with 80 mg of atorvastatin and 101 mg/dL with 10 mg of atorvastatin.
- The Incremental Decrease in End Points Through Aggressive Lipid Lowering (IDEAL) trial *(47)* studied patients with a history of a definite MI. The mean LDL-C level was reduced to 104 mg/dL in the simvastatin (20-mg treated group) and 81 mg/dL in the atorvastatin 80-mg group. A major coronary event occurred in 463 simvastatin patients (10.4%) and in 411 atorvastatin patients (9.3%) ($p =0 .07$). Nonfatal acute MI occurred in 321 (7.2%) and 267 (6.0%) in the two groups ($p = 0.02$).
- Ezetimibe in combination with a statin is a most welcome addition to our armamentarium for the management of refractory hyperlipidemia.

REFERENCES

1. Expert Panel. Grundy SM, Cleeman JI, Merz CN, et al. Implications of recent clinical trials for the National Cholesterol Education Program Adult Treatment Panel III guidelines. Circulation 2004;110:227–239. [Erratum, Circulation 2004;110:763.]
2. ASTEROID: Nissen SE, Nicholls SJ, Sipahi I, et al. Effect of very high-intensity statin therapy on regression of coronary atherosclerosis: The ASTEROID trial. JAMA 2006;295:1556–1565.
3. Cannon CP, Braunwald E, McCabe CH, et al. Intensive versus moderate lipid lowering with statins after acute coronary syndromes. N Engl J Med 2004;350:1495–1504.
4. Schwartz GG, Olsson AG, Ezekowitz MD, et al. for the Myocardial Ischemia Reduction with Aggressive Cholesterol Lowering (MIRACL) Study Investigators. Effects of atorvastatin on early recurrent ischemic events in acute coronary syndromes. The MIRACL STUDY: A randomized controlled trial. JAMA 2001;285:1711–1718.
5. Ridker PM, Cannon CP, Morrow D, et al. for the Pravastatin or Atorvastatin Evaluation and Infection Therapy-Thrombolysis in Myocardial Infarction 22 (PROVE IT–TIMI 22) Investigators. C-reactive protein levels and outcomes after statin therapy. N Engl J Med 2005;352:20–28.
6. Brown MS, Goldstein JL. A receptor-mediated pathway for cholesterol homeostasis. Science 1979;323: 361.
7. Gundersen T, Kjekshus J, Stokke O, et al. Timolol maleate and HDL cholesterol after myocardial infarction. Eur Heart J 1985;6:840.
8. Valimaki M, Maass L, Harno K, et al. Lipoprotein lipids and apoproteins during beta-blocker administration: Comparison of penbutolol and atenolol. Eur J Clin Pharmacol 1986;30:17.
9. Khan M Gabriel. Angina. Dyslipidemias. In: Heart Disease, Diagnosis and Therapy. Totowa, NJ, Humana Press, 2005.
10. Trustwell AS. End of a static decade for coronary disease? BMJ 1984;289:509.
11. Pietinen P, Huttunen JK. Dietary determinants of plasma high-density lipoprotein cholesterol. Am Heart J 1987;113:620.
12. Sanders TAB, Roshanai F. The influence of different types of n-3-polyunsaturated fatty acids on blood lipids and platelet function in healthy volunteers. Clin Sci 1983;64:91.

Table 17-2

Clinical Trials of Statins Indicating Reduction of Mortality and Nonfatal Infarctions With Points of Clinical Importance

Trial	*Patients*	*Events*	*Control*	*Treated*	*Percentage relative risk reduction*
CARE (pravastatin) *(45)*	Post MI TC 209 ± 17 mg/dL	Total mortality	196/2079 (9.4%)	180/2079 (8.7%)	9 $p = 0.37$*
		CAD deaths	119	96	20 $p = 0.10$
		Fatal MI	38	24	37 $p = 0.07$*
		Nonfatal MI	173	135	23 $p = 0.02$
		Breat cancer	1	12	$p = 0.002$*
45 (simvastatin) *(32)*	IHD	Total mortality	256/2223 (11.5%)	182/2221 (8.2%)	29 $p = 0.01$
	TC 210–310 mg/dL	Fatal MI	1891	111	41
West of Scotland (pravastatin) *(26)*	"Healthy" Scottish men	Total mortality	135/3293 (4.1%)	106/3302 (3.2%)	22 $p = 0.051$
	TC > 272 mg/dL	Nonfatal MI	204 (6.5%)	143 (4.6%)	31 $p = 0.001$
	LDL-C 174–232 mg/dL	Death from CAD	52 (1.7%)	38 (1.2%)	28 $p = 0.13$*
Helsinki Heart Study (gemfibrozil) *(42)*		Total mortality	42/2040 (2.1%)	45/2040 (2.2%)	–5.8*
		Nonfatal MI	61/2040 (3.0%)	40/2040 (2.0%)	34*

*Total mortality must be significantly reduced to be clinically meaningful. Most studies, except 45, show only a significant reduction of nonfatal MI that may be preventable with aspirin and lifestyle changes.

TC, total cholesterol; CAD, coronary artery disease; IHD, ischemic heart disease; MI, myocardial infarction.

13. Nestel PH, Connor WE, Reardon MF, et al. Suppression by diets rich in fish oil on very low density lipoprotein production in man. J Clin Invest 1984;74:82.
14. Illingworth DR, Harris WS, Connor WE. Inhibition of low density lipoprotein synthesis by dietary omega-3 fatty acids in humans. Arteriosclerosis 1984;4:270.
15. Singer P, Wirth M, Voigt S, et al. Blood pressure and lipid-lowering effect of mackerel and herring diet in patients with mild essential hypertension. Atherosclerosis 1985;56:223.
16. Van Lossonczy TO, Ruiter A, Bronsgeest-Schoute HC, et al. The effect of a fish diet on serum lipids in healthy human subjects. Am J Clin Nutr 1985;31:1340.
17. Fehily AM, Burr ML, Phillips KM, Deadman NM. The effect of fatty fish on plasma lipid and lipoprotein concentrations. Am J Clin Nutr 1983;38:349.
18. Hepburn FN, Exler J, Weihrauch JL. Provisional tables on the content of omega-3 fatty acids and other fat components of selected foods. J Am Diet Assoc 1986;86:788.
19. Exler J, Wehlrauch JL. Provisional table on the content of omega-3 fatty acids and other fat components in selected seafoods (Publication HNIS/PT-103). Washington, DC, US Department of Agriculture, 1986.
20. de Lorgeril M, Renaud S, Mamelle N, et al. Mediterranean alpha-linolenic acid rich diet in secondary prevention of coronary heart disease. Lancet 1994;343:1454.
21. de Lorgeril M, Salen P, Maril JL, et al. Mediterranean diet: Traditional risk factors, and the rate of cardiovascular complications after myocardial infarction: Final report of the Lyon Diet Heart Study. Circulation 1999;99:779.
22. Maxwell AJ, Zapien MP, Pearce GL, et al. Randomized trial of a medical food for the dietary management of chronic, stable angina. J Am Coll Cardiol 2002;39:37.
23. CARE: For the Cholesterol and Recurrent Events Trial Investigators. The effect of pravastatin on coronary events after myocardial infarction in patients with average cholesterol levels. N Engl J Med 1996; 335:1001.
24. Willett WC. Stamper MJ, Manson JE, et al. Intake of trans fatty acids and risk of coronary heart disease among women. Lancet 1994;341:581.
25. American Heart Association: Heart and Stroke Statistical Update. Dallas, AHA, 1997.
26. Shepherd J, Cobbe SM, Ford I, et al. Prevention of coronary heart disease with pravastatin in men with hypercholesterolemia. N Engl J Med 1995;333:1301.
27. Wierbicki AS, Lumb PJ, Semra YK, et al. Effect of atorvastatin on plasma fibrinogen. Lancet 1998;351: 569.
28. Oliver MF, for the MAAS Investigators. Effect of simvastatin on coronary atheroma: The Multi-Centre Anti-Atheroma Study (MAAS). Lancet 1994;344:633.
29. Hunninghake DB, Stein EA, Dujovne CA. The efficacy of intensive dietary therapy alone or combined with lovastatin in outpatients with hypercholesterolemia. N Engl J Med 1993;328:1213.
30. Tobert JA, Sheer CL, Chremos AN, et al. Clinical experience with lovastatin. Am J Cardiol 1990;65:23F.
31. O'Connor P, Freely J, Shepherd J. Lipid lowering drugs. BMJ 1990;300:667.
32. Scandinavian Simvastatin Survival Study Group. Randomised trial of cholesterol lowering in 4444 patients with coronary heart disease: The Scandinavian Simvastatin Survival Study (4S). Lancet 1994; 344:1383.
33. Pitt B, Mancini GBJ, Ellis SG, et al. Pravastatin limitation of atherosclerosis in the coronary arteries. J Am Coll Cardiol 1995;26:1133.
34. Hoeg JM, Maher MB, Bailey KR, et al. Comparison of six pharmacological regimens for hypercholesterolemia. Am J Cardiol 1987;59:812.
35. Vega GL, Grundy SM. Treatment of primary moderate hypercholesterolemia with lovastatin (mevinolin) and colestipol. JAMA 1987;2571:33.
36. Sommariva D, Bonfiglioli D, Tirrito M, et al. Probucol and cholestyramine combination in the treatment of severe hypercholesterolemia. Int J Clin Pharmacol Ther Toxicol 1986;24:505.
37. Jacobson TA, Chin MM, Fromell GJ, et al. Fluvastatin with or without niacin for hypercholeserolemia. Am J Cardiol 1994;74:149.
38. Murati EN, Peters TK, Leitersdorf E. Fluvastatin in familial hypercholesterolemia: A cohort analysis of the response to combination treatment. Am J Cardiol 1994;73:30D.
39. Rosenson RS, Frauenheim WA. Safety of combined pravastatin-gemfibrozil therapy. Am J Cardiol 1994; 74:499.
40. Lipid Research Clinics Coronary Primary Prevention Trial Results. I. Reduction in incidence of coronary heart disease. II. The relationship of reduction in incidence of coronary heart disease to cholesterol lowering. JAMA 1984;251:351.
41. Mullin GE, Greenson JK, Mitchell MC. Fulminant hepatic failure alter ingestion of sustained-release nicotinic acid. Ann Intern Med 1989;111:253.

42. Frick MH, Elo O, Haapa K, et al. Helsinki Heart Study: Primary-prevention trial with gemfibrozil in middle-aged men with dyslipidemia. N Engl J Med 1987;317:1237.
43. Effects of long-term fenofibrate therapy on cardiovascular events in 9795 people with type 2 diabetes mellitus (the FIELD study): Randomised controlled trial. The FIELD study investigators. Lancet 2005; 366:1849–1861.
44. PROVE IT-TIMI 22: Ray KK, Cannon CP, Cairns R, et al. for the PROVE IT-TIMI 22 Investigators. Relationship between uncontrolled risk factors and C-reactive protein levels in patients receiving standard or intensive statin therapy for acute coronary syndromes in the PROVE IT-TIMI 22 TRIAL. J Am Coll Cardiol 2005;46:1417–1424.
45. CARE: For the Cholesterol and Recurrent Events Trial Investigators. The effect of pravastatin on coronary events after myocardial infarction in patients with average cholesterol levels. N Engl J Med 1996;335: 1001.
46. TNT: Larosa JC, Grundy SM, Waters DD, et al. for the Treating to New Targets (TNT) Investigators. Intensive lipid lowering with atorvastatin in patients with stable coronary disease. N Engl J Med. 2005; 352:1425–1435.
47. IDEAL: Pedersen TR, Faergeman O, Kastelein JJP, et al. High-dose atorvastatin versus usual-dose simvastatin for secondary prevention after myocardial infarction: The IDEAL study: A randomized controlled trial. JAMA 2005;294:2437–2445.
48. LIPID Study Group. Prevention of cardiovascular events and death with pravastatin in patients with coronary heart disease and a broad range of initial cholesterol levels. N Engl J Med 1998;339:1349–1357.

SUGGESTED READING

Baigent C, Keech A, Kearney PM, et al. Efficacy and safety of cholesterol-lowering treatment: Prospective meta-analysis of data from 90,056 participants in 14 randomised trials of statins. Lancet 2005;366:1267–1278.

Cannon CP, Braunwald E, McCabe CH, et al. Intensive versus moderate lipid lowering with statins after acute coronary syndromes. N Engl J Med 2004;350:1495–1504.

Cannon CP, Steinberg BA, Murphy SA, et al. Meta-analysis of cardiovascular outcomes trials comparing intensive versus moderate statin therapy. J Am Coll Cardiol 2006;48:438–445.

Deedwania P, Barter P, Carmena R, et al. for the Treating to New Targets Investigators. Reduction of low-density lipoprotein cholesterol in patients with coronary heart disease and metabolic syndrome: Analysis of the Treating to New Targets study. Lancet 2006;368:919–928.

Gotto AM Jr. Statin therapy and the elderly. SAGE advise? Circulation 2007;115:681–683.

Griffin BP. Statins in aortic stenosis: new data from a prospective clinical trial. J Am Coll Cardiol 2007;49: 562–564.

Khush KK, Waters DD, Bittner V, et al. Effect of high-dose atrovastatin on hospitalization for heart failure: subgroup analysis of the treating to new targets (TNT) study. Circulation 2007;115:576–583.

Klein BE, Klein R, Lee KE, et al. Statin use and incident nuclear cataract. JAMA 2006;295:2752–2758.

Larosa JC, Grundy SM, Waters DD, et al. for the Treating to New Targets (TNT) Investigators. Intensive lipid lowering with atorvastatin in patients with stable coronary disease. N Engl J Med. 2005;352:1425–1435.

LIPID Study Group. Prevention of cardiovascular events and death with pravastatin in patients with coronary heart disease and a broad range of initial cholesterol levels. N Engl J Med 1998;339:1349–1357.

Nakamura H, Arakawa K, Itakura H, et al. for the MEGA Study Group. Primary prevention of cardiovascular disease with pravastatin in Japan (MEGA Study): A prospective randomized controlled trial. Lancet 2006; 368:1155–1163.

Nissen SE, Nicholls SJ, Sipahi I, et al. Effect of very high-intensity statin therapy on regression of coronary atherosclerosis: The ASTEROID trial. JAMA 2006;295:1556–1565.

Ramasubbu K, Mann DL. The emerging role of statins in the treatment of heart failure. J Am Coll Cardiol 2006; 47:342–344.

Scandinavian Simvastatin Survival Study Group. Randomised trial of cholesterol lowering in 4444 patients with coronary heart disease: The Scandinavian Simvastatin Survival Study (4S). Lancet 1994;344:1383.

Scirica BM, Morrow DA, Cannon CP. Intensive statin therapy and the risk of hospitalization for heart failure after an acute coronary syndrome in the PROVE IT-TIMI 22 study. J Am Coll Cardiol 2006;47:2326.

Setoguchi S, Glynn RJ, Avorn J, et al. Statins and the risk of lung, breast, and colorectal cancer in the elderly. Circulation 2007;115:27–33.

Shepherd J, Cobbe SM, Ford I, et al. Prevention of coronary heart disease with pravastatin in men with hypercholesterolemia. N Engl J Med 1995;333:1301.

18 Statin Controversies

HIGH-INTENSITY STATIN THERAPY CAUSES SIGNIFICANT REGRESSION OF CORONARY ATHEROMA: TRUE OR FALSE?

A Study to Evaluate the effect of Rosuvastatin On Intravascular ultrasound-Derived Coronary atheroma burden (ASTEROID) trial showed that very-high-intensity statin therapy resulted in significant regression of atherosclerosis for all three prespecified measures of disease burden *(1)*.

Percent atheroma volume (PAV) is believed to be the most rigorous intravascular ultrasound (IVUS) measure of disease progression and regression but is not a measure of hard clinical end points. In ASTEROID, 507 patients had a baseline IVUS examination. After 24 mo of rosuvastatin 40 mg, 349 patients had evaluable serial IVUS examinations. The mean (SD) change in PAV for the entire vessel was –0.98% (3.15%; $p < 0.001$ versus baseline). The mean (SD) change in atheroma volume in the most diseased 10-mm subsegment was –6.1 mm^3 (10.1 mm^3; $p < 0.001$ versus baseline). Change in total atheroma volume showed a 6.8% median reduction ($p < 0.001$ versus baseline). Each pair of baseline and follow-up IVUS assessments was analyzed in a blinded fashion. Rosuvastatin 40 mg/d achieved an average low-density lipoprotein cholesterol (LDL-C) of 60.8 mg/dL and increased high-density lipoprotein cholesterol (HDL-C) by 14.7% (*see* Chapter 17 for details of this trial).

Blumenthal and colleagues *(2)* point out, however, that shortfalls of the trial include

- Lack of a control group receiving a somewhat less intensive LDL-C-lowering regimen. However, the trialists firmly believe that controls were not necessary because the degree of obstructive atheroma was measured at commencement and the baseline findings serve as genuine controls.
- The absence of paired IVUS measurements in less diseased coronary segments to demonstrate reproducibility of atheroma volume measurements.
- Lack of definitive information regarding the relationship of LDL-C lowering and extent of atheroma regression to determine whether high-intensity treatment is necessary to obtain regression.

In addition, it is questionable whether the PAV reduction observed is clinically significant. Only a modest decrease in mean PAV was observed (from 39.6% to 38.6%), and mean AV in the most diseased 10-mm subsegment decreased from 65 to 59 mm^3. Would this degree of reduction of PAV result in reduced unfavorable cardiovascular disease (CVD) outcomes? Reduction of PAV might have no significant effect on the amelioration of plaque erosion and rupture, which dictate significant reduction of adverse CVD events. Regression is not synonymous with plaque stabilization, which is believed to be crucial in causing decreased events. The subjects studied were not a particularly high-risk group;

From: *Contemporary Cardiology: Cardiac Drug Therapy, Seventh Edition*
M. Gabriel Khan © Humana Press Inc., Totowa, NJ

they had significant but stable CAD, ASTEROID, however, is a remarkable trial and we now know that atheroma regression can be achieved.

LDL CHOLESTEROL: HOW LOW SHOULD IT BE FOR STABLE CAD PATIENTS?

The Pravastatin or Atorvastatin Evaluation and Infection Therapy-Thrombolysis in Myocardial Infarction (PROVE IT-TIMI) 22 trial findings *(3)* have laid the foundation for the achievement of low LDL-C levels, <70 mg/dL (1.8 mmol/L) in patients at high risk with acute coronary syndrome (ACS). The composite triple end point of death, myocardial infarction (MI), or rehospitalization with recurrent ACS at a mean follow-up of 2 yr occurred in 15.7% of patients assigned atorvastatin 80 mg and in 20.0% of patients assigned pravastatin 40 mg, reflecting a hazard risk reduction of 24% (HR = 0.76; 95% confidence interval [CI], 0.66–0.88; $p = 0.0002$; *see* Chapter 22).

Just how low a level should be advocated in stable patients with coronary artery disease (CAD) is controversial.

The Treating to New Targets (TNT) investigators *(4)* evaluated 10,001 patients with CAD who were randomly assigned to double-blind therapy and who received either 10 mg or 80 mg of atorvastatin per day; follow-up lasted for a median of 4.9 yr. The primary end point was the occurrence of a first major cardiovascular event, defined as death from CAD, nonfatal non-procedure-related MI, and fatal or nonfatal stroke.

- There was no difference between the two treatment groups in overall mortality. A primary event occurred in 434 patients (8.7%) receiving 80 mg of atorvastatin versus 548 patients (10.9%) receiving 10 mg of atorvastatin.
- Atorvastatin 80 mg caused a 22% relative reduction in the risk of nonfatal MI ($p = 0.004$) and a 25% relative reduction in the risk of fatal or nonfatal stroke ($p = 0.02$).
- The number of deaths from noncardiovascular causes in the 80-mg atorvastatin group was increased by 31. Although this nonsignificant excess in deaths from noncardiovascular causes could be owing to chance, it is a cause for concern, and larger, long-term randomized controlled trials (RCTs) beyond 5 yr are required to ensure safety from excess deaths and rhabdomyolosis caused by statin use, at any dose level.
- Atorvastatin 80 mg achieved a mean LDL cholesterol level of 77 mg/dL (2.0 mmol/L); the 10-mg dose achieved a mean level of 101 mg/dL (2.6 mmol/L). The incidence of persistent elevations in liver aminotransferase levels was 0.2% and 1.2% in the groups given 10 mg and 80 mg, respectively ($p < 0.001$).

The Incremental Decrease in End Points through Aggressive Lipid Lowering (IDEAL) trial *(5)* randomized 4439 patients with a history of acute MI to atorvastatin 80 mg/d and 4449 to simvastatin 20 mg/d, with a mean follow-up of 4.8 yr.

- A major coronary event occurred in 463 simvastatin patients (10.4%) and in 411 atorvastatin patients (9.3%) (HR, 0.89; 95% CI, 0.78–1.01). Thus the prespecified primary end point did not achieve statistical significance ($p = 0.07$).
- Also, there was no difference in all-cause or cardiovascular mortality.
- Significant myopathy occurred in 17 patients and rhabdomyolysis in 5 patients administered a statin.

RHABDOMYOLOSIS IS A CAUSE FOR ALARM: TRUE OR FALSE?

Graham et al. *(6)* assessed the incidence of hospitalized rhabdomyolysis in patients treated with lipid-lowering drugs. In 252,460 patients, treated 24 cases were identified.

Table 18-1
Statins: Pharmacokinetics and Drug Interactions

	Atorvastatin	*Fluastatin*	*Pravastatin*	*Rosuvastatin*	*Simvastatin*
Pharmacokinetics					
Lipophilic (L) or hydrophilic (H)	L	Both	H	Both	L
Renal excretion	No	~10% renal, ~90% fecal	~60%	~10% renal; ~90% fecal	No
Renal excretion, patient in a renal failure or elderly patient[a]	No	Yes, if GFR <30 mL/min	Yes; caution if GFR <50 mL/min	Yes, if GFR <30 mL/min: use cautiously if GFR is 31–60 mL/min	No
Cytochrome P-450	3A4	2C9	Not known (multiple pathways)	2C9	3A4
Drug interactions					
Warfarin—INR increased	No	Yes	No	Yes	No
Digoxin level increased	Yes (20%)	<10%	No	No	<10%
Macrolide[b] antibiotics	Yes	No	No	No	Yes
Antifungal agents	Yes	No	No	No	Yes
Antiviral agents	Yes	No	No	No	Yes
Cyclosporine	Yes	Yes	Yes	Yes	Yes
Fluoxetine and similar agents	Yes	No	No	No	Yes
Fibrates[c] or niacin[c]	Yes	Yes	Yes	Yes	Yes
Grapefruit juice	Yes	No	No	No	Yes
Phenytoin	No	Yes	No	Yes	No
Verapamil, diltiazem, or amiodarone	Weak	No	No	No	Weak

[a]Contraindicated if severe renal failure, GFR < 30 mL/min. Relatively contraindicated—the elderly (age > 70) often have diminished renal function yet a normal serum creatinine, yet GFR 50–60 mL/min.

[b]Erythromycin, clarithromycin, troleandomycin, azithromycin.

[c]**Caution:** myopathy and rare rhabdomyolysis (combination of statin and fibrate or nicotinic acid is not recommended by the author).

H, hydrophilic; INR, international normalized ratio; L, lipophilic.

Modified from Khan M Gabriel. On Call Cardiology. Philadelphia, Saunders-Elsevier, 2006, p. 441.

The average incidence per 10,000 person-years for monotherapy with atorvastatin, pravastatin, or simvastatin was 0.44. The incidence increased to 5.98 for combination with a fibrate. The number needed to treat to observe one case of serious rhabdomyolysis was 22,727 for statin monotherapy, but it was 484 for older patients with diabetes mellitus who were treated with statin combined with fibrate.

- Thus age, concomitant diseases (diabetes, hypothyroidism, renal and hepatic dysfunction, surgery), and combined therapy with fibrates, niacin, and other drugs that interact increase the risk considerably (*see* Table 18-1).
- Cases have been reported with the combination of statin and amiodarone and also with newer antidepressants (including **risperidone and cetirizine**). Simvastatin and atorvastatin are metabolized primarily by CYP3A4, and amiodarone is a recognized inhibitor of this enzyme.

Avoiding the concomitant use of drugs with the potential to inhibit CYP-dependent metabolism (e.g., amiodarone) or retard the elimination of statins may decrease the risk of statin-associated myopathy.

Alternatively, if drug therapy with a potent CYP-450 inhibitor is inevitable, choosing a statin without relevant CYP metabolism (e.g., pravastatin) should be considered provided there is normal renal function: GFR > 75 mL/min in patients younger than age 70, and >60 mL/min in patients age 70–80.

Rosuvastatin does not appear to interact with clopidogrel, an interaction that appears to occur with atorvastatin and simvastatin, which use the cytochrome P 450 pathway, and also appears to decrease the effectiveness of clopidogrel, but this association is controversial.

- **Warning: In patients with severe renal failure, GFR < 30 mL/min, there is a threefold increase in plasma concentration of rosuvastatin; also, a caution is advised in patients with GFR 41–50 mL/min and in individuals over age 70 who often have unrevealed renal dysfunction or diminution of function due to age.**
- Colchicine combined with statin can cause a myopathy with extremely high creatine kinase (CK; > 10,000–30,000).
- In the IDEAL study *(5)*, significant myopathy occurred in 17 patients and rhabdomyolysis in 5 of 8404 patients administered a statin.
- IN the TNT study *(4)* of 10,000 subjects, five cases of rhabdomyolysis were reported (two in the group given 80 mg of atorvastatin and three in the group given 10 mg of atorvastatin).

Cannon emphasizes *(7)* that although this class of drugs is safe, statin use mandates that physicians monitor patients for any adverse effects, which can occur in up to 5% of patients but are only rarely life-threatening. Cannon points out that in the CTT metaanalysis, 9 (0.023%) of 39,884 patients treated with statins versus 6 (0.015%) of 39,817 patients treated with placebo reported rhabdomyolysis, for a nonsignificant excess of 3 patients (0.01%) *(8)*.

WHAT ABOUT STATIN INTERACTIONS?

Statins are used worldwide in millions of individuals many of whom ingest several other medications and caution is required. Table 18-1 gives the pharmacokinetics and drug interactions of statins. Colchicine interaction was emphasized earlier. In addition, there is some controversy regarding the interaction of atorvastatin and clopidogrel; both agents are required after percutaneous coronary intervention (PCI) with stent deployment.

Consider the following:

- Myopathy may be caused by low-dose statin therapy (*see* TNT *[4]*). In IDEAL, simvastatin 20–40 mg caused 11 cases of myopathy and 3 cases of rhabdomyolosis versus high-dose atorvastatin (80 mg), which caused 9 and 2 cases respectively.
- Ethnicity: Chinese, those of African descent, and Asians appear to be more sensitive to lower doses of statins.
- Age over 70 poses an increased risk.
- Renal dysfunction, low thyroid, hepatic dysfunction, diabetes, excessive alcohol, trauma, pneumonias and other severe intercurrent illnesses, and surgery in addition to drug interactions are important triggers for myopathy. Importantly, individuals older than age 70 may have a normal serum creatinine but lowered creatinine clearance (estimated glomerular filtration rate [GFR] < 55 mL/min) because of normal loss of nephrons with aging.
- Mainly hydrophilic agents (pravastatin) and partially hepatically and renally eliminated agents (rosuvastatin and fluvastatin) should be avoided in patients older than age 75 and in all individuals with renal dysfunction: creatinine levels above normal or abnormal creatinine clearance (estimated GFR < 60 mL/ min). Importantly, the formula for estimated GFR is not reliable in patients > age 70; for African Americans, multiply by 1.2 (*see* Chapter 22).

- If muscle pain occurs with a statin, stop the drug.
- **It is advisable to give all patients treated with a statin a requisition for urgent assessment of CK and creatinine and a urinalysis if they develop unusual muscle pains for >2 d in the absence of an upper respiratory tract infection (URTI). In all cases of muscle pains, particularly if the patient complains of being unwell or has minimal weakness, evaluate serum creatinine, estimated GFR, and urinalysis for hemoglobinuria and myogloburinuria.**
- If the CK is two times normal, do not restart the drug. A 30-min treadmill workout and weight lifting can increase CK to >500. However, if the CK remains elevated for up to 5 d later, take care not to assume that the elevation is caused by the workout.

If drug is discontinued and pain disappears in the presence of normal CK, try another statin.

- If pain persists, assess the sedimentation rate, which if markedly elevated usually indicates polymyalgia rheumatica, although this is a rare disease.
- It is advisable to give patients order forms beforehand, so they can have these tests done if they feel ill with muscle pains; they should also be told to seek attention immediately.
- Ezetimibe can increase CK, with some muscle involvement. This is a problem of undetermined pathophysiology.

Statins for All With Heart Failure?

There is evidence from RCTs that statins reduce the incidence of heart failure (HF) in patients with known CAD by reducing coronary events. Ramasubbu and colleagues *(9)* noted that the RCT experience with statins in nonischemic cardiomyopathy is limited to small trials of <100 *(10)*. It is premature, therefore, to recommend the use of statins for all HF patients unless indicated by an elevated level of LDL cholesterol.

The COntrolled Rosuvastatin multiNAtional trial in heart failure (CORONA), the Gruppo Italiano per lo Studio della Sopravvivenza nell'Insufficienza Cardiaca (GISSI-HF; Italian Group for the Study of the Survival in Cardiac Insufficiency), and RosUvastatiN Impact on VEntricular Remodelling of lipidS and cytokines (UNIVERSE) are expected to provide some answers.

Statins for Malignant Arrhythmias

The Multicenter Automatic Defibrillator Implantation Trial (MADIT)-II found that statin use in patients with an implantable cardioverter defibrillator (ICD) was associated with a reduction in the risk of cardiac death or ventricular tachycardia or fibrillation (VT/VF), whichever occurred first, and was also associated with a reduction in VT/VF episodes *(11)*. These findings suggest that statins may have antiarrhythmic properties, and RCTs are evaluating this interesting finding.

DO FIBRATES HAVE A SMALL ROLE IN THE TREATMENT OF CVD?

After more than two decades of use, clofibrate was withdrawn in the early 1980s because of an increased mortality risk and increased cancer mortality *(12)*. Since then controversial reports have appeared on various fibrates (including gemfibrozil, bezafibrate, and fenofibrate) regarding reduction in CVD outcomes. Their combination with statins is fraught with danger because they cause an alarming risk for rhabdomyolysis, a risk that some clinicians and lipid clinics believe is justifiable. Endocrinologist believe fibrates play a role in the management of diabetic dyslipidemia.

The Fenofibrate Intervention and Event Lowering in Diabetes (FIELD) study *(13)* randomized 9795 diabetics who were not taking statin therapy. Subjects had a total cholesterol concentration of 3.0–6.5 mmol/L and a total cholesterol/HDL cholesterol ratio of 4.0 or more, or a plasma triglyceride count of 1.0–5.0 mmol/L. Micronized fenofibrate 200 mg daily (n = 4895) or matching placebo (n = 4900) was given.

Fenofibrate at approx 5-yr follow-up did not significantly reduce the risk of the primary outcome of CHD death or nonfatal MI: 5.9% (n = 288) of patients on placebo and 5.2% (n = 256) of those on fenofibrate had a coronary event (relative reduction of 11%; HR, 0.89, 95% CI, 0.75–1.05; p = 0.16). There was a nonsignificant increase in CHD mortality. Is this the end of the fibrate era? Many do not agree.

Targeting Cholesterol Ester Transfer Protein: A New Therapy for CVD

Barter and Kastelein, as well as others, believe the currently available data suggest that decreased cholesterol ester transfer protein (CETP) activity is antiatherogenic, particularly if associated with an increase in HDL-C levels *(14)*.

CETi-1 (JTT-705) is currently under investigation in humans. The failure of torcetrapid has been well advertised and represents a major setback in our endeavors to increase HDL-C.

CETi-1

The vaccine CETi-1 induces autoantibodies that specifically bind and inhibit the activity of endogenous CETP.

In a phase I human study with CETi-1, one patient at the highest dose (250 mg) of a total of 36 patients who received a single injection developed anti-CETP antibodies. In an extension study of 23 patients, 53% (8 of 15) who received a second injection of the active vaccine developed anti-CETP antibodies compared with 0% (0 of 8) in the placebo group *(15)*. The vaccine was well tolerated, and no significant laboratory abnormalities occurred. The effect of the vaccine on the concentration of HDL-C in humans has not yet been reported.

REFERENCES

1. Nissen SE, Nicholls SJ, Sipahi I, et al. Effect of very high-intensity statin therapy on regression of coronary atherosclerosis: The ASTEROID trial. JAMA 2006;295:1556–1565.
2. Blumenthal RS, Kapur NK. Can a potent statin actually regress coronary atherosclerosis? JAMA 2006;295: 1583–1584.
3. Ray KK, Cannon CP, Cairns R, et al. for the PROVE IT-TIMI 22 Investigators. Relationship between uncontrolled risk factors and C-reactive protein levels in patients receiving standard or intensive statin therapy for acute coronary syndromes in the PROVE IT-TIMI 22 trial. J Am Coll Cardiol 2005;46:1417–1424.
4. LaRosa JC, Grundy SM, Waters DD, et al. Treating to New Targets (TNT) Investigators. Intensive lipid lowering with atorvastatin in patients with stable coronary disease. N Engl J Med 2005;352:1425–1435.
5. Pedersen TR, Faergeman O, Kastelein JJP, et al. High-dose atorvastatin versus usual-dose simvastatin for secondary prevention after myocardial infarction: The IDEAL study: A randomized controlled trial. JAMA 2005;294:2437–2445.
6. Graham DJ, Staffa JA, Shatin D, Andrade SE. Incidence of hospitalized rhabdomyolysis in patients treated with lipid-lowering drugs. JAMA 2004;292:2585–2590.
7. Cannon CP. The IDEAL cholesterol: Lower is better. JAMA 2005;294:2492–2494.
8. Baigent C, Keech A, Kearney PM, et al. Efficacy and safety of cholesterol-lowering treatment: Prospective meta-analysis of data from 90,056 participants in 14 randomised trials of statins. Lancet 2005;366: 1267–1278.
9. Ramasubbu K, Mann DL.The emerging role of statins in the treatment of heart failure. J Am Coll Cardiol 2004;47:342–344.

10. Horwich TB, MacLellan WR, Fonarow GC. Statin therapy is associated with improved survival in ischemic and non-ischemic heart failure. J Am Coll Cardiol 2004;43:642–648.
11. Vyas AK, Guo H, Moss AJ, et al. for the MADIT-II Research Group. Reduction in ventricular tachyarrhythmias with statins in the Multicenter Automatic Defibrillator Implantation Trial (MADIT)-II. J Am Coll Cardiol 2006;47:769–773.
12. Research Group. Coronary Drug Project: Clofibrate and niacin in coronary heart disease. JAMA 1975; 231:360.
13. The Field Study Investigators. Effects of long-term fenofibrate therapy on cardiovascular events in 9795 people with type 2 diabetes mellitus (the FIELD study). Lancet 2005;366:1849–1861.
14. Barter PJ, Kastelein JJP. Targeting cholesteryl ester transfer protein for the prevention and management of cardiovascular disease. J Am Coll Cardiol 2006;47:492–499.
15. Davidson MH, Maki K, Umporowicz D, Wheeler A, Rittershaus C, Ryan U. The safety and immunogenicity of a CETP vaccine in healthy adults. Atherosclerosis 2003;169:113–120.

SUGGESTED READING

Barter PJ, Kastelein JJP. Targeting cholesteryl ester transfer protein for the prevention and management of cardiovascular disease. J Am Coll Cardiol 2006;47:492–499.

Blumenthal RS, Kapur NK. Can a potent statin actually regress coronary atherosclerosis? JAMA 2006;295: 1583–1584.

Setoguchi S, Glynn RJ, Avorn J, et al. Statins and the risk of lung, breast, and colorectal cancer in the elderly. Circulation 2007;115:27–33.

19 Antiplatelet Agents, Anticoagulants, and Specific Thrombin Inhibitors

ANTIPLATELET AGENTS

Antiplatelet agents are used in virtually all patients with coronary heart disease (CHD). Aspirin, the pioneer hallmark agent, is of proven value for the management of

- Acute myocardial infarction (MI).
- Post-MI prophylaxis.
- Unstable angina.
- Stable angina.
- Following coronary artery bypass graft (CABG) and coronary angioplasty.
- Coronary stents when combined with clopidogrel.
- Lone atrial fibrillation in individuals aged < 65 yr.
- Transient ischemic attacks (TIAs) or following nonhemorrhagic stroke.

Available antiplatelet agents include

- Aspirin.
- Ticlopidine.
- Clopidogrel.
- Dipyridamole + aspirin.
- Platelet glycoprotein IIb/IIIa receptor blockers.

The patient with CHD may have to face unstable angina, MI, and early cardiac death. There is now convincing evidence that antiplatelet agents and heparin (both unfractionated [UF] and low-molecular-weight [LMWH]), bivalirudin, and fondaparinux improve morbidity and mortality rates in patients with CHD. Oral anticoagulants in combination with low-dose aspirin have a role in some situations.

Coronary thrombosis is known to be the major cause of coronary artery occlusion resulting in acute MI. In a hallmark study by DeWood and colleagues *(1)*, coronary thrombus was present in 87% of 126 patients who had coronary arteriography performed within 4 h of the onset of symptoms and in 65% of those studied 12 h or more after the onset of symptoms.

Davies and Thomas *(2)* observed that, of patients with sudden cardiac ischemic death, 74 of 100 had coronary thrombi; 48 (65%) of the 74 thrombi were found at sites of preexisting high-grade stenosis. In patients with thrombi, the most common finding is an underlying fissured plaque *(2)*. The contents of the plaque and denuded endothelium are highly thrombogenic and initiate thrombosis, resulting in coronary occlusion. Thus, prevention of the atherosclerotic process, plaque rupture and thrombosis, and dissolution of thrombi with dilation of the stenotic lesions are important therapeutic goals.

From: *Contemporary Cardiology: Cardiac Drug Therapy, Seventh Edition*
M. Gabriel Khan © Humana Press Inc., Totowa, NJ

Antiplatelet agents (so called because they inhibit platelet aggregation) have a role in the prevention of coronary thrombosis, MI, and cardiac death. Platelets clump onto atherosclerotic plaques, causing occlusion of the artery, and/or embolize downstream, occluding coronary arterioles. This effect may induce fatal arrhythmias and precipitate death. Angioscopic studies *(3)* have confirmed the presence of platelet clumps on eccentric atheromatous plaques in patients with unstable angina and no such platelet aggregation in patients with stable angina. It is not surprising, therefore, that aspirin, a potent antiplatelet agent, has proved effective in preventing acute MI in patients with unstable angina. A small, but timely, trial by Lewis and colleagues *(4)* showed that aspirin 325 mg reduced nonfatal and fatal infarction rates by about 50% in patients with unstable angina. In the second International Study of Infarct Survival (ISIS-2), patients with acute MI administered aspirin 160 mg achieved a 25% reduction in the 35-d vascular mortality rate and a 50% decrease in the incidence of reinfarction *(5)*. The addition of aspirin to streptokinase enhanced thrombolytic efficacy, resulting in a 48% decrease in the 35-d vascular mortality rate over the period *(5)*.

Antiplatelet agents are not expected to prevent all forms of thrombotic events. Thrombi occurring in arteries are rich in platelets, so antiplatelet agents are effective. In **obstructed arteries**, with **low flow**, the thrombus consists mainly of red cells within a fibrin mesh and **very few platelets**. This situation is similar to venous thrombosis, in which platelets are not predominant. The contents of a ruptured plaque are highly thrombogenic. Aspirin is only partially effective in preventing coronary thrombosis following plaque rupture, the usual cause of acute MI (*see* Chapter 11) *(6)*. Thus, antiplatelet agents may not help sufficiently in this situation and direct thrombin inhibitors, such as bivalirudin, hirudin, hirulog, fondaparinux, and newer types of oral anticoagulants specific for thrombin and derivatives of atheromatous plaque contents, are receiving intensive study and clinical testing *(7)*.

This chapter emphasizes two antithrombins, bivaliuridin, and fondaparinux, that are welcome additions to the therapeutic armamentarium.

Drug name:	**Aspirin (acetylsalicylic acid)**
Supplied:	80, 81, 325 mg (US) 75, 100, 300 mg (UK) Noncoated or coated 75, 80, 81 mg chewable
Dosage:	75–325 mg daily for ischemic heart disease (IHD) prophylaxis **160–325 mg chewed and swallowed at onset of pain caused by a probable heart attack; *see* text**

Aspirin (acetylsalicylic acid; ASA) has rightly gained widespread use in the management of unstable angina *(4,8)* and acute MI and in the prevention of nonfatal and fatal MI during the years following infarction. Also, salutary effects have been demonstrated in patients with stable angina and cerebral TIAs and in the prevention of occlusion of CABGs (*see* indications, Table 19-1).

Historical Review

Although this text has not given historical reviews of pharmacologic agents, it would appear timely to document briefly a few of the historical details that led to the widespread acceptance of aspirin, a drug that can prolong life.

Table 19-1
Indications for Aspirin

Cardiovascular	*Comment*
1. Unstable angina	Proven
2. Stable angina	Proven
3. Acute-onset myocardial infarction	Proven, also enhances effect of thrombolytic agents
4. Post-MI	Proven effective
5. Silent ischemia	Strongly advisable
6. Coronary artery bypass surgery	May prevent graft occlusion
7. Post-coronary angioplasty	Modest decrease in reocclusion
8. Lone atrial fibrillation	As good as oral anticoagulants
9. Bioprosthetic valves	In combination with dipyridamole
10. Transient cerebral ischemic attacks	Proven in both men and women
11. Post-nonhemorrhagic strokes	
12. Patients over age 40 yr at risk	Strongly advisable; *see* Table 19-2
13. Diabetics at high risk for CHD	Advisable

CHD, coronary heart disease; MI, myocardial infarction.

- Hippocrates approx (400 BC) treated his patients for pain with willow bark, which contains salicylic acid.
- 1763: Reverend Stone of Chipping Norton described the benefit of willow bark for ague.
- 1853: Von Gerhardt of Bayer developed aspirin.
- 1899: Felix Hoffman, a Bayer chemist, treated his father for rheumatism with aspirin.
- 1948–1953: Lawrence Craven treated approx 1500 relatively healthy, overweight, sedentary men aged 40–65 yr to obviate coronary thrombosis and reported his findings in the *Mississippi Valley Medical Journal* ("In Those with Risk Factors for Coronary Artery Disease") *(9)*. Craven apparently started treating his patients with high doses of aspirin and finally concluded that one aspirin a day was sufficient because none of his 1500 or more patients given this low dose for approx 5 yr experienced a cardiac event.
- 1971: John Vane discovered that aspirin blocks the production of prostaglandins.
- 1974: Elwood and colleagues *(10)* reported negative results of a randomized trial of aspirin in the secondary prevention of mortality from MI. Aspirin was once more forgotten until it became clear that the clinical trial had studied patients who were given the drug 2, 3, and even 12 mo after infarction.
- 1972–1977: The Stroke Trial of Fields and associates *(11)* showed a favorable trend.
- 1978: Barnet and colleagues *(12)* reported that male patients with TIAs treated with aspirin showed a significant reduction in stroke rate. These investigators emphasized that aspirin did not have beneficial effects in women in their study, and this notion was perpetuated by others for several years. The trial had enrolled approximately 90% men; there was not a sufficient number of women to test the hypothesis.
- 1983: The timely randomized trial of Lewis et al. *(4)* showed conclusively that one Alka-Seltzer (ASA, 325 mg) produced a 49% reduction in nonfatal MI. Cairns and colleagues *(8)*, in a larger study, confirmed the observation using 1300 mg aspirin daily.
- 1988: ISIS-2 confirmed an increase in survival in patients given aspirin within 6 h of the onset of infarction. Aspirin enhanced the salutary effects of streptokinase and further improved survival rates (*see* Chapter 11) *(13)*.

Table 19-2
Patients at Risk, Aspirin Advisable

1. Hyperlipidemia: Total cholesterol level >240 mg/dL (5.2 mmol/L) especially if HDL-C < 35 mg/dL (0.9 mmol/L)
2. Mild hypertension[a]
3. Diabetes, except hemorrhagic retinopathy
4. Strong family history of vascular thrombosis:
   Myocardial infarction at age <60 yr, stroke at <70 yr
5. Refractory smokers with any one of the above factors strengthens indication
6. Following hip or knee surgery for 3 wk if oral anticoagulants not used

Dosage: Use aspirin 60–162 mg daily with food; or enteric coated, 81–325 mg daily.

[a]Not in severe hypertension, increased risk of hemorrhagic stroke.

- 1988: Primary prevention in 22,071 male physicians, aged 40–80 yr, randomly assigned to 325 mg aspirin on alternate days, resulted in a 44% reduction in fatal and nonfatal MI ($p < 0.0001$).
- 1989: The American College of Chest Physicians recommended *(14)* that aspirin, 325 mg daily, be considered for virtually all individuals with evidence of CHD and selected patients with risk factors for CHD.

The Swedish Angina Pectoris Aspirin Trial studied 2035 patients with chronic stable angina without infarction. **Aspirin 75 mg reduced the occurrence of infarction and sudden death by 34% in the treated patients versus placebo *(15)*.**

Table 19-1 gives the clinical indications for aspirin, and Table 19-2 defines patients at risk in whom aspirin is advisable.

The results of five randomized trials in patients with atrial fibrillation led to the following conclusions:

- Patients aged under 60 yr with lone atrial fibrillation (no risk factors and no structural heart disease) can be treated with aspirin 60–162 mg daily. They usually do not require oral anticoagulants for stroke prevention because the risk of stroke is low (<0.5% per yr).
- In patients aged 65–75 yr with lone atrial fibrillation, the stroke rate is also low (<2% per yr) and aspirin therapy is recommended by some *(16)*, but anticoagulant therapy should be individualized because there are no clear answers.
- In patients over age 75 yr, warfarin has proved more effective than aspirin, but most of this benefit was lost because of a high rate of intracranial hemorrhage caused by warfarin. In addition, the mean age of patients in these trials was 69 yr, and only about 25% were over age 75 yr *(17)*. Thus, until further trial results are available in patients older than 70 with lone atrial fibrillation, treatment should be individualized.

Actions

- Acetylsalicylic acid irreversibly acetylates the enzyme cyclooxygenase. This enzyme is necessary for the conversion of platelet arachidonic acid to thromboxane A_2. The latter is a powerful platelet-aggregating agent and vasoconstrictor.
- The conversion to thromboxane A_2 and platelet aggregation can be initiated by several substances, especially those released following the interaction of catecholamine or platelets with subendothelial collagen. Endothelial and smooth muscle cells, when stimulated by physical or chemical injury, cause cyclooxygenase to convert membrane arachidonic acid to prostacyclin (prostaglandin I_2, [PGI_2]), which is then released. Prostacyclin is a

powerful inhibitor of platelet aggregation as well as a potent vasodilator. Prostacyclin, therefore, may help keep the vessel wall clean.
- Prostacyclin production is greatly reduced in diseased arteries. Aspirin further reduces the formation of prostacyclin in the vessel wall, and this is an undesirable effect. Low-dose aspirin inhibits thromboxane A_2 synthesis and platelet aggregation and does not inhibit PGI_2 production significantly.

Dosage. Enteric-coated aspirin 75–325 mg daily is the dose recommended *(18)*. An 80- and 81-mg enteric-coated tablet is available in North America; 60–75 mg is often used in Europe; *chewable 80 mg is useful, 160–240 mg taken at the onset of symptoms of MI.*

Aspirin, 20–60 mg daily, inhibits serum thromboxane A_2 generation without affecting prostacyclin synthesis and completely suppresses platelet aggregation *(18)*. It is advisable not to exceed 325 mg daily; 60–80 mg appears to be optimal. In the Aspirin Reinfarction Study, although infarction rates decreased, sudden deaths were increased *(19)*. In addition, prostacyclin infusion has been shown to prevent ventricular fibrillation (VF) after circumflex artery occlusion in dogs. The importance of inhibition of prostacyclin by doses higher than 325 mg cannot be dismissed. The inhibition of prostacyclin synthesis by aspirin 1 g daily may increase the risk of sudden death during acute infarction.

The cardiovascular indications for aspirin are listed in Table 19-1.

Drug name:	**Dipyridamole**
Trade names:	Persantine, Persantin, Persantin Retard
Supplied:	25, 50, and 75 mg; Retard 200 mg
Dosage:	50–75 mg three times; Retard 200 mg twice daily

The drug is useful only when combined with aspirin. It inhibits platelet adhesion to vessel walls and surfaces but has a low effect on platelet aggregation.

Caution:

- The drug may increase ischemia and angina owing to coronary steal and is contraindicated in unstable angina and immediately after MI.
- Thus, the combination of dipyridamole and aspirin for the management of stroke and TIA is not advisable in patients with CHD because angina or ischemia may be precipitated.

Interaction. The drug causes an accumulation of adenosine; thus, severe hypotension may occur if IV adenosine is given for supraventricular tachycardia; the dose of adenosine should be halved.

Indications

1. **Prosthetic heart valves.** The combination of dipyridamole and warfarin has been shown to be more effective than oral anticoagulants alone in preventing embolization in patients at risk (i.e., those with previous embolism). The drug may be added to warfarin and aspirin if thromboembolism persists. This is an indication approved by the Food and Drug Administration (FDA) for dipyridamole, but an indication for stroke prevention should emerge; see point 3. The drug appears to be effective on foreign, nonbiological surfaces, such as prosthetic valves.
2. Patients with tissue valves who show evidence of embolization.
3. Dipyridamole combined with aspirin (Aggrenox) appears to provide beneficial effects for secondary prevention after stroke *(21)*. Dipyridamole should be added to aspirin if TIAs

occur during aspirin therapy; the author has recommended the combination since 1974 and welcomes the scientific proof. A recent randomized controlled trial (RCT) indicated that dipyridamole (slow-release formulation, 200 mg plus aspirin 50 mg twice daily) resulted in a highly significant reduction in the occurrence of stroke ($p < 0.001$). The risk reduction for aspirin and dipyridamole for stroke was 37% versus 15% for dipyridamole alone and 18% for aspirin alone. *At present, the combination of aspirin and dipyridamole or clopidogrel appears to be the most effective and safest therapy for secondary prevention of stroke,* but see **caution** given above.

Drug name:	**Clopidogrel**
Trade name:	Plavix
Supplied:	75 mg
Dosage:	75 mg daily with or without food

The drug has rendered ticlopidine obsolete, except in countries where clopidogrel is unavailable.

Clopidogrel is an analog of ticlopidine and inhibits platelet aggregation by inhibiting ADP-induced platelet activation. Like ticlopidine, clopidogrel is a thienopyridine derivative. These agents are selective antagonists of ADP-induced platelet aggregation and inhibit platelet fibrinogen binding. The drug is more effective than ticlopidine but with fourfold lower toxicity.

Clinical Trials With Clopidogrel

In the Clopidogrel versus Aspirin in Patients at Risk for Ischemic Events (CAPRIE) study *(22)*, clopidogrel was marginally better than aspirin ($p = 0.045$). This drug may be employed if aspirin cannot be used because of allergy or intolerable side effects.

The drug is indicated for the reduction of atherosclerotic events (MI, stroke, and vascular death) in patients with atherosclerosis documented by recent stroke. Clopidogrel is associated with a 2% incidence of gastrointestinal hemorrhage versus 2.7% for aspirin. The incidence of intracranial hemorrhage was 0.4% for clopidogrel and 0.5% for aspirin. In the CAPRIE study, neutropenia < 450 was observed in six patients taking clopidogrel and in two receiving aspirin, **but two patients receiving clopidogrel had neutrophil counts of zero**.

Thrombotic thrombocytopenia, a dangerous complication of ticlopidine, may occur with clopidogrel, albeit rarely *(23)*, so caution is required.

The conclusion of the Clopidogrel in Unstable Angina to Prevent Recurrent Events (CURE) trial was that "clopidogrel has beneficial effects in patients with acute coronary syndrome [ACS] without ST elevation [NSTEMI]. However, the risk of major bleeding is increased among patients treated with clopidogrel" and "for every 1000 patients treated, 6 will require a transfusion" *(24)*. The drug has replaced ticlopidine for prevention of stent occlusion *(25)*; a loading dose is required.

The Clopidogrel for the Reduction of Events During Observation (CREDO) trial showed that clopidogrel administered 6–24 h prior to PCI and continued with aspirin daily for 1 yr significantly reduced cardiac events *(26)*.

The PCI-Clopidogrel as Adjunctive Reperfusion Therapy (PCI-CLARITY) study *(27)* showed conclusively that pretreatment with clopidogrel significantly reduced the incidence of cardiovascular death, MI, or stroke following PCI (34 [3.6%] versus 58 [6.2%];

$p = 0.008$). Pretreatment with clopidogrel also reduced the incidence of MI or stroke prior to PCI (37 [4.0%] versus 58 [6.2%]; $p = 0.03$). Overall, pretreatment with clopidogrel resulted in a highly significant reduction in cardiovascular death, MI, or stroke from randomization through 30 d (70 [7.5%] versus 112 [12.0%]); $p = 0.001$; number needed to treat = 23). There was no significant excess in the rates of Thrombolysis in Myocardial Infarction (TIMI) major or minor bleeding (18 [2.0%] versus 17 [1.9%]; $p > 0.99$) *(27)*.

- **Caution:** Despite guideline recommendations in the United States, most NSTEMI ACS patients treated with acute clopidogrel needing CABG have their surgery within ≤5 d of treatment. A failure to delay surgery for >5 d is associated with increased blood transfusion requirements.

In the Clopidogrel and Metoprolol in Myocardial Infarction Trial/Second Chinese Cardiac Study (COMMIT/CCS-2) *(28)*, patients with acute MI received aspirin and were randomized to receive clopidogrel 75 mg/d or placebo. Clopidogrel caused a significant reduction in death, reinfarction, or stroke (9.2% versus 10.1%; relative risk reduction, 9%; $p = 0.002$; *see* Chapter 22).

Lev et al. studied the role of dual drug resistance *(29)* and found that regardless of which aspirin resistance definition was used, about 50% of patients who were aspirin resistant were also resistant to clopidogrel, and about 20% of aspirin-sensitive patients were clopidogrel resistant ($p \leq 0.02$) *(29)*.

Lev and colleagues *(29)* emphasized that the lower response to clopidogrel among aspirin-resistant patients is of importance, because clopidogrel has been suggested as alternative therapy for aspirin-resistant patients. This may be inappropriate, and other platelet inhibitors acting on additional targets (other than cyclooxygenase-1 and P2Y12) should be developed and investigated *(29)*.

The Clopidogrel for High Atherothrombotic Risk and Ischemic Stabilization, Management, and Avoidance (CHARISMA) trial *(30)* showed that clopidogrel plus aspirin administered to patients with stable CHD was not significantly more effective than aspirin alone in reducing the rate of MI, stroke, or death from cardiovascular causes *(30)* (*see* Chapter 22).

- Gebel points out that clinical studies provide little evidence that clopidogrel, with or without aspirin, is more efficacious for the prevention of strokes than aspirin alone *(31)*. The increased risk of bleeding episodes with clopidogrel and aspirin in combination probably outweighs any small reductions in secondary event risk. In contrast, extended-release dipyridamole (ER-DP) plus aspirin reduces secondary stroke risk to a significantly greater extent (23% relative risk reduction) than aspirin alone. Available trial data support the use of ER-DP plus aspirin, but not clopidogrel plus aspirin, to prevent secondary vascular events after stroke or TIA *(31)* (*see* discussion of the ESPIRIT trial Chapter 22).

Platelet Glycoprotein IIb/IIIa Receptor Blockers

There are approx 75,000 glycoprotein IIb/IIIa receptors on the surface of each platelet. Antagonism of these receptors blocks the final common pathway for platelet aggregation —the binding of fibrinogen to the platelet glycoprotein receptors. Blockade of these receptors prevents the platelet aggregation caused by thrombin, thromboxane A_2, ADP, collagen, and catecholamines, as well as shear-induced platelet aggregation.

Properties of antiplatelet agents are given in Table 19-3.

Platelets may be activated by a myriad of agonists (thrombin, epinephrine, collagen, thromboxane, serotonin, adenosine-5'-diphosphate, von Willebrand factor, and so on) through various receptors involving complex signaling pathways *(32)*. Platelet aggrega-

Table 19-3
Properties of Intravenous GP IIb/IIIa Antagonists

	Abciximab	*Eptifibatide*	*Tirofiban*	*Lamifban*
Commercial name	ReoPro	Integrilin	Aggrastat	—
Supplier	Centocor/Eli Lilly	COR/Schering-Plough	Merck	Roche
Year of approval	1995	1998	1998	—
Structure	Antibody Fab fragment	Cyclic heptapeptide	Synthetic nonpeptide	Synthetic nonpeptid
Integrin selectivity	$\alpha_{IIb}\beta_3$ and $\alpha_v\beta_3$	$\alpha_{IIb}\beta_3$	$\alpha_{IIb}\beta_3$	$\alpha_{IIb}\beta_3$
Molecular weight (kDa)	48	0.83	<0.5	<0.5
Plasma half-life	10–30 min	approx 2.5 h	approx 2 h	approx 2 h
Excretion	Unknown	approx 50% renal	40–70% renal	90% renal
Approved indications	PCI Refractory unstable angina, if PCI is to be performed within 24 h	NSTE ACS	NSTE ACS	Not approved
Approved dose	PCI: Bolus: 0.25 mg/kg Infusion: 0.125 μg/kg/min (max 10 μg/min) ACS + PCI (within 24 h): Same as above, for 12–24 h	ACS: Bolus: 180 μg/kg Infusion: 2.0 μg/kg/min × 72–96 h PCI: Bolus: 135 μg/kg Infusion: 0.5 μg/kg/min × 20–24 h ESPRIT: Bolus: 2 × 180 μg/kg (10 min apart), then 2.0 μg/k/min × 18–24 h	ACS: 0.4 μg/kg/min × 30 min, then 0.1 μg/kg/min × 48–108 h	Not approved
Major clinical trials	EPIC, EPILOG, CAPTURE, EPISTENT, RAPPORT, ADMIRAL, CADILLAC TARGET, GUSTO-IV, GUSTO-V	PURSUIT IMPACT-II	PRISM PRISM-PLUS RESTORE TARGET	PARAGON A PARAGON B

NSTE, non-ST-segment elevation; PCI, percutaneous coronary intervention; ACS, acute coronary syndrome.
From Cannon CP. Management of Acute Coronary Syndromes, 2nd ed., Totowa, NJ, Humana Press, 2003, p. 500.

tion, the occurrence of crosslinking between platelets to form a "white thrombus," requires the activation of a common final pathway, the glycoprotein (GP) IIb/IIIa receptor-mediated linking of one platelet to another by binding to fibrinogen and in high-shear-stress conditions to von Willebrand factor. Given that platelets may be activated by multiple pathways but aggregate through a single pathway, the GP IIb/IIIa receptor emerged *(33)*.

- Ori Ben-Yehuda *(34)* points out that despite an American College of Cardiology/American Heart Association (ACC/AHA) class I indication, the use of platelet GP receptor blockers in NSTEMI patients is only approx 20% because of a substantial bleeding risk and uncertainty over the best time to initiate therapy (upstream or in the catheterization laboratory). In addition, the increasing use of clopidogrel as a proven alternative antiplatelet agent, and the development of direct thrombin inhibitors such as bivalirudin and fondaparinux, which cause less major bleeding *(34)*, will further retard the use of platelet GP receptor blockers. These agents cause an increase in bleeding time and may cause mild mucosal membrane bleeding and increased bleeding at arterial access sites, particularly in patients administered heparin. Increased bleeding and transfusion requirement are major disadvantages.

Platelet glycoprotein receptor blockers used IV include abciximab, tirofiban, and eptifibatide.

It is essential to use a low-dose weight-adjusted heparin regimen or LMWH and to pay careful attention to access sites. Most important, abciximab paralyzes platelets present in the body at the time of administration and not newly infused platelets. Oral agents, however, have a systemic effect and therefore can be counteracted only with hemodialysis. This is a major defect of new oral agents that are under investigation.

Clinical trials, however, have not shown benefit for oral agents *(35)*.

- The Sibrafiban versus aspirin to Yield Maximum Protection from ischemic Heart events post-acute cOroNary syndromes (SYMPHONY) trial found that Sibrafiban was no better than aspirin and caused an excess mortality including sudden death *(35)*. An increase in mortality of approx 30% occurred.

Drug name:	**Abciximab**
Trade name:	ReoPro
Dosage:	When PCI is planned within 24 h, give 0.25 mg/kg IV bolus over at least 1 min, immediately followed by IV infusion: 0.125 μg/kg/min for 18–24 h (max. 10 μg/min), concluding 1 h after PCI. The half-life is 10–30 min

Aspirin 325 mg should be continued as well as heparin IV to keep the activated partial thromboplastin time (aPTT) at 60–85 s during the abciximab (ReoPro) infusion. Safety has been investigated only with concomitant administration of heparin and aspirin. ReoPro decreases morbidity and mortality when used as indicated in the Chimeric 7E3 Antiplatelet Therapy in Unstable Refractory Angina (CAPTURE) *(36)*, Evaluation of 7E3 for the Prevention of Ischemic Complications (EPIC) *(37)*, and Evaluation of PTCA to Improve Long-Term Outcome with Abciximab Glycoprotein IIb/IIIa Blockade (EPILOG) trials *(38)*. The drug has never been indicated for ACS patients not scheduled for PCI. The Global Use of Streptokinase and Tissue Plasminogen Activator for Occluded Arteries (GUSTO) IV trial *(39)* showed no benefit; this trial result is considered surprising by some, but the drug was used inappropriately. Anderson et al. *(40)* showed *this drug saved lives and decreased morbidity in a large population of ACS patients who requied PCI and in whom the drug is correctly indicated.*

The use of in-laboratory abciximab is still appropriate in patients who have not received a GP IIb/IIIa upstream.

- It remains the GP IIb/IIIa of choice in STEMI patients treated with primary PCI. (It should be started prior to arrival in the catheterization laboratory if possible.)

Drug name:	**Eptifibatide**
Trade name:	Integrilin
Supplied:	IV bolus prior to PCI
Dosage for ACS:	• Intravenous bolus of 180 μg/kg as soon as possible after diagnosis • Follow by continuous infusion of 2 μg/kg/min for a further 20–24 h after PCI • If the patient is to undergo CABG, eptifibatide should be discontinued before surgery

Eptifibatide was shown in the Enhanced Suppression of the Platelet IIb/IIIa Receptor with Integrilin Therapy (ESPRIT) trial *(41)* at 48 h to cause a 40% relative risk reduction for the composite end points of death, MI, and urgent revascularization ($p = 0.0015$). The trial was prematurely terminated after 2064 patients were enrolled owing to significant beneficial effects of eptifibatide and the absence of safety concerns. The study dose was a bolus of 180 μg/kg, followed immediately by an infusion of 2 μg/kg/min, and then a second 180-μg/kg bolus 10 min after the first. There was a trend toward increased risk of major and minor bleeding with the study drug.

In the Platelet IIb/IIIa Underpinning the Receptor for Suppression of Unstable Ischemia Trial (PURSUIT) *(42)*, the drug resulted in significant benefit in patients who underwent PCI within 72 h ($p = 0.01$) but no benefit at 30 d in those without PCI *(42)*.

Drug name:	**Tirofiban**
Trade name:	Aggrastat
Dosage:	Two-stage infusion: 0.40 μg/kg/min for 30 min; then 0.1 μg/kg/min for up to 48–108 h (*see* product monograph); half-life 2 h.

A meta-analysis of these three agents excluding abciximab used as indicated for PCI planned within 24 h indicated that nondiabetic patients had no survival benefit *(43)*.

At most institutions in the United States, the cost of treating a 75-kg patient with abciximab is approx $1350, compared with a cost of $350 with tirofiban. This difference in cost fueled the hope that the efficacy of the two agents would be similar, but the Do Tirofiban And ReoPro Give Similar Efficacy Trial (TARGET) did not prove this to be the case *(44)*.

Patients were assigned to receive either tirofiban or abciximab before undergoing PCI with the intent to perform stenting. The primary end point (a composite of death, nonfatal MI, or urgent target-vessel revascularization at 30 d) occurred in 7.6% in the tirofiban group versus 6.0% in the abciximab group, demonstrating the superiority of abciximab over tirofiban ($p = 0.038$) *(44)*. The difference in the incidence of MI between the tirofiban group and the abciximab group was significant (6.9% and 5.4%, respectively; $p = 0.04$). The relative benefit of abciximab was consistent regardless of age, sex, the presence or absence of diabetes, or the presence or absence of pretreatment with clopidogrel. The trial demonstrated that tirofiban offered less protection from major ischemic events than did abciximab *(44)*.

Tirofiban and abciximab differ significantly in the way in which they antagonize GP IIb/IIIa receptors, and this difference may account for the findings. Tirofiban is a small, nonpeptide molecule, with a short half-life and marked specificity for the GP IIb/IIIa receptor. Abciximab is a large monoclonal antibody directed against β_3 integrin, has a prolonged half-life, and also binds to the $\alpha_v\beta_3$ integrin (vitronectin) receptor (found on endothelial and smooth-muscle cells) and to white-cell $\alpha_M\beta_2$ integrin receptors. Thus, only abciximab has the potential to influence the adhesion of platelets and endothelial cells and of platelets and white cells, as demonstrated in several studies *(45–48)*, whereas both agents are highly effective in blocking interactions between platelets in the final common pathway of platelet aggregation.

The Platelet Receptor inhibition in Ischemic Syndrome Management in Patients Limited by Unstable Signs and symptoms (PRISM-PLUS) trial *(49)* was stopped prematurely for the group receiving tirofiban alone because of excess mortality at 7 d (4.6% versus 1.1% for heparin alone). The rates of the composite end point in the tirofiban-plus-heparin group were not significantly lower than those in the heparin-only group at 6 mo (12.3% versus 15.3%; $p = 0.06$) *(49)*.

The Treat Angina with Aggrastat and determine Cost of Therapy with an Invasive or Conservative Strategy (TACTICS)-TIMI 18 trial *(50)* compared early invasive and conservative strategies in patients with unstable coronary syndromes treated with the GP IIb/IIIa inhibitor tirofiban and showed superiority of an invasive strategy in patients with non-ST elevation ACS. Patients with acute NSTEMI as defined by positive troponin levels benefited the most; the drug was beneficial only in patients with ACS treated with an early invasive strategy (*see* Chapter 22 for outcomes of invasive and conservatives strategies in TACTICS-TIMI 18 according to troponin T level).

ANTICOAGULANTS

Drug name:	**Warfarin**
Trade names:	Coumadin, Marevan (UK)
Supplied:	1, 2, 2½, 4, 5, 7½, 10 mg
Dosage:	10 mg on d 1, and 5 mg on d 2 (*preferably at bedtime*), with adjustment of dosage on the third day to about 3–7.5 mg depending on the INR; *see* text for further advice

For less urgent anticoagulation, give 5 mg daily for 4 d, and then go to International Normalized Ratio (INR) 2–3. (Note that the 10 mg for 2 d starting dose used commonly in the 1980s can cause gangrene of the limbs, albeit rarely.) Warfarin is the most commonly used coumarin oral anticoagulant.

Dosage (Further Advice)

Adjustment of dosage to maintain an INR 2–3. An INR of 2–3 for deep vein thrombosis and pulmonary or systemic embolism is appropriate.

Bleeding owing to oral anticoagulant is reversed by vitamin K_1 2–5 mg or fresh frozen plasma 15 mL/kg.

For interactions see Table 19-4.

Foods and the Clotting Cascade

A decrease in oral anticoagulant response has been reported with dietary sources of vitamin K_1 including Ensure Plus and broccoli *(51)*. Foods with high vitamin K content include

Table 19-4
Oral Anticoagulant-Drug Interactions

1. Drugs that may enhance anticoagulant response

Alcohol
Allopurinol
Aminoglycosides
Amiodarone
Ampicillin
Anabolic steroids
Aspirin

Cephalosporins
Chloral hydrate
Chloramphenicol
Chlorpromazine
Chlorpropamide
Chlortetracycline
Cimetidine
Clofibrate (fibrates)
Co-trimoxazole

Danazol
Dextrothyroxine
Diazoxide
Dipyridamole
Disulfiram

Ethacrynic acid
Erythromycin

Fenclofenac
Fenoprofen
Flufenamic acid
Fluconazole

Isoniazid

Ketoconazole
Ketoprofen

Liquid paraffin

Mefenamic acid
Methotrexate
Metronidazole
Monoamine oxidase inhibitors

Nalidixic acid
Naproxen
Neomycin

Omeprazole

Penicillin (large doses IV)
Phenformin
Phenylbutazone
Propylthiouracil

Quinidine

Rosuvastatin

Sulfinpyrazone
Sulfonamides

Tamoxifen
Tetracyclines
Tolbutamide
Thyroxine
Tricyclic antidepressants
Trimethoprim-sulfamethoxazole

Verapamil

2. Drugs that may decrease antocoagulant response

Antacids
Antihistamines

Barbiturates

Carbamazepine
Cholestyramine
Colestipol
Corticosteroids
Cyclophosphamide

Dichloralphenazone
Disopyramide

Glutethimide
Griseofulvin

Mercaptopurine

Oral contraceptives

Pheneturide
Phenytoin
Primidone

Rifampicin

Vitamins K_1 and K_2

Food	μg/100 g
Turnip greens	650
Broccoli	200
Lettuce	129
Cabbage	125
Spinach	89
Green peas	14
Potatoes	3

Drug name:	**Heparin**
Dosage:	60-U/kg bolus (max. 4000 U) as an immediate bolus and then a continuous infusion of 12 U /kg (1000 U/h) to maintain the aPTT at 1.5–1.9 times baseline or 70 s. The aPPT is assessed Q 6 h until in the target range, then every12 h.

Action. Anticoagulant activity requires a cofactor, antithrombin III. Heparin binds to lysine sites on antithrombin III and converts the cofactor from a slow inhibitor to a very rapid inhibitor of thrombin. The heparin-antithrombin complex inactivates thrombin and thus prevents thrombin-induced activation of factors V and VIII. The reaction also inactivates factor X, other coagulation enzymes, and thrombin-induced platelet aggregation. The half-life is 30–60 min after a 75-U/kg IV bolus.

Adverse Effects. Apart from bleeding, heparin-induced thrombocytopenia (HIT) occurs in 3–5% between d 5 and 10 of IV use; assess platelet from d 3. Continuous infusion of heparin is superior to intermittent bolus, as the latter causes

- Peaks of activity and therefore a greater potential for hemorrhage in patients who are at risk of bleeding.
- Confusion about the exact time to draw blood for the activated aPTT estimation, leading to errors in interpretation. The aPTT can be estimated at any time when one is using continuous infusion because experimentally this level of activity usually results in arrest of the thrombotic process.

Caution. **Heparin use with thrombolytics: There continues to be an excessive number of hemorrhagic strokes and deaths reported in RCTs.** In the tenecteplase versus alteplase trial (Assessment of the Safety and Efficacy of a New Thrombolytic 2 [ASSENT-2]), patients >67 kg received heparin 5000 U at a 1000-U infusion rate and those <67 kg received 4000 U at 800 U/h *(52a)*. The 30-d *mortality rates in patients were: for PTT > 75 s, 5.8%; 50–75 s, 3.4%; <50 s, 3%.* In ASSENT 3 the heparin dosage was that given in the table above and the rate of major in-hospital bleeding ws 2.2% *(52b)* versus 4.7% in ASSENT 2.

Low-Molecular-Weight Heparin

Drug name:	**Enoxaparin**
Trade name:	Lovenox
Supplied:	Prefilled syringes: 30, 40 mg Graduated prefilled syringes: 60, 80, 100 mg Ampules: 30 mg
Dosage:	1 mg/kg every 12 h SC; plus aspirin 100–325 mg daily for a minimum of 2 d (*see* Chapters 11 and 22)

LMWH (enoxaparin) is available as a sterile solution for injection. Enoxaparin (1 mg/kg every 12 h subcutaneously) and regular heparin IV bolus and continuous infusion were tested in an RCT in patients with unstable angina and non-Q-wave MI *(53)*. The number of deaths, MI, or recurring angina was lower in the enoxaparin group and was sustained for up to 30 d. Enoxaparin appears to be the most beneficial LMWH, based on two positive RCTs for it versus one for dalteparin. Several RCTs have shown that LMWHs are as effective as regular heparin; the subcutaneous route is a major advantage. There is no need for PTT measurements, and the use of the agent is associated with bleeding similar to or less than that with standard IV heparin. Also, the incidence of HIT is lower.

The Enoxaparin and Thrombolysis Reperfusion for Acute Myocardial Infarction Treatment-Thrombolysis in Myocardial Infarction (EXTRACT-TIMI) 25 trial *(54)* studied enoxaparin versus UF heparin. *At 30 d follow-up,* the primary end point occurred in 12.0% of patients in the UF heparin group versus 9.% in the enoxaparin group (17% reduction in relative risk; $p < 0.001$). Nonfatal MI occurred in 4.5% and 3.0%, respectively (33% reduction in relative risk; $p < 0.001$); there was no difference in total mortality *(54)*.

- Major bleeding occurred in 1.4% with UF heparin versus 2.1% enoxaparin ($p < 0.001$).
- The dose of LMWH should be reduced in patients over age 70 and given once daily in those with creatinine clearance (estimated GFR) 30–50 mL/min and avoided in those with estimated GFR < 30 mL/min (*see* Chapter 22).
- The adjustment of dosage based on weight, age, and renal function is vital to reduce the in-creased risk of bleeding caused by LMWH.

SPECIFIC THROMBIN INHIBITORS

The composition of the material that causes coronary occlusion and, thus, acute MI is complex. The thrombogenic properties of ruptured atheromatous plaques cannot all be nullified by aspirin, platelet IIb/IIIa receptor blockers, and standard thrombolytic agents (t-Pa, streptokinase). Novel specific thrombin inhibitors are being sought. Direct thrombin inhibitors such as bivalirudin, fondaparinux, and hirudin do not need a cofactor to inhibit thrombin.

Bivalirudin

Bivalirudin binds reversibly to thrombin. The drug cleaves to thrombin then drops off, which may explain the short half-life of 25 min and the lower adverse effects compared with hirudin and heparin. Bivalirudin proved beneficial during PCI *(55)* and reduced the risk of death or MI by approx 30% at 50 d with significant reduction in major bleeding.

- In the Acute Catheterization and Urgent Intervention Triage Strategy (ACUITY) trial *(56)*, ischemic complications were suppressed in the bivalirudin (non-heparin, non-GP receptor blocker) arm just as effectively as in the heparin plus glycoprotein receptor blocker or bivalirudin GP receptor arms, but bivalirudin was associated with half of the major bleeding (*see* Chapter 22 for details).

Hirudin

Hirudin is a naturally occurring specific thrombin inhibitor. This 65-amino-acid polypeptide was isolated from the saliva of the leech (*Hirudo medicinalis*) more than 30 yr ago. Recombinant techniques have provided the form that is used clinically.

Advantages compared with heparin include *(57)*

- Hirudin neutralizes free thrombin directly. This effect does not require an intermediary molecule such as antithrombin III.

- It inhibits clot-bound thrombin.
- Heparins are inactivated by antiheparin proteins, e.g., platelet factor 4. Hirudin is not affected.
- Hirudin inhibits thrombin-mediated platelet activation and generation of fibrin.
- Hirudin inhibits thrombus-induced platelet activation but heparin does not.

The Global Utilization of Streptokinase and Tissue Plasminogen Activator for Occluded Arteries (GUSTO) IIb trial *(58)* indicated that the combination of hirudin and streptokinase (SK) is a promising alternative to t-PA with heparin. Death or reinfarction occurred in 8.6% of hirudin-treated patients versus 14.4% for heparin ($p = 0.004$). Hirudin interacts favorably with SK but not t-PA *(58)*.

Fondaparinux

Fondaparinux is a synthetic pentasaccharide that selectively inhibits factor Xa. Fondaparinux can be administered once daily without laboratory monitoring. In small dose-ranging studies, a low dose of fondaparinux (2.5 mg) had similar efficacy to higher doses of fondaparinux and the standard dose of enoxaparin, with a similar or lower risk of bleeding *(59)*.

- The Fifth Organization to Assess Strategies in Acute Ischemic Syndromes (OASIS-5) investigators compared fondaparinux and enoxaparin in acute coronary syndromes *(60)*. Fondaparinux was associated with a significantly reduced number of deaths at 30 d (295 versis 352; $p = 0.02$) and at 180 d (574 versus 638; $p = 0.05$).
- In OASIS-6, which involved patients with STEMI, particularly those not undergoing primary PCI, fondaparinux significantly reduced mortality and reinfarction without increasing bleeding and strokes *(61)*.

Gibbons and colleagues emphasized that the specific anti-factor Xa activity of fondaparinux, compared with the antithrombin and anti-factor Xa effect of enoxaparin, may in part be responsible for its safer profile *(59)*. Fondaparinux inhibits factor Xa within the clot, preventing thrombus progression and thus enhancing effectiveness, but does not inhibit platelet function, thus enhancing safety *(59; see* Chapter 22 for details of the RCTs).

- These recent large RCTs have endorsed fondaparinux as a leading antithrombotic drug in the treatment of ACS *(60,61)*. There is no evidence that fondaparinux is inferior to either UF heparin or LMW heparin for management of ACS.
- The once-daily dose and absence of the need for dose adjustment are major advantages over UF heparin and LMWH *(62)*.

Oral thrombin inhibitors are being tested. Specific thrombin inhibitors or nullifiers of atheromatous plaque contents may emerge as important additions to our armamentarium in the management of ACS.

REFERENCES

1. DeWood MA, Spores J, Notske R, et al. Prevalence of total coronary occlusion during the early hours of transmural myocardial infarction. N Engl J Med 1980;303:897.
2. Davies MJ, Thomas A. Thrombosis and acute coronary artery lesions in sudden cardiac ischemic death. N Engl J Med 1984;310:1137.
3. Sherman CT, Litrack F, Grundfest W, et al. Coronary angioscopy in patients with unstable angina pectoris. N Engl J Med 1986;315:913.
4. Lewis HD, Davis JW, Archibald DG, et al. Protective effects of aspirin against acute myocardial infarction and death in men with unstable angina: Results of a Veterans Administration Cooperative Study. N Engl J Med 1983;309:396.

5. ISIS-2 (Second International Study of Infarct Survival) Collaborative Group. Randomized trial of intravenous streptokinase, oral aspirin, both, or neither among 17,187 cases of suspected acute myocardial infarction: ISIS-2. Lancet 1988;2:350.
6. Clarke RJ, Mago G, Fitzgerald G, et al. Combined administration of aspirin and a specific thrombin inhibitor in man. Circulation 1991;83:1510.
7. Khan M Gabriel, Topol EJ. Complications of myocardial infarction. In: Heart Disease, Diagnosis and Therapy. Baltimore, Williams & Wilkins, 1996.
8. Cairns JA, Gent M, Singer J, et al. Aspirin, sulfinpyrazone or both in unstable angina. N Engl J Med 1986; 313:1369.
9. Craven LL. Experiences with aspirin (acetylsalicylic acid) in the non-specific prophylaxis of coronary thrombosis. Miss Valley Med J 1953;75:38.
10. Elwood PC, Cochrane AL, Burr ML, et al. A randomized controlled trial of acetylsalicylic acid in the secondary prevention of mortality from myocardial infarction. BMJ 1974;1:436.
11. Fields WS, Lemak NA, Frankowski RF, et al. Controlled trial of aspirin in cerebral ischemia. Stroke 1977; 8:301.
12. Canadian Cooperative Study Group. A randomized trial of aspirin and sulfinpyrazone in threatened stroke. N Engl J Med 1978;299:53.
13. ISIS-2 (Second International Study of Infarct Survival) Collaborative Group. Randomised trial of intravenous streptokinase, oral aspirin, both, or neither among 17,187 cases of suspected acute myocardial infarction. Lancet 1988;2:349.
14. Resnekov L, Chekiak J, Hirsh J, et al. Antithrombotic agents in coronary artery disease. Chest 1989;95: 528.
15. Juul-Moller S, Edvardsson N, Jhnmatz B, et al. Double-blind trial of aspirin in primary prevention of myocardial infarction in patients with stable chronic angina pectoris. Lancet 1992;40:1421.
16. Albers GW. Atrial fibrillation and stroke: Three new studies, three remaining questions. Arch Intern Med 1994;154:1443.
17. Atrial Fibrillation Investigators. Risk factor for stroke and efficacy of antithrombotic therapy in atrial fibrillation: Analysis of pooled data from 5 randomized controlled trials. Arch Intern Med 1994;154:1449.
18. Patrono C, Wood AJJ. Aspirin as an anti-platelet drug. N Engl J Med 1994;330:1287.
19. Aspirin Myocardial Infarction Study Research Group. A randomized, controlled trial of aspirin in persons recovered from myocardial infarction. JAMA 1980;243:661.
20. Keltz TN, Innerfield M, Gilter B, et al. Dipyridamole-induced myocardial ischemia. JAMA 1987;257:1516.
21. The ESPS Group. The European Stroke Prevention Study. Principal end points. Lancet 1987;2:1352.
22. CAPRIE Steering Committee. A randomized, blinded, trial of clopidogrel versus aspirin in patients at risk of ischemic events (CAPRIE). Lancet 1996;348:1329.
23. Bennett R, Connors JM, Carwile JM, et al. Thrombotic thrombocytopenic purpura associated with clopidogrel. N Engl J Med 2000;342:1773.
24. CURE: The Clopidogrel in Unstable Angina to Prevent Recurrent Events trial investigators. Effects of clopidogrel in addition to aspirin in patients with acute coronary syndromes without ST segment elevation. N Engl J Med 2001;345:494.
25. Bhatt DL, Bertrand ME, Berger PB, et al. Meta analysis of randomized and registry with clopidogrel after stenting. J Am Coll Cardiol 2002;39:9.
26. CREDO: Steinhubl SR, Berger PB, Mann JT, et al. for the CREDO investigators. Early and sustained dual oral anti-platelet therapy following percutaneous coronary intervention. JAMA 2002288:2411.
27. Sabatine MS, Cannon CP, Gibson CM. Effect of clopidogrel pretreatment before percutaneous coronary intervention in patients with ST-elevation myocardial infarction treated with fibrinolytics. JAMA 2005; 294:1224–1232.
28. COMITT-2 (ClOpidogrel and Metoprolol in Myocardial Infarction Trial) Collaborative Group. Addition of clopidogrel to aspirin in 45,852 patients with acute myocardial infarction: Randomised placebo-controlled trial. Lancet 2005;366:1607–1621.
29. CHARISMA: Lev EI, Patel RT, Maresh KJ. The role of dual drug resistance. J Am Coll Cardiol 2006; 47:27–33.
30. Bhat DL, Keith AA, Fox KAA, Hacke W, for the CHARISMA Investigators. Prevention of atherothrombotic events. N Engl J Med 2006;354:1706–1717.
31. Gebel JM Jr. Secondary stroke prevention with antiplatelet therapy with emphasis on the cardiac patient. A neurologist's view. J Am Coll Cardiol 2005;37:2059–2065.
32. Ben-Yehuda O. Anti-platelet therapies In: Chien K, ed. Molecular Basis of Cardiovascular Disease, A Companion to Braunwald's Heart Disease. Philadelphia, WB Saunders, 2004.

33. Coller BS. Blockade of platelet GP IIb/IIIa receptors as an antithrombotic strategy. Circulation 1995;92: 2373–2380.
34. Ben-Yehuda O. Editorial Comment: Upstream/downstream glycoprotein IIb/IIIa in non–ST-segment elevation myocardial infarction. J Am Coll Cardiol 2006;47:538–540.
35. SYMPHONY Investigators. A randomized comparison of sibrafiban, an oral platelet glycoprotein IIb/IIIa receptor antagonist, with aspirin for acute coronary syndromes. Lancet 2000;355:337.
36. CAPTURE Investigators. Randomized placebo-controlled trial of abciximab before and during coronary intervention in refractory unstable angina: The CAPTURE study. Lancet 1997;349:1429.
37. EPIC Investigators. Use of a monoclonal antibody directed against the platelet glycoprotein IIb/IIIa receptor in high-risk coronary angioplasty. N Engl J Med 1994;330:956.
38. EPILOG Investigators. Platelet glycoprotein IIb/IIIa receptor blockade and low-dose heparin during percutaneous coronary revascularization. N Engl J Med 1997;226:1689.
39. Simoons ML. Effect of glycoprotein IIb/IIIa receptor blocker abciximab on outcome in patients with acute coronary syndromes without early coronary revascularisation: The GUSTO IV-ACS randomised trial. Lancet 2001;357:1915.
40. Anderson RM, Califf RM, Stone GW. Long term mortality benefit with abciximab in patients undergoing percutaneous coronary intervention. J Am Coll Cardiol 2001;37;2059–2065.
41 ESPRIT: Novel dosing regimen of eptifibatide in planned coronary stent implantation: A randomized placebo controlled trial. Lancet 2000;356:2037.
42. PURSUIT: Inhibition of platelet glycoprotein IIb/IIIa with eptifibatide in patients with acute coronary syndromes. The PURSUIT Trial Investigators. Platelet Glycoprotein IIb/IIIa in Unstable Angina: Receptor Suppression Using Integrilin Therapy. N Engl J Med 1998;339:436.
43. Roffi M, Chew P, Mukherjee D, et al. Platelet glycoprotein IIb/IIIa inhibitors reduce mortality in diabetic patients with non ST segment elevation acute coronary syndromes. Circulation 2001;104:2767.
44. Topol EA, Moliterno DJ, Herrmann HC, et al. Comparison of two platelet glycoprotein IIb/IIIa inhibitors, tirofiban and abciximab, for the prevention of ischemic events with percutaneous coronary revascularization. N Engl J Med 2001;344:1888.
45. Kaul DK, Tsai HM, Liu XD, Nakada MT, Nagel RL, Coller BS. Monoclonal antibodies to $\alpha_v\beta_3$ (7E3 and LM609) inhibit sickle red blood cell-endothelium interactions induced by platelet-activating factor. Blood 2000;95:368–374.
46. Thompson RD, Wakelin MW, Larbi KY, et al. Divergent effects of platelet-endothelial cell adhesion molecule-1 and B_3 integrin blockade on leukocyte transmigration in vivo. J Immunol 2000;165:426–434.
47. Mickelson JK, Ali MN, Kleiman NS, et al. Chimeric 7E3 Fab (ReoPro) decreases detectable CD11b on neutrophils from patients undergoing coronary angioplasty. J Am Coll Cardiol 1999;33:97–106.
48. Neumann F-J, Zohlnhöfer D, Fakhoury L, Ott I, Gawaz M, Schömig A. Effect of glycoprotein IIb/IIIa receptor blockade on platelet-leukocyte interaction and surface expression of the leukocyte integrin Mac-1 in acute myocardial infarction. J Am Coll Cardiol 1999;34:1420–1426.
49. PRISM-PLUS: Platelet Receptor Inhibitor in Ischemic Syndrome Management in Patients Limited by unstable Signs and Symptoms (PRISM-PLUS) Study Investigators. Inhibition of the platelet glycoprotein IIb/IIIa receptor with tirofiban in unstable angina and non-Q-wave myocardial infarction. N Engl J Med 1998;338:1488.
50. Cannon CP, Weintraub WS, Demopoulos LA, et al. Comparison of early invasive and conservative strategies in patients with unstable coronary syndromes treated with the glycoprotein IIb/IIIa inhibitor tirofiban. N Engl J Med 2001;344:1879.
51. Kempin SJ. Warfarin resistance caused by broccoli. N Engl J Med 1983;308:1229.
52a. ASSENT-2: Single-bolus tenecteplase compared with front-loaded alteplase in acute myocardial infarction: the ASSENT-2 double-blind randomized trial. Lancet 1999;354:716–722.
52b. Efficacy and safety of tenecteplase in combination with enoxaparin, abciximab, or unfractionated heparin: The ASSENT-3 randomized trial in acute myocardial infarction. Lancet 2001;358:605–613.
53. Cohen M, Demers C, Gurfinkel EP, et al. A comparison of low-molecular-weight heparin with unfractionated heparin for unstable coronary artery disease. N Engl J Med 1997;337:447.
54. Antman EM, Morrow DA, McCabe CH, et al. Enoxaparin versus unfractionated heparin with fibrinolysis for ST-elevation myocardial infarction for the ExTRACT-TIMI 25 Investigators. N Engl J Med 2006; 354:1477–1488.
55. Kong D, Topol E, Bittl J, et al. Clinical outcomes of bivalirudin for ischemic heart disease. Circulation 1999;100:2049.
56. ACUITY: Stone GW, Bertrand M, Colombo A, et al. Acute Catheterization and Urgent Intervention Triage strategY (ACUITY) trial: Study design and rationale. Am Heart J 2004;148:764–775.

57. Olson RE. Vitamin K. In: Goodhart RS, Shils ME (eds). Modern Nutrition in Health and Disease, 6th ed. Philadelphia, Lea & Febiger, 1980, p 170.
58. Jang IK, Gold HK, Zisking AA, et al. Prevention of platelet-rich arterial thrombosis by selective thrombin inhibition. Circulation 1990;81:219.
59. Gibbons RJ, Fuster, V. Therapy for patients with acute coronary syndromes—new opportunities. N Engl J Med 2006;354:1524–1527.
60. The OASIS-5: The Fifth Organization to Assess Strategies in Acute Ischemic Syndromes Investigators. Comparison of fondaparinux and enoxaparin in acute coronary syndromes. N Engl J Med 2006;354: 1464–1476.
61. The OASIS-6 Trial Group. Effects of fondaparinux on mortality and reinfarction in patients with acute ST-segment elevation myocardial infarction. The randomized trial. JAMA 2006;295:1519–1530.
62. Califf RM. Fondaparinux in ST-segment elevation myocardial infarction. The drug, the strategy, the environment, or all of the above? JAMA 2006;295:1579–1580.

SUGGESTED READING

Antman EM, Morrow DA, McCabe CH, et al. Enoxaparin versus unfractionated heparin with fibrinolysis for ST-elevation myocardial infarction for the ExTRACT-TIMI 25 Investigators. N Engl J Med 2006; 354:1477–1488.

Bavry AA, Lincoff AM. Is clopidogrel cardiovascular medicine's double-edged sword? Circulation 2006; 113:1638–1640.

Ben-Yehuda O. Editorial comment: Upstream/downstream glycoprotein IIb/IIIa in non-ST-segment elevation myocardial infarction. J Am Coll Cardiol 2006:47:538–540.

Califf RM. Fondaparinux in ST-segment elevation myocardial infarction. The drug, the strategy, the environment, or all of the above? JAMA 2006;295:1579–1580.

Eisenstein EL, Anstrom KJ, Kong DF, et al. Clopidogrel use and long-term clinical outcomes after drug-eluting stent implantation. JAMA 2007;297:159–168.

Mehta RH, Roe MT, Mulgund J, et al. Acute clopidogrel use and outcomes in patients with non-ST-segment elevation acute coronary syndromes undergoing coronary artery bypass surgery. J Am Coll Cardiol 2006; 48:281–286.

Stevens LA, Coresh J, Greene T. Assessing kidney function—measured and estimated glomerular filtration rate. N Engl J Med 2006;354:2473–2483.

20 Cardiac Drugs During Pregnancy and Lactation

Most cardiovascular agents (like all other drugs) must be avoided in the first trimester of pregnancy because they may produce congenital malformations, especially from the 3rd to the 11th week of pregnancy.

When used during the second and third trimesters, several cardiac drugs may affect growth and functional development of the fetus or cause toxic effects on fetal tissues. Also, some agents must be avoided just before parturition as they may have adverse effects on labor or in the newborn.

Cardiovascular drugs are discussed mainly with an emphasis on their safety for the fetus or newborn.

The physician is commonly called to manage the following hazardous heart conditions in pregnancy:

- Acute severe hypertension caused by preeclampsia.
- Mitral stenosis and pulmonary edema that can be fatal.
- Arrhythmias that may be bothersome.
- Pulmonary hypertension that may cause sudden death.
- Peripartum cardiomyopathy causing heart failure.

ANTIHYPERTENSIVE AGENTS IN PREGNANCY

Fortunately, because of the vasodilating properties of early pregnancy, patients with mild hypertension often do not need drug therapy until after wk 20 of pregnancy.

The relatively safe agents commonly used from wk 16 to delivery include

- Methyldopa.
- Beta-adrenergic blockers (except atenolol; reserve for short-term use, weeks only, because of potential adverse effects).
- Hydralazine: short term, emergencies.
- Labetalol: short term, emergencies.

Caution is necessary with the following agents:

- Thiazide diuretics: short term only.
- Nifedipine: short-term hypertensive crisis: fulminating preeclampsia.

Agents that are contraindicated include

From: *Contemporary Cardiology: Cardiac Drug Therapy, Seventh Edition*
M. Gabriel Khan © Humana Press Inc., Totowa, NJ

- Angiotensin-converting enzyme (ACE) inhibitors.
- Nitroprusside.
- Reserpine.
- Furosemide.
- Diltiazem and verapamil.

Achievement of blood pressure control does not eliminate a risk for the patient or baby. Intensive maternal and fetal monitoring is mandatory irrespective of successful control of blood pressure, as a risk of abruption, seizures, and disseminated intravascular coagulopathy still prevails.

Drug name:	**Methyldopa**
Trade name:	Aldomet
Supplied:	125, 250, 500 mg
Dosage:	250 mg twice daily, increasing if needed to max. 1.5 g daily

Methyldopa was the most widely used agent for the long-term management of hypertension in pregnancy for over 30 yr until about 1990; since then, beta-blockers have often replaced methyldopa because depression (approx 22%), sedation, and postural hypotension cause problems with compliance and lead to approx 15% of patients stopping treatment. Also, the drug causes a positive direct Coombs test, and problems may occur with cross-matching the patient's blood. The long track record of efficacy and the preservation of fetal well-being, especially the absence of neurologic effects, have established a proven role for this old drug. Several newer agents have been tried for the chronic management of hypertension, and all but beta-blocking agents have fallen aside because of various adverse effects on the fetus. Notably, most studies of antihypertensive agents in pregnancy have been used in only a few patients and with age at entry later than w 24 of gestation. Caution is therefore necessary even with relatively safe agents used early in pregnancy. Thus, it is necessary, when possible, to avoid the use of all antihypertensive drugs during the first trimester of pregnancy.

In one study, only one (0.9%) fetal death occurred in 117 methyldopa-treated patients, and 9 (7.2%) fetal deaths occurred in the control group of 125 women *(1)*. Methyldopa is known to be relatively safe; it does not cause a decrease in uteroplacental blood flow. A 7-yr follow-up of children born to mothers treated with methyldopa showed no significant differences *(2)*. Other randomized trials, however, have failed to show any benefit from treatment compared with beta-blockers or no treatment *(3)*.

Methyldopa is the recommended agent for the treatment of severe hypertension (diastolic pressure >105 mmHg) associated with severe preeclampsia, remote from delivery. Occasionally, intravenous therapy is required, 250 mg diluted in 100 mL 5% dextrose in water, given over 30–60 min, repeated every 6 h.

Adverse Effects

Adverse effects include orthostatic hypotension, sedation, dizziness, fatigue, Coombs positivity; depression occurs in approx 22%.

Caution: Avoid methyldopa after parturition because the drug may precipitate depression (*see* Chapter 8).

The combination of methyldopa and beta-blockers is not advisable because both agents act centrally.

Beta-Adrenergic Blockers

Beta-blockers are relatively safe and effective agents in controlling hypertension during pregnancy from the 16th week prior to labor. Although they have been used effectively in patients within 48 h before labor and during delivery, other agents are preferred during this period. Blood pressure control, if required, just prior to delivery is best achieved with the use of methyldopa or hydralazine or the combination of hydralazine and a very low dose of atenolol.

Beta-blockers have advantages over methyldopa for prolonged treatment of chronic hypertension during the last trimester. These agents do not usually cause orthostatic hypotension, somnolence, or significant depression. Also, methyldopa must be taken two or three times daily as opposed to beta-blockers, which are given once daily. The most common beta-blockers used during pregnancy, *labetalol, atenolol, and pindolol,* are effective. Atenolol caused no fetal adverse effects in 120 pregnant women; neonates showed a minor incidence of transient bradycardia not requiring therapy, and a 1-yr follow-up gave results similar to those observed with methyldopa, with no differences in development or growth indices *(4)*. In another study, 4-yr follow-up revealed all normal infants *(5)*. Chronic atenolol therapy does not increase the incidence of neonatal respiratory distress syndrome. In one study, no child in the actively treated group required ventilation, as opposed to seven infants in the control group requiring ventilation for the respiratory distress syndrome *(6)*.

However, other studies with atenolol have found significantly lower infant birth and placental weights compared with the nontreatment arm *(7)*, and the concern appears to be unique to atenolol used for long-term but not for short-term treatment *(8)*.

Adverse effects of beta-blockers used during pregnancy include

- Fetal or neonatal bradycardia.
- Premature or prolonged labor.
- Delayed spontaneous breathing in the newborn, mainly observed with IV use.
- Rarely neonatal hypoglycemia.

Drug name:	**Atenolol**
Trade name:	Tenormin
Supplied:	25, 50, 100 mg
Dosage:	25–50 mg once daily, increasing if needed to max. 100 mg daily Doses of 200 mg have been used for short periods, but this is not advisable

Intrauterine growth retardation is often mentioned, and low infant birth weight may occur only with long-term treatment *(7,8)*. The author agrees with the cautious use of atenolol in pregnancy but does not recommend this beta-blocker for primary hypertension.

Drug name:	**Metoprolol**
Trade names:	Betaloc, Lopressor, Toprol XL
Supplied:	50, 100 mg
Dosage:	50 mg twice daily, max. 200 mg

The dosages of metoprolol and pindolol are much lower than those advised by the respective manufacturers.

Drug name:	**Labetalol**
Trade names:	Normodyne, Trandate
Supplied:	50, 100, 200 mg
Dosage:	Oral: 100 mg twice daily with food, increasing over 2–4 wk to 200 mg twice daily; max. 600 mg For hypertensive crises in pregnancy: IV slow bolus 20–50 mg, or infusion 20 mg/h titrated slowly with continuous BP monitoring to 30–160 mg/min The combination with hydralazine allows lower doses of both agents with fewer side effects

Labetalol is a beta-adrenergic blocking agent with alpha$_1$-blocking properties, and thus it causes vasodilation. The latter effect may result in orthostatic hypotension. **The drug may also cause fatal or life-threatening hepatic necrosis.** Labetalol is as effective as methyldopa in controlling hypertension during pregnancy. **The drug is extremely useful in the acute short-term management of severe resistant hypertension just before labor or during delivery, but there is concern about maternal hepatotoxicity;** ***the drug can cause hepatic necrosis.*** **Avoid in asthmatics. Some state that labetalol is generally safer and preferable to atenotol** ***(7).***

Adverse Effects

Adverse effects include about a 27% incidence of intrauterine growth retardation. The pregnant woman may experience perioral numbness, tingling and itching of the scalp, and rarely a lupus-like illness, a lichenoid rash; a rare association is retroplacental hemorrhage *(9)*. Also, *a rare but life-threatening complication is acute hepatic necrosis (8). These serious side effects are not caused by other beta-adrenergic blockers.*

The drug has a role in the management of severe resistant hypertension (diastolic blood pressure > 110 mmHg) associated with preeclampsia occurring just before or during delivery. Labetalol given intravenously appears to be more effective than IV hydralazine or methyldopa. The blood pressure-lowering effect is more predictable, and the drug causes less tachycardia and appears to cause less fetal distress than hydralazine.

Drug name:	**Hydralazine**
Trade name:	Apresoline
Supplied:	25 mg
Dosage:	25 mg twice daily, increasing to three times daily; max. 100 mg daily before the addition of a beta-blocking drug For hypertensive crisis: IV bolus 5–10 mg

Hydralazine is a pure arteriolar vasodilator and has been used extensively for acute control of severe hypertension in the third trimester of pregnancy. The drug is, however, teratogenic in animals. Safety for chronic use is not as secure as that observed with methyldopa or beta-blockers.

The drug causes reflex tachycardia and sodium and water retention, which may necessitate the use of a diuretic or a beta-blocker to blunt tachycardia as well as to enhance the antihypertensive effect.

The drug has a role in the short-term management of severe hypertension during late pregnancy unresponsive to methyldopa or beta-blockers. Acute lowering of blood pressure is necessary in severe preeclampsia to prevent cerebral hemorrhage, the main cause of the increase in maternal mortality seen in preeclampsia. The drug is very useful when a modest dose is combined with a low dose of a beta-blocking drug, such as atenolol 50 mg daily, or as an adjunct to methyldopa; combination therapy prevents tachycardia and headaches caused by hydralazine.

Adverse Effects

The chronic use of the drug is limited by adverse effects that include fetal thrombocytopenia, although this occurrence is rare. The mother may experience dizziness, postural hypotension, a lupus syndrome, palpitations, and edema.

Hydralazine for Hypertensive Emergencies and Pregnancy

Hydralazine is the mainstay of therapy for the treatment of acute severe hypertension (blood pressure > 170/110 mmHg) occurring just before labor, during labor, or at delivery. Hydralazine remains the agent of choice, given as boluses *(10)*; the drug:

- Acts quickly.
- Reduces blood pressure in a fairly well-controlled manner, although labetalol IV appears to be a reasonable alternative to hydralazine, producing a more predictable and controlled decrease in blood pressure. Also, nitroprusside is more effective but is contraindicated because of serious potential risks to the neonate.
- Does not decrease cardiac output.
- Preserves uteroplacental blood flow.
- Does not produce serious adverse maternal or neonatal effects.

Dosage. IV 5–10-mg bolus over 1–2 min, repeated in 20 min and then as often as necessary over several hours. The maximal effect of hydralazine is observed in 20 min. Duration of action is 6–8 h. Dosage is by IV infusion 5 mg/h increasing slowly, if necessary, to 10 mg/h, maximum 15 mg/h, with continuous evaluation of heart rate and blood pressure and fetal monitoring.

If hydralazine fails to control blood pressure adequately, the addition of methyldopa is advisable. Although beta-blockers potentiate the action of hydralazine and blunt sinus tachycardia, these agents are not considered as safe as methyldopa or hydralazine during labor, especially as IV beta-blockers may rarely cause delay in spontaneous respiration in the newborn.

As indicated earlier, labetalol IV bolus or infusion appears to be a reasonable alternative for hydralazine-resistant hypertension. If nifedipine is chosen, caution is necessary not to give magnesium sulfate concomitantly because severe hypotension may ensue.

Thiazide Diuretics

Because hypertension of pregnancy and preeclampsia are associated with reduced plasma volume, diuretics are not indicated. Fetal outcome is usually worse in women with preeclampsia who fail to expand plasma volume.

Adverse Effects

Thiazides may cause neonatal thrombocytopenia, albeit rarely. Also, diuretics may exacerbate maternal carbohydrate intolerance. A metaanalysis of randomized trials involving more than 7000 pregnant women indicated no increased incidence of adverse fetal effects *(11)*. Other studies have shown fetal and neonatal jaundice as well as thrombocytopenia. **(Furosemide is contraindicated during pregnancy; see later discussion of heart failure.)**

Calcium Antagonists

Calcium antagonists are teratogenic in animals. These agents have not been adequately tested except in a few small studies in late pregnancy for severe or accelerated hypertension in which nifedipine 5–10 mg orally has proved extremely effective without adverse consequences *(12)*.

Nifedipine is useful in severe hypertension or preeclampsia and has been used over a 4- to 6-wk period without adverse effects. Nifedipine given in late pregnancy to women with accelerated severe hypertension resulted in an average fall in blood pressure of 26/20 mmHg within 20 min of oral dosing *(12)*.

An increase in diastolic blood pressure > 110 mmHg uncontrolled by methyldopa and a beta-blocker should prompt cessation of methyldopa and commencement of the short-term use of nifedipine 25–50 mg.

Dosage. Long-acting 30–60 mg once daily. The drug is best combined with atenolol 50 mg daily or pindolol 5 mg daily. The combination used for 1–2 wk during the last trimester of pregnancy should suffice to smother the peaking of blood pressure, and maintenance therapy with a beta-adrenergic blocking agent, with or without combination of hydralazine, may be necessary.

Nifedipine has a role to play in the management of fulminating preeclampsia and severe hypertension resistant to therapy occurring in the last few weeks of pregnancy and for acute hypertensive emergencies, for which controlled clinical trials are necessary to establish indications and overall safety. Clinicians should check whether the drug is approved for these indications.

Caution. Do not use nifedipine or calcium antagonists concomitantly with magnesium sulfate because catastrophic lowering of blood pressure may occur. Magnesium sulfate is commonly used to prevent seizures in patients with severe preeclampsia in association with resistant hypertension.

Dosage. Nifedipine 5–10 mg three times daily or nifedipine sustained-release preparation 10 or 20 mg twice daily or once-daily formulation 30 mg daily. For the acute lowering of very severe hypertension, the oral capsule should lower blood pressure within 30 min and is preferable to the commonly used sublingual preparation, which lowers blood pressure in 10–20 min. The sublingual preparation is not approved by the Food and Drug Administration (FDA), although it is widely used. The oral capsule is preferred because the peak hypertensive effect is not significantly different from that obtained with sublingual usage.

ACE Inhibitors

ACE inhibitors are contraindicated during pregnancy. They may adversely affect fetal and neonatal blood pressure control and renal function. They may cause skull defects and oligohydramnios. These agents are teratogenic in animals and are associated with a high incidence of intrauterine death. **Acute renal failure with catastrophic consequences has been noted in neonates of mothers given ACE inhibitors in the third trimester.**

Magnesium Sulfate

Magnesium sulfate causes only a mild and transient lowering of blood pressure. The drug remains the most useful agent for the prevention of seizures associated with severe preeclampsia *(13)*. Magnesium sulfate is a neuromuscular blocker and appears to prevent the end-organ consequences of prolonged hypoxemia that may occur with concomitant seizure activity.

Dosage. IV dose of 4 g diluted in 100–200 mL of intravenous solution, given over 20 min. Maintenance 2 g/h with careful monitoring of blood pressure and urine output.

Caution. Magnesium sulfate is contraindicated in renal failure and hepatic dysfunction and should not be used concomitantly with calcium antagonists because severe hypotension may occur. The drug should not be used primarily for its antihypertensive effect.

DRUG THERAPY FOR HEART FAILURE IN PREGNANCY

Drugs are used to provide hemodynamic stability and reduce symptoms prior to prompt correction and treatment of the cause of heart failure or pulmonary edema.

The common causes of heart failure or pulmonary edema in pregnancy are

- Mitral stenosis and rarely other valvular heart disease. Mitral stenosis is the most common cause of pulmonary edema in pregnancy. Heart failure develops in more than 70% of patients during the third trimester and early puerperium.
- Systemic hypertension associated with preeclampsia.
- Pulmonary hypertension.
- Very rarely, peripartum cardiomyopathy.

Beta-Blockers

Beta-blockers are the cornerstone of treatment for the medical management of mitral stenosis during pregnancy *(14–16)*, particularly for prevention of pulmonary edema in pregnant patients with mitral stenosis. Left atrial pressure rises as diastolic blood flow through the tight mitral valve is slowed. In addition, cardiac output and intravascular volume reach a peak by wk 20–24. The heart rate increases an average of 10 beats/min. Increase in heart rate causes a shortened ventricular filling period and a marked increase in left atrial pressure. Sinus tachycardia, thus, may precipitate pulmonary edema, which may be fatal. Reduction in the resting heart rate from a mean of 86 to 78 beats/min was associated with a marked clinical improvement *(14–16)*. The dose of beta-blockers is titrated according to the patient's symptoms and heart rate. Also, with atrial fibrillation, beta-blockers are most useful to achieve a ventricular rate < 80/min. Digoxin does not slow the heart rate sufficiently. If pulmonary edema develops, diuretics are added to beta-blocker therapy.

Digoxin

Digoxin is of no value in the management of pulmonary edema caused by pure mitral stenosis but has a small role in hypertensive heart failure and in patients with dilated cardiomyopathy or other conditions associated with poor left ventricular systolic function. The drug is not advisable except when poor left ventricular function is proved, preferably by echocardiographic evaluation.

No teratogenic or untoward adverse fetal effects, except for digitalis toxicity, have been reported with the chronic use of digoxin *(17)*. Serum digoxin levels are similar in the mother and neonate *(18)*, but there is about a 50% reduction in digoxin serum levels in the pregnant, as opposed to the nonpregnant, state *(18)*.

Caution. Fetal deaths as a result of maternal digitalis toxicity have been reported *(19)*. **Digoxin levels must be maintained 0.6 to maximum 1.0 ng/mL. Toxicity can be avoided by the watchful physician; *see* Chapter 12.**

Diuretics

Diuretics have been discussed earlier in this chapter under antihypertensive agents. For the management of heart failure, especially in the crisis of pulmonary edema related to mitral stenosis, short-term thiazide diuretic therapy over a few days is indicated for symptomatic relief along with oxygen and morphine until mitral stenosis can be corrected by balloon valvuloplasty or by surgery. Thiazides rarely cause fetal or neonatal jaundice or thrombocytopenia, but their use is justifiable for the treatment of pulmonary edema and hypertension associated with preeclampsia. The anticipated benefit must be weighed against the possible hazards to the fetus or neonate exposed to short-term therapy. A randomized trial showed no untoward effects on the fetuses or neonates of >1000 pregnant women given hydrochlorothiazide 50 mg daily *(20)*. Also, thiazides increase serum urate concentration, which is used to monitor the progress of preeclampsia.

Caution. Furosemide is contraindicated because it causes fetal abnormalities, but it can be used for pulmonary edema in the last weeks of pregnancy and in the puerperium to manage life-threatening pulmonary edema.

Vasodilators

ACE inhibitors are contraindicated at all stages of pregnancy. If afterload reduction is deemed necessary for the management of heart failure, hydralazine may be used in the third trimester of pregnancy. The manufacturer indicates hydralazine toxicity and teratogenic effects in animal studies, and this agent must be avoided during the first trimester.

ANTIARRHYTHMIC AGENTS IN PREGNANCY

Adenosine

Adenosine is the drug of choice for the management of atrioventricular nodal reentrant tachycardia (AVNRT; *see* Chapter 14) *(21)*. The drug causes no significant change in fetal heart rate because it has a half-life of only a few seconds. A bolus of 6 mg followed by 12 mg is effective.

Amiodarone

Amiodarone has not been adequately tested during pregnancy. There is a possible risk of neonatal goiter because amiodarone is about 40% iodine by weight. Two studies indicate no adverse effects in neonates of women given amiodarone *(22,23)*. Amiodarone is not advised during pregnancy except for the management of life-threatening arrhythmias (ventricular tachycardia/fibrillation) unresponsive to other anti-arrhythmic agents. The dosage of amiodarone is given in Chapter 14.

Beta-Adrenergic Blockers

Beta-blocking agents are of proven value in the management of bothersome arrhythmias during pregnancy, mainly because other antiarrhythmic agents may pose hazards for the fetus or neonate.

Acute termination of paroxysmal supraventricular tachycardia (PSVT) is achieved with the use of intravenous esmolol or atenolol and provokes few or no adverse effects in the fetus. IV beta-blockers should be avoided if possible during labor and delivery because respiratory depression may occur in the neonate, albeit rarely. See earlier discussion of beta-blockers for hypertension. The dosage of IV beta-blockers is given in Chapter 14.

Beta-blockers are the safest antiarrhythmic agents available for the management of:

- Bothersome recurrent PSVT (chronic management); in these patients the beta-blocking agent may be used in combination with digoxin if needed.
- Bothersome ventricular premature contractions.
- Ventricular tachycardia: beta-blockers should be tried before the use of other antiarrhythmic agents.

Disopyramide

The drug crosses the placenta and may induce labor. Sufficient data are not available to allow a firm conclusion to be made.

Lidocaine

Lidocaine crosses the placenta and does not appear to be teratogenic. Sufficient data covering use in the first trimester are not available. There is evidence of its safety during the second and third trimesters.

Minimize the dose close to delivery to decrease the potential for fetal respiratory depression.

The drug is indicated for life-threatening ventricular arrhythmias.

Adverse Effects

Adverse effects include fetal acidosis, respiratory depression, apnea, and bradycardia in infants.

Phenytoin

Phenytoin given to pregnant women in the first trimester has resulted in infants with intellectual impairment, cleft palate, craniofacial malformation, ventricular septal defect, and other congenital heart defects. The drug is not approved by the FDA. Phenytoin is no longer indicated for the management of digitalis toxicity *(24)*. The drug should be considered obsolete for the management of arrhythmias *(24)*.

Quinidine

Quinidine has been used successfully to treat ventricular tachycardia in pregnancy without fetal adverse effects in small-group, short-term studies *(17,25)*. A general recommendation as to safety cannot be made. Quinidine crosses the placental barrier, and toxicity may precipitate spontaneous abortion, premature labor, and fetal cranial nerve damage.

Quinidine is a poorly effective antiarrhythmic agent with high proarrhythmic effects. The drug is indicated only for life-threatening ventricular arrhythmias after an adequate trial of beta-blocking agents and other antiarrhythmics. The benefits of therapy and efficacy of the drug must outweigh the potential risk to the fetus.

CARDIAC DRUGS DURING LACTATION

Virtually all maternally ingested drugs are excreted into breast milk, usually in amounts less than 2% of the maternal dose. The concentration in the milk is occasionally sufficient to cause adverse pharmacologic effects in the infant. Caution is necessary because there is insufficient evidence to provide guidance on all cardiac drugs and it is advisable to administer these agents to the lactating mother only if deemed absolutely necessary.

The best time to take the drug, if administered, is immediately after a feeding. The mother is advised to express and discard the morning breast milk, which usually contains the highest concentration of the drug, and to feed the infant at least 1–2 h after the drug is given.

Factors affecting drug excretion into breast milk include:

1. **Protein binding:** Drugs that are poorly protein bound are excreted into breast milk, for example, atenolol (only 5% bound) achieves sufficient concentration in breast milk to cause adverse effects in the infant, albeit rarely. *Atenolol, acebutolol, nadolol, and sotalol are contraindicated with breastfeeding.*
2. **Lipid solubility:** Because breast milk is an excretory pathway for lipophilic substances, which are not effectively metabolized by the body, cardiac agents that are lipophilic should be expected in higher concentration, and their use should be avoided unless alternatives are not available. Propranolol is lipophilic but is protein bound and *achieves low concentration in milk.*
3. **Molecular weight** is not an impediment to excretion into milk except for very large molecular weight agents, such as heparin and insulin, that are unable to gain passage to milk.
4. **Volume of breast milk:** Because the quantity of breast milk is greatest in the morning, transfer of the drug is maximal at this time. Consequently, this feed should be avoided if a drug that is excreted is indicated in therapy.
5. **pH of the milk:** Milk is usually acidic, with a pH of 6.35–7.65. Drugs that are weak bases, such as beta-adrenergic blockers, are trapped in the milk, but their concentration is fortunately low.

A high milk-to-plasma (MP) ratio implies an increased intake of a drug by the infant. The MP ratio may be altered by several factors, however, and is insufficiently accurate to serve as a reliable guide for prescribing most cardiac drugs. For example, a 240-mg daily dose of diltiazem achieves a concentration of about 200 ng/mL in breast milk with an MP ratio of only 1.0. Diltiazem is contraindicated with breastfeeding. Atenolol, 100 mg daily, achieves a milk concentration of about 0.6 μg/mL, MP ratio 3, and is also contraindicated. However, several agents with MP ratios of up to 3 have not indicated evidence of toxicity in infants.

The concentration of a drug in breast milk can be estimated and, when possible, agents with minimal concentrations should be prescribed. Specific drug concentrations in milk and their relation to toxicity in infants have not yet been established, and caution is required.

Drugs in breast milk may, at least theoretically, result in hypersensitivity in the infant even when drug concentration in the infant is too low to initiate a pharmacologic or toxic effect.

In addition, drugs to the mother must be avoided if the infant is premature or if either mother or infant is suspected of having hepatic or renal impairment because most drugs are metabolized or eliminated by the kidney.

Advice is given only for commonly used cardiac drugs.

ACE Inhibitors

The average concentration of captopril in breast milk is 5 μg/mL with an MP ratio of 0.1. The effect on a nursing infant has not been studied adequately, although a few reports have indicated no adverse effects. Until further information is available, ACE inhibitors should not be used during lactation except for the management of severe heart failure with poor systolic function, and breastfeeding should then be discontinued.

Adenosine

Because it has a half-life of less than 5 s, adenosine is safe during breastfeeding.

Amiodarone

Amiodarone is contraindicated during lactation because iodinated compounds attain high concentrations in breast milk, and there is a theoretical hazard from release of iodine, which causes hypothyroidism or goiter.

Anticoagulants

Warfarin is the most commonly used oral anticoagulant, has minimal transfer into breast milk, and rarely causes bleeding in the infant. Caution is necessary with dosing. Breastfeeding should be discontinued if the infant is premature and warfarin is deemed necessary.

Ethyl biscoumacetate and phenindione are contraindicated because they are associated with a high incidence of bleeding.

Aspirin

Acetylsalicylic acid appears in breast milk. Although the concentration is low, aspirin should be avoided because interference with platelet function and metabolic acidosis may rarely occur. Also, it is necessary to avoid the rare risk of Reye's syndrome.

Beta-Blockers

Because beta-blockers are weak bases, these agents become trapped in breast milk. **In addition, hydrophilic beta-blockers, atenolol, acebutolol, nadolol, and sotalol, are weakly protein bound and their concentration in the milk is much greater than that of propranolol, metoprolol, and timolol.** Levels of the lipophilic agents are about 30% lower than those of hydrophilic, loosely bound, agents *(26,27)*.

A case of atenolol toxicity in a full-term newborn infant has been reported. The mother was treated with atenolol for hypertension. Bradycardia, poor peripheral perfusion, and cyanosis were observed in the infant. Atenolol serum levels taken 48 h after cessation of breastfeeding were in the potentially toxic range for an adult *(28)*.

Caution is necessary in the use of hydrophilic beta-blockers, especially if renal dysfunction is present, as these agents are eliminated by the kidney. If a beta-blocker is deemed necessary, it is advisable to administer propranolol during lactation because this drug attains an average concentration in milk of 50 ng/mL, MP ratio of 0.6, and no adverse effects have been noted. Metoprolol attains an average concentration of 1.7 μg/mL plus an MP ratio of 3, but sufficient information is not available.

Pindolol and timolol attain low concentrations, but these drugs are partially excreted by the kidney and are partially lipophilic and hydrophilic; although they are not expected to be harmful, **propranolol has been well tested**. The American Academy of Pediatrics considers beta-blocker treatment to be compatible with breastfeeding *(29)*. **The author recommends only propranolol.**

Calcium Antagonists

Diltiazem is contraindicated because the average concentration is 200 ng/mL, MP ratio 1. Dihydropyridines have not been studied sufficiently during lactation, but nitrendipine attains a milk concentration of 5 ng/mL, MP ratio 2.5, and the concentration is believed to be too low to be harmful to the infant.

Verapamil attains an average milk concentration of about 20 μg/mL, MP ratio 0.4. The level in healthy infants has not caused adverse effects and is believed to be too low to be harmful. Accumulation and toxicity may occur, however, in the premature infant or in mothers with liver dysfunction.

Digoxin

Digoxin is excreted in breast milk; infant toxicity does not occur if care is taken in dosing relative to renal function. Average concentration in milk is 1.5 ng/mL, MP ratio 1.5. Digoxin is administered if indicated, with the usual precautions to avoid toxicity, and is compatible with breastfeeding.

Disopyramide

Disopyramide concentration in breast milk is believed to be too small to be harmful. Average concentration in milk is 3 μg/mL, MP ratio 0.9, with the mother receiving disopyramide 200 mg three times daily for several weeks *(30)*.

Lidocaine; Lignocaine

Lidocaine is excreted in breast milk in high concentrations: up to 40% of the maternal level *(31)*. If IV lidocaine is required for the management of ventricular tachycardia, breastfeeding should cease at least 12 h after use of the drug, with the breast milk during that period being discarded. Harm to the infant is not expected. The American Academy of Pediatrics considers lidocaine treatment to be compatible with continued breastfeeding.

Methyldopa

Methyldopa is frequently used during pregnancy to control hypertension and may be required up to delivery. Concentration in breast milk averages 1 μg/mL, MP ratio 0.3. The amount in breast milk does not appear to cause adverse effects in infants and is believed to be too small to be harmful. **Other agents, beta-blockers or ACE inhibitors, are preferred after delivery because methyldopa may cause depression.**

Mexiletine

Mexiletine appears in breast milk in small amounts, concentration 1.7 μg/mL, MP ratio 3, and is insufficient to cause toxicity in the infant. **Caution** is required, however, if hepatic or renal dysfunction exists in the mother. The drug is contraindicated in the premature infant.

Diuretics

Thiazides appear in breast milk. The concentration is low and usually not harmful to the infant. If large doses of thiazides beyond 25 mg daily are required, suppression of lactation may occur. The concentration of hydrochlorothiazide in breast milk is approximately 100 ng/mL, MP ratio 0.4. Because transfer to the infant is extremely small, thiazides are not contraindicated for the management of heart failure with pulmonary edema. In such a serious setting, however, breastfeeding is usually discontinued. Furosemide is more effective than thiazides for pulmonary edema.

Lastly, an update of selected cardiac and noncardiac drugs that can be used safely during pregnancy is given in a review article (32).

REFERENCES

1. Redman GWG, Beillin LJ, Bonnar J, et al. Fetal outcome in trial of anti-hypertensive treatment in pregnancy. Lancet 1976;2:753.
2. Cockburn J, Moar VA, Ounsted M, et al. Final report of the study on hypertension during pregnancy: The effects of specific treatment on the growth and development of the children. Lancet 1982;1:647.

3. Gallery EDM, Saunders DM, Hunyor SN, et al. Randomized comparison of methyldopa and oxprenolol for the treatment of hypertension in pregnancy. BMJ 1997;I:1591.
4. Reynolds B, Butters L, Evans J, et al. The first year of life after atenolol in pregnancy associated hypertension. Arch Dis Child 1984;59:1061.
5. Olofsson P, Montan S, Sartor G, et al. Effects of beta$_1$-adrenergic blockade in the treatment of hypertension during pregnancy in diabetic women. Acta Med Scand 1986;220:321.
6. Rubin PC, Butters L, Clark DM, et al. Placebo-controlled trial of atenolol in treatment of pregnancy-associated hypertension. Lancet 1983;1:431.
7. Churchill D, Beevers DG. Hypertension in pregnancy. BMJ Books 1999;70–77.
8. Clarke JA, Zimmerman HF, Tanner LA. Labetalol hepatoxicity. Ann Intern Med 1990;113:210.
9. Lindheimer MD, Katz AI. Hypertension in pregnancy. N Engl J Med 1985;313:675.
10. Patterson-Brown S, Robson SC, Redfern N, et al. Hydralazine boluses for the treatment of severe hypertension. Br J Obstet Gynaecol 1994;101:409.
11. Collins R, Yusuf S, Peto R. Overview of randomized trials of diuretics in pregnancy. BMJ 1985;290:17.
12. Walters BNJ, Redman GWG. Treatment of severe pregnancy-associated hypertension with calcium antagonist nifedipine. Br J Obstet Gynaecol 1984;91:330.
13. Saunders K, Hammersley V. Magnesium for eclampsia. Lancet 1995;346:788.
14. Al-Kasab S, Sabag T, Al-Zaibag M, et al. Beta-adrenergic receptor blockage in the management of pregnant women with mitral stenosis. Am J Obstet Gynecol 199;0163:37.
15. Narasimtian C, Joseph G, Singh TC. Propranolol for pulmonary edema in mitral stenosis. Int J Cardiol 1994;44:178.
16. Frishman WH, Chesner M. Use of beta adrenergic blocking agents in pregnancy. In: Maternal and Fetal Disease, 2nd ed. New York, Alan R. Liss, 1990, p 351.
17. Rotmensch HH, Elkayam Y, Frishman W. Antiarrhythmic drug therapy during pregnancy. Ann Intern Med 1983;98:47.
18. Rogers MC, Willerson JT, Goldblatt A, et al. Serum digoxin concentrate in the human fetus, neonate and infant. N Engl J Med 1972;287:1010.
19. Schumann JL, Locke RV. Transplacental neonatal digitalis intoxication. Am J Cardiol 1960;6:834.
20. Kraus GW, Marchese JR, Yen SS. Prophylactic use of hydrochlorothiazide in pregnancy. JAMA 1966; 198:128.
21. Harrison JK, Greefield RA, Warton JM. Termination of acute supraventricular tachycardia by adenosine during pregnancy. Am Heart J 1992;123:1386.
22. McKenna WJ, Harris L, Roland E, et al. Amiodarone therapy during pregnancy. Am J Cardiol 1983;51: 1231.
23. Robson DJ, Raj MVJ, Story GCA, et al. Use of amiodarone during pregnancy. Postgrad Med J 1985; 61:75.
24. Khan M Gabriel. Heart Disease, Diagnosis and Therapy. Baltimore, Williams & Wilkins, 1996.
25. Hill LM, Malkasian GD. The use of quinidine sulphate throughout pregnancy. Obstet Gynecol 1979;54: 366.
26. White WB. Management of hypertension during lactation. Hypertension 1984;6:297.
27. Riant P, Urein S, Albergres E, et al. High plasma protein binding as a parameter in the selection of beta-blockers for lactating women. Biochem Pharmacol 1986;24:4579.
28. Schmimmel MS, Eidelman AI, Wilschanski MA, et al. Toxic effects of atenolol consumed during breast-feeding. J Pediatr 1989;114:476.
29. Committee on Drugs, American Academy of Pediatrics. The transfer of drugs and other chemicals into human milk. Pediatrics 1994;93:137.
30. Barnett DV, Hudson BA, McBurney A. Disopyramide and its *N*-mono desalkyl metabolite in breastmilk. Br J Clin Pharmacol 1982;14:310.
31. Zeisler JA, Gaarder TD, Demesquita SA. Lidocaine excretion in breast milk. Drug Intell Clin Pharm 1986; 20:691.
32. Koren G, Pastuszak A, Ito F. Drugs in pregnancy. N Engl J Med 1998;338:1128.

SUGGESTED READING

Ramin SM, Gilstrap III LC. Pregnancy chronichypertension. In: Willansky S, Willerson JT (eds.). Heart disease in women. Philadelphia, Churchill Livingstone, 2002, pp. 471–474.

Witlin AG, Belfort M. Pre-eclampsia and eclampsia. In: Willansky S, Willerson JT (eds.). Heart disease in women. Philadelphia, Churchill Livingstone, 2002, p. 474.

21 Effects of Drug Interactions

Several cardiac drugs manifest some form of interaction with each other or with noncardiac drugs. It is of paramount importance for the physician to be aware of these interactions, which may be potentially harmful to patients or may negate salutary effects. In addition, the prescribing physician must be conscious of these interactions so as to avoid errors that may provoke medicolegal action.

The number of cardiac drugs available to the clinician has increased by more than 100% over the past 20 yr. Also, the drug armamentarium for the treatment of psychiatric, rheumatic, neurologic, infectious, and gastrointestinal (GI) diseases has expanded greatly. Consequently, drug interactions have increased.

Although drug interactions may have been briefly described for drug groups in earlier chapters, this chapter gives a structured summary of interactions. *This chapter deals with:*

- The interactions that occur between cardiac drugs.
- The interaction of cardiovascular drugs with agents used for treating diseases of other system and other agents with pharmacologic properties, such as caffeine, alcohol, and tobacco.
- The adverse cardiovascular effects of noncardiac drugs.

Drug interactions are usually:

1. **Pharmacodynamic:** Occurring between drugs that have similar or opposite pharmacologic effects or adverse effects; for example, these effects may occur because of competition at receptor sites or action of the drugs on the same physiologic system. In some instances, the hemodynamic effects of one agent increase or decrease the hemodynamic effects of another agent.
2. **Pharmacokinetic:** Occurring when one drug alters the absorption, distribution, metabolism, or excretion of another.

INTERACTIONS OF CARDIOVASCULAR DRUGS

Each cardiac drug, (or drug group) interaction is discussed under the following categories:

1. Cardiovascular effects:
   a. Vasodilator (arterial or venous, afterload or preload reduction), hypotension, presyncope.
   b. Inotropic: Positive or negative; alteration of ejection fraction (EF); propensity to precipitate congestive heart failure (CHF).
   c. On the sinoatrial (SA) or atrioventricular (AV) node.
   d. On the conduction system.
   e. Proarrhythmic.
2. Cholinergic effects.
3. Plasma levels.

From: *Contemporary Cardiology: Cardiac Drug Therapy, Seventh Edition*
M. Gabriel Khan © Humana Press Inc., Totowa, NJ

Table 21-1
Angiotensin-Converting Enzyme Inhibitors: Potential Interactions

- Aspirin: Appears to decrease salutary effects
- Potassium-sparing diuretics: amiloride, Moduretic, Moduret, triamterene, Dyazide, Dytide, spironolactone (Aldactone), Aldactazide
- Preload-reducing agents:
  Diuretics
  Nitrates
  Prazosin
- Renally excreted cardioactive agents
  Antiarrhythmics; beta-blockers (atenolol, sotalol, nadolol)
- Digoxin
- Agents that may alter immune status:
  Allopurinol
  Acebutolol
  Hydralazine
  Pindolol
  Procainamide
- Tocainide
- Furosemide
- Probenecid
- NSAIDs
- Lithium
- Cyclosporine
- Phenothiazis
- Imipramine

NSAIDs, nonsteroidal antiinflammatory drugs.

4. Renal clearance of the drug; effect on renal function and serum potassium (K^+) concentration.
5. Hematologic, including anticoagulant activity and/or immune effects.
6. Hepatic and GI.

ACE Inhibitors/ARBs

Cardiovascular Effects

When angiotensin-converting enzyme (ACE) inhibitors are used in combination with vasodilators, hypotension may occur. Preload-reducing agents, such as nitrates or prazosin, may cause syncope or presyncope (Table 21-1). Diuretics stimulate the renin-angiotensin system (RAS) and enhance the antihypertensive effects, producing a salutary interaction in hypertensive individuals, but hypotension may ensue in patients with CHF. The hypotensive effects are longer lasting with long-acting ACE inhibitors.

Renal Effects

- ACE inhibitors and ARBs may decrease glomerular filtration rate (GFR) in some patients with renal dysfunction and may result in decreased clearance of other cardiac drugs that are eliminated by the kidney. Interaction may occur with renally excreted beta-blockers, nadolol, atenolol, sotalol, and antiarrhythmic agents.
- Serum K+ may increase to dangerous levels if potassium-sparing diuretics **(amiloride, eplerenone, triamterene, spironolactone, Moduretic, Moduret, Dyazide)** are used concurrently. This occurrence is enhanced in patients with renal dysfunction. A normal serum creatinine level in patients with a lean body mass may not reflect underlying renal dysfunction, and **caution** is necessary, particularly in the elderly.

Table 21-2
Adenosine: Potential Interactions

• Carbamazepine
• Dipyridamole: **Caution**
• Methylxanthines (theophylline)
• Caffeine

- These agents may decrease the diuretic effect of furosemide *(1)*.
- **Probenecid** inhibits the tubular excretion of ACE inhibitors and increases the blood levels of these agents.
- ACE inhibitors may cause a 20–30% decrease in digoxin clearance and an increase in digoxin levels.
- Interaction with cyclosporine may cause hyperkalemia.

Hematologic/Immune

The risk of immune adverse effects may increase with concurrent use of agents that alter the immune status: assess antinuclear antibody levels and also assess for neutropenia with concurrent use of acebutolol, allopurinol, hydralazine, pindolol, procainamide, and tocainide.

Gastrointestinal

The absorption of fosinopril is reduced by antacids.

ANTIARRHYTHMIC AGENTS

Adenosine

The electrophysiologic effects of adenosine are competitively antagonized by methylxanthines (theophylline) and are potentiated by dipyridamole, which inhibits its cellular uptake, and **severe hypotension may occur** (Table 21-2).

Amiodarone

Cardiovascular Effects

- Amiodarone has a mild vasodilator effect, and interaction may occur with antihypertensive agents, causing hypotension. This interaction is more prominent with intravenous amiodarone.
- Because of a mild inotropic effect, CHF may be precipitated, especially when amiodarone is combined with agents that possess negative inotropism (e.g., beta-blocking agents, verapamil, or diltiazem).
- Combination with verapamil or diltiazem may cause sinus arrest or AV block (Table 21-3).
- The proarrhythmic effect of amiodarone is low, but interaction may occur and may increase the risk of torsades de pointes when amiodarone is used concurrently with the following agents: diuretics, which cause hypokalemia, class IA agents (quinidine, disopyramide, procainamide), sotalol, tricyclics, phenothiazines, and erythromycin.

Oral Anticoagulants

Their activity is increased.

Plasma Levels

Digoxin levels may double because amiodarone decreases renal clearance of digoxin. Flecainide and procainamide levels increase.

Table 21-3
Amiodarone: Potential Interactions

- Antihypertensive agents
- Drugs that are negatively inotropic: Verapamil, diltiazem, beta-blockers
- Agents that inhibit SA and AV node conduction: Diltiazem, verapamil
- Agents that ↑ the QT interval
  Class IA agents: quinidine, disopyramide, procainamide
  Sotalol
  Tricyclic antidepressants
  Phenothiazines
  Erythromycin (other macrolides)
  Pentamidine
  Zidovudine
- Agents that decrease serum K^+ concentration (diuretics)
- Agents that are renally eliminated: digoxin, flecainide, procainamide
- Anticoagulants
- Cimetidine

AV, atrioventricular; SA, sinoatrial.

Disopyramide

Cardiovascular Effects

The negative inotropic effect of disopyramide is increased by beta-blocking agents, **verapamil, diltiazem, and flecainide**. Proarrhythmic effects, in particular torsades de pointes, are increased with agents that prolong the QT interval or cause hypokalemia. Sinus and AV node effects may occur when disopyramide is used concurrently with drugs that depress the sinus node (verapamil, diltiazem, digitalis).

Cholinergic Effects

Because disopyramide inhibits muscarinic receptors, the anticholinergic activity may cause constipation. Thus, the drug should not be combined with verapamil. Disopyramide may precipitate glaucoma, and this effect may be counteracted by timolol or betaxolol.

Flecainide

Cardiovascular Effects

The powerful, negative, inotropic effect of flecainide is worsened by negative inotropic agents; interaction occurs with **verapamil, diltiazem, beta-blockers, and disopyramide**; intraventricular conduction defects may occur when the drug is combined with class IA agents.

Plasma Levels

Plasma levels increase with concomitant **amiodarone** administration; thus, the flecainide dose should be decreased. Flecainide causes an increase in **digoxin** levels.

Lidocaine; Lignocaine

Plasma Levels

- Lidocaine is metabolized in the liver. An increase in plasma levels may occur with decreased hepatic blood flow caused by **beta-blocking agents** *(2)*: **caution** is necessary to avoid lidocaine toxicity, which may occur when lidocaine and beta-blockers are administered to patients with acute myocardial infarction.

- Lidocaine plasma levels decrease with **phenytoin**, which stimulates the hepatic oxidase system, resulting in accelerated breakdown of hepatically metabolized cardiovascular agents.

Mexiletine

Cardiovascular Effects

Hypotension may occur when mexiletine is combined with vasoactive agents that reduce blood pressure. AV block may worsen with the concomitant use of **amiodarone, verapamil, diltiazem, or beta-blocking drugs**.

Plasma Levels

Because the drug is partly metabolized in the liver, **phenytoin** decreases plasma levels.

Phenytoin

Phenytoin activates the hepatic oxidase system and thus accelerates the breakdown of hepatically metabolized cardiac agents, resulting in a decrease in their plasma levels: **lidocaine, hepatically metabolized beta-blockers (propranolol, metoprolol, labetalol), diltiazem, verapamil, nifedipine** (and other **dihydropyridine calcium antagonists**), **mexiletine**, and **quinidine**. Aspirin metabolism is increased; thus, phenytoin decreases the effects of aspirin.

Propafenone

Cardiovascular Effects

Hypotension may be precipitated by drugs that lower blood pressure. A prominent negative inotropic effect may be increased by other negative inotropic agents. Sinus node suppression may occur when the drug is combined with **verapamil** or **diltiazem**. AV block or conduction defects may increase with class IA agents. Digoxin level and warfarin are enhanced.

Plasma Levels

Digoxin levels are increased.

Hematologic

Oral anticoagulant activity is increased.

Procainamide

The **negative inotropic effects** of oral procainamide are increased by other negative inotropic agents. **Torsades de pointes** may be precipitated when procainamide is combined with agents that increase the QT interval. **ACE inhibitors** may enhance immune effects; both agents may cause neutropenia or agranulocytosis.

Quinidine

Hypotension

Because alpha-receptors are inhibited by quinidine, other vasoactive agents that decrease blood pressure may precipitate hypotension (e.g., **prazosin**, **verapamil**).

Intraventricular Conduction Defects

These increase when quinidine is combined with class IC agents (**flecainide**, **encainide**, **propafenone**, **lorcainide**).

Proarrhythmic Effects

Drugs that prolong the QT interval and diuretics that cause hypokalemia may precipitate torsades de pointes.

Hematologic

Oral anticoagulant activity may increase.

Plasma Levels

Quinidine levels decrease with phenytoin or nifedipine and increase with verapamil *(3)* or **diltiazem** administration. Digoxin levels increase because quinidine decreases clearance of digoxin.

ANTIPLATELET AGENTS/ANTICOAGULANTS

Anticoagulants have several interactions with cardiac and noncardiac drugs (*see* Table 19-4).

Aspirin. The metabolism of aspirin is increased by agents such as **phenytoin**, **barbiturates**, and **rifampin** that induce the hepatic oxidase system. Phenytoin, therefore, decreases the effects of aspirin. The risk of bleeding is increased with concurrent administration of anticoagulants. Aspirin and thiazide **diuretics** inhibit urate excretion, whereas ACE inhibitors and sulfinpyrazone increase renal urate excretion.

Clopidogrel interacts unfavorably with atorvastatin and simvastatin, *which use the hepatic cytochrome pathway, and its beneficial effect on intracoronary stent occlusion is probably reduced;* rosuvastatin does not appear to interact, but further investigations are needed to clarify this important area of concern.

BETA-BLOCKERS

Cardiovascular Effects

- Hypotension may be precipitated when beta-blockers are combined with calcium antagonists and other antihypertensive agents. Hypertension may ensue with concurrent use of vasoactive agents that are sympathomimetic (e.g., phenylpropanolamine).
- Effects on the SA and AV nodes: Electrophysiologic interaction occurs with **verapamil**, **diltiazem**, and **amiodarone**; severe bradycardia, complete heart block, or asystole may be precipitated (Table 21-4).
- Inotropic effects: Other negative inotropic agents (**verapamil**, **diltiazem**, **flecainide**, **disopyramide**, **procainamide**, **propafenone**) increase the risk of CHF.
- Proarrhythmic effects: Sotalol, because of its unique class III activity, is the only beta-blocking agent with proarrhythmic effects, and it can induce torsades de pointes, especially if the serum K^+ level is low. Avoid K^+-losing diuretics. Do not combine sotalol with agents that prolong the QT interval.

Plasma Levels

Metoprolol and propranolol plasma levels are increased by verapamil. Atenolol, sotalol, and nadolol plasma levels are not increased because they are not hepatically metabolized beta-blockers. Nifedipine plasma levels increase.

Table 21-4
Beta-Adrenergic Blockers: Potential Interactions

- Antiarrhythmics: amiodarone, disopyramide, flecainide, lidocaine, procainamide, propafenone
- Calcium antagonists: diltiazem, verapamil, nifedipine
- Sympathomimetics (phenylpropanolamine)
- Phenytoin
- K^+-losing diuretics (sotalol only)
- Cimetidine-like agents (hepatically metabolized; metoprolol, propranolol; *see* Chapter 1)
- NSAIDs
- Fluvoxamine
- Tobacco smoking (propranolol)

Table 21–5
Calcium Antagonists: Potential Interactions

- Amiodarone
- Beta-blockers
- Cyclosporin
- Digoxin
- Phenytoin
- Quinidine
- t-PA (diltiazem *[4,5]*)
- Magnesium IV
- Cimetidine
- Lithium
- Carbamazepine
- Quinine, chloroquine
- Grapefruit juice
- Tobacco (smoking): hepatically metabolized agents

t-PA, tissue plasminogen activator.

Immune Effects

Acebutolol and pindolol may alter immune status. The risk is additive when these agents are used concomitantly with hydralazine, procainamide, or ACE inhibitors.

CALCIUM ANTAGONISTS

Antihypertensive agents interact favorably to lower blood pressure, but hypotension may occur. The combination of magnesium sulfate may cause severe hypotension. Verapamil decreases the hepatic metabolism of prazosin, and concurrent use may cause hypotension. The combination of verapamil and quinidine may cause hypotension because of combined inhibition of peripheral alpha-receptors.

Negative Inotropic Agents

Added to verapamil or diltiazem. these agents may precipitate CHF (Table 21-5).

Table 21-6
Digoxin: Potential Interactions

Agents that increase serum levels:
- Atorvastatin >10%
- Ranolazine increases levels
- Quinidine displaces digoxin at binding sites, decreases renal elimination (quinine, chloroquine)
- Verapamil, diltiazem, nicardipine, felodipine, amiodarone, flecainide, propafenone, prazosin, and ACE inhibitors may decrease renal elimination
- NSAIDs decrease renal elimination
- Lomotil, probanthine decrease intestinal motility
- Erythromycin, tetracycline eliminate *Eubacterium lentum*
- Spironolactone: Digoxin assay falsely raised

Agents that decrease serum levels or bioavailability:
- Antacids, metoclopramide, cholestyramine, colestipol, Metamucil, neomycin, phenytoin, phenobarbital, salicylazosulfapyridine
- Electrophysiologic interactions may occur with amiodarone, diltiazem, verapamil

ACE, angiotensin-converting enzyme; NSAIDs, nonsteroidal antiinflammatory drugs.
From Khan M Gabriel. Heart failure. In: Heart Disease, Diagnosis and Therapy. Baltimore, Williams & Wilkins, 1996.

Sinoatrial and AV Nodal Effects

Verapamil and diltiazem have electrophysiologic actions on the SA and AV node that are increased by beta-blocking drugs, digoxin, amiodarone, and quinidine.

Plasma Levels

Nifedipine plasma levels are increased by agents that decrease hepatic blood flow (beta-blockers). Verapamil increases metoprolol plasma levels but does not increase the levels of atenolol, sotalol, and nadolol because these agents are not metabolized in the liver. Verapamil and diltiazem interaction with digoxin results in a substantial increase in digoxin levels. Verapamil and diltiazem increase quinidine levels. Verapamil, diltiazem, and nicardipine increase cyclosporine levels. Phenytoin stimulates the hepatic oxidase system and decreases plasma levels and the activity of calcium antagonists. **Mibefradil (Posicor)**, a calcium antagonist, has been withdrawn because of serious and potential interactions with a host of cardiac drugs that are influenced by the action of cytochrome P-450 3A4. Torsades de pointes and rhabdomyolysis have been noted (*see* above). **Clinicians should be cautious with combinations of agents that interfere with cytochrome P-450.**

Hematologic

An important interaction between diltiazem and tissue plasminogen activator (t-PA) has been observed. Experimentally, the combination of t-PA and diltiazem (3 d) resulted in significantly more blood loss than when t-PA was used alone *(4)*. In the Thrombolysis in Myocardial Infarction (TIMI) phase II study, an increased risk of intracerebral hemorrhage was observed in patients who were administered calcium antagonists at study entry *(5)*.

DIGOXIN

Digoxin interacts with several cardiac and noncardiac drugs, resulting in either an increase or decrease in digoxin levels (Table 21-6). Digoxin interacts with several cardiac drugs that have electrophysiologic effects on the SA and AV nodes. Diuretics interact by causing hypokalemia and increased sensitivity to digoxin. Cardioactive agents that decrease renal clearance of digoxin and increase digoxin plasma levels include amiodarone, flecainide, propafenone, quinidine, diltiazem, verapamil, and some dihydropyridine calcium antagonists, and ACE inhibitors. Prazosin displaces digoxin at binding sites and increases digoxin levels.

DIURETICS

Diuretics that cause hypokalemia interact with sotalol, amiodarone, and class IA agents and may precipitate torsades de pointes. Digoxin toxicity is enhanced. K^+-sparing diuretics administered with ACE inhibitors may cause an increase in serum K^+ levels. Ethacrynic acid increases the anticoagulant effect of warfarin. Both diuretics and dobutamine cause hypokalemia. Thus, caution is required when IV furosemide is administered concurrently with an infusion of dobutamine.

NITRATES

Nitroglycerin and other nitrates are preload-reducing agents and may increase the preload effect of ACE inhibitors and prazosin, resulting in syncope. High-dose IV nitroglycerin interacts with heparin, and this interaction may be important in patients with unstable angina who are treated with both agents; nitroglycerin presumably alters the antithrombin-3 molecule. Thus, a higher dose of heparin may be required. Also, excretion of heparin is increased by IV nitrates.

LIPID-LOWERING AGENTS

Statins

Fluvastatin and rosuvastatin interact with anticoagulants and cause a modest rise in INR. Administration of statins with nicotinic acid, gemfibrozil, other fibrates, cyclosporin, or erythromycin may cause myalgia, and increase in creatinine kinase levels, myopathy, rhabdomyolysis, and possible renal failure. Fluvastatin does not alter digoxin pharmacokinetics *(6)*, but atorvastatin and simvastatin increase digoxin levels approx 20% and <10%, respectively (*see* **Table 18-1**).

Bile acid sequestrants: Cholestyramine and colestipol decrease the absorption of digoxin, coumarin anticoagulants, diuretics, beta-blockers, HMG-CoA reductase inhibitors, L-thyroxine, and other vasoactive agents. These agents must be given 1 h before or 4 h after resin administration. **Probucol** may prolong the QT interval *(7)*; combination with a thiazide diuretic or class IA or III antiarrhythmic agent may precipitate torsades de pointes.

THROMBOLYTIC AGENTS

t-PA

The thrombolytic efficacy of t-PA is impaired by nitroglycerin. Diltiazem combined with t-PA appears to cause an increased risk of cerebral hemorrhage; beta-blockers appear to decrease the risk.

INTERACTIONS OF CARDIAC AND NONCARDIAC DRUGS

Antibiotics

Erythromycin and other macrolides may increase the QT interval and interact with cardiac agents that cause QT prolongation with the precipitation of torsades de pointes. Erythromycin may enhance the effects of digoxin (*see* Table 21-6).

Rifampin can induce the hepatic oxidase system, accelerating the metabolism of several cardiovascular drugs and thus resulting in decreased drug levels of these agents.

Cephalosporins or aminoglycoside antibiotics interact with furosemide and may increase nephrotoxicity; the effects of oral anticoagulants are increased.

The antifungal agent pentamidine and the antiviral **zidovudine** may prolong the QT interval, may interact with cardiac drugs that increase the QT interval, and may precipitate torsades de pointes. **Amphotericin** with diuretics causes an increase in hypokalemia.

Antihistamines

Administered with class IA and class III antiarrhythmics, they increase the risk of ventricular tachyarrhythmias, particularly torsades de pointes. Astemizole and terfenadine should not be used concomitantly with sotalol, amiodarone, class I antiarrhythmics, erythromycin, and other macrolides.

Antimalarials

Halofantrine increases the QT interval; cardioactive agents that cause QT prolongation may precipitate torsades de pointes.

Mefloquine and calcium channel blockers may interact to cause bradycardia. Bradycardia may be increased with digoxin.

Quinine, chloroquine, and hydroxychloroquine raise plasma concentrations of digoxin. Bradycardia may occur with diltiazem and verapamil.

Anticonvulsants

The effects of carbamazepine are enhanced by verapamil and diltiazem. The effects of nifedipine and isradipine are reduced by carbamazepine, phenobarbitone, primidone, and phenytoin. Carbamazepine may increase the degree of heart block caused by adenosine.

Cimetidine binds to the hepatic oxidase system, inhibits the breakdown of hepatically metabolized cardiovascular agents, and thus increases blood levels of the following agents:

- Hepatically metabolized beta-blockers (metoprolol, propranolol, labetalol).
- Lidocaine (lignocaine).
- Procainamide (but cimetidine also decreases renal clearance of procainamide).
- Verapamil and diltiazem.
- Nifedipine and other dihydropyridines.
- Amiodarone and flecainide, propafenone, quinidine.
- Enhances the effect of oral anticoagulants and several other drugs.

Drugs that affect urate excretion: Urate excretion is increased by ACE inhibitors, sulfinpyrazone, and probenecid. Urate excretion is decreased by diuretics and aspirin. Therefore, favorable or untoward interactions may occur. Also, probenecid decreases renal tubular secretion of captopril and may increase blood levels of ACE inhibitors.

Cyclosporin

Hyperkalemia may occur with concurrent use of ACE inhibitors or K^+-sparing diuretics. Plasma cyclosporin concentrations are reduced by concurrent rifampin administration and increased by nicardipine, diltiazem, and verapamil. Cyclosporin appears to increase plasma levels of nifedipine. Hyperkalemia may occur with the use of K^+-sparing diuretics. Myopathy or rhabdomyolysis may occur with coadministration of HMG-CoA reductase inhibitors or mibefradil (Posicor) (*see* above).

Lithium

Both loop diuretics and thiazides decrease sodium reabsorption in the proximal tubules and may cause an increased resorption of lithium, which may result in lithium toxicity. ACE inhibitors reduce excretion of lithium, resulting in increased plasma lithium concentration. Diltiazem and verapamil interact with lithium, and neurotoxicity may occur without an increase in plasma lithium levels.

Nonsteroidal Antiinflammatory Drugs (NSAIDs)

These agents block the production of vasodilator prostaglandins and reduce the antihypertensive effectiveness of ACE inhibitors, diuretics, and perhaps beta-blockers. NSAIDs decrease the diuretic effect of furosemide. There is an increased risk of hyperkalemia with K^+-sparing diuretics and precipitation of renal failure when indomethacin is administered with triamterene.

Psychotropic Agents

Phenothiazines, especially thioridazine, have quinidine-like effects on the heart; QT prolongation and interaction with amiodarone, sotalol, and class LA agents may induce torsades de pointes. Phenothiazines may interact with ACE inhibitors to cause severe postural hypotension.

Tricyclic antidepressants have a class I antiarrhythmic action. The quinidine-like effect may prolong the QT interval and induce torsades when combined with agents, such as sotalol, amiodarone, and others, that increase the QT interval.

These agents have anticholinergic properties (atropine-like) and interact with cardioactive agents with anticholinergic effects. Tricyclics antagonize the hypotensive effects of clonidine and increase the risk of rebound hypertension on clonidine withdrawal. Imipramine and possibly other tricyclics increase plasma concentration of diltiazem and verapamil. Because tricyclics produce a dry mouth, the effect of sublingual nitrates may be reduced.

Selective serotonin reuptake inhibitors (SSRIs): fluvoxamine, fluoxetine, sertraline. SSRIs are highly protein bound and may interact with cardioactive agents that are highly protein bound, causing a shift in plasma levels of these agents, particularly warfarin and digoxin. Sinus node slowing has been reported *(8–10)*.

Sinus bradycardia and syncope have been observed. Thus, interaction may emerge with agents that inhibit sinus node function or cause bradycardia (amiodarone, diltiazem, verapamil). Fluvoxamine increases plasma concentration of propranolol; the same interaction is likely to occur with other hepatically metabolized beta-blockers and other SSRIs.

Monoamine oxidase inhibitors: These agents may cause hypertensive crises with tyramine (in cheese) sympathomimetics. They increase the hypotensive effects of diuretics. They inhibit the hepatic drug metabolism enzymes. Thus, blood levels and effects of hepatically metabolized cardioactive agents may be increased.

Theophylline

Theophylline interacts with several cardioactive and noncardioactive agents (Table 21-7). Diltiazem and verapamil enhance effects of theophylline.

Thyroxine

The metabolism of propranolol and other hepatically metabolized beta-blockers is increased, causing reduced effect.

Table 21-7
Theophylline: Potential Interactions

Drug	*Effect* [a]	*Response*
Adenosine	↓effects of adenosine	
Allopurinol	↓theophylline clearance	↓dose of theophylline
Barbiturates	↑theophylline clearance	↓dose of theophylline
Carbamazepine	↑theophylline clearance	↑dose of theophylline
Corticosteroids	Variable metabolic effects	Monitor theophylline levels
Coumarins	Interferes with assay method for serum level resulting in falsely low values	No adjustment in dose necessary
Diltiazem	Slight ↓ in theophylline clearance	Possible ↓ in theophylline dose
Erythromycin	↓theophylline clearance	↓dose of theophylline
Estrogens	↓theophylline clearance	↓dose of theophylline
H_2-blockers		
Cimetidine	↓theophylline clearance	↓dose of theophylline
Ranitidine	No effect	No adjustment
Famotidine	No effect	No adjustment
Influenza vaccine	↓theophylline clearance	↓dose of theophylline
Interferon	↓theophylline clearance	↓dose of theophylline
Isoniazid	↓theophylline clearance	↓dose of theophylline
Isoproterenol	↑theophylline clearance	↑dose of theophylline
Lithium	↑lithium clearance	↑dose of lithium
Mexiletine	↓theophylline clearance	↓dose of theophylline
Nicorette	No effect	No response
Oral contraceptives	↓theophylline clearance	↓dose of theophylline
Pancuronium	↓pancuronium responsiveness	↑dose of pancuronium
Phenytoin	↑theophylline clearance	↑dose of theophylline
Quinolones	↓theophylline clearance	↓dose of theophylline
Tobacco smoking	↑theophylline clearance	↑dose of theophylline
Troleandomycin	↓theophylline clearance	↓dose of theophylline
Verapamil	↓theophylline clearance	↓dose of theophylline
Vidarabine	↓theophylline clearance	↓dose of theophylline

[a] ↑, increase; ↓, decrease.
From Khan M Gabriel. Cardiac and Pulmonary Management. Philadelphia, Lea & Febiger, 1993.

CARDIAC EFFECTS OF NONCARDIAC DRUGS

The cardiac effects of selected noncardiac drugs are summarized in Table 21-8.

Antibiotics

Erythromycin blocks a K^+ current important in cardiac repolarization. This action can predispose to early after-depolarizations and ventricular arrhythmias *(11)*.

Erythromycin IV has been reported to cause QT prolongation and, along with other macrolides, may precipitate torsades de pointes, albeit rarely. In addition, erythromycin inhibits the metabolism of astemizole and terfenadine; the increased plasma levels of terfenadine may precipitate torsades de pointes.

Spiramycin has been noted to cause QT prolongation and cardiac arrest in a newborn infant *(12)*.

Table 21-8
Cardiac Effects of Noncardiac Drugs

Drug	*Cardiac effect*
Antimicrobials	
Erythromycin (macrolides)	↑QT interval, ↑risk of torsades de pointes
Co-trimoxazole	↑risk of torsades de pointes (rare)
Ketoconazole	↑risk of torsades de pointes
Pentamidine	↑risk of torsades de pointes
Itraconazole	↑risk of torsades de pointes
Spiramycin	↑risk of torsades de pointes
Histamine H_1-antagonist	↑QT interval, ↑risk of torsades de pointes
Astemizole	↑risk of torsades de pointes
Terfenadine	↑QT interval, ↑risk of torsades de pointes
Amantadine	↑risk of torsades de pointes
Antimalarials	
Halofantrine	↑QT interval, ↑risk of torsades de pointes Mobitz I, II block
Chloroquine	SHMD
Tricyclic antidepressants	Arrhythmias: SVT, VPBs, RBBB, conduction defect, ↑QT interval, ↑risk of torsades de pointes
Cocaine	Hypertension; LVH, arrhythmias, MI
Sumatriptan	Chest pain 3–5%, risk of MI (rare)
Agents for treatment of AIDS	
Foscarnet (trisodium phosphate)	Acute reversible cardiac dysfunction
Zidovudine	SHMD
Pentamidine	Torsades de pointes
Cancer chemotherapeutic agents (*see* Table 21-10)	

AIDS, acquired immunodeficiency syndrome; LVH, left ventricular hypertrophy; MI, myocardial infarction; SHMD, specific heart muscle disease.

Antimalarials

Chloroquine has caused "cardiomyopathy."

Halofantrine: High-dose therapy has been reported to cause cardiac death *(13)*. Also, Mobitz type I and II block, prolongation of the QT interval, and torsades de pointes may be precipitated.

Histamine H_1-Antagonists

Astemizole and terfenadine have been reported to cause torsades de pointes and sudden cardiac death, albeit rarely. Terfenadine blocks the outward rectifier K^+ current. Increased terfenadine blood levels prolong the QT interval. Concomitant administration of agents that inhibit the hepatic oxygenase cytochrome P-450 system (erythromycin, clarithromycin, and other macrolide antibiotics; imidazole antifungal medications, such as ketoconazole or itraconazole) may further prolong the QT interval and precipitate torsades de pointes *(14, 15)*. In addition, patients with hepatic dysfunction, hypokalemia, or hypo-magnesemia, including patients with diarrhea, are at increased risk for torsades de pointes when treated with H_1-antagonists.

Antidepressants

Tricyclics: These agents predispose to a number of arrhythmic complications *(16)*: ventricular premature beats (VPBs), supraventricular arrhythmias, right bundle branch block (RBBB), other intraventricular conduction delay, QT prolongation, and the risk of torsades de pointes.

SSRIs: There have been rare reports of sinus bradycardia; VPBs and complete heart block have been reported with trazodone. Monoamine oxidase inhibitors may cause VPBs, ventricular tachycardia, and hypertensive crises (particularly when combined with tyramine).

Other Agents

Corticosteroids: Palpitations have been reported in up to 47% of patients given steroid pulse therapy *(17)*. Sudden cardiac death has been reported following large doses of steroids; VPBs may be precipitated by corticosteroid administration *(14,17)*.

Organophosphates may cause prolonged episodes of enhanced parasympathetic tone, QT alterations, ST-T wave changes, conduction defects, ventricular tachycardia, and fibrillation *(14)*.

Sumatriptan: This agent, used for migraine and cluster headache, may cause tightness in the chest in 3–5% of patients *(18)*. Acute myocardial infarction has been reported, including a case in a 47-yr-old woman *(18)*.

Ergotamine is known to cause coronary vasospasm and an increase in angina.

Metoclopramide: This frequently used antiemetic has few side effects; supraventricular arrhythmias may occur, albeit rarely. Two cases of bradycardia and complete heart block have been reported *(19)*.

Beta$_2$-agonists: Albuterol (salbutamol), terbutaline. These agents stimulate beta-receptors (some beta$_2$-receptors are present in the heart) and cause tachycardia. They may cause transient, but important, lowering of serum K^+ levels, which may trigger life-threatening ventricular arrhythmias, including ventricular fibrillation in patients with status asthmaticus treated with high-dose beta$_2$-agonists.

Foscarnet has been reported to cause reversible cardiac dysfunction in a patient treated for cytomegalovirus infection *(20)*.

Cancer Chemotherapeutic Agents

Cardiotoxicity may occur early or late during the administration of these agents (Table 21-9). Early complications include arrhythmias, left ventricular dysfunction, electrocardiographic changes, pericarditis, myocarditis, myocardial infarction, and sudden cardiac death. Late or chronic effects include sinus tachycardia, pericardial effusion, left ventricular dysfunction, CHF, and specific heart muscle disease (cardiomyopathy).

Doxorubicin: Early cardiotoxicity may manifest by the occurrence of nonspecific ST-T wave changes, arrhythmias, left ventricular dysfunction, pericarditis, or sudden cardiac death *(21)*. These changes may occur within the first week or two of drug administration. Late cardiotoxicity: Cardiomyopathy is caused by cumulative effects of the drug at high doses. CHF may be precipitated. The incidence of specific heart muscle disease with doxorubicin is about 2%, and that with daunorubicin is 5% *(21)*.

Cyclophosphamide: Cardiac effects usually occur during acute treatment: Low voltage in the electrocardiogram, acute pericarditis, supraventricular arrhythmias, and nonspecific ST-T wave changes.

Table 21-9
Cardiac Effects of Cancer Chemotherapeutic Agents

Chemotherapeutic agent	*Cardiac effect*
Busulfan	Pulmonary hypertension owing to pulmonary fibrosis
Cisplatinum	Coronary artery spasm: ischemia
Cyclophosphamide	Acute SHMD, pericarditis, CHF
Doxorubicin	Early: arrhythmias, ST-T changes Late: SHMD 2% *(20)*, refractory CHF
Daunorubicin	SHMD (5%)
5-Fluorouracil	Coronary vasospasm, ischemia (angina), myocardial infarction (rare)
Interferon-alpha	Cardiomegaly, CHF, pericardial effusion
Methotrexate	ST-T changes
Vincristine	Coronary vasospasm, ischemia

CHF, congestive heart failure; SHMD, specific heart muscle disease.

5-Fluorouracil may cause myocardial ischemia or chest pain owing to coronary artery spasm *(22)*.

Cisplatin, bleomycin, vincristine, and vinblastine may cause vasospasm similar to that observed with 5-fluorouracil *(22)*, myocardial ischemia, and, rarely, myocardial infarction.

Miscellaneous

Cisapride (Prepulsid) interacts with sotalol, quinidine, procainamide, other class I and class III agents, and noncardiac drugs that increase the QT interval; torsades de pointes and other life-threatening arrhythmias and sudden death may occur. **Caution** is required with the concomitant use of diuretics (e.g., thiazides, furosemide) because depletion of electrolytes may result in cardiac arrhythmias induced by Prepulsid. The drug is contraindicated in patients with arrhythmias, bradycardia, sinus node dysfunction, ischemic heart disease, valvular heart disease, CHF, QT prolongation associated with diabetes, and family history of sudden death. The drug was withdrawn in 2001.

Sildenafil (Viagra) coadministration with nitrates increases the risk of life-threatening hypotension, and nitrates must not be taken within 48 h of sildenafil. Less than 15% of all associated cardiovascular deaths reported occurred in men who were using nitrates. Caution is required with the use of antihypertensive agents. Interaction may occur with drugs that are metabolized by or that inhibit cytochrome P-450 3A4: amlodipine, amiodarone, diltiazem, disopyramide, felodipine, losartan, mibefradil, nifedipine, ranolazine or similar agents, quinidine, verapamil, clarithromycin or similar antibiotics, antifungals, and statins (except Pravachol), cimetidine, Prepulsid.

Saint John's wort (*Hypericum perforatum*) has been reported to cause a fall in cyclosporine serum levels that has been responsible for two cases of acute heart transplant rejection. A reduced anticoagulant effect of warfarin (decreased INR) also occurs. This and other herbal remedies induce drug-metabolizing enzymes of the cytochrome P-450 system. Thus, all herbal remedies must now be screened for interaction with prescribed medications.

Grapefruit juice (naringenin) inhibits the P-450 system and should be avoided with many medicines that use the P-450 pathways.

Herbal drugs and digoxin: Milkweed, lily of the valley, Siberian ginseng, oleander, squill, and hawthorne berries contain digoxin-like substances. Kushen exhibits digoxin-like properties. Kyushin and chan-su, used in Japan, cross-react with digoxin assays and cause spuriously high digoxin levels *(23)*. Also, ginseng may falsely elevate digoxin levels. Licorice and opium increase the risk of digoxin toxicity. Saint John's wort may reduce digoxin levels.

A review article on the benefits, adverse effects, and drug interactions of herbal therapies with cardiovascular effects is included in the Suggested Reading list.

REFERENCES

1. McLay JS, McMurray JJ, Bridges AB, et al. Acute effects of captopril on the renal actions of furosemide in patients with chronic heart failure. Am Heart J 1993;126: 879.
2. Ochs HR, Carstens G, Greenblatt DJ. Reduction in lidocaine clearance during continuous infusion and by coadministration of propranolol. N Engl J Med 1980303:373.
3. Trohman RG, Estes DM, Castellanos A, et al. Increased quinidine plasma concentration during administration of verapamil: A new quinidine-verapamil interaction. Am J Cardiol 1986;57:706.
4. Becker RC, Caputo R, Ball S, et al. Hemorrhagic potential of combined diltiazem and recombinant tissue-type plasminogen activator administration. Am Heart J 126: 11, 1993.
5. Gore JM, Sloan M, Price TR, et al. and the TIMI Investigators. Intracerebral hemorrhage, cerebral infarction, and subdural hematoma after acute myocardial infarcttion and thrombolytic therapy in the Thrombolysis in Myocardial Infarction study. Circulation 1991;83:448.
6. Blum CB. Comparison of properties of four inhibitors of 3-hydroxy-3-methylglutaryl-coenzyme A reductase. Am J Cardiol 1994;73:3D.
7. Browne KF, Prystowsky EN, Neger JJ, et al. Prolongation of the QT interval induced by probucol: Demonstration of a method for determining QT interval change induced by a drug. Am Heart J 1984;107:680.
8. Ellison JM, Milofsky JE, Ely E. Fluoxetine-induced bradycardia and syncope in two patients. J Clin Psychiatry 1990;51:385.
9. Buff DD, Brenner R, Kirtane SS, Gilboa R. Dysrhythmia associated with fluoxetine treatment in an elderly patient with cardiac disease. J Clin Psychiatry 1991;52:174.
10. Feder R. Bradycardia and syncope induced by fluoxetine. J Clin Psychiatry 1991;52:139.
11. Zipes DP. Unwitting exposure to risk. Cardiol Rev 1993;1:1.
12. Stramha-Badiale M, Guffanti S, Porta N, et al. QT interval prolongation and cardiac arrest during antibiotic therapy with spiramycin in a newborn infant. Am Heart J 1993;126:740.
13. Nosten F, terKuile FO, Luxemburger C. Cardiac effects of anti-malarial treatment with halofantrine. Lancet 1993;341:1054.
14. Martyn R, Somberg JC, Kerin NZ. Proarrhythmia of nonanti-arrhythmia drugs. Am Heart J 1993;126: 201.
15. Simons FER, Simons KJ, Wood AJJ. The pharmacology and use of H_1-receptor-antagonist drugs. N Engl J Med 1994;330:1663.
16. Glassman AH, Roose SP, Bigger JT. The safety of tricyclic antidepressants in cardiac patients. JAMA 1993;269:2673.
17. Belmonte MA, Cequiere A, Roig-Escofet D. Severe ventricular arrhythmia after methylprednisone pulse therapy in rheumatoid arthritis. J Rheumatol 1986;13:477.
18. Ottervanger JP, Paalman HJA, Boxma GL, et al. Transmural myocardial infarction with sumatriptan. Lancet 1993;341:861.
19. Esselink RAJ, Gerding MN, Brouwers PJAM, et al. Total heart block after intravenous metoclopramide. Lancet 1994;343:182.
20. Brown DL, Sather S, Cheitlin MD. Reversible cardiac dysfunction associated with foscarnet therapy for cytomegalovirus esophagitis in an AIDS patient. Am Heart J 1993;125:1439.
21. Lipshultz SE, Colan SD, Gelber RD, et al. Late cardiac effects of doxorubicin therapy for acute lymphoblastic leukemia in childhood. N Engl J Med 1991;324:808.
22. Baker WP, Dainer P, Lester WM, et al. Ischemic chest pain after 5-fluorouracil therapy for cancer. Am J Cardiol 1986;57:497.
23. Cheng TO. Interaction of herbal drugs with digoxin. J Am Coll Cardiol 2002;40:838.

SUGGESTED READING

Jhund P, McMurray JJV. Does aspirin reduce the benefit of an angiotensin-converting enzyme inhibitor?: Choosing between the Scylla of observational studies and the Charybdis of subgroup analysis. Circulation 2006;113:2566–2568.

O'Gara PT. Common drug interactions in cardiology. ACC Curr J Rev Jul/Aug:1, 2002.

Valli G, Giardina EV. Benefits, adverse effects and drug interactions of herbal therapies with cardiovascular effects. J Am Coll Cardiol 2002;39:1083.

22 Hallmark Clinical Trials

Results that dictate a reduction in end points observed in a few hallmark and other recent randomized clinical trials (RCTs) are given. *The appropriate reference source is given so that the reader can explore the details of the RCT if required.* Because of the constraints of available space, only a brief comment is given in the text regarding the results and their implications.

Prior to the assessment of these RCTs, the reader may wish to review the following brief points that relate to the interpretation of clinical trials:

Questions to ask when reading and interpreting the results of a clinical trial include *(1)*

- The "gold standard" statistical test of treatment effect is the determination of the p value using the χ^2 or Fisher exact test. Although a p value < 0.05 is at the significant level, in clinical medicine it is advisable to use $p \leq 0.02$ as a level of significant treatment effect.
- Statements describing treatment effect *(2)*: relative risk (RR), relative risk reduction, odds ratio (OR), and *absolute risk difference (ARD)*.
- An RR, relative risk reduction, or OR < 1 indicates treatment benefit. However, an RR reduction may give the impression of a greater treatment effect if the ARD and number needed to treat, the (1/ARD), is not given: the number of lives saved per 1000 patients treated.
- Metaanalysis: Data pooling or quantitative review provides partial answers that may receive support from some and skepticism from others. One rule must be invoked when one is assessing the results derived from clinical metaanalysis: do not accept information based on subgroup analysis unless the primary end point, particularly the effect on all-cause mortality or cardiovascular mortality, showed a significant treatment effect.
- Are the results of the study valid?: Was the assignment of patients to treatment randomized? Were all patients who entered the trial properly accounted for at its conclusion? Was follow-up complete and patients analyzed in the groups to which they were randomized?

ACUTE CORONARY SYNDROME RCTs

OASIS-5: Comparison of Fondaparinux and Enoxaparin in Acute Coronary Syndromes

The Fifth Organization to Assess Strategies in Acute Ischemic Syndromes (OASIS-5) investigators assigned 20,078 patients with acute coronary syndrome (ACS) to either fondaparinux (2.5 mg daily) or enoxaparin (1 mg/kg twice daily) for a mean of 6 d *(3)*. Patients were age 66.6 ± 11 yr. The primary outcome was death, myocardial infarction (MI), refractory ischemia major bleeding, and their combination at 9 d and 6 mo *(3)*.

At 6-mo follow-up, the number of patients with primary-outcome events was similar in the two groups (579 with fondaparinux [5.8%] versus 573 with enoxaparin [5.7%]; hazard ratio [HR] in the fondaparinux group, 1.01), with no significant differences at 30 d.

From: *Contemporary Cardiology: Cardiac Drug Therapy, Seventh Edition*
M. Gabriel Khan © Humana Press Inc., Totowa, NJ

- However, the rate of major bleeding at 9 d was 47% lower with fondaparinux than with enoxaparin (217 events [2.2%] versus 412 events [4.1%]; HR, 0.52; $p < 0.001$) *(3)*.

The trialists were concerned regarding the bleeding safety profile of enoxaparin and should have used more stringent safety ground rules for the use of low-molecular-weight heparin (LMWH). Patients, particularly cardiac patients, older than age 72 often have a creatinine clearance (estimated glomerular filtration rate [GFR]) < 55 mL/min, and enoxaparin should be given once daily in patients with creatinine clearance 40–55 mL/min; patients in this category received enoxaparin twice daily. In addition patients, 75 yr and older should be given 0.75 mg/kg twice daily, but if the estimated GFR is <55, LMWH should be given once daily.

Unfortunately, patients with a creatinine clearance < 30 mL/min were given LMWH 1 mg /kg once daily; LMWH should be avoided in patients with creatinine clearance < 30 mL/min if bleeding is to be minimized.

OASIS-6: Effects of Fondaparinux on Mortality and Reinfarction in Patients With Acute ST-Segment Elevation Myocardial Infarction (STEMI)

OASIS-6 was an RCT of fondaparinux versus usual care in 12,092 STEMI patients. A 7–8-d course of fondaparinux was compared with either no anticoagulation or unfractionated (UF) heparin (75% received unfractionated heparin for <48 h). Streptokinase was the main fibrinolytic used (73% of those who received lytics) *(4)*. The primary outcome was a composite of death or reinfarction at 30 d.

- **Conclusion:** In patients with STEMI, particularly those **not** undergoing primary percutaneous coronary intervention (PCI), fondaparinux significantly reduced mortality and reinfarction without increasing bleeding and strokes *(4)*.

Since most STEMI patients in North America undergo PCI as preferred therapy, it appears that fondaparinux would play a small role. However, in countries where PCI is not readily available, the drug can be used with streptokinase without any form of heparin administration. In addition, the one dose of fondaparinux with no adjustments for weight is a great advance in developing or developed countries.

Califf *(5)* points out that a reasonable conclusion from this trial is that fondaparinux is highly beneficial in patients in whom the noninterventional approach has been predetermined and will be more preferred in settings in which the use of angiographic-based reperfusion is not routine. In addition, the absence of the need for dose adjustment is remarkable *(5)*. These two large RCTs have endorsed fondaparinux as a leading antithrombotic drug in the treatment of ACS. There is no evidence that fondaparinux is inferior to either UF heparin or LMWH for management of ACS *(5)*. The reduction in bleeding in the fondaparinux group compared with the group receiving no antithrombotic therapy should give clinicians some confidence that at the dose used, fondaparinux has a desirable margin of safety *(5)*. Also, heparin-induced thrombocytopenia (HIT) can be avoided. Caution with dosage is needed, however, in patients with significant renal dysfunction (estimated GFR < 50 mL/min).

ExTRACT-TIMI 25: Enoxaparin Versus Heparin in Acute MI

Enoxaparin and Thrombolysis Reperfusion for Acute Myocardial Infarction Treatment-Thrombolysis in Myocardial Infarction (EXTRACT-TIMI) 25 RCT *(6)* compared enoxaparin with heparin. A total of 20,506 patients with STEMI treated with thrombolytics received enoxaparin or weight-based UF heparin for at least 48 h. The primary efficacy end point was death or nonfatal recurrent MI *(6)*.

- **At 30-d follow-up:** The primary end point occurred in 12.0% of patients in the UF heparin group versus 9.9% in the enoxaparin group (17% reduction in RR; $p < 0.001$). Nonfatal MI occurred in 4.5% and 3.0%, respectively (33% reduction in RR; $p < 0.001$); there was no difference in total mortality *(6)*.
- Major bleeding occurred in 1.4% with UF heparin versus 2.1% with enoxaparin ($p < 0.001$) *(6)*.
- The exclusion of men with a creatinine level > 2.5 mg/dL (220 μmol/L) and women with a creatinine level > 2.0 mg/dL (177 μmol/L) was an important adjustment to prevent bleeding.
- This curtailment could have been adjusted further, however, using the suggested cut off: for estimated GFR of 30–55 mL/min, give the 0.75-mg/kg dose once daily.

LMWH and Major Bleeding: Advice

- *For the conversion of serum creatinine in mg/dL, multiply × 88 (= mmol/L). The serum creatinine is only a rough measure of renal function and must not be relied on, particularly in patients older than age 70.*
- *Use the creatinine clearance estimated GFR rather than serum creatinine levels, but note that some electronic formulas are inaccurate in patients older than age 70 and must be adjusted in blacks (for African Americans, the laboratory-reported estimated GFR should be multiplied by a factor of 1.21 and reinterpreted accordingly).*
- Patients, particularly cardiac patients, older than age 70 with a serum creatinine in the upper normal range of 1–1.2 mg/dL (88–106 μmol/L) often have a lowered GFR because of the underlying normal diminution of GFR with age. A substantial number of nephrons are lost annually beyond age 70, and in many elderly patients renal disease coexists.
- For patients older than age 75, enoxaparin 0.75 mg/kg once daily is an easy dose to recall, but it might be preferable to use the lower age cutoff: >70 yr of age.
- Enoxaparin and other LMWHs should be given once daily in patients with a GFR, creatinine clearance of 40–55 mL/min. Patients in this category received enoxaparin twice daily in several RCTs; unfortunately, patients with a creatinine clearance < 30 mL/min were given 1 mg/kg once daily in some RCTs.
- Importantly, if major bleeding is to be minimized in patients with ACS, LMWH should be avoided if the creatinine clearance is <30 mL/min. An estimated GFR of <30 mL/min, reflects poor renal function. Clinicians most often use a creatinine clearance < 15 mL/min to indicate severe renal failure. This information is correct, but end-stage renal failure (GFR < 15 mL/min) should be regarded as very severe renal failure, and drugs that have a potential to cause major bleeding must be used only with justification. Use in patients with ACS is not justifiable because alternative therapies are available.
- Do not switch from UF heparin to LMWH and vice versa in the management of a patient with ACS.
- Guidelines need to be rewritten concerning the use of LMWH, with consideration of the aforementioned points: in patients aged > 70 yr, use 0.75 mg/kg, and in all patients with creatinine clearance 30–50 mL/min dose once daily and avoid if the estimated GFR is <30 mL/min.

ACUITY: Heparins Versus Bivalirudin for ACS

The Acute Catheterization and Urgent Intervention Triage Strategy (ACUITY) RCT evaluated the use of bivalirudin as a replacement for UF heparin and LMWH administered in the emergency department and continuing through the catheterization laboratory *(6a,b)*. The control arm of ACUITY comprised patients treated with the heparins combined with platelet glycoprotein (GP) IIb/IIIa receptor blockers. A second arm studied bivalirudin

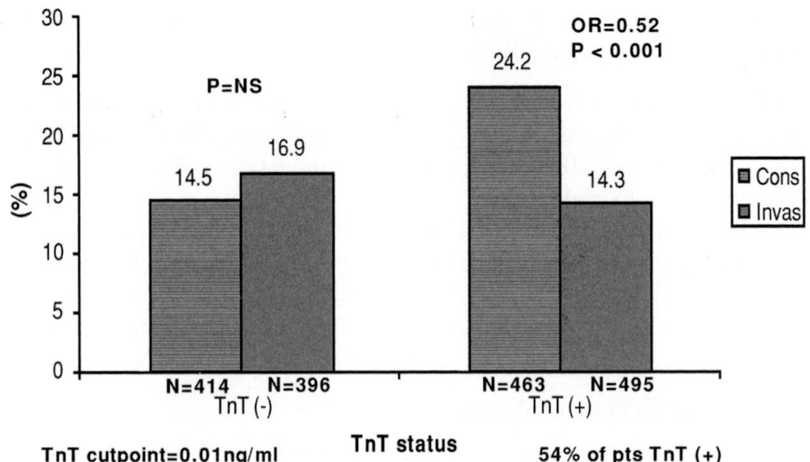

Fig. 22-1. Outcomes of invasive and conservative strategies in TACTICS-TIMI 18 according to troponin level. (From Cannon CP. Management of Acute Coronary Syndromes, 2nd ed. Humana Press, Totowa, NJ, 2003.)

with added GP IIb/IIIa receptor blockers; the third arm studied bivalirudin alone as monotherapy. (In the third arm, approx 7% of study patients received GP receptor blockers.)

- Patients who received the combination of bivalirudin with GP IIb/IIIa blockers (compared with a heparin-based regimen) had equivalent rates of bleeding and ischemia; overall patient outcomes were also equivalent.
- Bivalirudin monotherapy suppressed ischemic complications just as effectively as heparins plus GP IIb/IIIa blockers but was associated with half of the major bleeding, resulting in a significant improvement in overall patient outcomes.

TACTICS-TIMI 18: Invasive Versus Conservative Strategy in ACS Patients Treated With Tirofiban

The Treat Angina with Aggrastat and determine Cost of Therapy with an Invasive or Conservative Strategy-Thrombolysis in Myocardial Infarction (TACTICS-TIMI) 18 trial evaluated the superiority of an invasive strategy (stenting and use of the platelet inhibitor tirofiban) in patients with non-ST elevation ACS (unstable angina or STEMI) *(7)*. Coronary angiography was completed within 4–48 h, and PCI was accomplished in the invasive arm.

- The cumulative incidence of the primary end point of death, nonfatal MI, or rehospitalization for an ACS during the 6-mo follow-up period was lower in the invasive-strategy group than in the conservative-strategy group (15.9% versus 19.4%; OR, 0.78; 95% confidence interval [CI], 0.62–0.97; $p = 0.025$). Patients with positive troponin levels achieved the greatest benefit from an early invasive strategy (14.3% versus 24.2%; $p < 0.001$; *see* Fig. 22-1) *(7)*.

Thus, only patients with NSTEMI (as defined by positive troponin levels) benefited significantly. Patients with unstable angina with or without ischemic electrocardiographic (ECG) changes and negative troponin levels showed no significant benefit with an invasive strategy. It appears, therefore, that patients with unstable angina and negative troponin levels should not be considered to have ACS but simply unstable angina. These patients have not sustained infarctions and are a heterogenous group with a markedly different prognosis compared with non-STEMI patients, a pure group with a well-defined prognosis.

CAPRICORN: Carvedilol in Postinfarct Patients

In the Carvedilol Postinfarct Survival Controlled Evaluation (CAPRICORN) trial, patients with acute MI and ejection fraction (EF) < 40% (mean 32.8), 1–21 d prior to randomization, treated with an angiotensin-converting enzyme (ACE) inhibitor, were randomly assigned; the treatment arm received carvedilol 6.25 mg, which was increased progressively to 25 mg twice daily in 74% of treated patients *(8)*.

- Carvedilol caused a significant 23% reduction in all-cause mortality in patients with acute MI observed for 2.5 yr (mortality 116 [12%] in the treated versus 151 [15%] in the placebo arm; $p = 0.031$) *(8)*.
- The absolute reduction in risk was 2.3%: 43 patients need to be treated for 1 yr to save one life; this reduction is virtually the same as that observed in a metaanalysis of three ACE inhibitor trials, SAVE, AIRE, and TRACE.
- Notably, the reduction by carvedilol is in addition to those of ACE inhibitors alone.

HEART FAILURE RCTs

COPERNICUS: Carvedilol in Severe Chronic HF

The Carvedilol Prospective Randomized Cumulative Survival Study (COPERNICUS) *(9)* involved 2289 patients with severe heart failure (HF; EF 19.8 ± 4%).

- There were 190 deaths in placebo recipients and 130 in those given carvedilol, a 35% decrease in the risk of death ($p = 0.0014$). The dose of carvedilol was 6.25 mg, with a slow increase to 25 mg twice daily. An ACE inhibitor, *digoxin,* and spironolactone were used in 97%, 66%, and 20% of patients, respectively *(9)*.
- The 35% lower risk in the carvedilol group was significant: $p = 0.00013$ (unadjusted) and $p = 0.0014$ (adjusted) *(9)*.

MERIT-HF: Metoprolol CR/XL in Chronic Heart Failure

The Metoprolol CR/XL Randomized Intervention Trial in Congestive Heart Failure (MERIT-HF) trial *(10)* studied metoprolol succinate (not tartrate) in patients with class II and III HF (mean EF 0.28). An ACE inhibitor or angiotensin receptor blocker (ARB) and digoxin were used in 95% and 64% of patients, respectively.

- Metoprolol caused significant reductions in the primary outcomes *(10)*.

CHARM: Candesartan in Chronic HF

The Candesartan in HF Assessment of Reduction in Mortality and Morbidity (CHARM-Alternative) trial *(13)* ($n = 2028$) examined the effects of the ARB, candesartan in patients with reduced left ventricular EF < 40% who were ACE inhibitor intolerant. Treated patients received candesartan 4–8 mg titrated to 32 mg once daily plus the treatment given to placebo patients: standard antifailure therapy that included diuretics, a beta-blocker, digoxin, and spironolactone (85%, 54%, 45%, and 24%, respectively).

- After 33.7 mo, patients given candesartan were 23% less likely to experience cardiovascular death or HF hospitalization compared with those who received placebo (40% versus 33%; $p = 0.0004$) *(13)*.

A-HeFT: Isosorbide Dinitrate and Hydralazine in Blacks with HF

In the African American Heart Failure Trial (AHeFT) *(14)*, 1050 black patients who had class III or IV HF with dilated ventricles were randomly assigned to receive 37.5 mg of hydralazine hydrochloride and 20 mg of isosorbide dinitrate three times daily. The dose was increased to two tablets three times daily, for a total daily dose of 225 mg of hydralazine hydrochloride and 120 mg of isosorbide dinitrate. (It is surprising that nitrate tolerance did not alter the results.)

- The study was terminated early (at 18 mo) because of a significantly higher mortality rate in the placebo group than in the group given isosorbide dinitrate plus hydralazine (10.2% versus 6.2%; $p = 0.02$). There was a 43% reduction in the rate of death from any cause (HR, 0.57; $p = 0.01$) and a 33% relative reduction in the rate of first hospitalization for HF (16.4% versus 22.4%; $p = 0.001$) *(14)*.

ALDOSTERONE ANTAGONIST TRIALS

RALES: Spirinolacatone in Severe HF Patients

Significant results were obtained in the Randomized Aldactone Evaluation Study (RALES) trial *(11)* with the use of spironolactone (Aldactone) in patients with severe HF class III and IV (EF 25 ± 6.8). ACE inhibitors and digoxin were used in 95% and 74% of patients, respectively.

- Spironolactone (Aldactone) is a major addition to our HF armamentarium.

EPHESUS: Eplerenone in Post-Acute MI

The Eplerenone Post-Acute MI and HF Efficacy and Survival Study (EPHESUS) *(12)* showed that eplerenone, a selective aldosterone blocker, added to optimal medical therapy in patients with acute MI and heart failure (EF < 35%), significantly reduced mortality and morbidity. The trial randomized 6600 patients. An eplerenone dose of 25 mg was titrated up to 50 mg daily. Gynecomastia was not observed, but significant hyperkalemia occurred in 5.5% and 3.9% of patients in the treated and placebo groups, respectively ($p = 0.002$) *(12)*.

Caution: This useful replacement for spironolactone should not be used in patients with serum creatinine > 1.5 mg/dL (133 μmol/L), particularly in patients older than age 72 or in type 2 diabetics and in all patients with GFR < 50 mL/min because hyperkalemia may be precipitated. Most important, the serum creatinine does not reflect creatinine clearance, particularly in the elderly, who are most often treated for HF.

ACE Inhibitor RCT

The Heart Outcomes Prevention Evaluation (HOPE) trial *(15)* studied high-risk patients (diabetes 38%, MI 52%, angina 80%, peripheral vascular disease [PVD] 43%, hypertension 47%) without known significant left ventricular dysfunction.

- Ramipril significantly reduced the rates of death, MI, and stroke The RR of the composite outcome in the ramipril group compared with the placebo group was 0.78 (95% CI, 0.70–0.86). Treatment of 1000 patients for 4 yr prevents approx 150 events in approx 70 patients.

HYPERTENSION TRIALS

ALLHAT: ACE Inhibitor or Calcium Channel Blocker Versus Diuretic to Prevent HF

The Antihypertensive and Lipid-Lowering Treatment to Prevent Heart Attack Trial (ALLHAT) is a hallmark clinical trial *(16)*.

A total of 33,357 hypertensive patients (mean age, 67) were randomized to receive chlorthalidone, 12.5–25 mg/d ($n = 15,255$); amlodipine, 2.5–10 mg/d ($n = 9048$); or lisinopril, 10–40 mg/d ($n = 9054$), with a follow-up of 4.9 yr. There was good representation for women (47%) and blacks (35%); 36% were diabetics.

The primary outcome, combined fatal CHD or nonfatal MI, occurred in 2956 participants, with no difference between treatments. All-cause mortality did not differ between groups *(16)*.

- **The doxazosin arm of the trial was halted because of a marked occurrence of HF (47%) caused by doxazosin. No significant increase in cholesterol was caused by chlorthalidone.**
- The primary outcomes for amlodipine versus chlorthalidone, were similar except for a higher 6-yr rate of HF with amlodipine *(16)*.
- **The 6 yr rate for HF with amlodipine was 10.2% versus 7.7% with chlorthalidone; a 32.5% higher risk of HF ($p < 0.001$) *(16)* with a 6-yr absolute risk difference of 2.5% and a 35% higher risk of hospitalized/fatal HF ($p < 0.001$). Elderly patients had a higher incidence of HF, which was even greater in black individuals *(16)*.** Importantly, because BP goal was achieved with chlorthalidone monotherapy in <30% of patients, added therapy was atenolol 25–100 mg, and in some reserpine or clonidine. It appears that a beta-blocker was used in >605 of patients in this arm of this study.

STATIN RCTs

PROVE IT-TIMI 22: Early and Late Benefits of High-Dose Atorvastatin in ACS Patients

Cannon and colleague *(17)* strongly advocate intensive versus moderate lipid lowering with statins for patients admitted with ACS. In the Pravastatin or Atorvastatin Evaluation and Infection Therapy (PROVE IT) TIMI 22 trial *(17)*, 4162 patients with NSTEMI-ACS were randomized to receive atorvastatin 80 mg (intensive statin therapy) or pravastatin 40 mg (standard therapy).

The composite triple end point of death, MI, or rehospitalization for recurrent ACS at 30 d occurred in 3.0% of patients receiving atorvastatin 80 mg versus 4.2% of patients receiving pravastatin 40 mg (HR, 0.72; 95% CI, 0.52–0.99; $p = 0.046$) *(17)*.

- In stable patients, atorvastatin 80 mg was associated with a composite event rate of 9.6% versus 13.1% in the pravastatin 40 mg group (HR, 0.72; 95% CI, 0.58–0.89; $p = 0.003$).
- From 6 mo after ACS to the end of the study, the primary end point occurred in 15.1% of patients receiving intensive therapy versus 17.7% of patients on pravastatin, resulting in an 18% reduction in events (HR, 0.82; 95% CI, 0.69–0.99; $p = 0.037$) *(18)*.
- At 1 yr after ACS to the end of follow-up, there was an absolute event rate of 5.6% with intensive therapy versus 8.0% with standard therapy (HR, 0.72; 95% CI, 0.54–0.95; $p = 0.02$).

Cannon and colleagues indicated that, based on this RCT, ACS patients should be started in-hospital and continued long-term on intensive statin therapy *(17)*. Ridker et al. *(19)* noted that patients who had low C-reactive protein (CRP) levels after statin therapy had better clinical outcomes than those with higher CRP levels, regardless of the resultant level of low-density lipoprotein cholesterol (LDL-C). Patients who had LDL cholesterol levels < 70 mg/dL and CRP levels < 1 mg/L after statin therapy had the lowest rate of recurrent events (1.9 per 100 person-years) *(19)*. Perhaps strategies to lower cardiovascular risk with statins in selected individuals should include monitoring CRP as well as cholesterol *(19)*.

ASTEROID: High-Intensity Statins for Atheroma Regression

A Study to Evaluate the Effect of Rosuvastatin on Intravascular Ultrasound-Derived Coronary Atheroma Burden (ASTEROID) *(20)* assessed whether very intensive statin administration could regress coronary atheroma as evaluated by intravascular ultrasound (IVUS) imaging using percent atheroma volume (PAV), the most rigorous IVUS measure of disease progression and regression. A baseline IVUS examination was done on 507 patients who received rosuvastatin 40 mg daily. After 24 mo, 349 patients had serial IVUS examinations *(20)*. Two primary efficacy parameters were prespecified: the change in PAV and the change in nominal atheroma volume in the 10-mm subsegment with the greatest disease severity at baseline. Findings at 24 mo were as follows:

- The mean (SD) change in PAV for the entire vessel was –0.98% (3.15%), with a median of –0.79% (97.5% CI, –1.21% to –0.53%; $p < 0.001$ versus baseline). The mean (SD) change in atheroma volume in the most diseased 10-mm subsegment was –6.1 (10.1) mm^3, with a median of –5.6 mm^3 (97.5% CI, –6.8 to –4.0 mm^3; $p < 0.001$ versus baseline). Change in total atheroma volume showed a 6.8% median reduction, with a mean (SD) reduction of –14.7 (25.7) mm^3 and a median of –12.5 mm^3 (95% CI, –15.1 to –10.5 mm^3; $p < 0.001$ versus baseline) *(20)*.
- The mean (SD) baseline LDL-C level of 130.4 (34.3) mg/dL was reduced to 60.8 (20.0) mg/dL (53.2%; $p < 0.001$) *(21)*. The mean (SD) high-density lipoprotein cholesterol (HDL-C) level at baseline was 43.1 (11.1) mg/dL; it increased to 49.0 (12.6) mg/dL (14.7%; $p < 0.001$) *(20)*.
- Adverse events were infrequent and similar to those of other statin trials.

Nissen and colleagues concluded that very high-intensity statin therapy with rosuvastatin 40 mg/d achieved an average LDL-C of 60.8 mg/dL and increased HDL-C by 14.7%. This marked amelioration of lipid levels caused significant regression of atheroma for all three prespecified IVUS measures of disease burden *(20)*. Blumental et al. *(21)*, however, stated that the trial has some concerns, including lack of a control group receiving a somewhat less intensive LDL-C-lowering regimen and the absence of paired IVUS measurements in less diseased coronary segments to demonstrate reproducibility of atheroma volume measurements. The study does not provide definitive information regarding the relationship of LDL-C lowering and extent of atheroma regression to determine whether high-intensity treatment is necessary to obtain regression. Nonetheless, it is the first clear evidence that coronary atheroma can regress significantly when LDL-C is markedly lowered.

ASTEROID *(20)*, PROVE IT-TIMI 22 *(17)*, and the RCTs discussed in Chapter 18, Statin Controversies, indicate that guidelines need to be reviewed *(22)*.

MRC/BHF Heart Protection Study: Cholesterol Lowering to Reduce Event Risk

The MRC/BHF Heart Protection Study *(23)* indicates that in vascular high-risk patients, 40 mg simvastatin safely reduced the risk of heart attack, of stroke, and of revascularization by at least one-third. Notably, cholesterol lowering proved of benefit in reducing major events irrespective of cholesterol levels, sex, or age. Among the 4000 patients with a total cholesterol < 5 mmol/L (200 mg/dL), a clear reduction in major events was observed *(23)*.

- All-cause mortality was significantly reduced (1328 [12.9%] deaths among 10,269 allocated simvastatin versus 1507 [14.7%] among 10,267 allocated placebo; $p = 0.0003$), owing to a highly significant 18% (SE 5) proportional reduction in the coronary death rate (587 [5.7%] versus 707 [6.9%]; $p = 0.0005$). There were highly significant reductions of about one-fourth in the first-event rate for fatal and nonfatal MI (898 [8.7%] versus 1212 [11.8%]; $p < 0.0001$), for nonfatal or fatal stroke (444 [4.3%] versus 585 [5.7%]; $p < 0.0001$) and for coronary or noncoronary revascularization (939 [9.1%] versus 1205 [11.7%]; $p < 0.0001$) *(23)*.

PROSPER: Pravastatin in the Elderly

In the Prospective Study of Pravastatin in the Elderly at Risk (PROSPECT) *(24)*, pravastatin 40 mg was administered to 5804 randomized elderly patients aged 70–82. At the short, 3.5-yr follow-up, there was no difference in the number of strokes, but CHD death was reduced by 24% *(24). There were 245 new cases of cancer in the pravastatin group, versus 199 in the placebo group. Breast and gastrointestinal cancers showed the largest increases.* New cancer diagnoses were more frequent on pravastatin than on placebo (HR, 1.25; 95% CI, 1.04–1.51, $p = 0.020$) *(24). **Caution** is required because in the CARE study (25) there were 12 cancers in the pravastatin-treated patients versus 1 in the control group* (*see* Chapter 18, Statin Controversies).

LIPID: Pravastatin for Prevention

This RCT compared the effects of 40 mg pravastatin with those of a placebo in 9014 patients with past MI, hospitalization for unstable angina, and cholesterol levels of 155–271 mg/dL who were 31–75 yr of age. Both groups received advice on following a cholesterol-lowering diet. The primary study outcome was mortality from coronary heart disease *(26)*.

- In these 31–75-yr-old patients, at a mean follow-up of 6.1 yr, overall mortality was 14.1% in the placebo group and 11.0% in the pravastatin group (relative reduction in risk, 22%; 95% CI, 13–31%; $p < 0.001$). Death from CHD occurred in 8.3% of the patients in the placebo group and 6.4% of those in the pravastatin group, a relative reduction in risk of 24% (95% CI, 12–35%; $p < 0.001$) *(26)*. Importantly, there were no differences in cancer deaths (128 for pravastatin versus 141 for placebo) *(26)*.

ARRHYTHMIA RCTs

AFFIRM: Rate Versus Rhythm Control in Atrial Fibrillation

The Atrial Fibrillation Follow-up Investigation of Rhythm Management (AFFIRM) was a well-run rate versus rhythm control RCT with 2–5 yr of follow-up *(27)*. The conclusions were as follows:

- Rate control is an acceptable primary therapy. In the rate control arm, 51% received digoxin and 49% a beta-blocker. At 2 yr of follow-up, the perceived benefit of restoring and maintaining sinus rhythm did not alter mortality. Patients in the rhythm control arm still required warfarin (70%); mortality, stroke rate, and hospitalizations were slightly increased, and bradycardiac arrest and torsades de pointes were of concern *(27)*. Amiodarone was used in approx 39%, sotalol in approx 33%, and propafenone in approx 10% to maintain rhythm control, which required frequent changes in drug and dosing schedule.

An RCT conducted in The Netherlands in patients with persistent atrial fibrillation < 1 yr randomly assigned to electrical conversion and rhythm control versus rate control indicated that rate control was not inferior to rhythm control. Nonfatal end points were slighter greater in the rhythm control group; cardiovascular mortality was the same in both groups.

BETA-BLOCKERS AND DIABETES

GEMINI: Beta-Blockers for Hypertensive Diabetics

The Glycemic Effects in Diabetes Mellitus: Carvedilol-Metoprolol Comparison in Hypertensives (GEMINI) trial *(28)* addressed concerns regarding the increased incidence of type 2 diabetes caused by beta-blockers. Carvedilol is a unique beta-blocker with properties that are subtly different from other beta-blockers. This randomized, double-blind, parallel-group trial compared the effects of carvedilol and metoprolol tartrate on glycemic control in the context of cardiovascular (CDV) risk factors in 1235 individuals with hypertension and type 2 diabetes mellitus (glycosylated hemoglobin [HbA_{1c}], 6.5–8.5%) who were receiving ACE inhibitors or ARBs. Patients were randomized to receive a 6.25–25-mg dose of carvedilol or 50–200-mg dose of metoprolol tartrate each twice daily *(28)*.

- At 35 wk of follow-up, the mean (SD) HbA_{1c} increased with metoprolol (0.15% [0.04%]; $p < 0.001$) but not carvedilol (0.02% [0.04%]; $p = 0.65$).
- **Insulin sensitivity improved with carvedilol (–9.1%; $p = 0.004$) but not metoprolol (–2.0%; $p = 0.48$)** ***(28).***
- **Carvedilol treatment had no effect on HbA_{1c} (mean [SD] change from baseline to end point, 0.02% [0.04%]; 95% CI, –0.06–0.10%; $p = 0.65$), whereas metoprolol increased HbA_{1c} (0.15% [0.04%]; 95% CI, 0.08–0.22%; $p < 0.001$** ***(28).***
- Blood pressure was similar between groups. Metoprolol increased triglycerides (13%, $p < 0.001$), whereas carvedilol had no effect. Significant weight gain was observed in the metoprolol group (mean [SD], 1.2 [0.2] kg for metoprolol, $p < 0.001$ versus 0.2 [0.2] kg for carvedilol, $p = 0.36$) *(28).*

CLOPIDOGREL

PCI-CLARITY: Clopidogrel Before PCI

PCI-Clopidogrel as Adjunctive Reperfusion Therapy (PCI-CLARITY) *(29)* was an RCT of the 1863 patients undergoing PCI after mandated angiography in CLARITY-TIMI, an RCT of clopidogrel. All patients received aspirin and were randomized to receive either clopidogrel (300 mg loading dose and then 75 mg once daily) or placebo initiated with thrombolytics and given until coronary angiography was performed 2–8 d after initiation of the study drug. For patients undergoing coronary artery stenting, it was recommended that open-label clopidogrel (including a loading dose) be administered after the diagnostic angiogram. The primary outcome was the incidence of the composite of CVD death, recurrent MI, or stroke from PCI to 30 d after randomization.

- Pretreatment with clopidogrel significantly reduced the incidence of CVD death, MI, or stroke following PCI (34 [3.6%] versus 58 [6.2%]; adjusted OR, 0.54; (95% CI, 0.35–0.85; $p = 0.008$). Pretreatment with clopidogrel also reduced the incidence of MI or stroke prior to PCI (37 [4.0%] versus 58 [6.2%]; OR, 0.62; (95% CI, 0.40–0.95; $p = 0.03$). Overall, pretreatment with clopidogrel resulted in a highly significant reduction in cardiovascular death, MI, or stroke from randomization through 30 d (70 [7.5%] versus 112 [12.0%]; adjusted OR, 0.59; (95% CI, 0.43–0.81; $p = 0.001$; number needed to treat = 23). There was no significant excess in the rates of bleeding *(29).*

CLOPIDOGREL/BETA-BLOCKERS

COMMIT: Clopidogrel + Aspirin in Acute MI

In the Clopidogrel and Metoprolol in Myocardial Infarction Trial (COMMIT) *(30)*, clopidogrel was added to aspirin in 45,852 patients with acute MI (a randomized placebo-controlled trial).

- Clopidogrel caused a significant reduction in death, reinfarction, or stroke (9.2% versus 10.1%; relative risk reduction, 9%; $p = 0.002$). Clopidogrel was equally effective with or without thrombolytic therapy *(30)*.

COMMIT/CCS-2: IV and Then Oral Metoprolol in Acute MI

COMMIT/Second Chinese Cardiac Study (CCS-2) *(31)* is the second largest trial ever conducted on the emergency treatment of STEMI patients. Patients received aspirin and were randomized to receive clopidogrel 75 mg/d or placebo; within these two groups, patients were then randomized to metoprolol (*15 mg IV in three equal doses followed by 200 mg/d oral*) or placebo. Patients were randomized within 24 h of suspected acute MI and demonstrated ST elevation or other ischemic abnormality and excluded if they were undergoing PCI. The primary end point varied between study drugs: for clopidogrel, it was death or the combination of death, reinfarction, or stroke up to 4 wk in the hospital or prior to discharge; for metoprolol, it was death or death, reinfarction, or cardiac arrest/ ventricular fibrillation (VF) up to 4 wk in the hospital or prior to discharge.

- Metoprolol produced a significant 18% relative risk reduction in reinfarction (2.0% versus 2.5%; $p = 0.001$) as well as a 17% relative risk reduction in ventricular fibrillation (2.5% versus 3.0%; $p = 0.001$), there was no effect on mortality (7.7% versus 7.8%).
- Metoprolol significantly increased the relative risk of death from cardiogenic shock by 29%, with the greatest risk of shock occurring primarily on d 0–1 *(31)*. Cardiogenic shock understandably was more evident in patients in Killip class II and III; this adverse effect was largely iatrogenic because the dose of metoprolol was excessive. Oral beta-blocker therapy is preferred, and the IV use is cautioned against.
- Importantly. metoprolol IV was administered to patients who were hemodynamically unstable, a situation that must be avoided. (*See* Chapter 2, Beta-Blocker Controversies.)

CHARISMA: Clopidogrel and Aspirin Versus Aspirin Alone for the Prevention of Atherothrombotic Events

The Clopidogrel for High Atherothrombotic Risk and Ischemic Stabilization, Management, and Avoidance *(32)* study assigned 15,603 patients with either clinically evident CVD or multiple risk factors to receive clopidogrel (75 mg/d) plus low-dose aspirin (75–162 mg/ d) or placebo plus low-dose aspirin. Patients were followed for a median of 28 mo. The primary efficacy end point was a composite of MI, stroke, or death from cardiovascular causes.

- At 28 mo of follow-up, the rate of the primary efficacy end point was 6.8% with clopidogrel plus aspirin and 7.3% with placebo plus aspirin ($p = 0.22$). Clopidogrel plus aspirin was not significantly more effective than aspirin alone in reducing CVD outcomes *(32)*.
- It must be emphasized that the trial studied patients with stable CHD. The combination therapy provides salutary effects in patients with ACS and in patients undergoing PCI.
- The trial did not study sufficient numbers of patients with recent transient ischemic attack or recent stroke. The combination may have a role and needs to be tested in RCTs.

FOLIC ACID/B_6, B_{12}

HOPE-2: Homocysteine Lowering

The Heart Outcomes Prevention Evaluation (HOPE) study *(33)* randomly assigned 5522 patients 55 yr of age or older who had vascular disease or diabetes to treatment either with the combination of 2.5 mg of folic acid, 50 mg of vitamin B_6, and 1 mg of vitamin B_{12} or with placebo.

- At 5-yr follow-up, this therapy did not reduce the risk of major CVD events in patients with vascular disease *(33)*.
- Mean plasma homocysteine levels decreased by 2.4 μmol/L (0.3 mg/L) in the active-treatment group and increased by 0.8 μmol/L (0.1 mg/L) in the placebo group.
- Primary outcome events occurred in 519 patients (18.8%) assigned to active therapy and 547 (19.8%) assigned to placebo (RR, 0.95; 95% CI, 0.84–1.07; $p = 0.41$) *(33)*.

This extensive, well-run RCT should convince clinicians and the public that lowering homocysteine levels does not decrease risk for CVD.

REFERENCES

1. Guyatt GH, Sackett DL, Cook DJ. The medical literature: Users' guide to the medical literature: II. How to use an article about therapy or prevention: A. Are the results of the study valid? JAMA 1993;270:2590–2601; B. What were the results and will they help me in caring for my patients? JAMA 1994;271:59–63.
2. Antman EM, Califf RM, Kupersmith J. Tools for assessment of cardiovascular tests and therapies. In: Antman EM. Cardiovascular Therapeutics, 2nd ed. Philadelphia, WB Saunders, 2002, pp. 1–19.
3. The Fifth Organization to Assess Strategies in Acute Ischemic Syndromes Investigators. Comparison of fondaparinux and enoxaparin in acute coronary syndromes. N Engl J Med 2006;354:1464–1476.
4. The OASIS-6 Trial Investigators. Effects of fondaparinux on mortality and reinfarction in patients with acute ST-segment elevation myocardial infarction. The OASIS-6 randomized trial. JAMA 2006;295: 1519–1530.
5. Califf RM. Fondaparinux in ST-segment elevation myocardial infarction. The drug, the strategy, the environment, or all of the above? JAMA 2006;295:1579–1580.
6. Antman EM, Morrow DA, McCabe CH, et al. Enoxaparin versus unfractionated heparin with fibrinolysis for ST-elevation myocardial infarction for the ExTRACT-TIMI 25 Investigators. N Engl J Med 2006; 354:1477–1488.

6a. Stone GW, Bertrand M, Colombo A, et al. Acute Catheterization and Urgent Intervention Triage strategY (ACUITY) trial: Study design and rationale. Am Heart J 2004;148:764–775.

6b. ACUITY: Stone GW, McLaurin BT, Cox DA, et al. for the ACUITY Investigators. Bivalirudin for patients with acute coronary syndromes. N Engl J Med 2006;355:2203–2216.

7. TACTICS-TIMI-18 Investigators. Comparison of early invasive and conservative strategies in patients with unstable coronary syndromes treated with the glycoprotein IIb/IIIa inhibitor tirofiban. N Engl J Med 2001;344:1879–1887.
8. CAPRICORN Investigators. Effect of carvedilol on outcome after MI in patients with left ventricular dysfunction; The CAPRICORN randomized trial. Lancet 2001;357:1385–1390.
9. Carvedilol Prospective Randomized Cumulative Survival Study Group. Effect of carvedilol on survival in severe chronic heart failure. N Engl J Med 2001;344:1651–1658.
10. MERIT-HF Study Group. The Metoprolol CR/XL Randomized Intervention Trial in CHF. Effects of controlled-release metoprolol on total mortality, hospitalizations and well-being in patients with heart failure. JAMA 2000;283:1295–1302.
11. RALES: The Randomized Aldactone Evaluation Study Investigators. The effect of spironolactone on morbidity and mortality in patients with severe heart failure. N Engl J Med 1999;341:709–717.
12. EPHESUS: Pitt B, Remme W, Zannad F, et al. for the Eplerenone Post-Acute Myocardial Infarction Heart Failure Efficacy and Survival Study Investigators. Eplerenone, a selective aldosterone blocker, in patients with left ventricular dysfunction after myocardial infarction. N Engl J Med 2003;348:1309–1321.
13. CHARM: Granger CB, McMurray JJV, Yusuf S, et al. for the CHARM Investigators and Committees. Effects of candesartan in patients with chronic heart failure and reduced left ventricular systolic function intolerant to angiotensin converting enzyme inhibitors; the CHARM-Alternative trial. Lancet 2003;362: 772–776.
14. A-HeFT: Taylor AL, Ziesche S, Yancy C, et al. Combination of isosorbide dinitrate and hydralazine in blacks with heart failure. N Engl J Med 2004;351:2049–2057.
15. HOPE: Heart Outcomes Prevention Evaluation Study Investigators. Effects of an angiotensin-converting enzyme inhibitor, ramipril, on cardiovascular events in high risk patients. N Engl J Med 2000;342: 145–153.
16. The ALLHAT Officers and Coordinators for the ALLHAT Collaborative Research Group. Major outcomes in high-risk hypertensive patients randomized to angiotensin-converting enzyme inhibitor or

calcium channel blocker vs diuretic. The Antihypertensive and Lipid-Lowering Treatment to Prevent Heart Attack Trial (ALLHAT). JAMA 2002;288:2981–2997.
17. Cannon CP, Braunwald E, McCabe CH, et al. Intensive versus moderate lipid lowering with statins after acute coronary syndromes. N Engl J Med 2004;350:1495–1504.
18. PROVE IT-TIMI 22: Ray KK, Cannon CP, McCabe CH, et al. for the PROVE IT-TIMI 22 Investigators. Early and late benefits of high-dose atorvastatin in patients with acute coronary syndromes: Results from the PROVE IT-TIMI 22 trial. J Am Coll Cardiol 2005;46:1405–1410.
19. Ridker PM, Cannon CP, Morrow D, et al. for the Pravastatin or Atorvastatin Evaluation and Infection Therapy-Thrombolysis in Myocardial Infarction 22 (PROVE IT-TIMI 22) Investigators. C-reactive protein levels and outcomes after statin therapy. N Engl J Med 2005;352:20–28.
20. ASTEROID: Nissen SE, Nicholls SJ, Sipahi I, et al. Effect of very high-intensity statin therapy on regression of coronary atherosclerosis: The ASTEROID trial. JAMA 2006;295:1556–1565.
21. Blumenthal RS, Kapur NK. Can a potent statin actually regress coronary atherosclerosis? JAMA 2006; 295:1583–1584.
22. Grundy SM, Cleeman JI, Merz CNB, et al. Implications of recent clinical trials for the National Cholesterol Education Program Adult Treatment Panel III guidelines. Circulation 2004;110:227–239.
23. Heart Protection Study Collaborative Group. MRC/BHF Heart Protection Study of cholesterol lowering with simvastatin in 20,536 high-risk individuals: A randomised placebo-controlled trial. Lancet 2002; 360:7–22.
24. Shepherd J, Blauw GJ, Murphy MB, et al. Pravastatin in elderly individuals at risk of vascular disease: A randomised controlled trial. Lancet 2002;360:1623–1630.
25. CARE: For the Cholesterol and Recurrent Events Trial Investigators. The effect of pravastatin on coronary events after myocardial infarction in patients with average cholesterol levels. N Engl J Med 1996;335:1001.
26. LIPID Study Group. Prevention of cardiovascular events and death with pravastatin in patients with coronary heart disease and a broad range of initial cholesterol levels. N Engl J Med 1998;339:1349–1357.
27. AFIRM: The Atrial Fibrillation Follow-up Investigation of Rhythm Management Investigators. A comparison of rate control and rhythm control in patients with atrial fibrillation. N Engl J Med 2002;347: 1825.
28. GEMINI: Bakris GL, Fonseca V, Katholi RE, et al. Metabolic effects of carvedilol vs metoprolol in patients with type 2 diabetes mellitus and hypertension: A randomized controlled trial. JAMA 2004;292: 2227–2236.
29. Sabatine MS, Cannon CP, Gibson CM. Effect of clopidogrel pretreatment before percutaneous coronary intervention in patients with ST-elevation myocardial infarction treated with fibrinolytics. JAMA 2005; 294:1224–1232.
30. COMMIT (ClOpidogrel and Metoprolol in Myocardial Infarction Trial) Collaborative Group. Addition of clopidogrel to aspirin in 45,852 patients with acute myocardial infarction: Randomised placebo-controlled trial. Lancet 2005;366:1607–1621.
31. COMMIT/CCS-2 (Clopidogrel and Metoprolol in Myocardial Infarction Trial) Collaborative Group. Early intravenous then oral metoprolol in 45,852 patients with acute myocardial infarction: Randomised placebo-controlled trial. Lancet 2005;366:1622–1632.
32. CHARISMA: Bhatt DL, Fox KAA, Hacke W, for the CHARISMA Investigators. Clopidogrel and aspirin versus aspirin alone for the prevention of atherothrombotic events. N Engl J Med 2006;354:1706–1717.
33. HOPE 2: The Heart Outcomes Prevention Evaluation (HOPE) 2 Investigators. Homocysteine lowering with folic acid and B vitamins in vascular disease. N Engl J Med 2006;354:1567–1577.

SUGGESTED READING

ACUITY: Stone GW, McLaurin BT, Cox DA, et al. for the ACUITY Investigators. Bivalirudin for patients with acute coronary syndromes. N Engl J Med 2006;355:2203–2216.

Cannon CP, Braunwald E, McCabe CH, et al. Intensive versus moderate lipid lowering with statins after acute coronary syndromes. N Engl J Med 2004;350:1495–1504.

COMMIT (Clopidogrel and Metoprolol in Myocardial Infarction Trial) Collaborative Group. Early intravenous then oral metoprolol in 45,852 patients with acute myocardial infarction: Randomised placebo-controlled trial. Lancet 2005;366:1622–1632.

COMMIT (Clopidogrel and Metoprolol in Myocardial Infarction Trial) Collaborative Group. Addition of clopidogrel to aspirin in 45,852 patients with acute myocardial infarction: Randomised placebo-controlled trial. Lancet 2005;366:1607–1621.

Davis BR, Piller LB, Cutler JA, et al. for the Antihypertensive and Lipid-Lowering Treatment to Prevent Heart Attack Trial (ALLHAT) Collaborative Research Group. Role of diuretics in the prevention of heart failure: The Antihypertensive and Lipid-Lowering Treatment to Prevent Heart Attack Trial. Circulation 2006;113:2201–2210.

Rahman M, Pressel S, Davis BR, et al. for the ALLHAT Collaborative Research Group. Cardiovascular outcomes in high-risk hypertensive patients stratified by baseline glomerular filtration rate. Ann Inter Med 2006;144:172–180.

Stevens LA, Coresh J, Greene T. Assessing kidney function—measured and estimated glomerular filtration rate. N Engl J Med 2006;354:2473– 2483.

Tu K, Gunraj N, Mamdani M. Is ramipril really better than other angiotensin-converting enzyme inhibitors after acute myocardial infarction? 2006;98 6–9.

Appendix I: Infusion Pump Charts

Dopamine Infusion Pump Chart
(Dopamine 400 mg in 500 mL [800 μg/mL][a]

Dosage (μg/kg/min)	*Rate (mL/h [pump] or drops/min [microdrip])[b] for different body weights (kg)*						
	40	*50*	*60*	*70*	*80*	*90*	*100*
1.0	3	4	5	5	6	7	8
1.5	5	6	7	8	9	10	11
2.0	6	8	9	11	12	14	15
2.5	8	9	11	13	15	17	19
3.0	9	11	14	16	18	20	23
3.5	11	13	16	18	21	24	26
4.0	12	15	18	21	24	27	30
4.5	14	17	20	24	27	30	34
5.0	15	19	23	26	30	34	38
6.0	18	23	27	32	36	41	45
7.0	21	26	32	37	42	47	53
8.0	24	30	36	42	48	54	60
9.0	27	34	41	47	54	61	68
10.0	30	38	45	53	60	68	75
12.0	36	45	54	63	72	81	90
15.0	45	56	68	79	90	101	113
20.0	60	75	90	105	120	135	150
25.0	75	94	113	131	150	169	188

[a]The above rates apply only for an 800 mg/L concentration of dopamine. If a different concentration must be used, appropriate adjustments in rates should be made. Start at 1 μg/kg/min; ideal dose range 5–7.5 μg/kg/min. Maximum suggested 10 μg/kg/min. Dopamine should be given via a central line.

[b]Use chart for (1) pump (mL/h) or (2) microdrip (drops/min). Example: 60-kg patient at 2.0 μg/kg/min: (1) set pump at 9 mL/h; (2) run microdrip solution at 9 drops/min.

From: *Contemporary Cardiology: Cardiac Drug Therapy, Seventh Edition*
M. Gabriel Khan © Humana Press Inc., Totowa, NJ

Nitroprusside Infusion Pump Chart
(Nitroprusside 50 mg [1 vial] in 100 mL [500 mg/mL][a]

Dosage	Rate (mL/h) for different body weights (kg)						
(μg/kg/min)	40	50	60	70	80	90	100
0.2	1	1	1	2	2	2	2
0.5	2	3	4	4	5	5	6
0.8	4	5	6	7	8	9	10
1.0	5	6	7	8	10	11	12
1.2	6	7	9	10	12	13	14
1.5	7	9	11	13	14	16	18
1.8	9	11	13	15	17	19	22
2.0	10	12	14	17	19	22	24
2.2	11	13	16	18	21	24	26
2.5	12	15	18	21	24	27	30
2.8	13	17	20	23	27	30	34
3.0	14	18	22	25	29	32	36
3.2	15	19	23	27	31	35	38
3.5	17	21	25	29	34	38	42
3.8	18	23	27	32	36	41	46
4.0	19	24	29	34	38	43	48
4.5	22	27	32	38	43	49	54
5.0	24	30	36	42	48	54	60
6.0	29	36	43	50	58	65	72

[a] The above rates apply only for a 500 mg/L concentration of nitroprusside. If a different concentration must be used, appropriate adjustments in rates should be made. Start at 0.2 μg/kg/min. Increase slowly. Average dose 3 μg/kg/min. Usual dose range 0.5–5.0 μg/kg/min.

Continuous Infusion Heparin[a]

Rate (mL/h)		Units (/h)	Units (/24 h)	Volume (mL/24 h)
1.	21	840	20,160	
2.	25	1000	24,000	600
3.	28	1120	26,880	
4.	30	1200	28,800	
5.	32	1280	30,720	
6.	34	1360	32,640	
7.	36	1440	34,560	
8.	38	1520	36,480	912
9.	40	1600	38,400	
10.	42	1680	40,320	
11.	44	1760	42,240	

[a] 20,000 heparin in 500 mL 5% dextrose; 1 mL = 40 units. Start with infusion no. 1 for patients < 67 kg for acute MI, and choose no. 2 for patients > 67 kg. Choose the appropriate alternative depending on the PTT value. Nos. 3 to 10 are mainly for pulmonary embolism and massive DVT.

Start with infusion no. 2 and choose the appropriate alternative depending on the once-daily PTT value.

Appendix II: Drug Index

The Drug Index gives the generic drug name in lowercase; the pharmaceutical trade names begin with a capital letter. C, Canada when different from USA; F, France; G, Germany.

USA	UK	Europe	Japan
ACE inhibitors			
benazepril Lotensin		benazepril Briem (F), Cibace Cibacin Lotensine	benazepril
captopril Capoten	captopril Capoten	captopril Captolane (F) Lopril (F) Loprin (G) Tensobon (G)	captopril Captopril
cilazapril Inhibace	cilazapril Vascace	cilazapril Dynorm (G)	cilazapril
enalapril Vasotec	enalapril Innovace	enalapril Pres (G) Renitec (F) Xanef (G)	enalapril Renivace
fosinopril Monopril	fosinopril Staril	fosinopril Dynacil (G) Eliten (I)	fosinopril
lisinoporil Prinivil Zestril	lisinopril Carace Zestril	lisinopril Longes Zestril (F)	lisinopril
moexipril	moexipril	moexipril	

From: *Contemporary Cardiology: Cardiac Drug Therapy, Seventh Edition*
M. Gabriel Khan © Humana Press Inc., Totowa, NJ

USA	UK	Europe	Japan
ACE inhibitors (continued)			
Univasc	Perdix		
perindopril	perindopril	perindopril	perindopril
Coversyl	Coversyl	Acertil	
		Coversum	
		Pexum	
quinapril	quinapril	quinapril	quinapril
Accupril	Accupro	Accuprin	
		Acuitel	
		Korec (F)	
ramipril	ramipril	ramipril	rarnipril
Altace	Tritace	Delix	
		Ramace	
		Triatec (F)	
		spirapril	spirapril
		Renpress	
		Sandopril	
trandolapril	trandolapril	trandolapril	trandolapril
Mavik	Gopten	Gopten	
	Odrik		
		zefenopril	zefenopril
Angiotensin II receptor blockers			
candesartan	candesartan		candesartan
Atacand	Amias		
eprosartan	eprosartan		
Teveten			
irbesartan	irbesartan		
Avapro	Aprovel		
losartan	losartan	losartan	losartan
Cozaar	Cozaar	Cozaar	
olmesartan	olmesartan	olmesartan	
Benicar			
telmisartan	telmisartan	telmisartan	telmisartan
Micardis			
valsartan	valsartan	valsartan	valsartan
Diovan	Diovan	Diovan	

USA	UK	Europe	Japan
Antiarrhythmics			
adenosine Adenocard	adenosine Adenocor	adenosine	adenosine
amiodarone Cordarone	amiodarone Cordarone X	amiodarone	amiodarone
disopyramide Norspace Rythmodan	disopyramide Dirythmin SA Rythmodan	disopyramide	disopyramide
flecainide Tambocor	flecainide Tambocor	flecainide	flecainide
mexiletine Mexitil	mexiletine Mexitil	mexiletine	mexiletine
procainamide Pronestyl	procainamide Pronestyl	procainamide	procainamide
propafenone Rythmol	propafenone Arythmol	propafenone Rytmonorm	propafenone
quinidine	quinidine	quinidine	quinidine
sotalol Betapace Sotacor	sotalol Beta-cardone Sotacor	sotalol Sotacor	sotalol
Anticoagulants			
dalteparin Fragmin	dalteparin	dalteparin	
enoxaparin Lovenox	enoxaparin Clexane	enoxaparin	enoxaparin
warfarin Coumadin	warfarin Marevan	warfarin	warfarin
Antiplatelet agents			
abciximab ReoPro	abciximab ReoPro		
aspirin	aspirin	aspirin	aspirin
clopidogrel Plavix			

(continued)

USA	UK	Europe	Japan
Antiplatelet agents (continued)			
dipyridamole	dipyridamole	dipyridamole	dipyridamole
Persantine	Persantine	Persantine	
	Persantin	Cardoxin	
	Retard		
ebtifibatide			
Integrilin			
tirofiban			
Aggrastat			
Beta-blockers			
acebutolol	acebutolol	acebutolol	acebutolol
Sectral	Sectral	Prent	
Monitan		Neptall	
		Sectral	
atenolol	atenolol	atenolol	atenolol
Tenormin	Tenormin	Tenormine (F)	
		Tenormin	
		Bêtatop	
betaxolol	betaxolol	betaxolol	betaxolol
Kerlone	Kerlone	Kerlone	
bisoprolol	bisoprolol	bisoprolol	bisoprolol
Zebeta	Emcor		
(Ziac)	Monocor		
carteolol		carteolol	carteolol
Catrol			
carvedilol	carvedilol		carvedilol
Coreg	Eucardic		
	celiprolol	celiprolol	celiprolol
	Celectol	Celector	
		Celectol (F)	
esmolol	esmolol	esmolol	
Brevibloc	Brevibloc	Brevibloc	
labetalol	labetalol	labetalol	labetalol
Normodyne	Trandate	Trandate	Trandate
metoprolol	metoprolol	metoprolol	metoprolol
Betaloc	Betaloc		

USA	UK	Europe	Japan
Beta-blockers (continued)			
Lopressor Toprol XL	Lopressor	Lopressor Metohexal Séloken	
nadolol Corgard	nadolol Corgard	nadolol Corgard Solgol (G)	nadolol
nebivolol Nebilit	nebivolol Nebilit	nebivolol Nebilit	nebivolol
propranolol Inderal	propranolol Inderal Inderal-LA	propranolol Angilol Avolacardyl (F) Berkolol Dociton (G) Efektolol	propranolol
sotalol Sotacor	sotalol Sotacor	sotalol Sotacor	sotalol
Betapace	Beta-Cardone	Sotalex (G) Sotalex (F)	
timolol Blocadren	timolol Blocadren Betim	timolol Timacor (F) Temserin	timolol
Calcium antagonists			
amlodipine Norvasc	amlodipine Istin	amlodipine Amlor (F) Norvasc	amlodipine
diltiazem Cardizem CD Tiazac	diltiazem Adizem XL Tildiem LA Viazem XL	diltiazem Dilrene (F) Dilzem Herbesser	diltiazem
felodipine Plendil Renedil	felodipine Plendil	felodipine Flodil (F)	felodipine
isradipine	isradipine	isradipine	

(continued)

USA	UK	Europe	Japan
Calcium antagonists (continued)			
DynaCirc	Prescal	Flodil (F)	
	lacidipine	lacidipine	lacidipine
	Montens		
nicardipine	nicardipine		nicardipine
Cardene	Cardene		
Cardene SR	Cardene SR		
nifedipine	nifedipine	nifedipine	nifedipine
Adalat CC	Adalat LA	Adalat	
Adalat XL (C)	Nifensar XL		
Procardia XL			
nisoldipine	nisoldipine	nisoldipine	
Sular	Syscor	Baymycard	
		nitrendipine	
		Baypress	
verapamil	verapamil	verapamil	verapamil
Isoptin SR	Securon SR	Isoptin	
Calan SR	Univer	Isoptine	
Covera-HS	Cordilox	Arpamyl	
Chronovera (C)			
Digitalis			
digitoxin	digitoxin	digitoxin	digitoxin
digoxin	digoxin	digoxin	digoxin
Lanoxin	Lanoxin	Lanoxin	
		Lanoxine	
Diuretics			
bendrofluazide	bendrofluazide	bendrofluazide	
Naturetin	Aprinox		
	Neo-Naclex		
bumetanide	bumetanide	bumetanide	bumetanide
Bumex	Burinex		
Burinex			
chlorothiazide	chlorothiazide	chlorothiazide	
Diuril	Saluric	Saluric	
chlorthalidone	chlorthalidone	chlorthalidone	chlorthalidone
Hygroton	Hygroton	Hygroton	
	Cyclopentazide	Cyclopentazide	
	Navidrex	Navidrex	

USA	UK	Europe	Japan
Diuretics (continued)			
furosemide Lasix hydrochlorothiazide	frusemide Lasix hydrochlorothiazide	frusemide hydrochlorothiazide	furosemide hydrochlorothiazide
Esidrix Hydro Diuril	Esidrex Hydro Saluric		
indapamide Lozol Lozide (C)	indapamide Natramid Natrilix	indapamide Natrillix	indapamide
metolazone Zaroxolyn	metolazone Metenix	metolazone Diulo	
spironolactone Aldactone	spironolactone Aldactone		
torsemide Demadex	torasemide Torem		
Combination drugs			
hydrochlorothiazide plus amiloride Moduretic Moduret (C)	co-amilozide Amil-Co Moduret 25 Moduretic		hydrochlorothiazide plus amiloride
hydrochlorothizide plus triamterene Dyazide	hydrochlorothizide plus triamterene Dyazide		hydrochlorothizide plus triamterene
Lipid-lowering agents			
Statins			
atrovastatin Lipitor	atrovastatin Lipitor	atrovastatin	atrovastatin
fluvastatin Lescol	fluvastatin Lescol	fluvastatin Lipur (F)	fluvastatin
lovastatin Mevacor			
pravastatin Pravachol	pravastatin Lipostat	pravastatin Elisor Vasten	pravastatin
rosuvastatin Crestor	rosuvastatin Crestor	rosuvastatin Cresto	rosuvastatin

(continued)

USA	UK	Europe	Japan
Lipid-lowering agents (continued)			
Statins			
simvastatin	simvastatin	simvastatin	simvastatin
Zocor	Zocor	Zocor	
		Lodales	
Resins			
cholestyramine	cholestyramine	cholestyramine	cholestyrarnine
Questran	Questran	Questran	
	Questran Light	Cuemrid	
colestipol	colestipol	colestipol	
Colestid	Colestid		
Fibrates			
bezafibrate	bezafibrate	bezafibrate	bezafibrate
Bezalip	Bezalip		
Bezalip Mono	Bezalip Mono		
fenofibrate	fenofibrate	fenofibrate	fenofibrate
Lipidil	Lipantil Micro		
gemfibrozil	gemfibrozil	gemfibrozil	gemfibrozil
Lopid	Lopid	Lopid	
		Lipur (E)	
Nitrates			
isosorbide dinitrate	isosorbide dinitrate	isosorbide dinitrate	isosorbide dinitrate
Isordil	Cedocard Retard		
	Isocard		
	Isordil		
	Sorbid SA		
	Sorbitrate		
isosorbide mononitrate	isosorbide mononitrate	isosorbide mononitrate	isosorbide mononitrate
Imdur	Imdur		
nitroglycerin	nitroglycerine	nitroglycerine	nitroglycerin
nitroglycerin	glyceryl trinitrate		
Nitrolingual spray	Nitrolingual spray		
	Coro-nitrospray		

INDEX

B

F

G

H

I

N

T

U

V